AF669516

Atlas of
Laparoscopic and Robotic
Urologic Oncological Surgery

Atlas of Laparoscopic and Robotic Urologic Oncological Surgery

Editor

Reza Ghavamian MD

Professor and Chairman
Department of Urology
Director of Genitourinary Oncology Program and Robotic Surgery
Montefiore Medical Center
Albert Einstein College of Medicine
Bronx, New York, USA

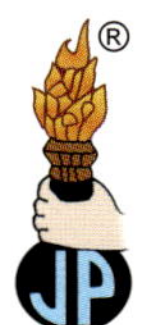

JAYPEE BROTHERS MEDICAL PUBLISHERS (P) LTD

New Delhi • Panama City • London • Dhaka • Kathmandu

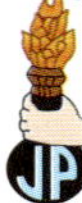

Jaypee Brothers Medical Publishers (P) Ltd

Headquarters
Jaypee Brothers Medical Publishers (P) Ltd
4838/24, Ansari Road, Daryaganj
New Delhi 110 002, India
Phone: +91-11-43574357
Fax: +91-11-43574314
Email: jaypee@jaypeebrothers.com

Overseas Offices

J.P. Medical Ltd
83, Victoria Street, London
SW1H 0HW (UK)
Phone: +44-2031708910
Fax: +02-03-0086180
Email: info@jpmedpub.com

Jaypee-Highlights Medical Publishers Inc.
City of Knowledge, Bld. 237, Clayton
Panama City, Panama
Phone: +507-301-0496
Fax: +507-301-0499
Email: cservice@jphmedical.com

Jaypee Brothers Medical Publishers (P) Ltd
17/1-B Babar Road, Block-B, Shaymali
Mohammadpur, Dhaka-1207
Bangladesh
Mobile: +08801912003485
Email: jaypeedhaka@gmail.com

Jaypee Brothers Medical Publishers (P) Ltd
Shorakhute, Kathmandu
Nepal
Phone: +00977-9841528578
Email: jaypee.nepal@gmail.com

Website: www.jaypeebrothers.com
Website: www.jaypeedigital.com

Inquiries for bulk sales may be solicited at: jaypee@jaypeebrothers.com

Atlas of Laparoscopic and Robotic Urologic Oncological Surgery

First Edition: **2013**

ISBN 978-93-5025-958-0

Printed at: Ajanta Offset & Packagings Ltd., New Delhi

Dedicated to

The nurses and surgical technologists of the urology and robotic surgical team at Montefiore Medical Center, whose dedication and commitment to detail have been vital to excellent patient care and outcomes.

A special thanks goes to all my past and present residents and fellows who make the art of teaching surgery stimulating and rewarding.

Finally, to all my patients, taking care of whom has been an honor and a privilege.

Contributors

Ronney Abaza MD FACS
Director, Robotic Urologic Surgery
Co-Director, Ohio State's Center for Advanced Robotic Surgery
Associate Professor, Department of Urology
The Ohio State University Comprehensive Cancer Center—Arthur G. James Cancer Hospital & Richard J Solove Research Institute
Columbus, OH, USA

Faris S Azzouni MBBS FEBU
Clinical Fellow in Uro-Oncology and Robotic Surgery
Department of Urology
Roswell Park Cancer Institute
Buffalo, New York, NY, USA

Aron Bruhn MD
Resident in Urology
New York University Langone Medical Center
New York, NY, USA

Jacob H Cohen MD
Fellow, Endourology
New York Medical College
Valhalla, New York, NY, USA

Jonathan A Coleman MD
Assistant Professor
Weill-Cornell Medical College
Memorial Sloan Kettering Cancer Center
New York, NY, USA

Jan Colli MD
Fellow, Tulane University School of Medicine
New Orleans, LA, USA

Douglas M Dahl MD FACS
Associate Professor of Surgery
Harvard Medical School
Chief, Division of Urologic Oncology
Massachusetts General Hospital
Boston, MA, USA

Brian D Duty MD
Attending Physician
The Arthur Smith Institute for Urology
Hofstra University, North Shore—Long Island Jewish Health System
Department of Urology
New Hyde Park, New York, NY, USA

Shadi Al Ekish MD
Fellow of Endourology
Alpert Medical School of Brown University
Providence, RI, USA

Boris Gershman MD
Resident in Urology
Massachussetts General Hospital
Boston, MA, USA

Reza Ghavamian MD
Professor and Chairman
Department of Urology
Director of Genitourinary Oncology Program and Robotic Surgery
Montefiore Medical Center
Albert Einstein College of Medicine
Bronx, New York, NY, USA

Ahmed Ghazi MD FEBU
Fellow in Urologic Laparoscopy and Robotic Surgery
University of Rochester Medical Center
Rochester, New York, NY, USA

Michael Grasso III MD
Professor and Vice Chairman
Department of Urology
New York Medical College
Valhalla, New York, NY, USA

Joseph A Graversen MD
Minimally Invasive Surgery and Endourology
Fellow, University of California, Irvine, USA

Khurshid A Guru MD
Director, Robotic Surgery
Robert P Huben Endowed Professor of Urologic Oncology
Department of Urology
Roswell Park Cancer Institute
Buffalo, New York, NY, USA

Ashok K Hemal MS MCh FACS FAMS FRCS (Glasg)
Professor, Department of Urology
Comprehensive Cancer Center
Professor, Institute for Regenerative Medicine
Director, Robotics and Minimally Invasive Surgery
Wake Forest Medical School & Baptist Medical Center, Medical Center Boulevard
Winston-Salem, NC, USA

Samay Jain MD
Fellow, Minimally Invasive & Robotic Urologic Surgery
Hackensack University Medical Center
Hackensack, NJ, USA

Jean Joseph MD MBA
Professor of Urology and Oncology
Head-Section of Urologic Laparoscopy and Robotic Surgery
Director-Center for Robotic Surgery and Innovation
University of Rochester Medical Center
Rochester, New York, NY, USA

David Y Josephson MD
Tower Urology
Cedars-Sinai Medical Center
Los Angeles, CA, USA

Louis R Kavoussi MD
Professor and Chairman
The Arthur Smith Institute for Urology
Hofstra University, North Shore—Long Island Jewish Health System
Department of Urology
New Hyde Park, New York, NY, USA

Chris R Kelly MD
Postdoctoral Residency Fellow
Department of Medicine
New York-Presbyterian Hospital/ Columbia University Medical Center
New York, NY, USA

Simon Y Kimm MD
Urologic Oncology Fellow
Memorial Sloan Kettering Cancer Center
Department of Surgery, Division of Urology
New York, NY, USA

Jaime Landman MD
Professor of Urology and Radiology
Chairman of the Dept. of Urology
University of California, Irvine, USA

Michael S Lasser MD
Fellow in Endourology, Laparoscopy and Urologic Robotic Surgery
Montefiore Medical Center
Albert Einstein College of Medicine
Bronx, New York, NY, USA

Philip Lebowitz MD
Professor of Clinical Anesthesiology
Montefiore Medical Center
Albert Einstein College of Medicine
Bronx, New York, NY, USA

Benjamin R Lee MD FACS
Professor of Urology & Medicine (Oncology)
Tulane University School of Medicine
New Orleans, LA, USA

Achim Lusch MD
Urology Research Fellow,
University of California, Irvine, USA

Michael B Marean MD
Resident, Department of Urology
New York Presbyterian Hospital - Weill Cornell Medical College
New York, NY, USA

Nishant Mishra
Research Assistant
Department of Urology
New York Presbyterian Hospital
Weill Cornell Medical College
New York, NY, USA

Phillip Mucksavage MD
Assistant Professor, University of Pennsylvania
Philadelphia, PA, USA

Ravi Munver MD, FACS
Associate Professor and Vice Chairman
Chief, Minimally Invasive & Robotic Urologic Surgery
Hackensack University Medical Center
Hackensack, NJ, USA

Rishi Nayyar MS MCh
IAUA fellow, Department of Urology
Wake Forest Medical School & Baptist Medical Center, Medical Center Boulevard
Winston-Salem, NC , USA

Gyan Pareek MD
Director, Division of Minimally Invasive Urologic Surgery
Alpert Medical School of Brown University
Providence, RI, USA

Kush Patel MD
Chief Resident
Tulane University School of Medicine
New Orleans, LA, USA

Joseph J Del Pizzo MD
Associate Professor of Urology and Transplantation Surgery
Director, Laparoscopic and Minimally Invasive Surgery
Weill Cornell Medical College of Cornell University
New York, NY, USA

James S Rosoff MD
Resident, Department of Urology
New York Presbyterian Hospital—Weill Cornell Medical College
New York, NY, USA

Ornob P Roy MD
Attending Physician
The Arthur Smith Institute for Urology
Hofstra University, North Shore—Long Island Jewish Health System
Department of Urology
New Hyde Park, New York, NY, USA

Iqbal Singh MS MCh DNB
Fellow and Instructor, Department of Urology
Wake Forest Medical School & Baptist Medical Center, Medical Center Boulevard
Winston-Salem, NC , USA

Prasanna Sooriakumaran BMedSci(Hons) BMBS(Hons) MRCS(Eng) PhD PGC(MedLaw) FRCS(Urol) ADC(Clinlnv)
Visiting Fellow in Urology
Karolinska Institute, Stockholm, Sweden

Abhishek Srivastava MD
Urology Resident, PGY1
Department of Urology
Montefiore Medical Center
Albert Einstein College of Medicine
Bronx, New York, NY, USA

Michael Stifelman MD
Associate Professor of Urology
Director of Robotic Surgery
New York University Langone Medical Center
New York, NY, USA

Ashutosh K Tewari MD MCh
Ronald P Lynch Professor of Urologic Oncology
Director, LeFrak Institute of Robotic Surgery and Director, Prostate Cancer Institute
Department of Urology
New York Presbyterian Hospital
Weill Cornell Medical College
New York, NY, USA

Raju Thomas MD FACS MHA
Professor and Chairman
Department of Urology
Tulane University School of Medicine
New Orleans, LA, USA

Praneeth Vemulapalli MD
Robotic Urologic Surgery Fellow
Clinical Instructor, Department of Urology
The Ohio State University Wexner Medical Center
Columbus, OH, USA

James G Widyn MD
Resident in Anesthesiology
Montefiore Medical Center
Albert Einstein College of Medicine
Bronx, New York, NY, USA

Stephen B Williams MD
Associated Urologists of Orange County, Division of Urologic Oncology,
The Center for Cancer Prevention and Treatment at St. Joseph Hospital
Orange, CA, USA

Steve K Williams MD
Resident in Urology
Montefiore Medical Center
Albert Einstein College of Medicine
Bronx, New York, NY, USA

Jennifer K Yates MD
Attending, Minimally Invasive & Robotic Urologic Surgery
Hackensack University Medical Center
Hackensack, NJ, USA

Preface

Over the last decade and a half, the field of Urology has experienced a "minimally invasive revolution". This started out with laparoscopy in the late 1990s gradually and culminated in the last few years with the dramatic and enthusiastic adoption of robotic urologic surgery. While urologists were late adopters of laparoscopy as compared to other surgical specialists, the introduction of robotic surgery has certainly changed the playing field. The widespread adoption of robotic surgery, by the urologic community, has placed urologists as the surgical specialists spearheading the robotic revolution in surgery. Urologists are the most experienced surgeons in their respective institutions in robotic surgery and often head their respective robotic programs.

The dramatic explosion in robotic urologic surgery is a remarkable story. Much of it has to do with the fact that despite the valiant efforts of many pioneers in laparoscopic urologic surgery in the United States, urologists were slow to adapt to and adopt laparoscopy. The reasons behind this are several fold. First, as a new surgical concept was brought about in this field, the few initial pioneers served to describe procedures and prove their feasibility. As these surgeons trained a second generation of "Laparoscopic Urologists", the number, indication and experience in laparoscopic urology incrementally increased. However, many common urologic oncological procedures were deemed quite complex to master laparoscopically except for a select few expert surgeons. Procedures such as laparoscopic radical prostatectomy and partial nephrectomy were performed in select institutions in the United States but were not widely adopted due to their steep learning curve.

The introduction of robotic urologic surgery, initially for radical prostatectomy, provided a platform for laparoscopically naive surgeons to be able to offer their patients minimally invasive surgery. It has now been proven to decrease the learning curve necessary for complex urologic cancer surgery. However, in many respects the procedures are still quite complex and are associated with a significant learning curve. The learning curve, however, is easier to overcome given the unique features of robotic surgery. These include dramatic magnification, three-dimensional visualization and the tremor-free dexterity afforded by the robotic surgical system facilitating complex extirpative and reconstructive urologic oncological surgery. Furthermore, tactile sensation is substituted by markedly improved visual cues.

Robotic urologic surgery provides the advantages of laparoscopic surgery, namely faster recovery, shorter length of stay and decreased pain for the patient. However, its main disadvantage is its increased cost. While the adoption of the robotic technology is widespread in the United States, this is certainly not the case worldwide due to this mere fact. It is for this reason that many common urologic cancer operations are and should still be performed purely laparoscopically. Simple extirpative procedures with no major reconstruction can be quickly and efficiently performed without a robot, as is the case for most radical nephrectomies and adrenalectomies for example.

It is for this reason that I decided to include the pure laparoscopic approach to all common urologic oncological procedures, as the pure laparoscopic approach will continue to play a valuable part in our surgical discipline. It is also crucial for the education and experience of residents and fellows in training. In this atlas, all common urologic oncological procedures are described in their pure laparoscopic and robotic forms in separate chapters. This atlas thus serves to educate residents and fellows in both techniques and approaches. In addition, it also serves to provide the expert in urologic laparoscopic surgery, the necessary tools to adopt the robotic approach and compare and contrast the procedures side by side in a single volume. All chapters are written by thought leaders in the field and include detailed intraoperative photographs depicting critical sequential procedural steps. There are valuable sections on instrumentation and surgical preparation and nuances of the procedures and procedural steps are discussed in select chapters.

It is my hope that the targeted readership, namely all urologic surgeons interested in adopting minimally invasive and robotic urologic surgery as well as residents and fellows in training, find this atlas a valuable educational adjunct.

Reza Ghavamian

Contents

SECTION 1 Anesthesia and Setup

SECTION 2 Upper Tract Surgery

SECTION 3 Lower Tract Surgery

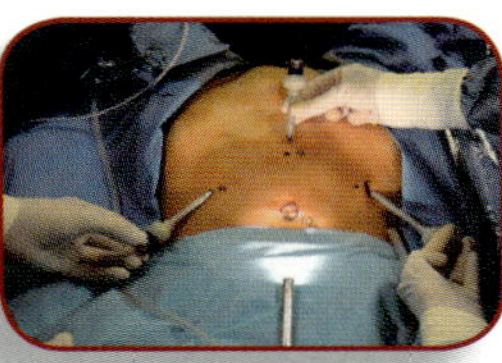

SECTION

1

Anesthesia and Setup

Anesthesia for Robotic Urological Surgery

James G Widyn, Philip Lebowitz

INTRODUCTION

The anesthetic plan for a patient undergoing robotic urological surgery requires careful consideration and close discussion with the surgical team. The patient will be subject to profound physiologic stressors and in order to provide the patient with the very best level of care, a patient-specific strategy for anesthetic management must be carefully constructed. Perhaps, the best way to think about the anesthetic plan for these patients is to break the plan down into three separate, but intertwined, components: preoperative evaluation, intraoperative management, and postoperative care.

PREOPERATIVE MANAGEMENT

All patients undergoing robotic urological surgery must have a preoperative evaluation performed by an anesthesiologist. This allows the anesthesiologist to obtain information regarding the patient's medical history, perform a physical examination, and review relevant labs and studies the patient has had done. This also affords the anesthesiologist the opportunity to suggest further testing, if required, before the patient undergoes his or her surgery. This evaluation can be done on the day of surgery or ideally earlier in an anesthesiology preoperative evaluation clinic.

During this evaluation, anesthesiologists assess patients according to the American Society of Anesthesiologists (ASA) Physical Status classification system that was developed in 1941.[1] The classification system, while simple, allows the anesthesiologist to stratify patients according to their overall state of health, and helps determine the level of concern the anesthesiologist should have regarding a patient's anesthetic plan. The classification system is constructed as follows:

ASA Physical Classification System

I. A normal healthy patient
II. A patient with mild systemic disease
III. A patient with severe systemic disease
IV. A patient with severe systemic disease that is a constant threat to life
V. A moribund patient who is not expected to survive without the operation
VI. A declared brain-dead patient whose organs are being removed for donor purposes
E. Emergency operation [appended to the foregoing, e.g. IIIE]

While this classification system may leave to debate what terms such as "mild disease" versus "severe disease" actually encompass, it is this system that forms the basis for the anesthesiologist's preoperative plan organization. Much like the anesthetic plan itself, the testing that a patient must have prior to surgery is entirely patient-specific. It is the job of the surgical team to refer the patient for the appropriate workup prior to the day of surgery. The extent and focus of the preoperative testing should reflect the patient's overall state of health, his or her comorbidities, and the urgency of the surgery. For example, young healthy patients often require minimal or no testing. Meanwhile, a patient with a history of coronary artery disease that required stent placement in the past may need to be seen by a cardiologist and have stress testing or more.

What constitutes an appropriate preoperative workup is also a product of the urgency of the procedure. Elective surgery provides the patient with time to see appropriate specialists, become medically optimized and undergo needed testing. Emergency surgery, on the other hand, limits the amount of medical optimization and testing that can take place. It is important to remember that despite the consults obtained over the course of the preoperative period, only an anesthesiologist can clear a patient for surgery on the day of the operation.

Surgeons should evaluate their patients preoperatively and make thoughtful decisions about what, if any, further testing each patient should undergo prior to surgery. If surgeons are unsure if their patient has undergone appropriate testing and medical optimization, the patient can be referred to an anesthesiology preoperative clinic where he or she will be evaluated and recommendations regarding further testing can be made.

In 2009, Fleischer et al. published the American College of Cardiology Foundation/American Heart Association (ACCF/AHA) Perioperative Guidelines for cardiac assessment.[2] These guidelines provide a stepwise approach to assessing a patient's cardiac risk for noncardiac surgery and are a valuable resource for both surgeons and anesthesiologists when caring for patients undergoing noncardiac surgery during the perioperative period.

Patients that need emergency noncardiac surgery should proceed to the operating room. In general, emergency situations do not allow for preoperative patient optimization, and cardiac conditions are no exception. Anesthesiologists will monitor these patients in the intraoperative and postoperative period and manage their cardiac comorbidities accordingly.

If the surgery is nonemergent, the next step is to assess for the presence of active cardiac conditions, which are defined as: unstable or severe angina, recent myocardial infarction, decompensated heart failure, significant arrhythmias, and severe valvular disease. Significant arrhythmias are defined as high-grade atrioventricular (AV) block, Mobitz Type II block, third degree AV block, symptomatic ventricular arrhythmias, supraventricular arrhythmias with uncontrolled ventricular response, symptomatic bradycardia, or newly recognized ventricular tachycardia. Severe valvular disease is defined as severe aortic stenosis or symptomatic mitral regurgitation.

These conditions should be treated according to the ACCF/AHA guidelines and the appropriate consultations should be made before proceeding with surgery.

If the patient does not have any active cardiac conditions, the next step is to determine if the surgery is considered to be low-risk. Fleischer et al. define low-risk surgery as procedures that have a less than 1% mortality rate, even in patients deemed to be high-risk. Examples of low-risk surgery include endoscopic procedures, superficial procedures, cataract surgery, breast surgery, or ambulatory surgery. They recommend that patients undergoing low-risk procedures should proceed with surgery, stating that cardiovascular interventions and investigations in these stable patients would have little impact on management.

If patients are not undergoing low-risk surgery, the next step is to assess their exercise tolerance. If the patient has an exercise tolerance of at least four metabolic equivalents (METs), often defined as the ability to walk four blocks or climb a flight of stairs, then the decision should be made to proceed with surgery.

If the patient does not have an exercise tolerance of four METs or has an unknown functional capacity, then the need for further testing will be determined by the presence of clinical risk factors. Fleischer et al. define clinical risk factors as any of the following conditions: diabetes mellitus, compensated or prior heart failure, renal insufficiency, cerebrovascular disease, or ischemic heart disease.

Patients with no clinical risk factors should proceed with the planned surgery. Patients with two clinical risk factors undergoing intermediate-risk surgery, defined as prostate surgery, orthopedic surgery, head and neck surgery, carotid endarterectomy, or intraperitoneal/intrathoracic surgery, or high-risk surgery, defined as major vascular surgery, should either proceed to the operating room with heart rate controlled by beta blockade or undergo further testing if the result might change management.

If patients have three or more clinical risk factors and are scheduled to undergo an intermediate-risk procedure should proceed with surgery with heart rate control with beta blockade, or undergo further testing the result might change patient management. If the patient has three or more risk factors and is going to have a major vascular procedure, the patient should undergo further testing if the result might change management.

Another area of concern in the preoperative period is the patient's NPO status (Latin for nil per os, or nothing by mouth), which refers to the last time the patient put anything into the stomach, including gastrostomy feeds. General anesthesia abolishes a patient's airway reflexes and consequently places the patient at a higher risk of pulmonary aspiration of gastric contents, should they be regurgitated during anesthetic induction or even during the surgery itself. With this in mind, the ASA has developed guidelines regarding what patients may consume during the preoperative period.[3] The recommendations suggest that patients need 2 hours to digest clear liquids, and thus clear liquids should not be consumed in the 2 hours preceding elective surgery. Further the guidelines recommend 4 hours to digest breast milk, and 6 hours to digest infant formula, nonhuman milk, or a light meal. If a patient consumes a meal containing fatty foods or meat, a greater interval—some say 8 hours—should elapse between the time of consumption and the induction of anesthesia. Because the time of surgery may change, patients are usually told to remain NPO after midnight preceding elective surgery. Despite these guidelines, practitioners will undoubtedly encounter patients that have been NPO for a period of time exceeding the ASA recommendations that still had partially digested food in the stomach, reminding us that these are only guidelines that serve to aid practitioners in their clinical decision-making.

INTRAOPERATIVE MANAGEMENT

Once a patient has been cleared for surgery, the anesthesiologist is faced with the challenge of developing the anesthetic plan that is both the safest for the patient and allows the urologist to perform the required surgery. Laparoscopic robotic urological surgeries require insufflation of the abdomen with carbon dioxide (and concomitant muscle relaxation), steep Trendelenburg positioning, and several hours to complete. These requirements make general anesthesia with mechanical ventilation typically the anesthetic of choice.

An anesthesiologist will proceed through many steps when inducing general anesthesia in a patient undergoing elective surgery who has adhered to the ASA-specified fasting guidelines. The first step is the placement of ASA-specified standard monitors, including a continuous electrocardiography, a blood pressure monitor, a pulse oximeter, and capnogram. A temperature monitoring device needs to be available and monitored if changes in temperature are anticipated. This is typically done after intubation using an esophageal stethoscope. The anesthesiologist will also place an intravenous catheter if the patient does not already have one. The anesthesiologist will also decide if additional monitors are necessary, such as an invasive blood pressure monitor or a central venous catheter. Patients are then preoxygenated with 100% oxygen for 3–5 minutes in order to fill the lungs with pure oxygen and rid them of other gases, principally nitrogen.[4] This prolongs the amount of time patients may remain apneic during laryngoscopy and intubation without decreasing their oxygen saturation.

Anesthesiologists will then administer a series of medications designed to induce general anesthesia. Often these include a benzodiazepine, which serves as an anxiolytic and causes anterograde amnesia, an opioid analgesic, and a sedative-hypnotic such as propofol or etomidate. Lidocaine is often administered prior to the sedative-hypnotic because drugs such as propofol and etomidate cause a burning sensation when administered via a peripheral IV catheter. After the patient becomes apneic, the anesthesiologist will attempt to mask ventilate the patient, looking for exhaled carbon dioxide on the capnogram, chest rise, and condensation in the mask. Once ventilation has been confirmed, the anesthesiologist will administer a muscle relaxant to paralyze the patient and help facilitate laryngoscopy and tracheal intubation. The eyes are taped prior to performing laryngoscopy in order to minimize the chance of corneal abrasions. Once intubation has been accomplished, lung auscultation is done to check for bilateral breath sounds, the endotracheal tube is secured with tape, and a volatile anesthetic is turned on. Then an esophageal temperature probe is inserted and antibiotics are administered.

Laparoscopic robotic urological surgeries present the anesthesiologist with a variety of challenges. To allow for the insertion of trocars and provide better visualization for the urologist, carbon dioxide is insufflated into the peritoneal or retroperitoneal space at the beginning of the operation. In order to accomplish this, the anesthesiologist administers neuromuscular blocking agents to relax the muscles of the abdominal wall. Adequate muscle paralysis is required for the duration of the case in order for the operative field to remain easily distended.

The use of insufflated carbon dioxide can result in marked respiratory acidosis as a result of carbon dioxide absorption.[5] In order to help rid the body of excess carbon dioxide, the anesthesiologist will frequently hyperventilate the patient to facilitate its respiratory excretion. The insufflated carbon dioxide can travel cephalad to the thorax and neck resulting in subcutaneous emphysema. Similarly, patients undergoing laparoscopic procedures are at risk for airway compromise as a result of pneumothoraces due to this cephalad migration of insufflated gas.[6]

The combination of pneumoperitoneum and steep Trendelenburg positioning has important pulmonary and circulatory implications as well. Lestar et al. have shown that patients undergoing robotic laparoscopic prostatectomy have up to a 50% decrease in pulmonary compliance.[7] This can result in increased peak airway pressures during mechanical ventilation and decreased functional residual capacity. Phong et al. have also reported that changes in intrathoracic pressure are reflected in central venous pressure (CVP) and pulmonary arterial (PA) pressures, sometimes increasing three-fold and two-fold respectively during these robotic surgeries.[8] The rise in CVP increases cardiac preload, end-diastolic volume, and myocardial oxygen consumption. The increased PA pressure affects fluid dynamics by increasing the hydrostatic pressure of the blood circulating through the lungs. Increased intravascular hydrostatic pressure can cause extravasation of fluid into the lungs, and pulmonary edema has been reported in patients undergoing robotic urological surgery. Pressure-controlled ventilation, in contrast to volume-controlled ventilation, with peak end-expiratory pressure (PEEP) can beneficially improve lung ventilation in patients positioned head-down for extended periods of time. A full discussion of this topic may be found in standard anesthesiology texts.[9]

Patients undergoing robotic urological surgery are also at risk for development of laryngeal edema, especially in the setting of prolonged procedures that require large amounts of fluid administration.[8] Steep Trendelenburg positioning and its associated gravitational gradient promotes the cephalad migration of interstitial fluid. This accumulation of fluid in the tissues of the head and neck is common and usually innocuous. However, it can result in significant airway edema. Anesthesiologists take this into consideration when determining if a patient should be extubated immediately at the conclusion of the procedure, or later in the post anesthesia care unit (PACU). If the anesthesiologist does not feel the patient meets criteria for extubation at the conclusion of the surgery, the patient can be transferred to the PACU tracheally intubated. There, the patient can remain on a ventilator, or breathing spontaneously with continuous positive airway pressure and pressure support, until the edema subsides and the anesthesiologist determines that it is safe to extubate the patient.

Robotic urologic surgery can have marked effects on a patient's heart rate. Insufflation and stretching of the peritoneum can cause a reflex increase in vagal tone. This can produce extreme bradycardia and even asystole, and the anesthesiologist must be prepared to deal with these consequences. The administration of an anticholinergic drug such as atropine can counteract the effects of this increase in vagal tone. The anesthesiologist may also ask the urologist to release the insufflated carbon dioxide to eliminate the vagal stimulus. These two interventions are usually curative.

Studies show that patients undergoing robotic urological surgery have significantly increased intraocular and intracranial pressure. Reports of increases in intraocular pressure as high as 13 mm Hg have been documented.[10] The combination of steep Trendelenburg positioning and insufflation with carbon dioxide that occurs during these procedures has been implicated as a potential source of decreased ocular perfusion. There are two instances in the literature of patients who experienced postoperative posterior ischemic optic neuropathy after undergoing robotic urological surgery.[11] Anesthesiologists take great care during these procedures to maintain both cerebral perfusion and ocular perfusion, but patients should be aware that these procedures carry a risk of cerebral ischemia. Awad et al. found that the two factors that contributed to increased intraocular pressure during robotic radical prostatectomy were elevated $ETCO_2$ and prolonged length of surgery.[12] They found that for every 1 mm Hg increase in $ETCO_2$, there was a corresponding 0.21 mm Hg increase in intraocular pressure. Further they found that for each minute of surgery in steep Trendelenburg positioning, intraocular pressure increased 0.05 mm Hg. These results suggest that shorter duration of surgery and prevention of hypercapnea may help prevent postoperative vision loss in patients undergoing robotic urological surgeries.

Traditionally, patients with glaucoma were considered to be at elevated risk for blindness during procedures requiring steep Trendelenburg positioning, due to their baseline elevated intraocular pressure. In the past, these patients were not considered candidates for procedures such as robot-assisted radical prostatectomies. However, Abaza recently presented research findings looking at 17 patients with well-controlled glaucoma who underwent robotic-assisted radical prostatectomies and found that these patients had no increased risk of postoperative visual disturbances.[13] All of these patients were referred for ophthalmology consults prior to undergoing surgery. This topic remains controversial and further investigations are currently underway to explore the safety of these procedures for patients with baseline increases in intraocular pressure.

POSTOPERATIVE CARE

As mentioned earlier, the combination of extreme Trendelenburg positioning and insufflation of the peritoneum during robotic urological surgery can cause swelling of the head and neck, including the airway structures. After surgery, the anesthesiologist will assess the patient's airway, the amount of fluid administered during the surgery, and the duration of the surgery before deciding if the patient meets criteria for extubation. If the larynx and vocal cords are thought to be edematous, the anesthesiologist will choose to leave the breathing tube in place until the edema resolves, so as not to induce upper airway obstruction upon removal of the endotracheal tube. Often, placing patients in the head-up position over the next several hours will be enough to help drain fluid in the caudad direction and greatly reduce airway edema, allowing tracheal extubation later that same day.

Also, since these patients require muscle relaxation to allow for distension of the abdomen during laparoscopy, the anesthesiologist will also assess the patient's strength before deciding if the patient can be safely extubated. Anesthesiologists will administer an anticholinesterase, such as neostigmine, to help increase the concentration of acetylcholine and reverse the effects of the neuromuscular block agents administered during the surgery and restore neuromuscular function. Concomitantly, the anesthesiologist will administer an anticholinergic drug, such as glyocopyrrolate, to counteract the side effects of the anticholinesterase, such as bradycardia and salivation. Patients that are extubated without adequate restoration of neuromuscular function are at risk for developing respiratory failure necessitating reintubation in the postoperative period.

Patients who do not meet criteria for extubation can be transferred to the postanesthesia care unit (PACU) tracheally intubated. There, they can be monitored closely by an anesthesiologist until they may be safely extubated.

REFERENCES

1. Saklad M. Grading of patients for surgical procedures. Anesthesiology 1941;2:281-4.
2. Fleisher LA, Beckman JA, Brown KA, et al. 2009 ACCF/AHA Perioperative Guidelines. J Am Coll Cardiol. 2009;54:e113-8.
3. Practice Guidelines for Preoperative Fasting and the Use of Pharmacologic Agents to Reduce the Risk of Pulmonary Aspiration: Application to Healthy Patients Undergoing Elective Procedures: A Report by the American Society of Anesthesiologists Task Force on Preoperative Fasting. [online] Available from journals.lww.com/anesthesiology/Fulltext/1999/03000/Practice_Guidelines_for_Preoperative_Fasting_and.34.aspx. [Accessed December, 2011].
4. Usharani N, Suvarchala DC, Salem MR, et al. (2001) Preoxygenation with Tidal Volume and Deep Breathing Techniques: The Impact of Duration of Breathing and Fresh Gas Flow. [online] Available from www.anesthesia-analgesia.org/content/92/5/1337.full.pdf. [Accessed December, 2011].
5. Weingram J, Sosa RE, Stein B, et al. Subcutaneous emphysema (SCE) during laparoscopic pelvic lymph node dissection (LPLND). Anesth Analg. 1993;76:S460.
6. Whiston RJ, Eggers KA, Morris RW et al. Tension pneumothorax during laparoscopic cholecystectomy. Br J Surg. 1991;78:1325.
7. Lestar M, Gunnarsson L, Lagerstrand L, et al. Hemodynamic Perturbations During Robot-Assisted Laparoscopic Radical Prostatectomy in 45° Trendelenburg Position. Anesth Analg. 2011;113:1069-75. Epub 2011 Jan 13.
8. Phong SV, Koh LK. Anaesthesia for robotic-assisted radical prostatectomy: considerations for laparoscopy in the Trendelenburg position. Anaesth Intensive Care. 2007;35:281.
9. Miller's Anesthesia. In: Miller RD (Ed). 7th edition. Philadelphia: Elsevier; 2010.
10. Awad H, Santilli S, Ohr M, et al. (2009). The Effects of Steep Trendelenburg Positioning on Intraocular Pressure During Robotic Radical Prostatectomy. [online] Available from www.anesthesia-analgesia.org/content/109/2/473.full. [Accessed December, 2011].
11. Weber ED, Colyer MH, Lesser RL, et al. Posterior ischemic optic neuropathy after minimally invasive prostatectomy. J Neuroophthalmol 2007;27:285-7.
12. Awad H, Santilli S, Ohr M, et al.. The Effects of Steep Trendelenburg Positioning on Intraocular Pressure During Robotic Radical Prostatectomy. Anesth Analg. 2009;109:473-8.
13. Available from www.aua2011.org/abstracts/process.cfm?ID=Ronney/Abaza&searchType=presenter&seachKey=Search+by+Presenter. [Accessed December, 2011].

Chapter 2 Laparoscopic and Robotic Instrumentation

Michael S Lasser, Reza Ghavamian

Smaller incisions, reduced blood loss, shortened hospital stay and time to convalescence, and reduced postoperative pain are the benefits of laparoscopy that have propelled the integration of laparoscopy into modern surgical practice. Laparoscopic approaches have gained momentum as the preferred treatment modality for many surgical diseases. This is especially true in the field of urology where minimally invasive approaches have become commonplace.

Despite the exponential growth of minimally invasive surgery, complex laparoscopic procedures remain a daunting task. In urology, this is particularly true with regard to pelvic surgery due to the small operative space, lack of depth perception secondary to 2-dimensional vision, and rigid instrumentation utilized in laparoscopy. As the utilization of laparoscopy increased, there has been an evolution of laparoscopic instrumentation. The integration of novel technologies has allowed for the expansion of minimally invasive surgical approaches to a vast array of disease states.

LAPAROSCOPIC INSTRUMENTATION

Camera System

Laparoscopy has been made possible through the pursuit of novel technologies. Among the most essential developments was the camera system. These systems have benefited from rapid advancement resulting in improved visual acuity for the surgeon.

Most camera systems consist of three components: camera head, control unit, and monitor. The control unit and monitor are situated within a surgical tower for improved mobility within the operative suite (Fig. 1). The camera head is a sterile component of the operative field that is attached to both the laparoscope and control unit (Fig. 2).

As technology has progressed, the incorporation of high-definition (HD) cameras has provided the surgeon with superior imaging. To fully appreciate the advantages of HD technology, however, one must utilize an HD capable camera, control unit and monitor.

Laparoscope

The previously described camera head connects directly to the laparoscope. Standard laparoscopes come in two diameters, 5 and 10 mm (Fig. 3) with a fixed lens at the distal end. The standard lens angulations available include 0°, 30°, and 45° (Fig. 4).

Intracorporeally, the laparoscope has a tendency to fog due to body and room temperature differential. This can be diminished through the utilization of a warming thermos or heated water bath (Fig. 5).

Trocars

Trocars are utilized to maintain both access and insufflation during laparoscopy. Trocars exist in two basic categories: bladed and nonbladed (Figs 6A and B). Nonbladed trocars spread the fascial fibers whereas bladed trocars cut the fascia to obtain access into the operative field. Bladed trocars consist of either an open or protected blade. Most modern bladed trocars have a protective covering that springs into place over the blade once access is achieved.

Nonbladed trocars dilate the fascia and as such can obviate the need to close the fascial defect.[1] There are several types of dilating trocars currently utilized in clinical practice. The least complex consists of a blunt cone-shaped tip that is manipulated in a twisting motion to enter the fascia. A modification of this system led to the development of the visual obturator. This afforded the surgeon the ability to place these trocars under direct visual guidance.

An additional system that the authors' utilizes is the Step trocar (Tyco) (Fig. 7). In this system, an outer sheath is placed with the veress needle under direct visual guidance. After appropriate positioning is obtained, either a 5 or 10 mm trocar is placed through the sheath. This sheath dilates as it is stretched by the trocar. One advantage of this system is the ability of the surgeon to rapidly change a 5 mm port to a larger 10 mm trocar intraoperatively through the existing sheath.

Hand-Assisted Devices

During hand-assisted surgery, the surgeon utilizes his/her hand in addition to laparoscopic instrumentation. To facilitate reentry and maintain insufflation, a hand-port device is utilized. Many devices

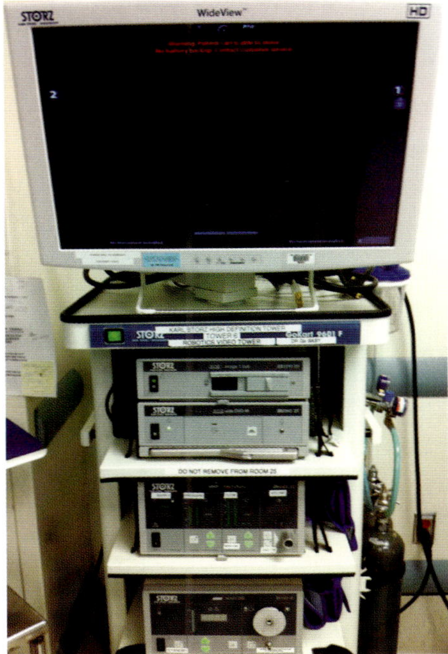

Fig. 1: Laparoscopic surgical tower

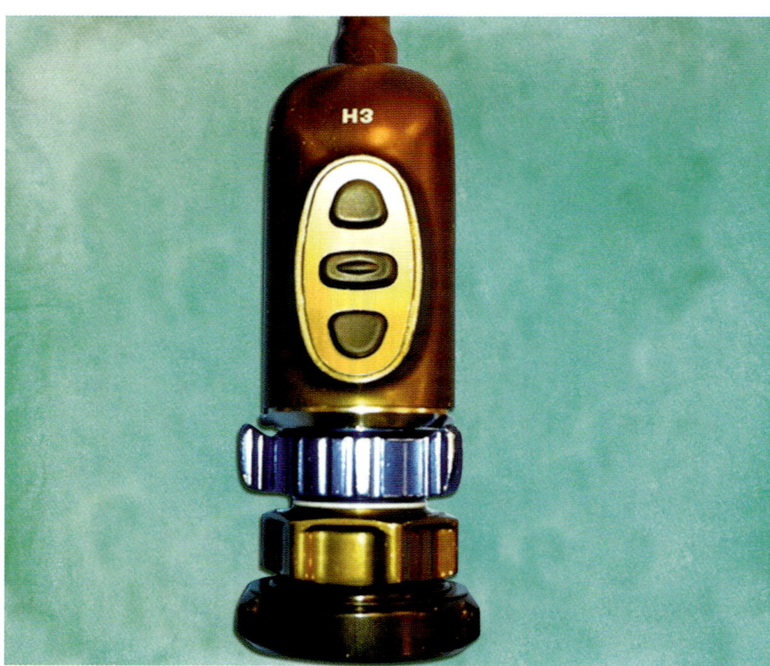

Fig. 2: Laparoscopic camera head

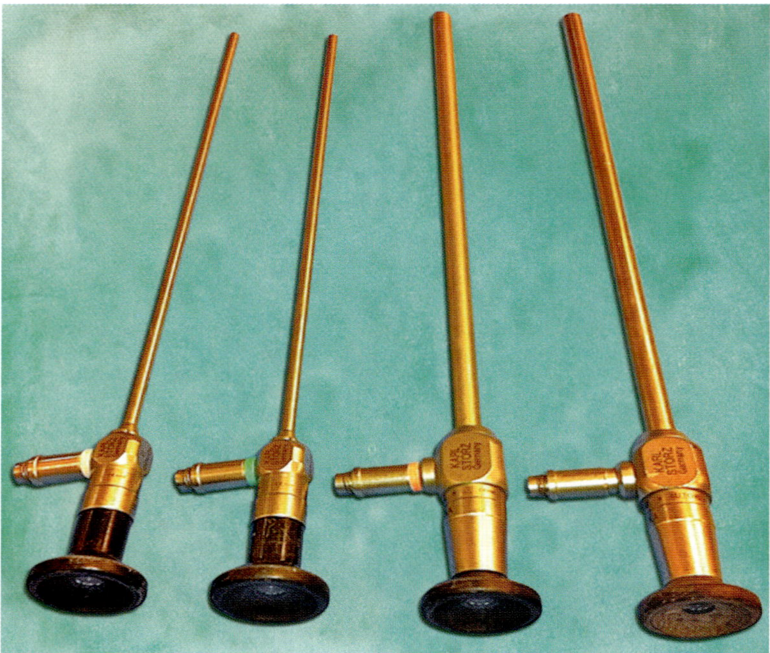

Fig. 3: 5 and 10 mm laparoscopes (*Source*: Karl Storz)

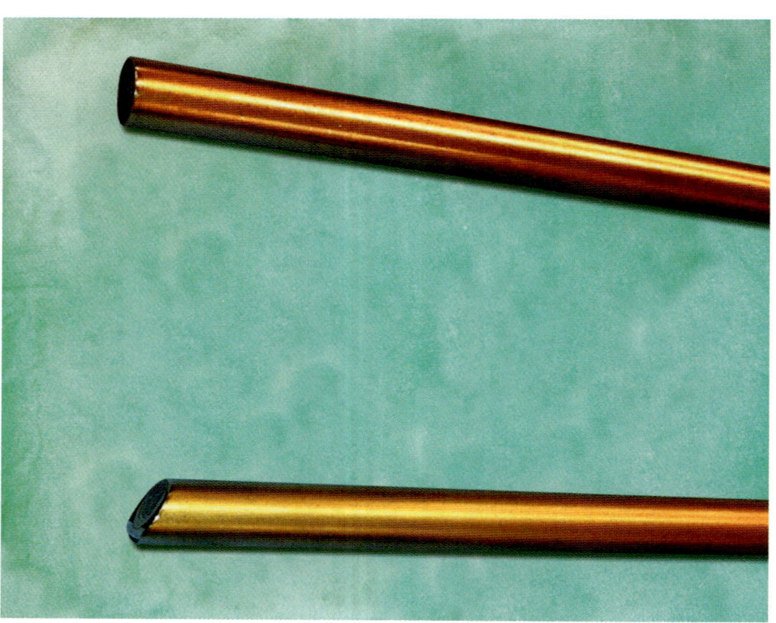

Fig. 4: 0°(top) and 30°(bottom) angled laparoscope lens (*Source*: Karl Storz)

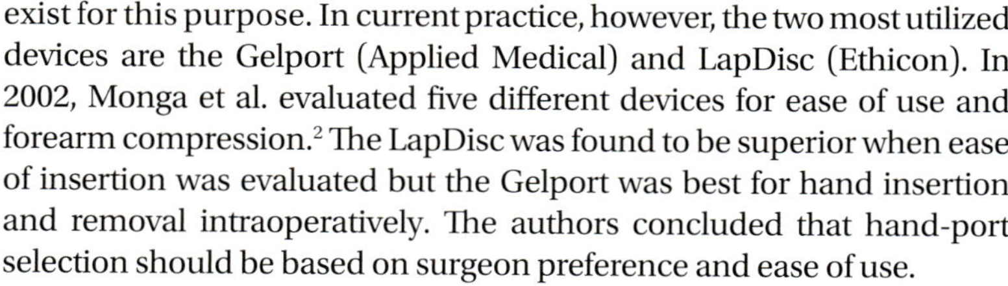

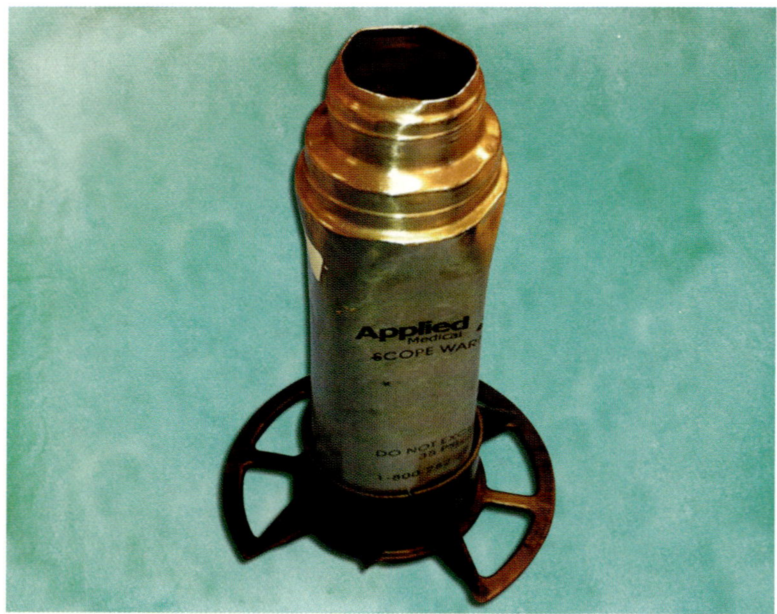

Fig. 5: Laparoscope warming thermos (*Source*: Applied Medical)

exist for this purpose. In current practice, however, the two most utilized devices are the Gelport (Applied Medical) and LapDisc (Ethicon). In 2002, Monga et al. evaluated five different devices for ease of use and forearm compression.[2] The LapDisc was found to be superior when ease of insertion was evaluated but the Gelport was best for hand insertion and removal intraoperatively. The authors concluded that hand-port selection should be based on surgeon preference and ease of use.

Suturing

During laparoscopic surgery, intracorporeal suturing is accomplished via the use of a laparoscopic needle holder (Fig. 8). The manipulation of sutures is difficult due to the 2-dimensional view and limited needle manipulation afforded by laparoscopic needle holders. Furthermore, intracorporeal knot tying is a skill that can prove particularly difficult.

The Lapra-Ty (Johnson and Johnson) was developed to facilitate intracorporeal suturing by eliminating the need for knot tying (Fig. 9). This device consists of vicryl clips that are applied to suture material to supplant the knot. The use of this device can save considerable time during laparoscopic surgery.

Dissection

During laparoscopy, the surgeon is tasked with the manipulation of viscera and dissection of surgical planes without the benefit of their hands. There are a plethora of instruments available to facilitate this task. These devices can be categorized as either active or passive dissectors. Active dissectors utilize an energy source to both dissect and achieve hemostasis whereas passive dissectors do not incorporate an energy source.

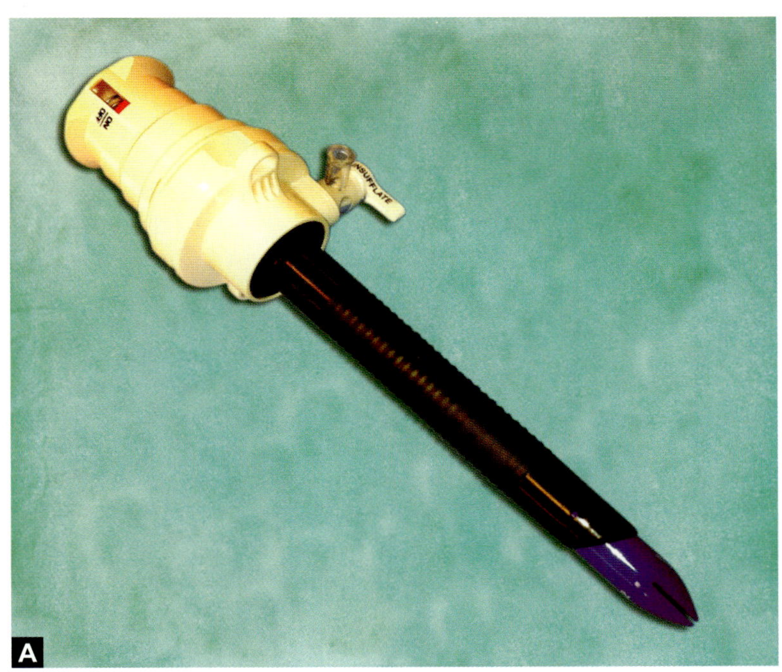
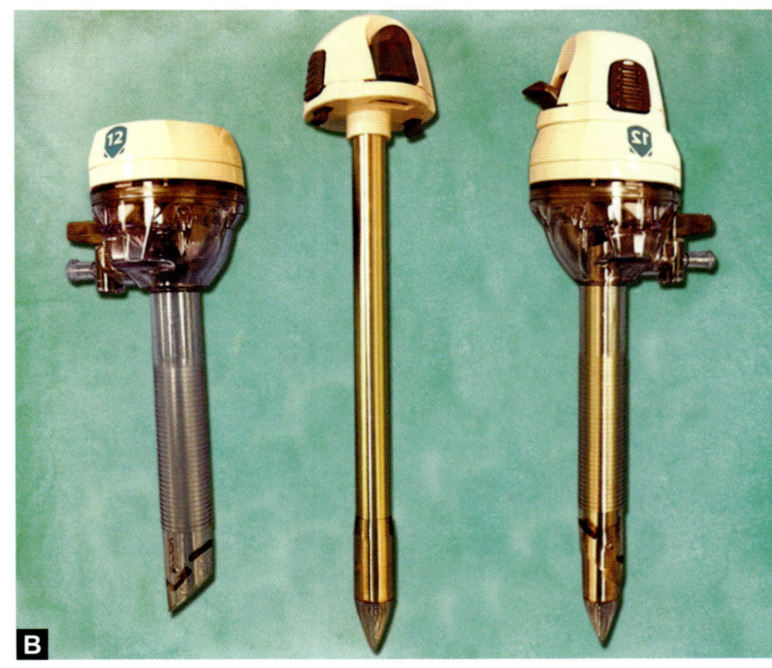

Figs 6A and B: (A) Versaport plus bladed 12 mm trocar (*Source*: Covidien Surgical); (B) Non-bladed 12 mm optical trocar (*Source*: Ethicon Endosurgery)

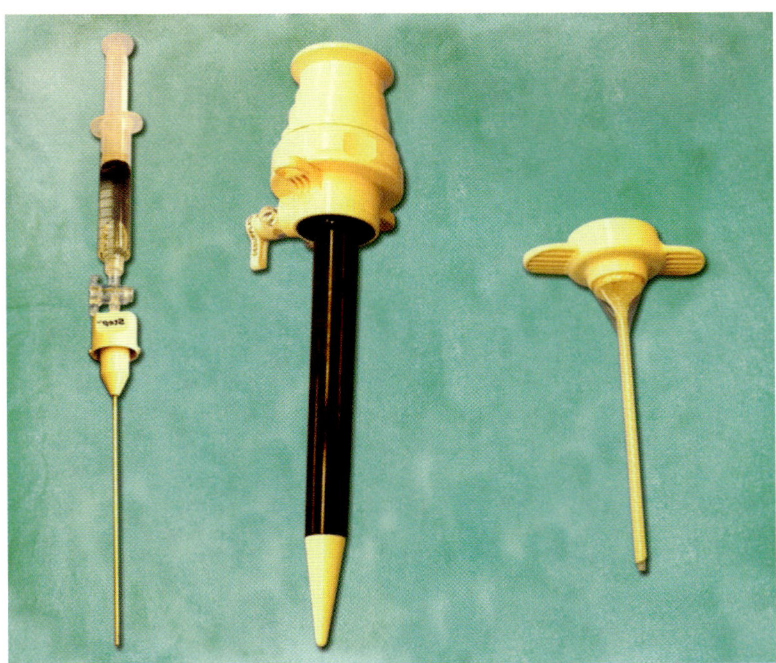

Fig. 7: VesaStep bladeless trocar system (*Source*: Covidien Surgical)

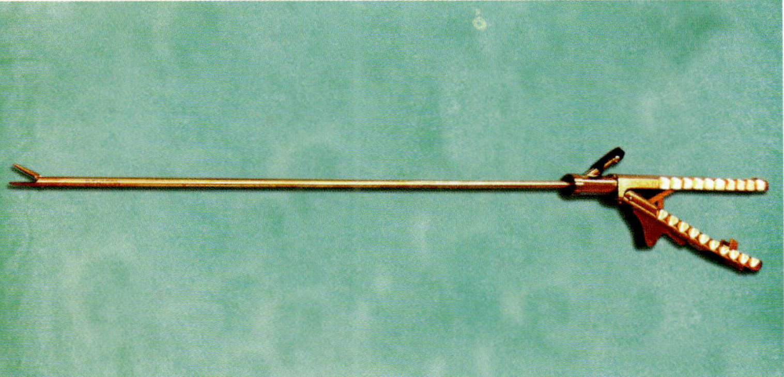

Fig. 8: Laparoscopic needle driver (*Source*: Ethicon Endosurgery)

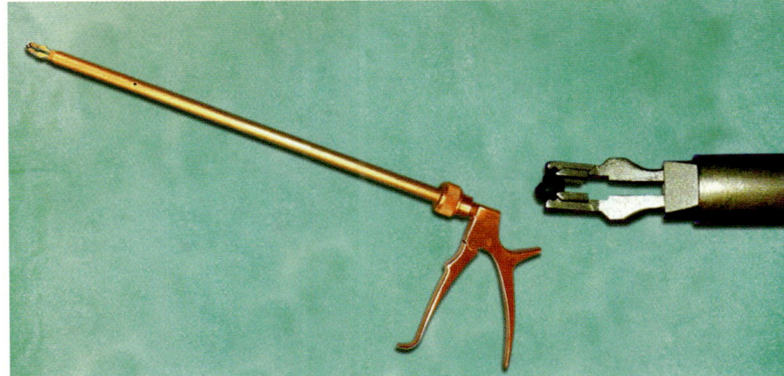

Fig. 9: Lapra-Ty absorbable suture clips (*Source*: Ethicon Endosurgery)

Many passive dissectors are currently available (Fig. 10) including the Maryland dissector, right-angle dissector, needle-nose dissector, and Kelly dissector. Within the category of passive dissectors, the authors also include graspers and scissors as they are often utilized for tissue manipulation and dissection. These include the babcock grasper, atraumatic bowel grasper, alligator grasper, fundus grasper, and allis grasper. Intraoperatively the most commonly utilized scissor is the curved metzenbaum scissor.

Active dissectors include the Harmonic scalpel (Ethicon Endosurgery), the Ligasure (Tyco Valleylab), and electrocautery (both monopolar and bipolar).

Monopolar electrocautery can be used as an adjunct with several of the passive dissectors, including the scissors and Maryland grasper, or via specialized instruments (Fig. 11). Care must be taken when this energy source is utilized as the current conducts in all directions for several millimeters and inadvertent visceral injury has been described.[3,4]

Bipolar electrocautery functions via passage of current between the instrument's arms. This facilitates hemostasis with a decreased risk of inadvertent visceral injury. Bipolar electrocautery can be delivered via several different devices including specialized graspers and the Ligasure (Figs 12A and B). This device functions via thermal energy to close vessels up to 7 mm in diameter. The incorporation of a blade provides tissue division upon adequate cauterization, further facilitating the surgical dissection.

The Harmonic scalpel utilizes ultrasonic energy to achieve hemostasis and tissue division (Fig. 13). In this device, electrical energy is converted to mechanical energy resulting in oscillation of the active limb at 55,000 Hz. This results in frictional heating and protein denaturation with minimal lateral transduction. This results in hemostasis and tissue division at higher temperatures than the Ligasure.[5]

Hemostasis

Despite the multitude of active dissectors available, there remains a potential for active bleeding. The use of energy-based dissectors may not prove adequate or may purposely be avoided to prevent injury to vital structures. It is this situation that mandates the use of surgical clips and staplers.

Surgical clips provide mechanical compressive force. Through this mechanism, they can control nearly any bleeding structures and vessels. Surgical clips are available in several forms. The most commonly utilized clip is the titanium clip (Fig. 14). These are available in 5 and 10 mm and can be utilized in both open and laparoscopic procedures.

In addition to the standard titanium clip, Hem-o-Lok clips (Teleflex Medical) can be applied laparoscopically (Fig. 15). These clips are composed of a permanent non-absorbable polymer and were initially designed for vessel ligation. Despite this, however, they have been implemented in multiple laparoscopic procedures including prostatectomy[6], partial nephrectomy[7,8], and nephrectomy.[9,10] They are available in three sizes: medium-large, large, and extra large (XL).

Laparoscopic staplers provide both mechanical compression, via six rows of staples, as well as tissue division, through the incorporation

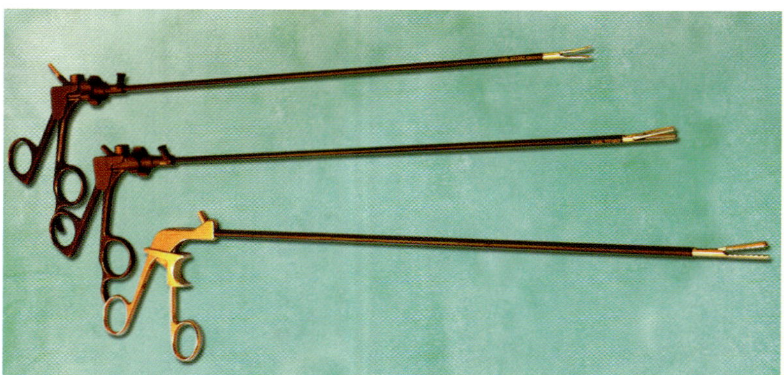

Fig. 10: Laparoscopic passive dissectors and graspers

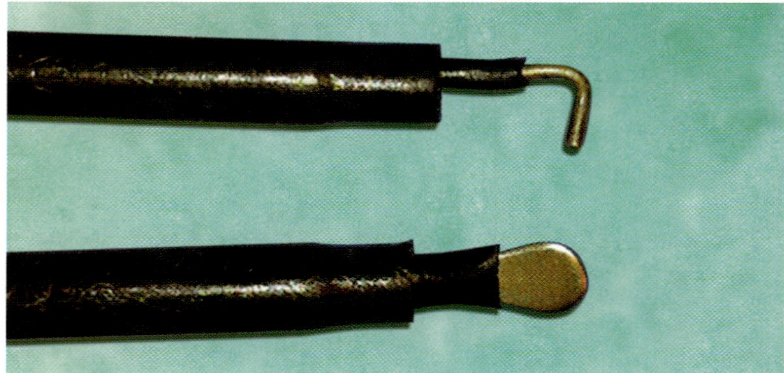

Fig. 11: Monopolar devices

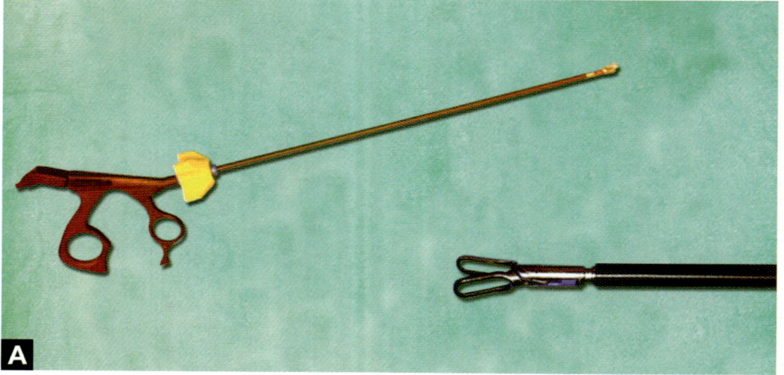

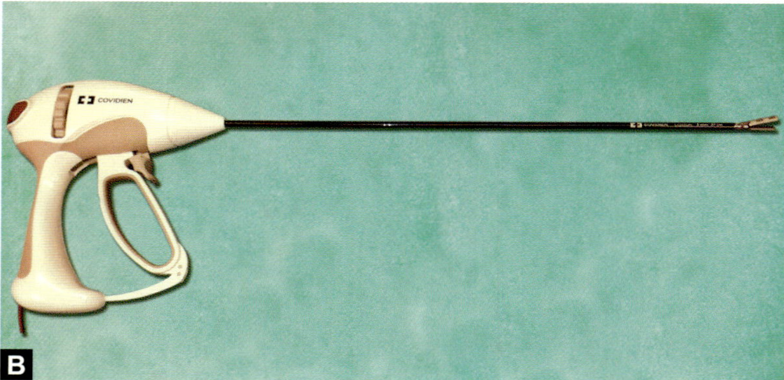

Figs 12A and B: (A) Laparoscopic bipolar dissector (*Source*: Aesculap); (B) Ligasure 5 mm laparoscopic instrument (*Source*: Covidien Surgical)

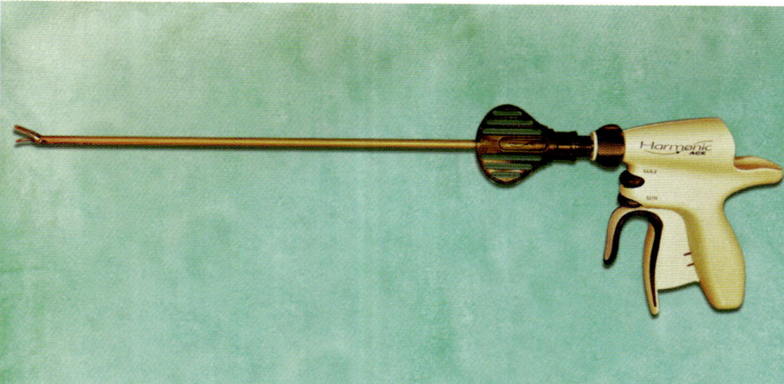

Fig. 13: Harmonic scalpel laparoscopic instrument (*Source*: Ethicon Endosurgery)

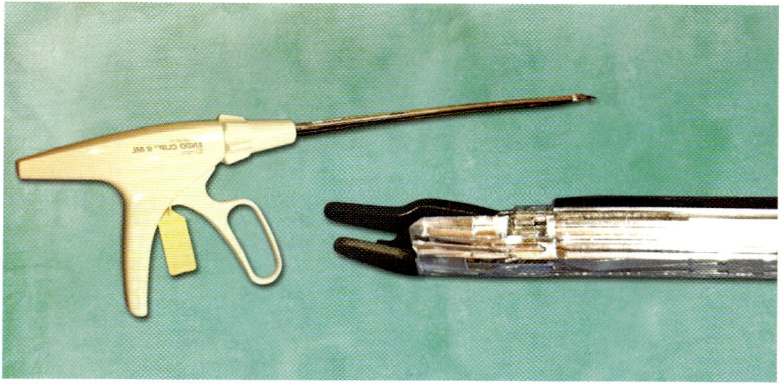

Fig. 14: Titanium clip laparoscopic applier (*Source*: Covidien Surgical)

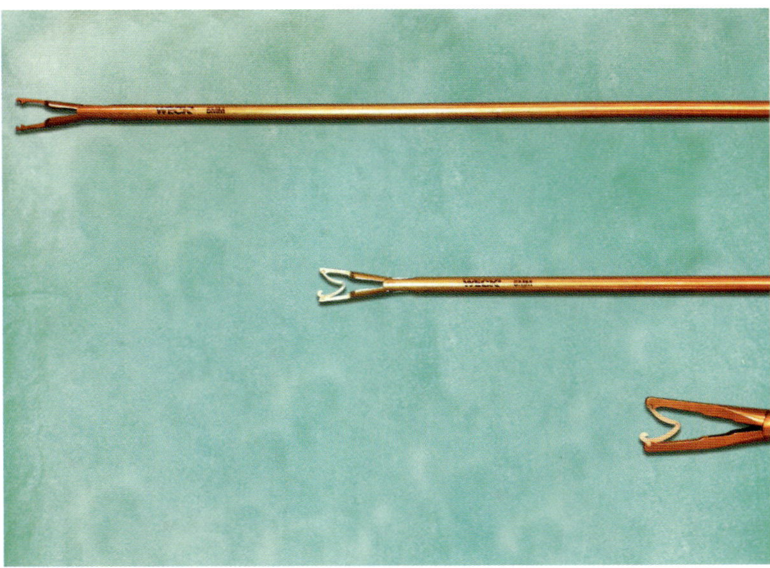

Fig. 15: Hem-o-Lok (WECK) clip laparoscopic applier (*Source*: Teleflex Medical)

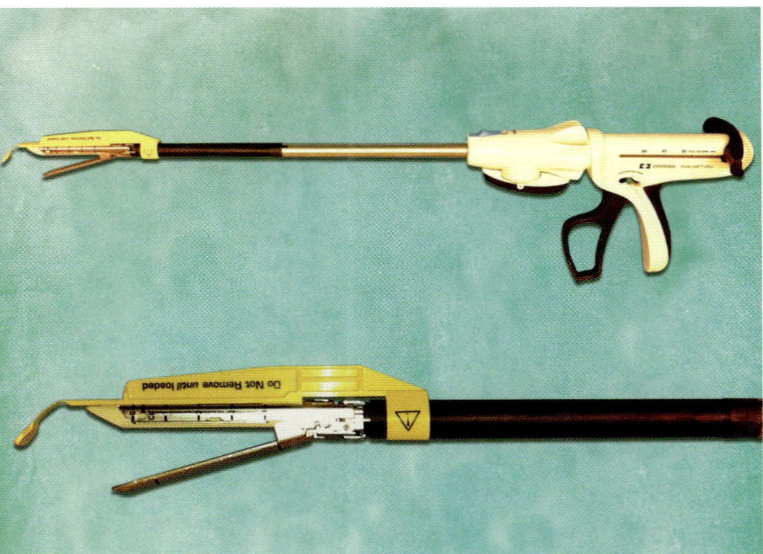

Fig. 16: Endo GIA ultra laparoscopic stapler (*Source*: Covidien Surgical)

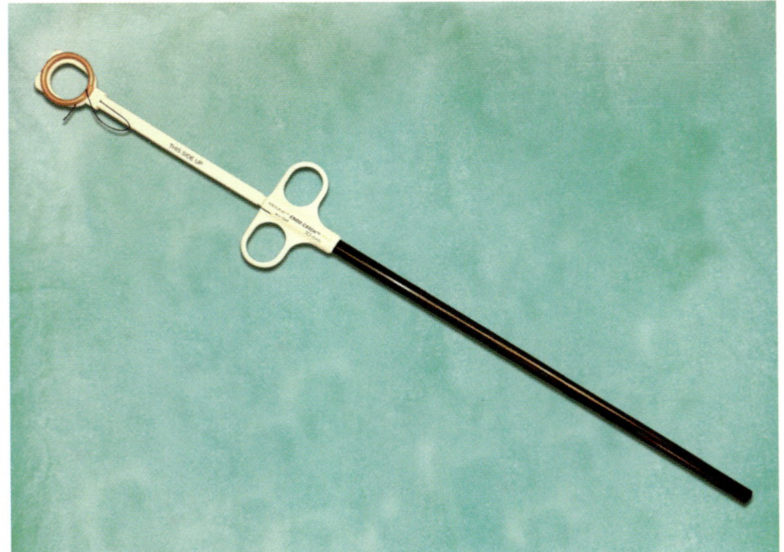

Fig. 17: 10 mm Laparoscopic specimen removal device (*Source*: Covidien Surgical)

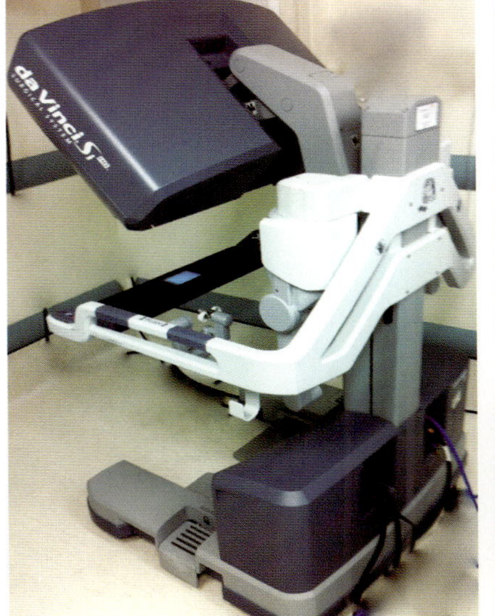

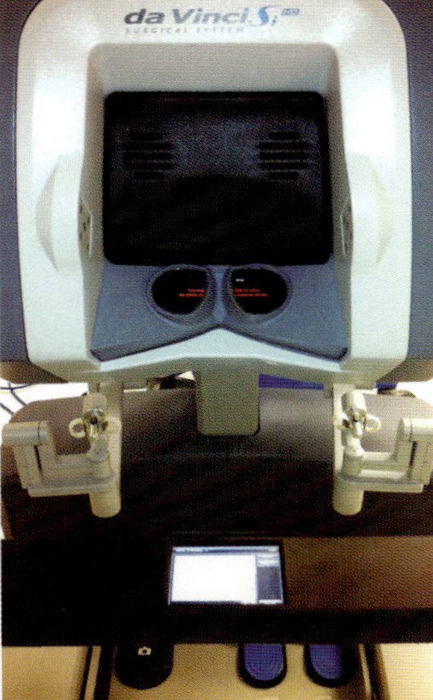

Fig. 18: Surgeon console

of a cutting blade. Staplers are available in several forms, i.e. vascular, etc. and sizes (45, 60, and 80 mm) (Fig. 16).

Specimen Removal

During laparoscopic procedures, small incisions are utilized. As a result, surgical specimens are often left within the surgical field until the procedure is complete. Laparoscopic specimen removal bags are utilized to facilitate removal, avoid the spread of infection, and prevent tumor implantation (Fig. 17).

ROBOTIC INSTRUMENTATION

To date, four da Vinci® robotic surgical systems (Intuitive Surgical) have been released: standard, streamlined (S), S-high definition (HD), and S incorporated (Si). The da Vinci® system consists of an operator console (Fig. 18) and a patient-side robotic cart (Fig. 19) that houses one camera arm and 2–3 surgical arms. The camera incorporates two separate lenses to provide a 3-dimensional visual field for the operating surgeon and also provides up to 10x magnification (Fig. 20). In addition to the improved visualization, the instrument arm's Endowrist® technology provides the surgeon with 7 degrees of freedom allowing for movements that mimic a human wrist (Fig. 21). These advantages help to filter out human tremors, provide the surgeon with a comfortable position from which he or she will operate, and provide for more facile intracorporeal suturing. It is through these advances that the incorporation of robotics into surgical procedures has helped to allay several of the limitations of standard laparoscopy.

The da Vinci® robotic system is an example of a master-slave system in which the surgeon resides at a console separate from the patient, but within the same operative suite, and directly manipulates the robot to perform the surgical procedure (Fig. 22).

During robot-assisted laparoscopic surgery, the surgeon performs all tasks other than suction, specimen entrapment, and at times clip placement. These tasks are accomplished through the use of multiple robotic instruments that incorporate Endowrist® technology. Preoperatively each robotic arm is fitted with a sterile drape specially designed for the robotic system (Figs 23A and B).

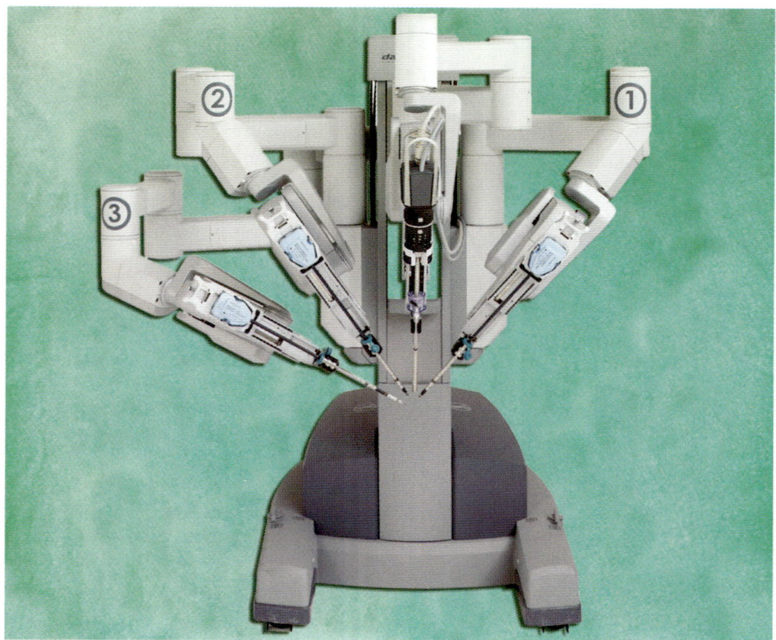

Fig. 19: da Vinci® Si HD surgical system patient cart (*Source*: Intuitive Surgical, Inc., 2010)

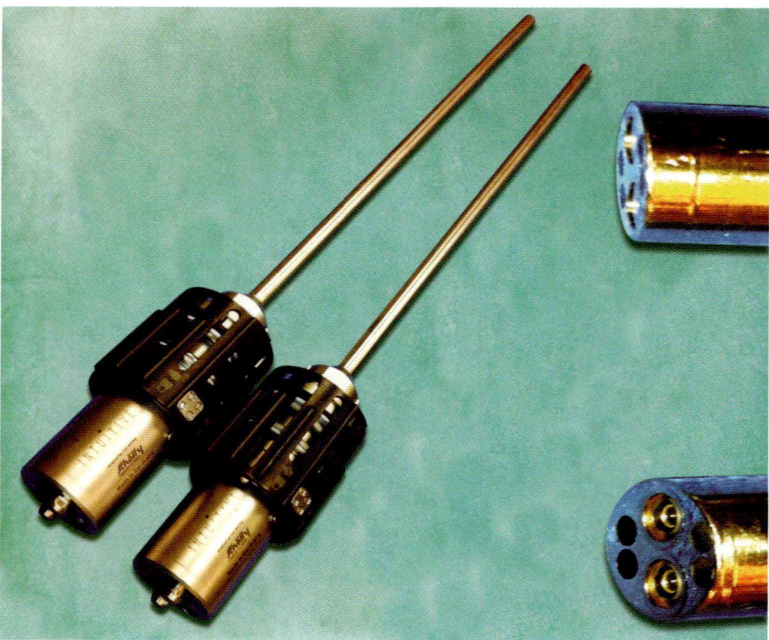

Fig. 20: da Vinci® Si HD surgical system camera, including both 30° and 0° lens

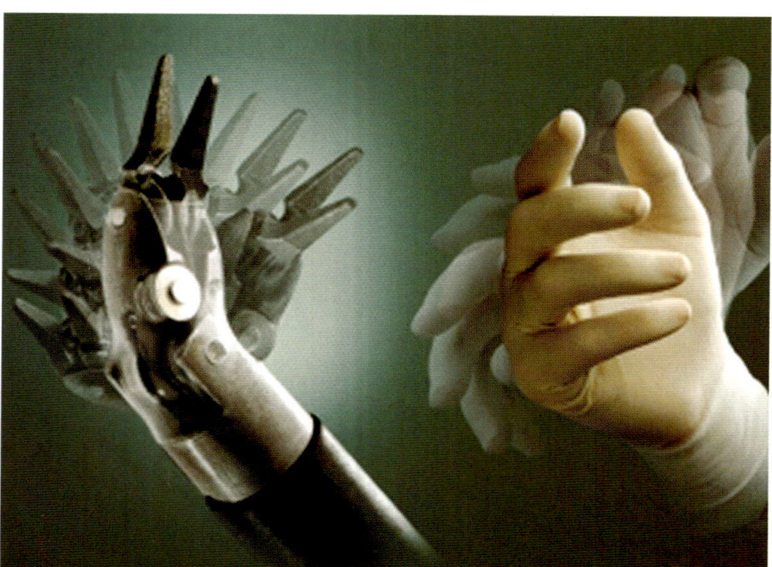

Fig. 21: Endowrist® articulated instruments with 7 degrees of freedom (*Source*: ©2005 Intuitive Surgical, Inc)

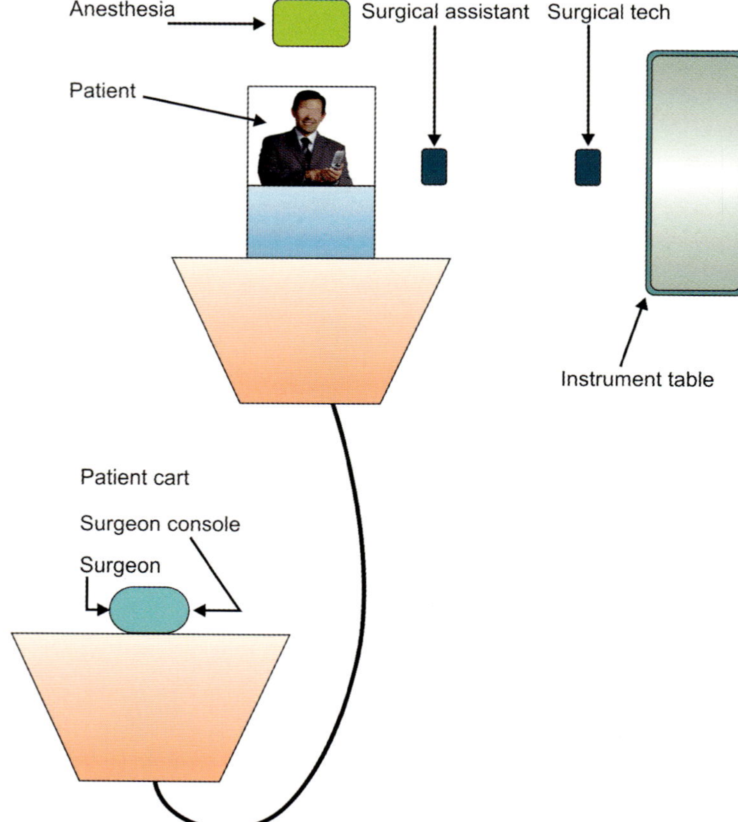

Fig. 22: Robotic surgery operating room organization

This system facilitates the interchange of robotic instruments throughout the course of the operation. A multitude of instruments have been developed for use with the surgical robot including Maryland forceps, bipolar dissector, etc (Fig. 24).

It is important to note that the robotic arms are only compatible with specific robotic trocars (Fig. 25). These trocars can be utilized with either sharp or blunt obturators.

CONCLUSION

The continuing advancement of technology has made both laparoscopic and robotic surgery a reality. As imaging is improved and instrumentation becomes more specialized, the urologist is afforded the ability to perform more complex procedures with minimally invasive technique.

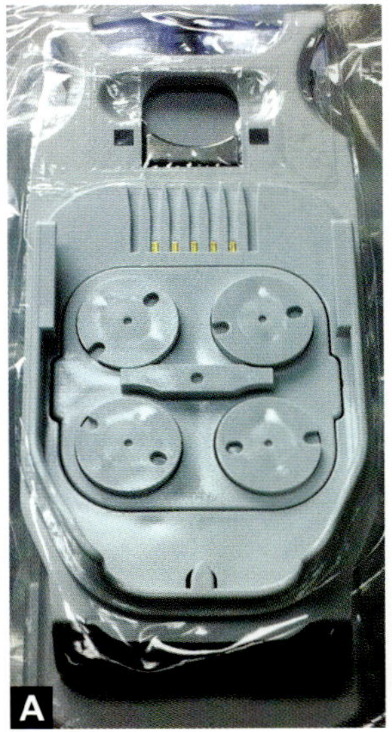

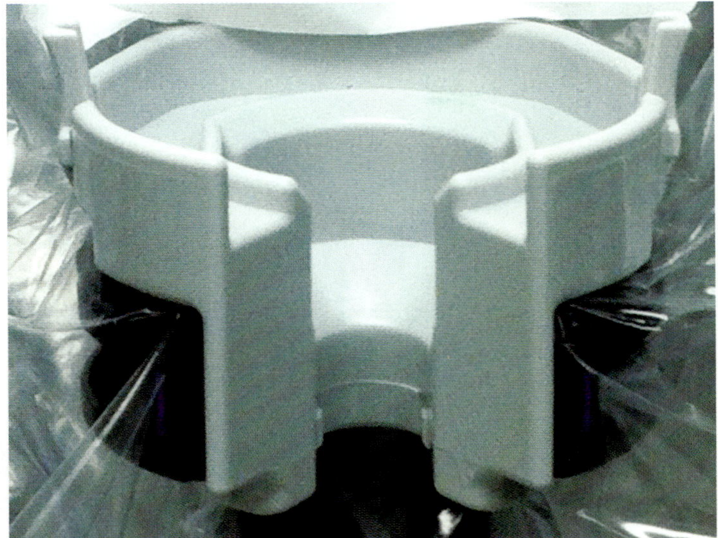

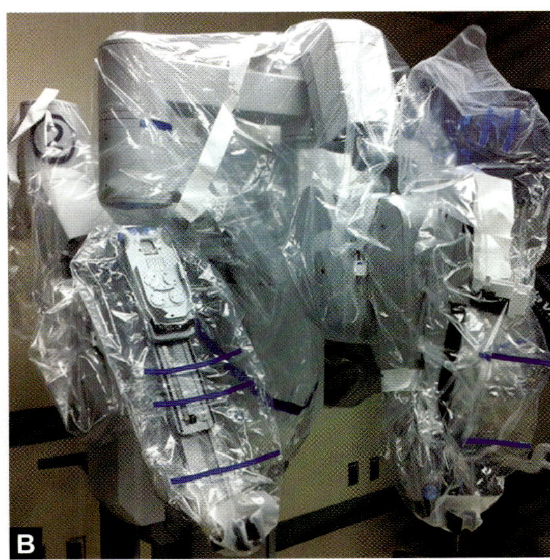

Figs 23A and B: (A) da Vinci® Si HD surgical system patient cart; (B) Patient cart prepped for surgery

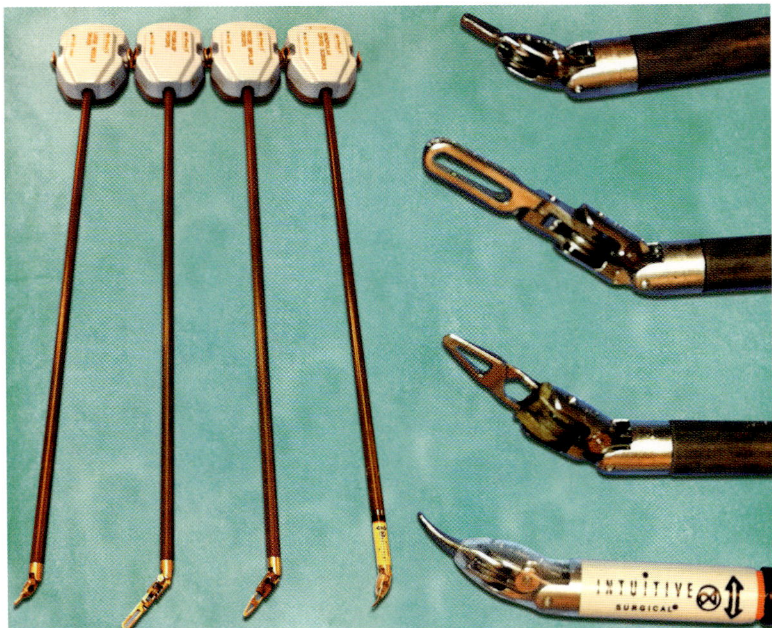

Fig. 24: Robotic Endowrist® instruments

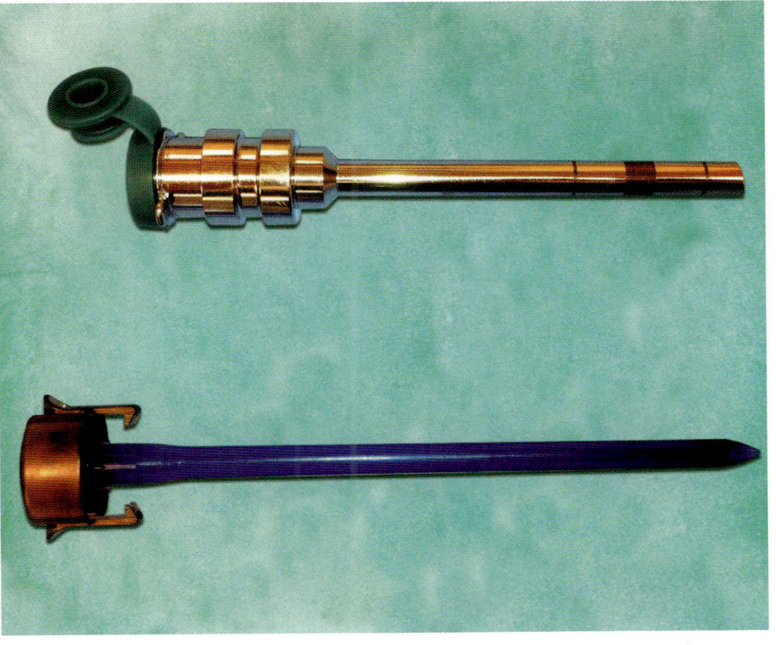

Fig. 25: Robot trocar with blunt obturator

REFERENCES

1. Shalhav AL, Barret E, Lifshitz DA, et al. Transperitoneal laparoscopic renal surgery using blunt 12-mm trocar without fascial closure. J Endourol, 2002;16:43-6.
2. Monga M, Premoli J, Skemp N, et al. Forearm compression by laparoscopic hand-assist devices. J Endourol. 2004;18:654-6.
3. Tsigris C, Tsechpenakis A, Nikiteas N, et al. Laparoscopic bowel injury: role of the site and the instrument type: study with an animal model. Surg Endosc. 2008;22:2164-7.
4. Bishoff JT, Bishoff JT, Allaf ME, et al. Laparoscopic bowel injury: incidence and clinical presentation. J Urol, 1999;161:887-90.
5. Kim FJ, Chammas MF, Gewehr E, et al. Temperature safety profile of laparoscopic devices: Harmonic ACE (ACE), Ligasure V (LV), and plasma trisector (PT). Surg Endosc. 2008;22:1464-9.
6. Blumenthal KB, Sutherland DE, Wagner KR, et al. Bladder neck contractures related to the use of Hem-o-lok clips in robot-assisted laparoscopic radical prostatectomy. Urology. 2008;72:158-61.
7. Canales BK, Lynch AC, Fernandes E, et al. Novel technique of knotless hemostatic renal parenchymal suture repair during laparoscopic partial nephrectomy. Urology. 2007;70:358-9.
8. Ho HS, Peschel R, Neururer R, et al. Another novel application of Hem-o-Lok clips for transient vascular occlusion in robot-assisted laparoscopic partial nephrectomy: an alternative to laparoscopic bulldog and Satinsky clamps. J Endourol, 2008;22:1677-80.
9. Eswar C, Badillo FL. Vascular control of the renal pedicle using the hem-o-lok polymer ligating clip in 50 consecutive hand-assisted laparoscopic nephrectomies. J Endourol. 2004;18:459-61.
10. Ponsky L, Cherullo E, Moinzadeh A, et al. The Hem-o-lok clip is safe for laparoscopic nephrectomy: a multi-institutional review. Urology. 2008;71:593-6.

SECTION

2

Upper Tract Surgery

3

Chapter

Laparoscopic Transperitoneal Radical Nephrectomy

Simon Y Kimm, Jonathan A Coleman

INTRODUCTION

Laparoscopic radical nephrectomy is an essential procedure to master for any urologic surgeon using minimally invasive techniques to address the upper urinary tract. Intimate knowledge of the renal anatomy as well as the surrounding retroperitoneal structures are required in order to safely and effectively dissect along the proper surgical planes. What follows is a simplified description of the techniques used for laparoscopic radical nephrectomy using a transperitoneal approach. Retroperitoneal approaches to the kidney have been described, but are less common and outside the scope of this chapter. To ensure the safety and success of this procedure, consideration must be given to patient factors such as significant comorbid conditions and prior history of abdominal surgery.

INDICATIONS

The primary indication for laparoscopic radical nephrectomy is a neoplasm of the kidney not amenable to partial nephrectomy. Other indications may include pathologic processes which involve the kidney necessitating its removal. A malignancy of urothelial origin also requires radical renal excision using the same principles, and in addition, requires removal of the ipsilateral ureter and ureteral orifice. This is often performed using a combination of laparoscopic and open approaches. Large tumor size, prior abdominal surgery, and obesity increase the challenge of the procedure, but are not contraindications to it. Relative contraindications include tumor thrombi requiring cavotomy and thrombectomy malignant involvement of adjacent major organs (e.g. bowel, pancreas, liver) and widespread metastatic disease with carcinomatosis. Absolute contraindications include abdominal sepsis, uncontrolled coagulopathy, and severe cardiopulmonary morbidity causing hemodynamic or pulmonary instability under conditions of pneumoperitoneum.

INSTRUMENTATION

- *Laparoscopic atraumatic bowel grasper*: For manipulating bowel during bowel mobilization.
- *Endoscopic shears*: For sharp dissection and application of electrocautery.
- *Suction/Irrigator*: Critical for adequate suction of the operative field. Often helpful as a blunt dissector and for lateral retraction of the kidney to expose the renal hilum.
- *Maryland dissector or Crile dissector*: Double-action fine tipped instrument for fine dissection of the vascular hilum. Particularly useful for dissecting between renal artery and vein and for lymph node dissection.
- *Harmonic scalpel (Ethicon) or 5 mm laparoscopic LigaSure (Covidien)*: For coagulating and dividing small caliber vessels (< 4–5 mm diameter) including the gonadal and lumbar vessels. Can also be used in a limited way for tissue manipulation including blunt dissection and grasper.
- *Endoscopic gastrointestinal anastomosis (GIA) stapler with vascular staple load*: Used for dividing renal artery, vein and vascular attachments between adrenal and upper pole or dividing the ureter with periureteral vessels.
- *Laparoscopic clip applier*: 5 mm and/or 10 mm instruments including disposable titanium clip appliers or Hem-o-lok (Weck) clip applier. Useful in ligating larger vessels (gonadal vessels, lumbar vessels) and lymphatics. May be used to secure the renal artery when space is limited (interaortocaval approach).
- *Laparoscopic bowel retractor*: 10 mm fan retractor or 5 mm snake retractor for the bowel or liver.
- *Crawford laparoscopic vascular clamp*: Useful for the immediate vascular control of large vessels such as the vena cava and aorta without need for specialized port.
- *Endocatch bag (Covidien)*: 15 mm specimen pouch.
- *Carter-Thomason CloseSure system (Cooper Surgical)*: Laparoscopic trocar site fascial closure system, consisting of a sharp suture passer and guide.

PATIENT PREPARATION

Patients are placed on a clear liquid diet the day prior to procedure and are kept nil per os (NPO) or nothing by mouth starting at midnight the day of surgery. An optional bowel preparation with one bottle of magnesium citrate can be given the day prior to surgery. Antibiotic prophylaxis is administered, typically a cephalosporin such as cefazolin. For the prophylaxis of deep vein thrombosis, pneumatic compression devices are applied to the legs and optionally, 5,000 units of subcutaneous heparin may be placed.

General endotracheal anesthesia is induced and the stomach decompressed with an orogastric tube. Surgical clippers are used to clear hair from the operative, extraction, and grounding pad sites. For a midline extraction incision, the skin should be marked while the patient is still supine. A urinary catheter may be placed if a long or complicated procedure is anticipated. Due to the hemodynamic changes that occur under laparoscopic conditions, the authors often seek to achieve euvolemia during this period by hydrating the patient with at least 750 cc of IV crystalloid solution before the initiation of pneumoperitoneum.

PATIENT POSITIONING

Close attention must be paid to patient positioning to minimize the risks of compression and positional injury.

The patient is carefully positioned in the modified flank position, utilizing approximately 50–60° of flank elevation (Fig. 1). The patient should be centered on the operating table with the upper brim of the iliac crest below the table break to avoid direct gluteal pressure. An axillary roll may be placed if necessary. The authors find that having the patient in the 50° position places the weight of the upper torso on the scapula, avoiding traction injury to the brachial plexus, and thereby rendering unnecessary the need for an axillary roll in most cases. Appropriate judgment, however, must be used in each case. Two large gel rolls are placed behind the back, one above and one below the break of the table. After rolling to the flank position, the legs are flexed and separated by two pillows, avoiding adduction strain on the upside leg. The leg in contact with the table is flexed to a greater degree with additional padding placed at the hip, knee, and ankle pressure zones.

The downside arm is cushioned on an armboard with the elbow flexed. A folded pillow is then placed between the arms and care is taken to minimize tension at the elbow and shoulder joint. The hands are placed in a neutral position (Fig. 1). Flexible foam tape is used to secure the arms.

The patient is first secured to the table at the hip with 2 inch fabric tape. Padding is used on the skin such that the adhesive surface of the tape does not come in contact with the skin. A padded safety strap is used to further secure the lower extremities. The operating table is flexed by 15–20° (Fig. 2). The upper body is secured with padded cloth tape applied over the thorax just below the axilla. It is important to secure the torso only after the table is flexed and not before since table flexion while the upper torso is secured will change the direction and pressure from the tape and may increase the risk of patient injury. When taping the torso, care is taken to minimize tension on the chest wall that would limit rib excursion and impact ventilation. A grounding pad is applied. Patient is then prepped and draped.

ACCESS

Pneumoperitoneum is established by use of a Veress needle at the umbilicus. The Veress is directed cephalad with 20–30° of angulation to help avoid placement of the tip in the preperitoneal space. To facilitate atraumatic insertion, the abdominal wall can be elevated by placing the thumb in the umbilicus and grasping the rectus muscle on one side and pulling anteriorly (Fig. 3). A drop test, injecting saline under gravity, may be used to check placement of the needle tip in the peritoneal space. Gas insufflation is provided slowly (2 liters/min) to an initial pressure of 12–15 mm Hg. If hemodynamic instability is noted during insufflation, the gas line should be immediately disconnected and gas is evacuated passively. If any difficulty is encountered using the Veress technique then direct visual entry into the peritoneum should be performed with cut-down technique. Direct cut-down entry may be preferred in patients with history of prior abdominal surgery or other risks for adhesions.

Several laparoscopic port configurations can be used. Demonstrated here (Figs 4A and B) is a typical triangular configuration with the 10 mm camera port placed lateral and cephalad to the umbilicus along the axial plane of the lowest extent of the rib cage. If needed, this can be facilitated by following a line drawn directly off the tip of the 11th rib toward the midline. Lateralizing the camera port placement is often helpful in avoiding interference from the bowel, particularly in patients with increased abdominal girth. A 5 mm or 10 mm port is then placed approximately 10 cm cephalad to the

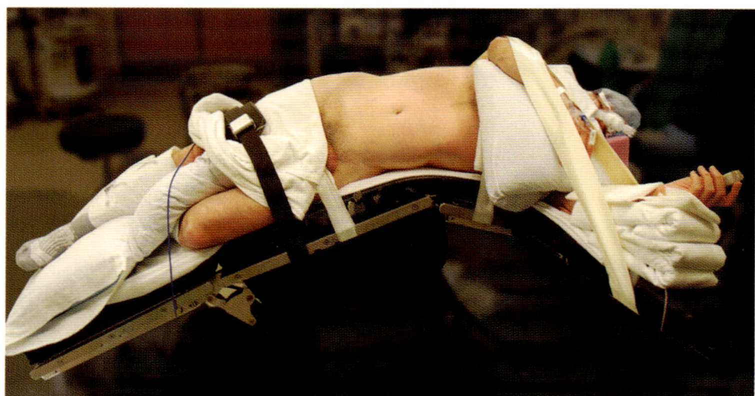

Fig. 2: The flexion point of the table must be above the bony pelvis to prevent pressure injury. The arm board may be angled toward the head. Fabric tape to secure the patient at the hip and torso is attached directly to the table railing. The arm is secured with crossed foam tape to the arm board in this manner without stretching the tape over the skin in order to avoid tape burn injury

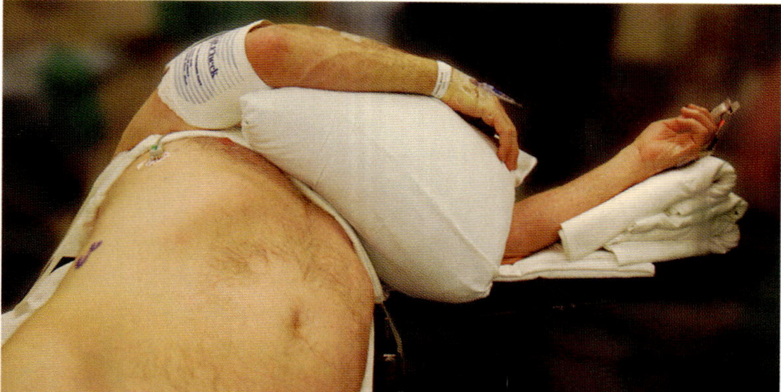

Fig. 1: Example of a right sided procedure. The arms are neutrally positioned, note elevation of contralateral forearm on the armboard and blood pressure cuff placement. The position of the arms is natural before they are secured

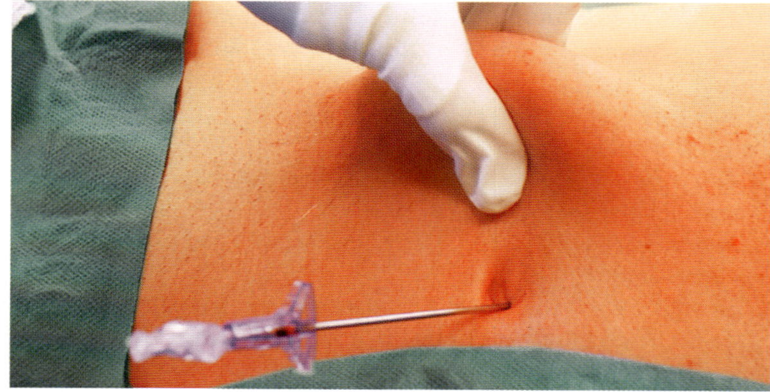

Fig. 3: Demonstration of Veress needle insertion through the umbilicus. Traction on the abdominal wall may be provided by grasping the rectus muscle as demonstrated. The needle tip is typically angled toward the head and, in most cases, only a single click from the needle is heard upon entering the peritoneum

camera port and a 10 mm or 12 mm port is placed between 8–10 cm along the line between the camera port and the anterior superior iliac spine. Optional accessory ports may be placed at the umbilicus (which can later be extended to a midline incision for extraction) or in the subxiphoid area for a liver retractor when operating on the right kidney. Smaller camera ports can be used when utilizing 5 mm lenses. Although the operation can be safely performed with small instruments and lenses through 5 mm ports, it is recommended that at least one 10 or 12 mm port be utilized (typically the most inferior lateral port) to allow use of a larger instrument at time of need including use of the surgical stapler. A 30-degree laparoscope may also be utilized in alternative port configurations including umbilical camera port access or with an offset configuration utilizing the superior most port for the laparoscope. It bears noting, however, that use of these lenses may be disorienting to an inexperienced camera operator. The authors typically utilize nonbladed, blunt dilating tip ports to minimize sharps-related injuries. All ports are placed under direct vision. After port placement, a careful inspection is carried out to evaluate the operative field and viscera for evidence of anatomic abnormalities or inadvertent injury.

RIGHT RADICAL NEPHRECTOMY

Initial Dissection

For surgery in the right upper quadrant, an additional 5 mm subxiphoid port is frequently required for liver retraction. A 5 mm grasper with a locking handle is used through this port, passed under the edge of the liver, and secured to the triangular ligament or sidewall, lifting the liver from the field (Fig. 5). When needed, the liver may be more completely mobilized in a cephalad manner by incising the peritoneum between the superior pole of the kidney and the liver, then dividing the fatty plane between liver and kidney with the LigaSure or stapler.

Compared to left-sided dissections, less mobilization of the colon is necessary on the right side to adequately expose the kidney. However, care must be taken to additionally recognize and mobilize the duodenum which lies behind the colon and often covers the renal hilum and cava.

The ascending colon is mobilized by incising the peritoneum lateral to the colon using the lateral border of the colon as a guide and incising 1 or 2 cm lateral to this (Fig. 6).

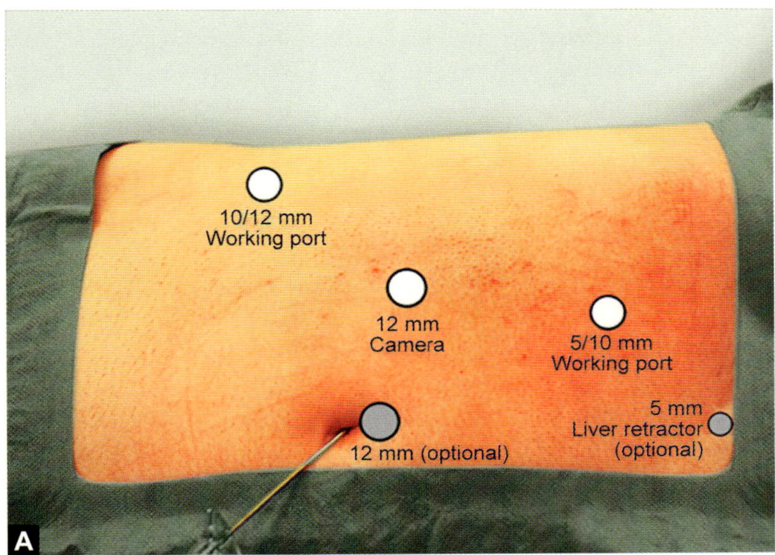

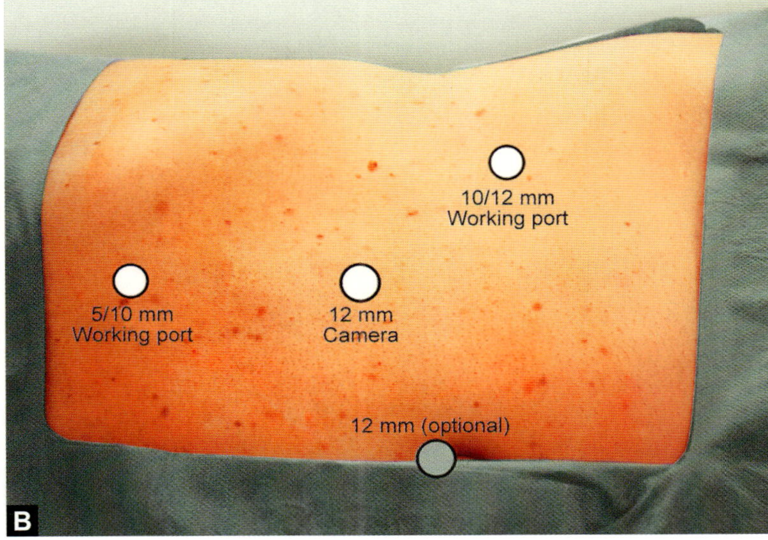

Figs 4A and B: (A) Right-sided triangular port arrangement; (B) Left-sided triangular port arrangement. Optionally, the camera port may be placed in the supraumbilical area or an optional port may be placed here for use of a bowel retractor. This area is often later used for midline incision and specimen extraction

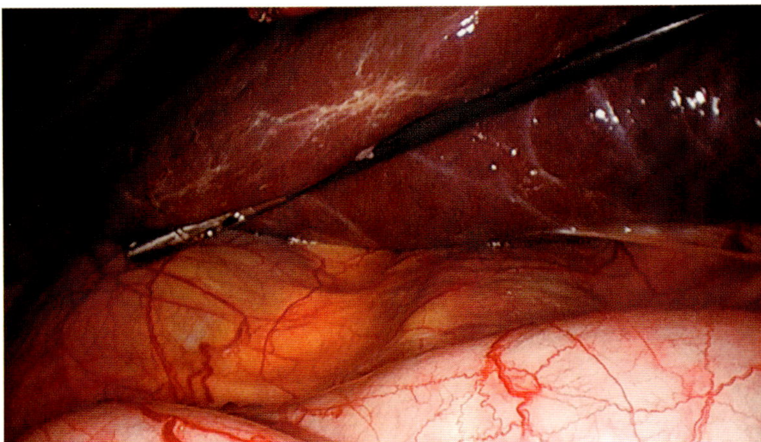

Fig. 5: An atraumatic grasper with a locking handle is passed under the liver to retract the liver in a cephalad manner

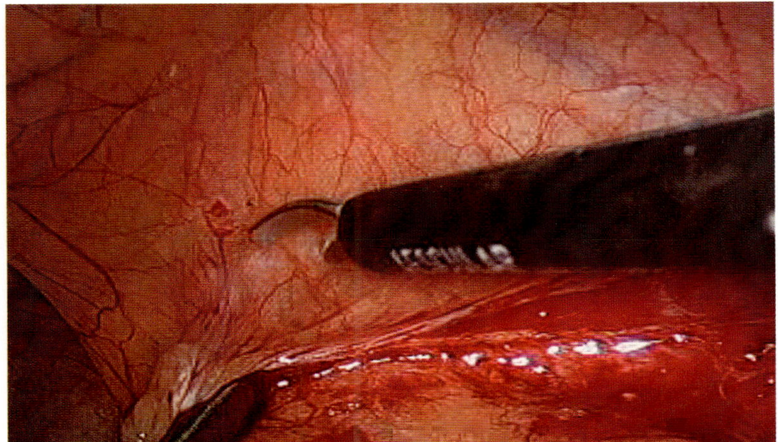

Fig. 6: The peritoneum in incised just lateral to the colon while a bowel grasper retracts the colon away to identify the proper plane

Anterior traction of the colon is provided by atraumatic grasping forceps. The plane is most easily identified below the lower pole of the kidney and this plane is developed cephalad and carried medially toward the inferior vena cava taking care to preserve the lateral attachments of the kidney to the abdominal wall. Preservation of these lateral attachments between kidney and abdominal wall facilitates the later dissection and control of the renal hilum by preventing the kidney from falling into the operative field. The hepatic flexure of the colon is released. The duodenum is mobilized by a Kocherization and sharp dissection, then gently retracted medially to expose the inferior vena cava and right renal hilum (Fig. 7).

Right Renal Hilar Control

Dissection is directed inferior to the lower pole of the kidney where the ureter and gonadal vein are identified. Gerota's fascia is entered medially to these structures, and a broad plane is developed by blunt dissection exposing the muscular plane of the psoas. The gonadal vein can be followed superiorly toward the cava sidewall before dividing it using either surgical clips or a thermal dissector (e.g. LigaSure, Harmonic scalpel, SonoSurg). The ureter and lower pole are retracted laterally, displacing the kidney away from the great vessels and stretching the renal hilar vessels, improving their exposure (Fig. 8).

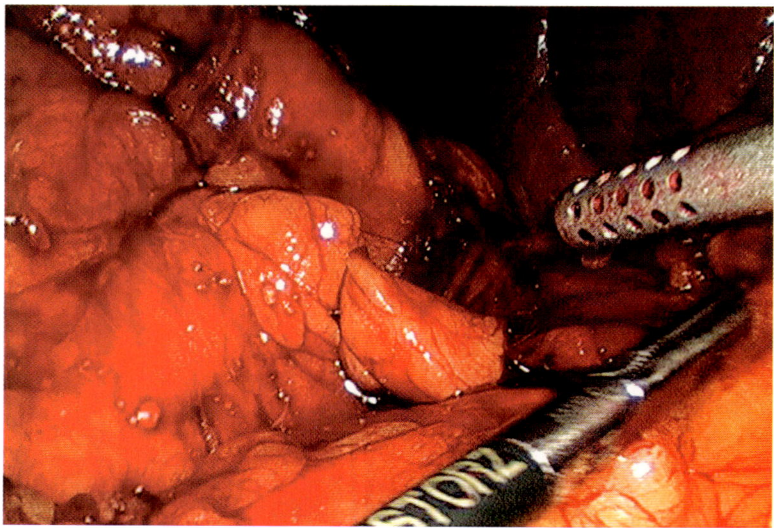

Fig. 7: After releasing the bowel and hepatic flexure, the colon is mobilized medially with a bowel grasper to expose the vena cava and duodenum

Dissection along the psoas muscle is continued toward the renal hilum until the renal vein is encountered (Fig. 9).

Division of the Right Hilar Vessels

Attention is then directed toward identifying the renal artery, usually situated behind the renal vein. Firm and steady lateral retraction of the kidney helps to facilitate this dissection, which is often easily performed with the use of the suction-irrigator behind the vessels. Once the artery is identified, it can be controlled by several means. Because we often perform lymph node dissection, it is often preferable to control the renal artery with selective ligation using surgical clips. Large metallic or Weck Hem-o-Lok clips can be used to secure the artery with two clips recommended on the side closest to the aorta. The authors often provide a single clip on the renal side prior to dividing the artery though this is not considered necessary since the renal artery is an end-artery with negligible backflow (Fig. 10).

A gastrointestinal anastomosis (GIA) stapler can also be used if space is sufficient although this may interfere with subsequent node dissection due to the excess metallic material deposited behind the hilum (Fig. 11). When space is limited, it is acceptable to place a single clip to secure the artery without dividing it (Fig. 10). This allows the vein to be taken, providing exposure for completing the dissection and division of the artery. This is particularly helpful when the right renal artery is taken in the interaortocaval location. The right adrenal gland is dissected free from the superior-medial aspect of the kidney.

The remaining superior and lateral attachments of the kidney are freed, often best completed with a thermal device (e.g. LigaSure). Care should be taken to avoid injury to the diaphragm in along this border between the upper pole and the liver and posteriorly (Fig. 12).

Inferiorly, the ureter is divided below the lower pole between Weck clips or with the GIA stapler (Fig. 13).

Extraction, Inspection and Closure

A 15 mm Endocatch bag is introduced into the abdomen. Due to its caliber, a 15 mm port is required or, alternatively, a 12 mm port may be removed and the instrument inserted under vision through this incision and deployed. To aid in this insertion, the bag may be advanced 2–3 cm from the tip to serve as a blunt obturator for the shaft of the device. Once the specimen is entrapped, the bag is then secured with the drawstring. If the specimen cannot be entrapped within the bag and it is necessary to deliver the specimen by hand,

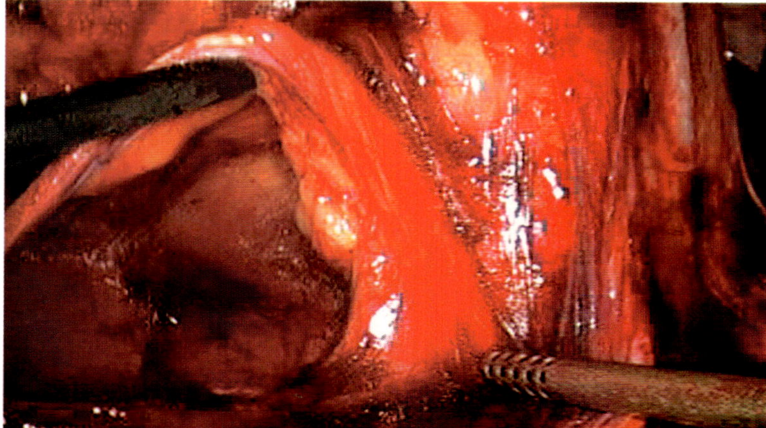

Fig. 8: After exposing the vena cava, dissection is directed under the lower pole of the kidney onto the psoas muscle. The lower pole and ureter are then elevated and displaced anteriorly to facilitate dissection toward the hilum

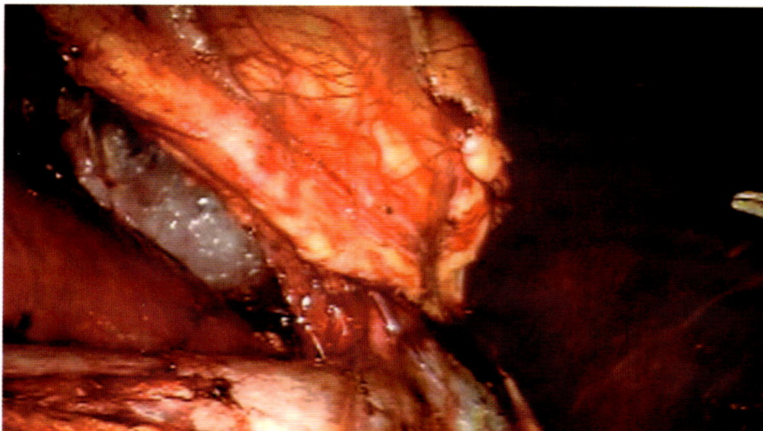

Fig. 9: Dissection is carried along the side of the vena cava toward the hilum while maintaining upward retraction of the kidney. Gentle but firm stretch on the renal hilum is critical to aid in dissection of the vessels

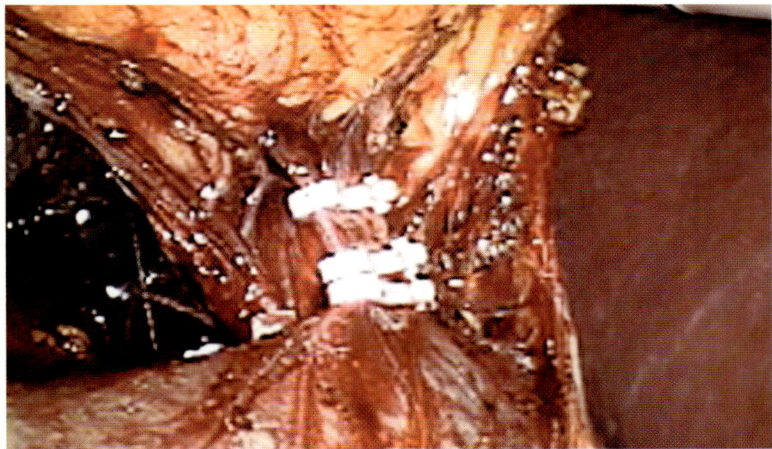

Fig. 10: The renal artery(ies) are dissected and should be controlled before the vein. Once the arterial supply is controlled, the vein may be clipped and divided. Here 1 clip is on the renal artery and multiple clips on the vein. After dividing the vein more proximal dissection on the artery can be performed to aid in retrocaval lymph node dissection

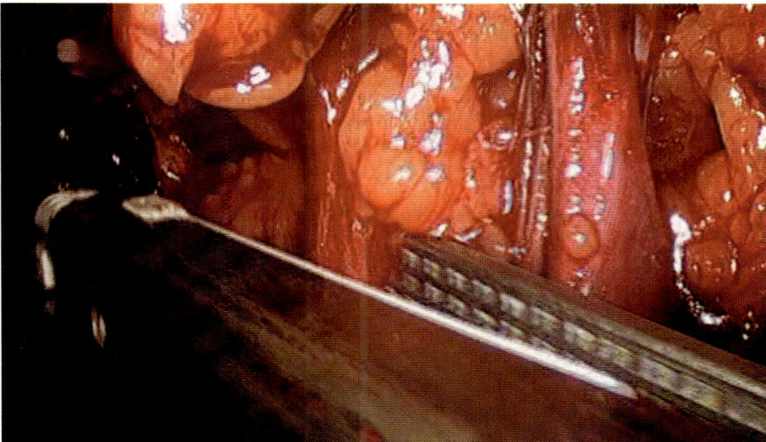

Fig. 11: In a separate case, the renal artery and surrounding tissue is taken entirely with a stapler. Surgical clips placed in the area prior to this can result in stapler malfunction if caught in the stapler jaws with devastating consequences

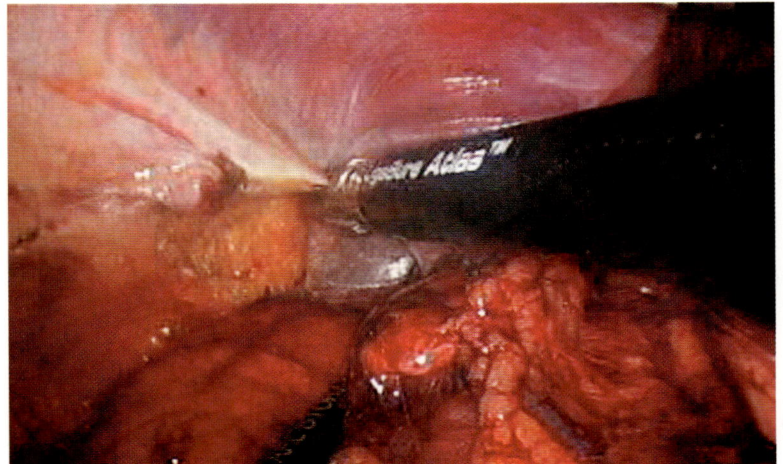

Fig. 12: The kidney is fully mobilized away from the abdominal wall by dividing the lateral peritoneal attachments. Notice the lower instrument providing anteromedial displacement of the kidney for adequate exposure

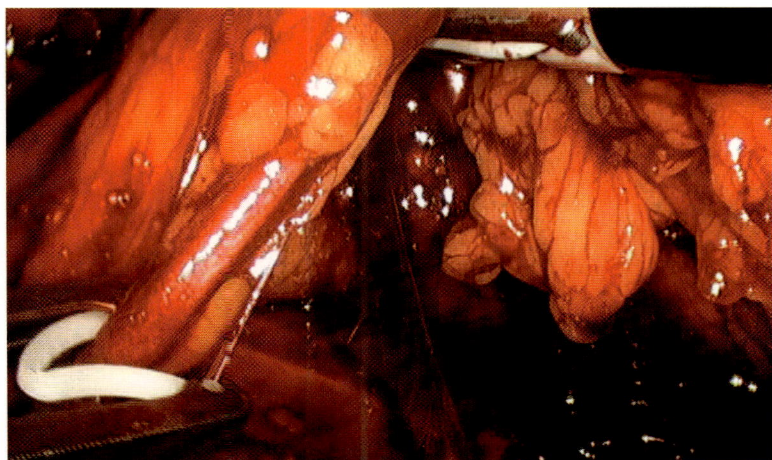

Fig. 13: The ureter is taken with a locking clip. The inferior envelope of Gerota's fascia lies lateral to this and should also be taken with respect for the vascular structures contained within

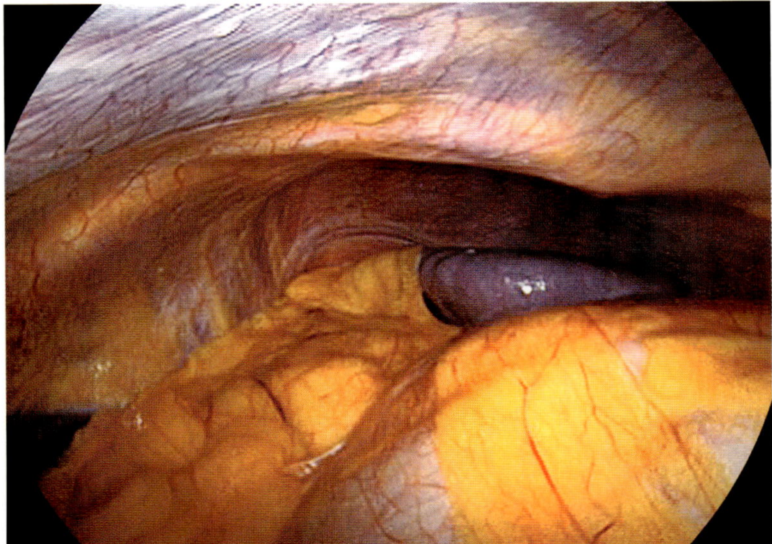

Fig. 14: The initial view of the left upper quadrant for approach to the left kidney. The kidney is typically obscured by the left colon, spleen and tail of the pancreas which must be mobilized carefully away

a generous incision should be used to avoid excessive manipulation of the specimen through the incision. A variety of extraction incisions may be used, most commonly employing muscle-splitting options including Gibson, midline or Pfannenstiel incisions.

A final laparoscopic inspection of the surgical site is performed prior to desufflation and extraction. Closure of any port sites using 2-0 or 0-Vicryl suture is performed at this time. A Carter-Thomason device may be used to facilitate port closure. Following extraction, inspection of the viscera may also be performed through the extraction site using standard open techniques. Port sites may be closed through this access as well. The skin is closed with subcuticular monocryl suture.

LEFT RADICAL NEPHRECTOMY

Initial Dissection

On the left side, the anterior aspect of Gerota's fascia is often obscured by the splenic flexure, spleen, and tail of the pancreas (Fig. 14).

The left colon requires more mobilization than on the right, and the peritoneal incision and dissection is extended more cranially on this side, typically beyond the lienorenal ligament to the diaphragm.

Dissection is initiated by dividing the sustentaculum coli and incising directly on the white line of Toldt while mobilizing the right colon with anteromedial traction. Great care must be taken to stay very superficial in this dissection plane behind the colon and anterior to Gerota's fascia in order to avoid detaching the lateral renal attachments or inadvertently dissecting through the mesentery to the colon (Fig. 15).

The colon is mobilized broadly and far inferiorly to facilitate exposure for the medial dissection (Fig. 16).

Once exposure over the lower pole is completed, dissection is carried cephalad over the hilum and superiorly with care taken to recognize the location of the tail of the pancreas in its association to the superomedial aspect of the kidney and adrenal. The pancreas and spleen are gently retracted medially (Fig. 17A) while dissecting the alveolar plane between these organs and the upper pole of the kidney. Great care should be taken to avoid injury to the spleen with the tip of the retracting instrument. This can best be avoided by passing the instrument tip beyond the spleen and not allowing it to press directly into the spleen or splenic hilum (Fig. 17B). As the dissection proceeds posteriorly along this plane, care should be taken to avoid the diaphragm or unnecessary use of cautery in the region of the pancreas or superior mesenteric artery, found medial to the adrenal. Medial mobilization of the spleen requires release of the splenocolic and splenophrenic ligaments, with care to prevent tearing the splenic capsule. Eventually, the splenorenal fascial attachments must be released, but these are often obscured until later in the dissection.

Left Renal Hilar Control

The left gonadal vein is identified inferiorly as it courses toward the left renal vein (Fig. 18). Posterior and lateral to this structure, the left ureter is identified. Similar to the right-sided dissection, a plane is broadly developed between the psoas muscle and the laterally retracted ureter and gonadal vein (Fig. 19). This lateral retraction aids in exposure by placing the renal hilum on stretch. Dissection proceeds carefully toward the hilum until the left renal vein is encountered.

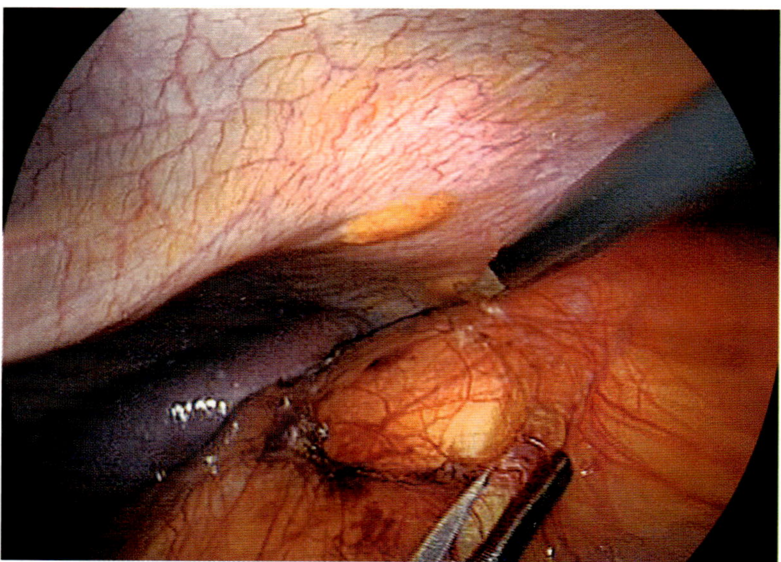

Fig. 15: Initial dissection is made sharply through the superficial most plane of peritoneum just lateral to the colon, exposing the anterior plane of Gerota's fascia. A grasper is used for gentle retraction

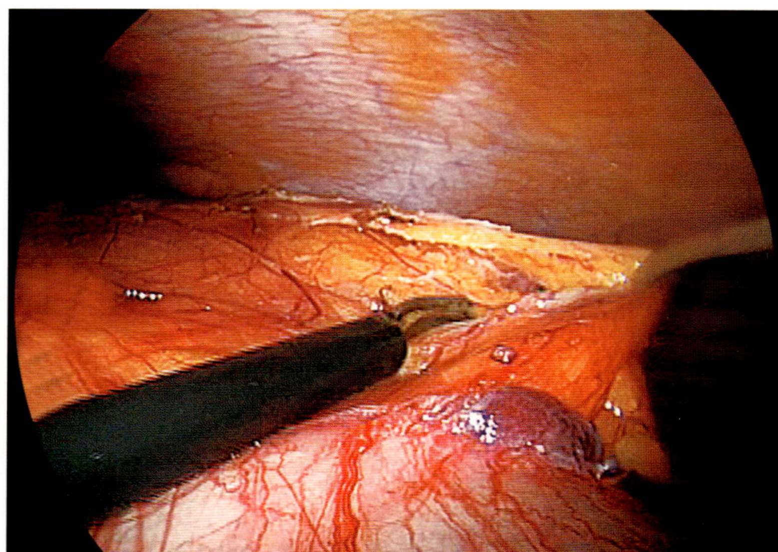

Fig. 16: Note the gentle use of a grasper applied to provide lifting (not downward) retraction of the tissue. The grasper is not in contact with the bowel. The scissor is used to first bluntly dissect the plane before dividing the lateral peritoneal attachments

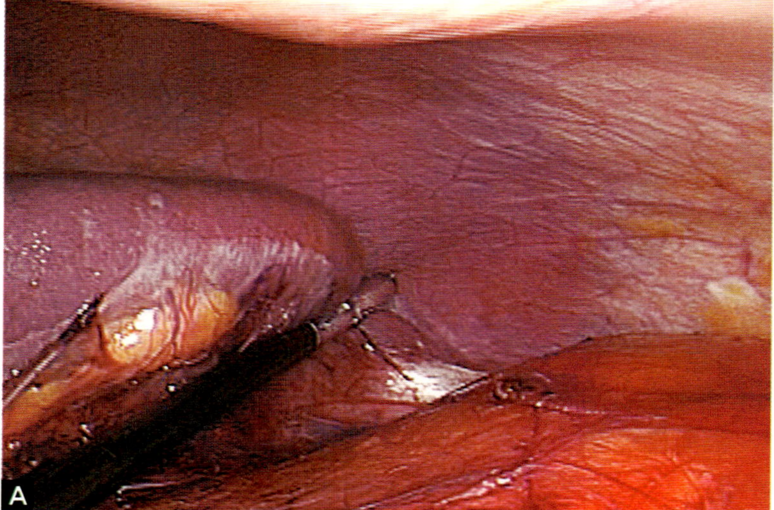

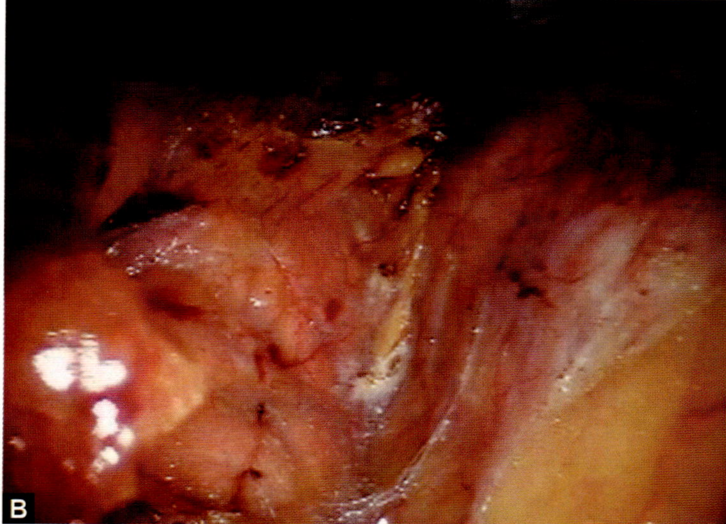

Figs 17A and B: The superior medial attachments to the spleen and pancreas are demonstrated by very gently retracting the spleen away. Note how the tip of this blunt ended grasper is passed beyond the edge of the spleen (A) to avoid injury caused by the instrument tip. A suction irrigator wand may also be found useful. After the initial dissection of the spleen, the tail of the pancreas (B) will be encountered and should be carefully dissected away by following the avascular plane between this and the medial portion of the renal upper pole to the and adrenal

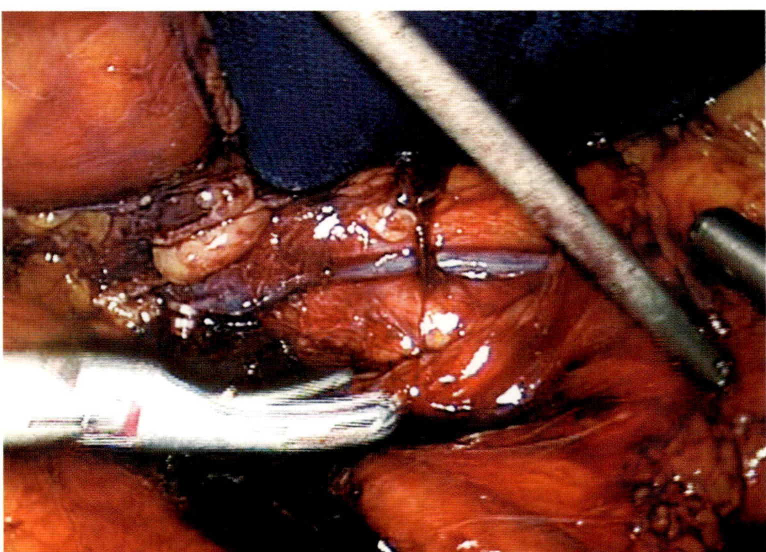

Fig. 18: The left gonadal vein may be used as a landmark to find the left renal vein by dissecting superiorly it along its course. This may be particularly helpful when the vasular hilum is obscured by fat or very large tumors

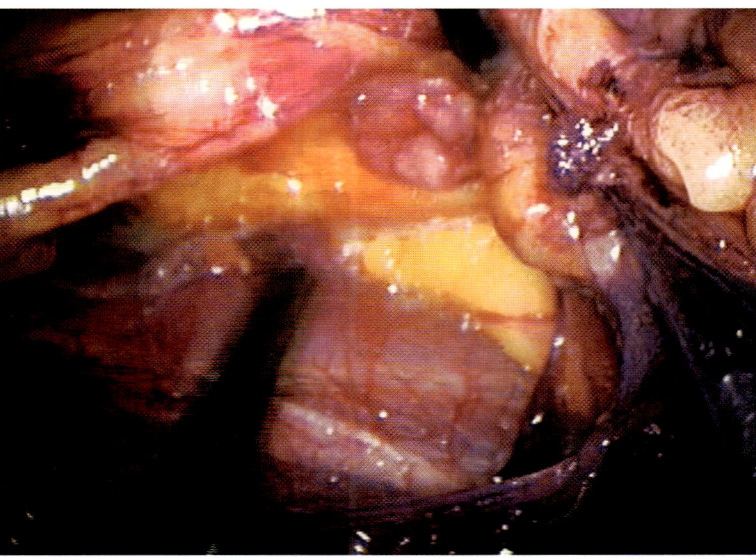

Fig. 19: Identifying and bluntly developing the posterior plane between the kidney and psoas is often a simple step, yet provides excellent means for lifting the kidney anteriorly to initiate the hilar dissection

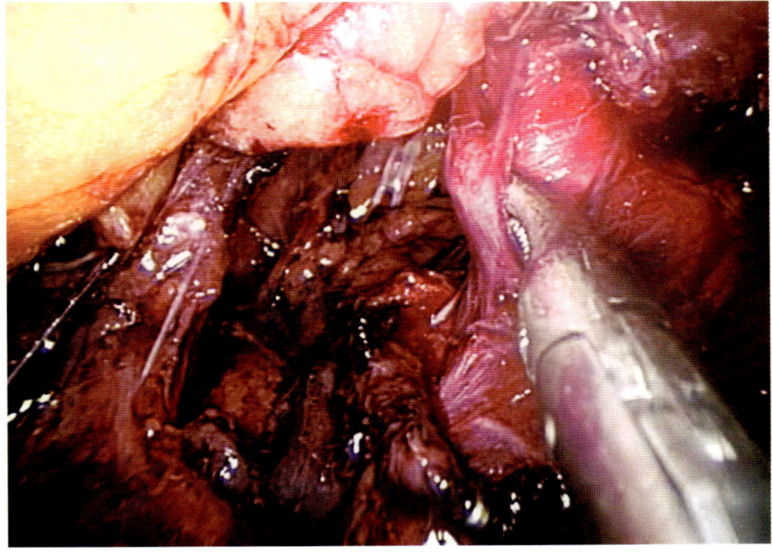

Fig. 20: A Maryland dissector is used for careful dissection of lymphatics from the renal artery

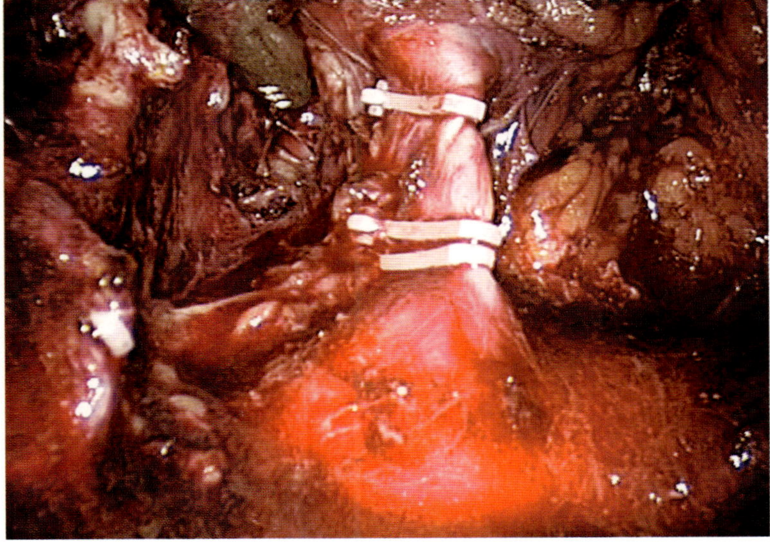

Fig. 21: The left renal artery is clipped with 2 locking Weck clips applied to the side closest to the aorta

Appropriate lateral retraction of the kidney is a key to success and staying in the proper orientation to the hilum. Excessive medial dissection is to be avoided where inadvertent injury may occur to the duodenum, mesenteric vessels, or chylous lymphatics.

Division of the Left Renal Hilar Vessels

After identification of the left renal vein, the left gonadal vein is divided and may be used to as a handle to provide anterior displacement of the renal vein. It is not uncommon to encounter a lumbar vein coming directly from the left renal vein that should be controlled and divided. Large lymphatics, coursing toward the receptaculum chyli behind the aorta, may be encountered with medial dissection and should be clipped to prevent chylous ascites. The left renal artery is identified posterior to the renal vein (Fig. 20).

The artery is controlled in similar fashion to the right side, with large metallic or Weck clips (Fig. 21). Two clips on the proximal or aortic side and a single clip on the specimen side are placed. The artery is then divided (Fig. 22). A GIA stapler can also be used if there is sufficient clearance. Again, when space is limited, it is acceptable

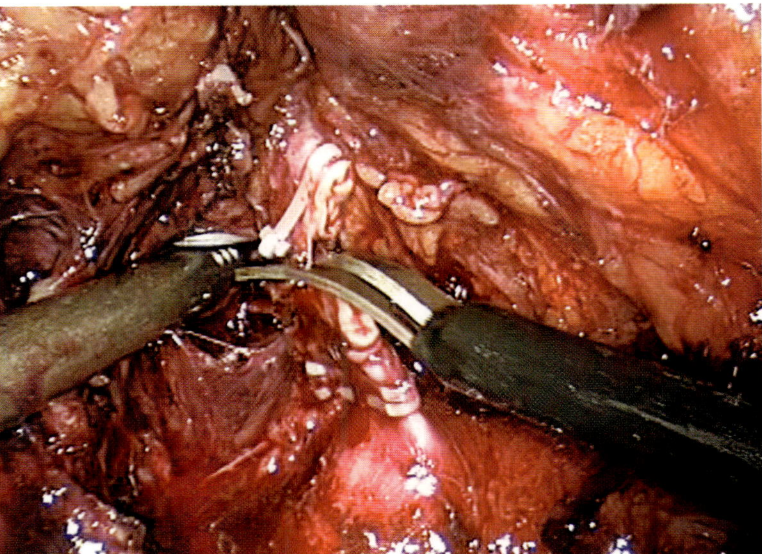

Fig. 22: When dividing the renal artery it is prudent to cut slowly and deliberately while leaving sufficient tissue around the clips. Cutting too close to a clip may risk having the clip work its way off the vessel

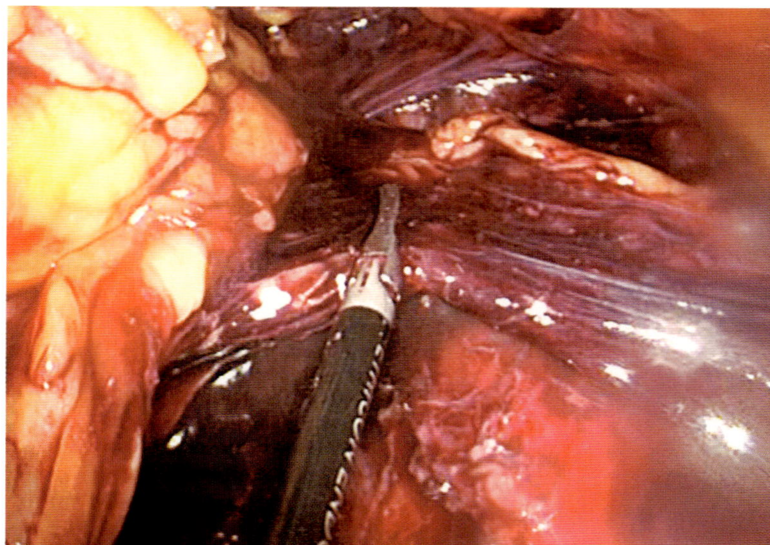

Fig. 23: An alternative is to divide the ureter with a thermal sealing device, in this case, the ultrasonic shears

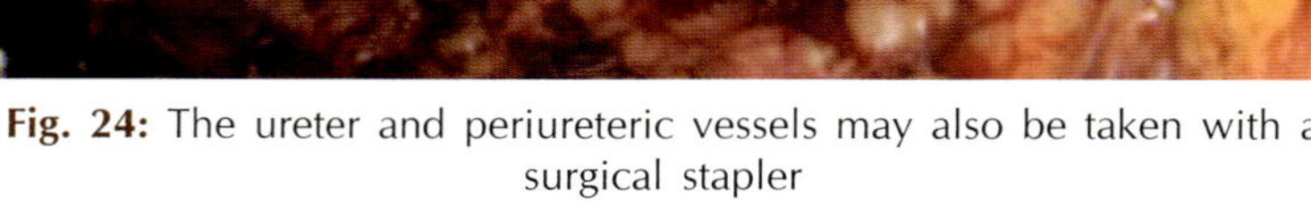

Fig. 24: The ureter and periureteric vessels may also be taken with a surgical stapler

to place a single clip to secure the artery, dividing the renal vein, and then completing the dissection and division of the artery after better exposure is obtained.

Specimen Mobilization

Dissection of the adrenal follows either the medial or lateral plane depending on the intention for adrenal preservation. A thermal ligation device (e.g. LigaSure) is useful in this area though care should be taken in the region of the mesenteric artery to avoid thermal injury to this vessel. The remaining superior and lateral attachments of the kidney are freed (Fig. 23). The ureter is divided below the lower pole between Weck clips or with a GIA stapler (Fig. 24). The specimen is placed in an Endocatch bag. Specimen extraction, inspection, and wound closure are performed in a similar fashion as the right kidney.

Chapter 4

Extraperitoneal Laparoscopic Radical Nephrectomy and Partial Nephrectomy

Jacob H Cohen, Michael Grasso III

INTRODUCTION

The extraperitoneal approach for laparoscopic radical nephrectomy (LRN) and laparoscopic partial nephrectomy (LPN) is an effective approach for a variety of benign and malignant conditions. Advantages of the extraperitoneal approach include prompt access to the renal vasculature without requiring manipulation of intraperitoneal bowel or solid viscera, and containment of either malignant or inflammatory processes to the retroperitoneum. The morbidly obese and those with a history of previous abdominal surgery or radiotherapy, where intra-abdominal adhesions are expected, are well served with this approach. Direct and prompt access to the great vessels and renal hilum are hallmarks of retroperitoneal access, especially when the retroperitoneum is distorted by lymphadenopathy and tumor neovascularity.

LRN is routinely performed for a variety of malignant and benign conditions. For malignant renal tumors, the decision to perform simultaneous adrenalectomy and regional lymphadenectomy is individualized based on radiological and intraoperative findings.[1] Extraperitoneal LRN for nonfunctioning, hydronephrotic kidneys associated with chronic pyelonephritis has the advantage of localizing the infectious process to a contained space.[2] Laparoscopic donor nephrectomy is also facilitated by an extraperitoneal approach, where direct access to the aorta and vena cava aid in developing adequate length of the renal vessels for transplantation.[3]

LPN is typically performed for renal tumors, but may also be performed for benign conditions, such as removing a nonfunctioning upper pole moiety of a duplicated system.[4,5]

LAPAROSCOPIC INSTRUMENTATION AND ESSENTIAL ACCESSORIES

Basic laparoscopic equipment is similar to transperitoneal renal surgery and includes a xenon light source, carbon dioxide insufflator, main and accessory monitors, varied diameter laparoscopic ports and laparoscopic lenses of various angulation of view. Accessory equipment is listed in Table 1. Creation of a sizeable surgical field is based on the development of the extraperitoneal space. Grauer in India first described the development of a pure retroperitoneal laparoscopic working space, created by filling a surgical glove placed bluntly into the retroperitoneum with hydrodistending saline.[6,7] This has been replaced by spherical or kidney shaped dissecting balloons placed through a small subcostal incision and directed adjacent to the belly of the psoas muscle. Self-sealing balloon working ports seal the access site and help maintain acceptable pneumoretroperitoneal pressures.

EXTRAPERITONEAL LAPAROSCOPIC RADICAL NEPHRECTOMY

Extraperitoneal LRN begins with induction of general anesthesia and placement of an oral gastric tube and Foley catheter for stomach and bladder decompression. The patient is positioned in full flank with the ipsilateral side up, employing and axillary roll and padding all potential pressure points. A kidney rest can be raised and the table gently flexed to broaden the space between the iliac crest and the costal margin for infracostal access (Fig. 1).

The retroperitoneal space is most commonly accessed via a 1 cm incision just medial and inferior to the tip of the 11th or 12th rib. Blunt dissection is employed to gently divide overlying fascia and musculature, down to and through the lumbodorsal fascia. A spherical balloon dissector is then placed adjacent to the belly of the psoas, expanding both in a cephalad and caudad direction to develop an adequate surgical field. A self-retaining, 10 mm balloon port is then employed to seal this access site, and pneumoretroperitoneum of 15 mm Hg is then established (Figs 2 and 3).

A 10 mm or 12 mm posterior port is then placed 1 cm below the 12th rib, adjacent to the paraspinous muscles, taking great care to avoid the intercostal neurovascular bundle. A 3rd anterior port, most commonly 5 mm in diameter, is placed under direct vision in the midaxillary line, avoiding the peritoneal reflection (Fig. 4).

After retroperitoneal insufflation, endoscopic dissection begins by defining surgical landmarks. Gerota's fascia is opened posteriorly and laterally, parallel to and along the psoas muscle. Other important landmarks include the great vessels (e.g. inferior vena

Table 1: Accessory equipment for extraperitoneal laparoscopic radical and partial nephrectomy
Atraumatic graspers
Right-angle laparoscopic clamps
Scissors
Dissectors (hook electrocautery, LigaSure or harmonic scalpel)
Specimen retrieval bags
Retroperitoneal balloon access device
Laparoscopic bulldog clamps
Clips (Weck and standard metal surgical clips)
Laparoscopic ultrasound
Absorbable suture (2-0 Vicryl on UR-5 and UR-6 needles)
Tissue sealants (SURGIFLO)
Absorbable hemostatic agents (SURGICEL, FIBRILLAR)

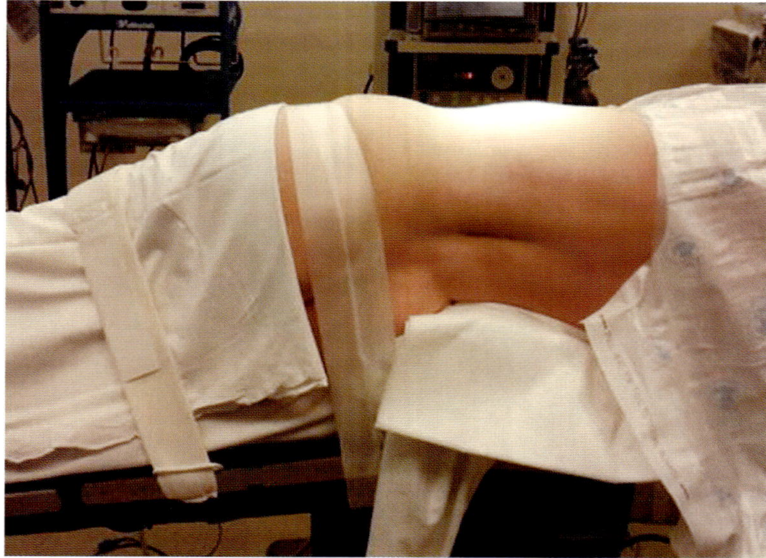

Fig. 1: The patient is positioned in full flank position with the ipsilateral side up

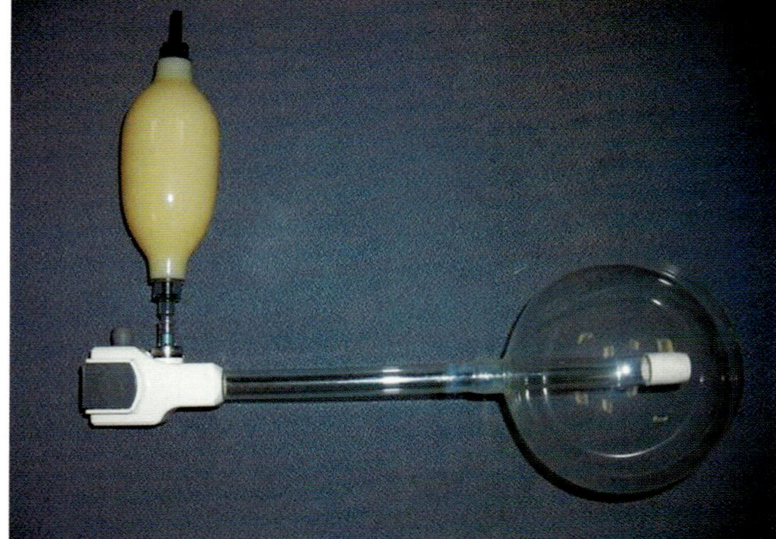

Fig. 2: A spherical balloon dissector is inflated to develop the retroperitoneal space

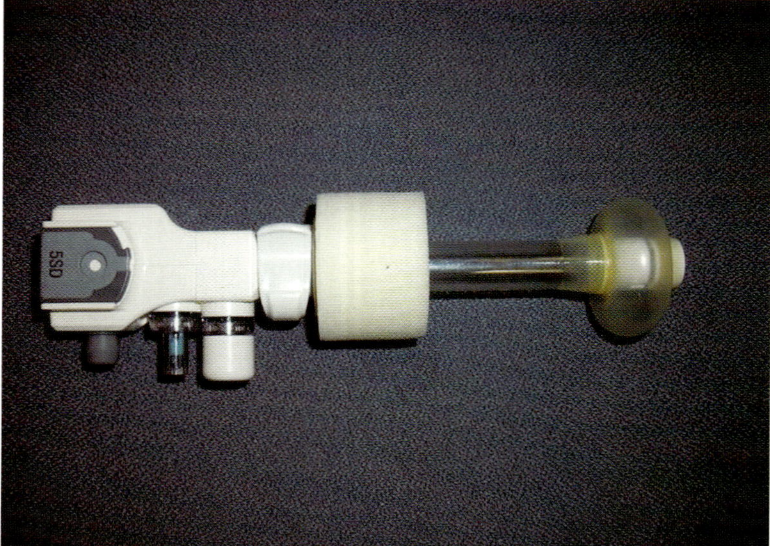

Fig. 3: A self-retaining, 10 mm balloon port seals the access site and allows for placement of the laparoscope

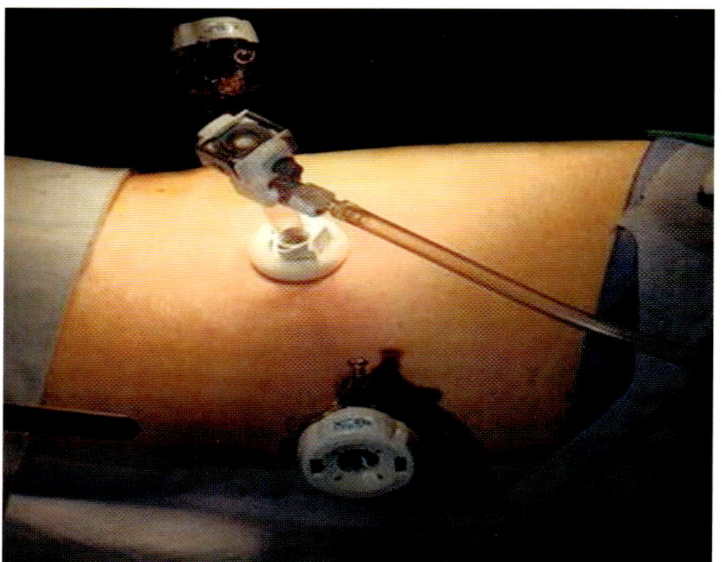

Fig. 4: An additional 10 or 12 mm posterior port and a 5 mm anterior port are placed

cava for right-sided tumors or pulsating aorta for left-sided tumors), diaphragmatic insertion, with the ureter and gonadal vessels inferiorly (Fig. 5).

Extraperitoneal renal hilar dissection is performed early, with identification and control of the renal artery first. The renal artery is meticulously cleared of surrounding adipose tissue, vasovasorum and lymphatics. Care is taken to define and ligate adjacent, often adherent, perforating lumbar vessels. Lymphadenopathy may also obscure the renal hilum with large, adherent nodes, requiring resection to gain access to the renal vasculature. If a lymph node dissection is planned with the nephrectomy, the associated lumbar vessels are ligated for hemostasis, developing the package along the respective great vessel above and below the renal vessels (Fig. 6).

The renal artery is secured with large Weck (10 or 15 mm) and/or metal surgical clips. Each has certain surgical advantages, with the application of sequential clips of each type affording excellent hemostasis (Fig. 7).

The renal vein is secured most commonly with an endovascular stapler employing six rows of interdigitating vascular staples. An unbladed stapler has the advantage of allowing the surgeon to inspect the staple line for adequacy of fire and proper position. Once properly secured, the vein may then be divided under direct vision with laparoscopic shears, leaving at least three rows on the specimen side. For left-sided nephrectomies, the gonadal, lumbar and adrenal veins are also secured with either clips or LigaSure seal and divided (Fig. 8).

After hilar control and renal vessel division, retroperitoneal dissection continues cephalic along the psoas and great vessels to the diaphragmatic insertion. For radical nephrectomy, hemostatic dissectors (i.e. LigaSure or harmonic scalpel) are employed to divide adrenal vessels as the adrenal gland is mobilized with the specimen. For right-sided tumors, the adrenal vein is clipped and divided at its origin from the inferior vena cava (Fig. 9).

The contents of Gerota's fascia are then mobilized anteriorly away from the peritoneum. Dissecting landmarks include the extraperitoneal liver and duodenum on the right and the spleen and pancreatic tail on the left (Fig. 10).

The ureter and remaining inferior attachments are divided leaving a completely free specimen. The specimen is bagged and extracted using a large, 15 mm port and a large entrapment sac (Fig. 11). The extraction

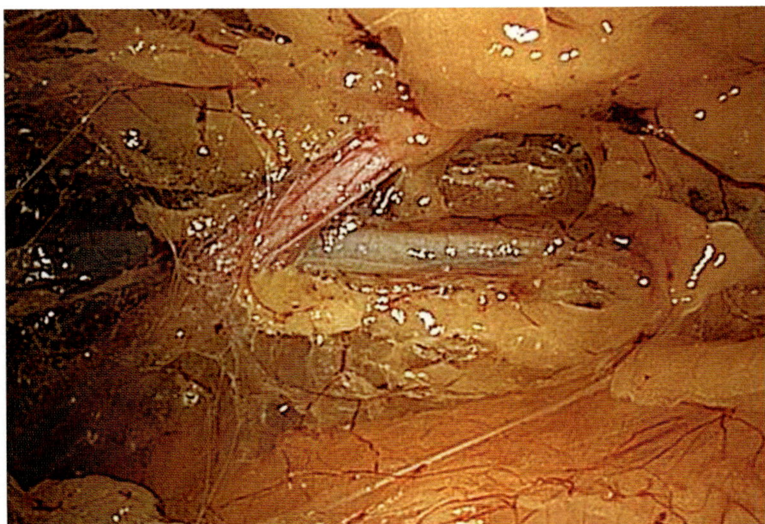

Fig. 5: View of the ureter crossing the gonadal vein in the retroperitoneum

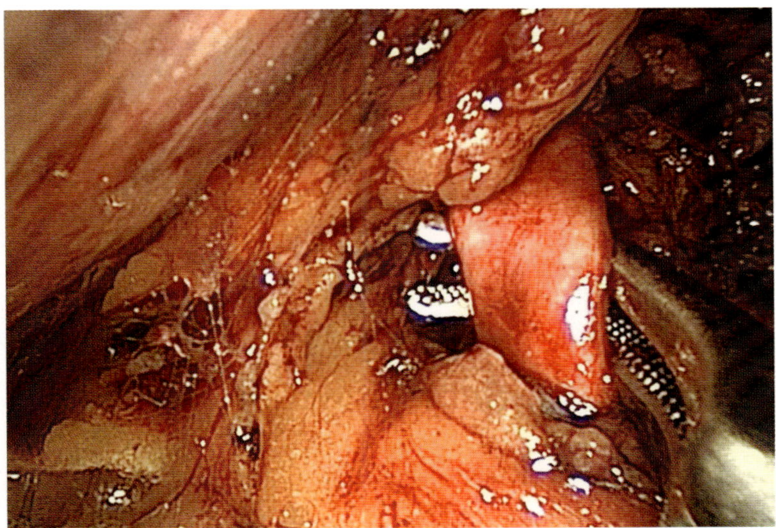

Fig. 6: The renal artery is cleared of overlying adipose and lymphatic tissue

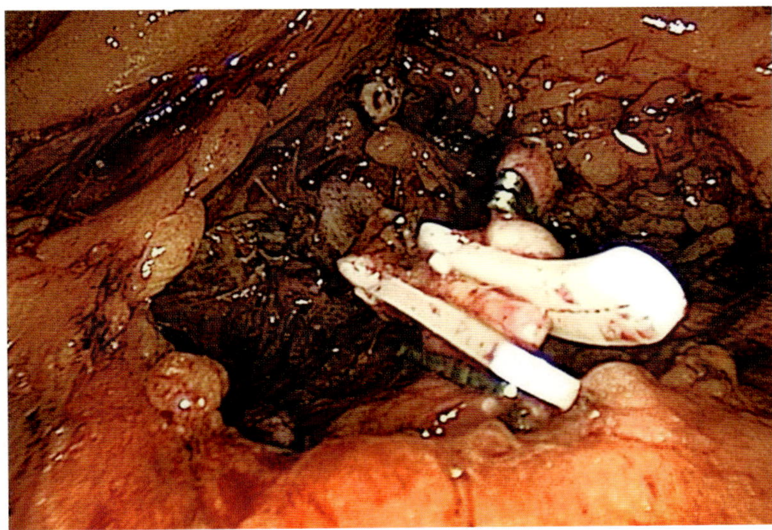

Fig. 7: The renal artery is secured with Weck (10 or 15 mm) and metal surgical clips

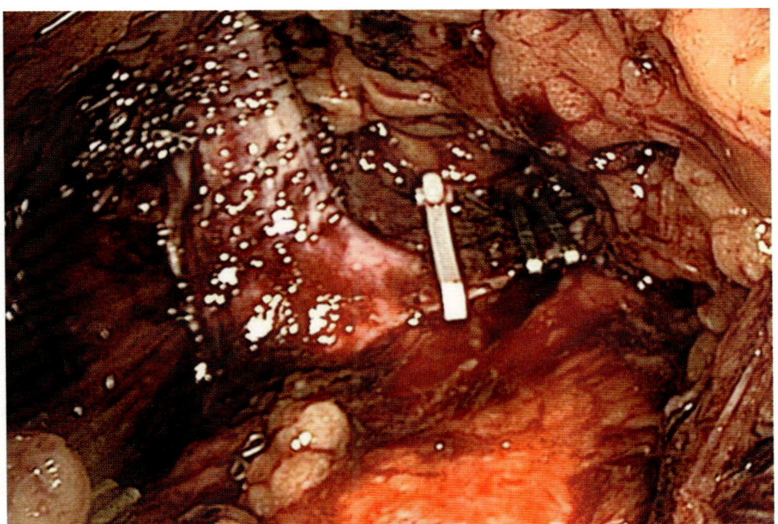

Fig. 8: The left renal vein is stapled, and the left adrenal vein is clipped and divided

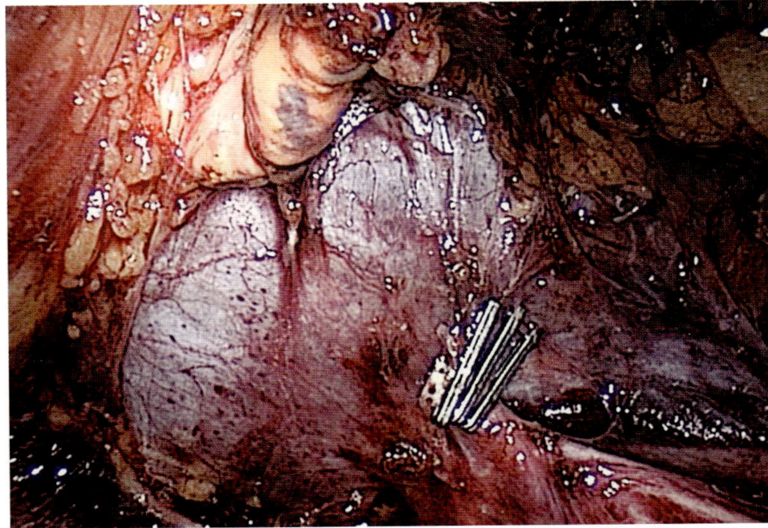

Fig. 9: The right adrenal vein is secured with metal clips just beyond its origin from the inferior vena cava

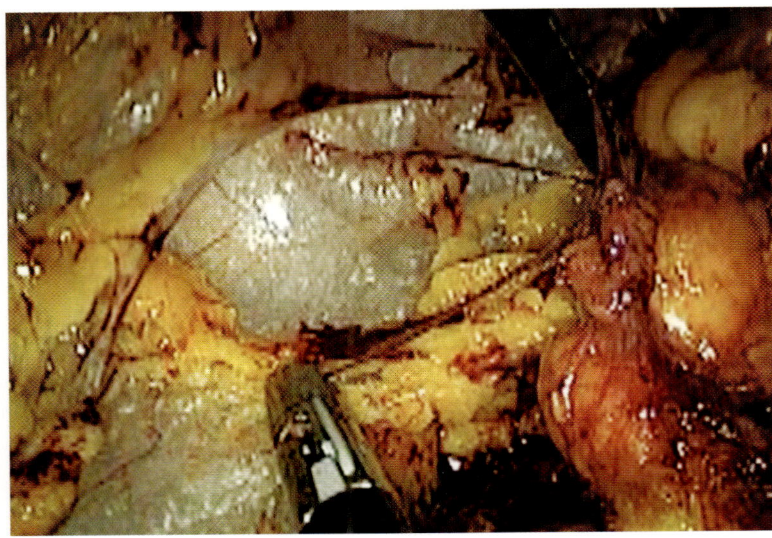

Fig. 10: The contents of Gerota's fascia are mobilized inferiorly

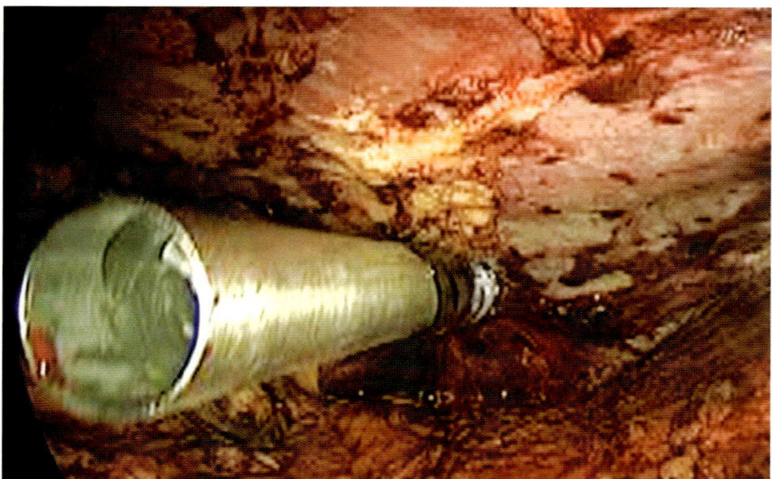

Fig. 11: The specimen is bagged and removed using a large, 15 mm port and a large entrapment sac

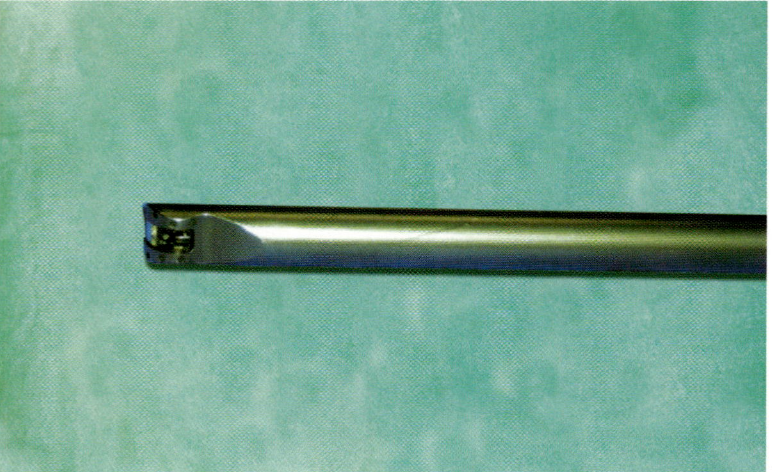

Fig. 12: A steerable, optical telescope with up to 120 degrees of deflection

port is placed extraperitoneally through a small groin or Gibson incision. This incision is closed in routine fashion. Laparoscopic port site closure after extraperitoneal dissection is also straightforward. Since the peritoneum is not violated, there is minimal risk of herniation of intraperitoneal contents. The larger port sites are closed with simple fascial sutures, and the skin with a subcuticular stitch.

EXTRAPERITONEAL LAPAROSCOPIC PARTIAL NEPHRECTOMY

Laparoscopic partial nephrectomy is routinely performed extraperitoneally for both solid and cystic malignancies. The retroperitoneal approach is uniquely suited for posterior lesions. In addition, steerable, optical telescopes with up to 120 degrees deflection facilitate complete resection of lesions in most parenchymal and hilar locations using this approach (Fig. 12).

Prophylactic ureteral stenting is performed routinely when large, hilar or endophytic tumors require resection. The stents can be placed cystoscopically at the procedural onset, especially when the collecting system may require significant repair. Stents are a useful landmark during hilar and lower pole dissection. As with LRN, initial dissection for LPN begins with identification of the renal hilar structures. The renal vessels are meticulously developed to facilitate partial or complete cross clamping during parenchymal dissection. Isotonic intravenous fluid and mannitol are administered early in the procedure in preparation for vascular clamping. The surgeon must be keenly aware of the potential for multiple and accessory vessels (Figs 13 and 14).

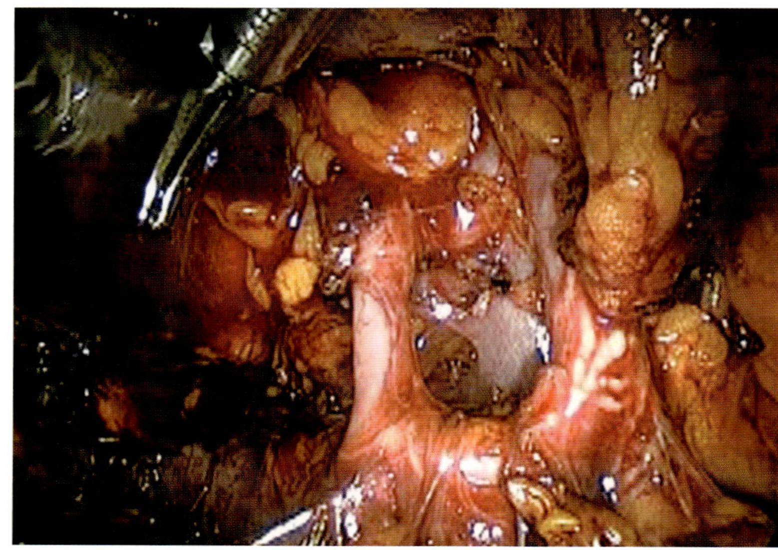

Fig. 13: Multiple renal arteries with renal vein

Renal parenchymal preparation begins by mobilizing Gerota's fascia and adjacent fat, exposing the renal capsule until the renal lesion is identified. A clear renal capsule is developed circumferentially around the tumor. Commonly the adherent fatty tissue is left attached to the exophytic tumor as a peripheral margin of resection (Fig. 15).

Intraoperative laparoscopic ultrasound is employed to define the endophytic tumor and the parenchymal margins of resection. Commonly, a 1 cm (10 MHz) articulating laparoscopic ultrasound probe is employed. Power Doppler imaging is particularly useful in defining the relationship between tumor and adjacent vasculature and collecting system in the renal sinus (Figs 16 and 17).

Using real time sonography as a guide, the parenchymal margins of resection are marked with electrocautery. A hook electrode is useful in both marking and incising the renal capsule prior to resection (Fig. 18).

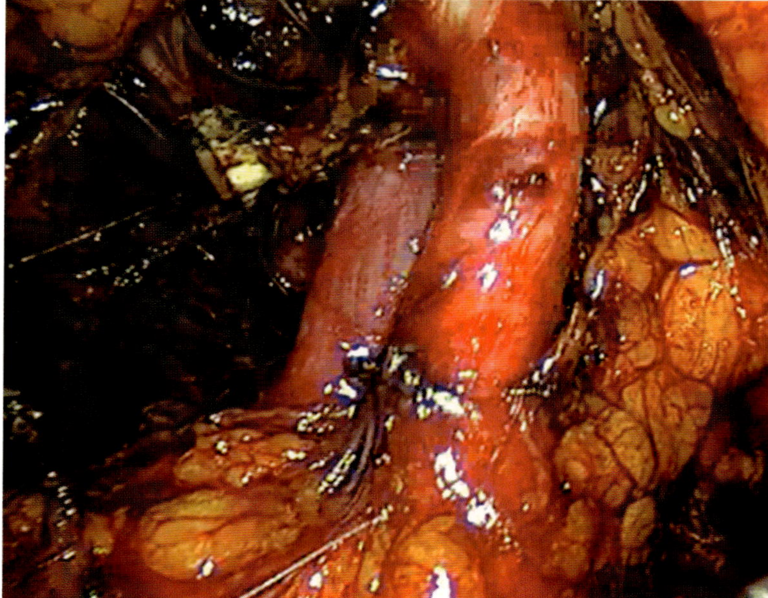

Fig. 14: Renal hilum cleared of adipose and lymphatic tissue

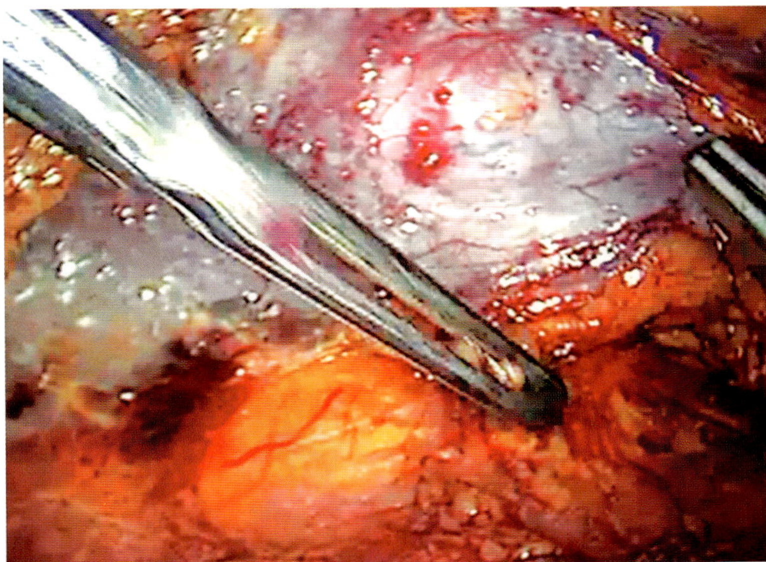

Fig. 15: The kidney is cleared of overlying fat to identify the tumor

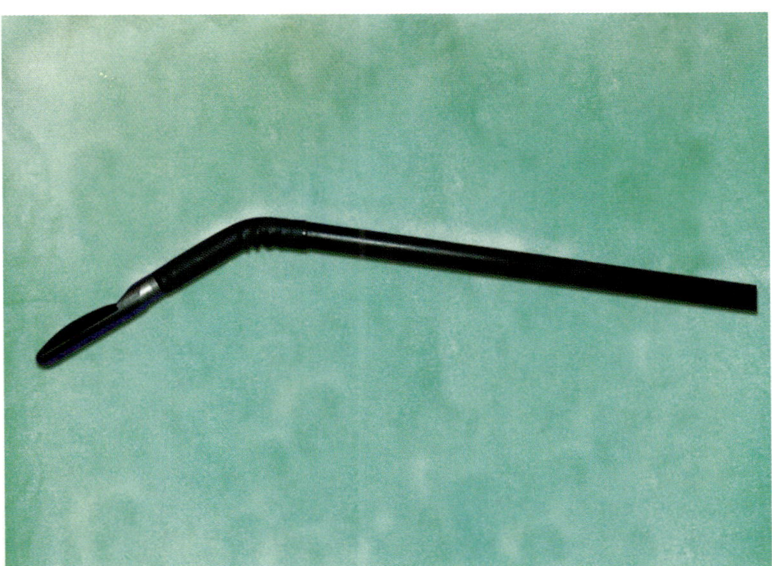

Fig. 16: A 1-cm, 10 MHz, laparoscopic ultrasound probe

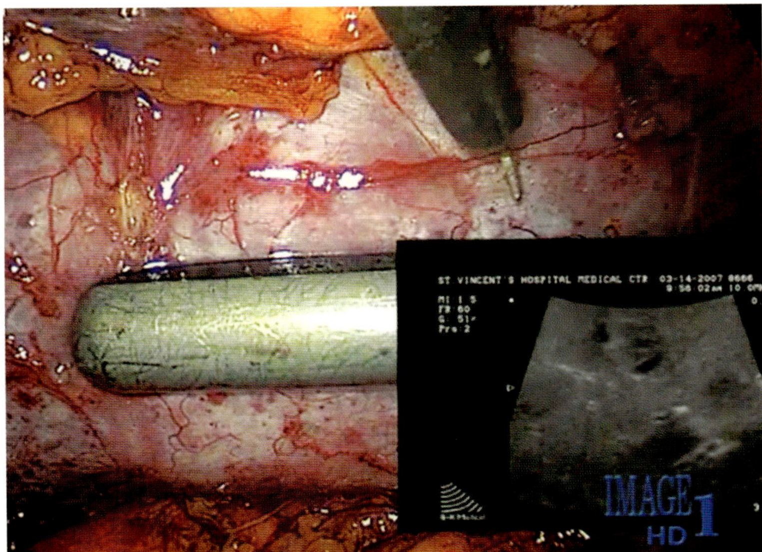

Fig. 17: The ultrasound probe is used to identify an endophytic tumor

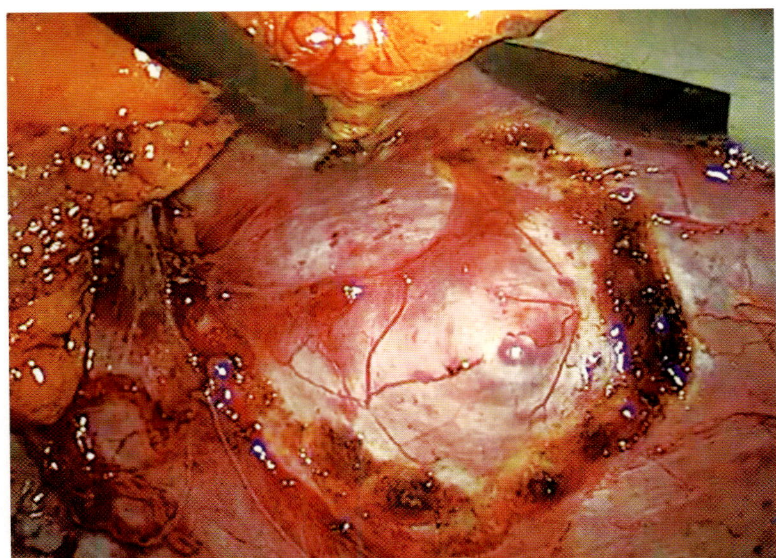

Fig. 18: Using real-time sonography, the parenchymal margins of resection are marked with electrocautery on a hook electrode

Depending on the depth of parenchymal penetration and whether renal sinus vasculature is adherent to or intimately associated with the tumor, an intraoperative plan is crafted with regard to renal hilar cross clamping. In cases of renal ectopy or horseshoe kidney, for example, only the segmental vessels associated with involved parenchymal segment require potential cross clamp. Here again intraoperative sonography with Doppler is useful in defining segmental vasculature. Directed by intraoperative parameters and just prior to parenchymal resection, the renal artery (with or without the renal vein) is clamped with noncrushing laparoscopic bulldog clamps. The decision on whether to clamp the renal vein with the artery is based on intraoperative finding including tumor involvement of venous tributaries and the venous plexus located in the renal sinus. Intraoperative ultrasound with Doppler can be employed to confirm vasculature control of the tumor and adjacent parenchyma. Persistent blood flow after clamping indicates either accessory artery inflow or incomplete arterial occlusion due to atherosclerotic disease. For the former, a search for an accessory artery is warranted, and for the latter, the application of a second arterial clamp proximal or distal will often facilitate better vessel wall coaptation (Fig. 19).

The actual tumor resection is based initially on sharp scissor dissection along the pre-marked parenchymal margin, employing suction circumferentially to clear the surgical field (Fig. 20). Intraoperative sonography is employed intermittently to better ensure proper direction of incisions.

Particularly with deep and endophytic lesions, the parenchymal is divided to sinus fat. The specimen is then gently rolled from side to side or lifted out of the sinus, with the adherent vasculature and collecting system meticulously developed and peripherally divided (Fig. 21).

Arterial perforators and venous sinus are suture ligated with short runs of absorbable suture. The peripherally collecting system is meticulously closed as well (Fig. 22).

The parenchyma is reconstructed by preplacing 2-0 Vicryl stitches across the defect, through the capsule and superficial parenchyma. These sutures are not placed deeply through the sinus to prevent inadvertent ligation of adjacent structures (Fig. 23).

Surgiflo or other topical hemostatic agents can be placed in the base of the parenchymal defect (Fig. 24).

The preplaced parenchymal reconstruction sutures are tied or clipped over an absorbable patch placed into the defect (Fig. 25). The patch facilitates a gentle compressive force to the resection defect for hemostasis. The kidney is then reperfused by removing the bulldog vascular clamps, with subsequent inspection of the patch and hilum for adequate hemostasis. Minor edge bleeding is commonly addressed with topical hemostatic agents.

The specimen is placed in a laparoscopic sac and removed either through the middle port site or through a small extraperitoneal groin incision for larger lesion, similar to the extraction technique described for radical nephrectomy (Fig. 26). A closed suction drain is commonly placed through the most posterior port and positioned next to the repair.

SUMMARY

Prompt access to the great vessels and renal hilum and avoidance of the intraperitoneal contents are among some of the advantages of performing an extraperitoneal LRN or LPN. This is particularly useful in those who have undergone prior intraperitoneal surgical interventions where adhesions are expected. Relative disadvantages of the retroperitoneal approach include a smaller working space and a longer learning curve. Once mastered, the extraperitoneal approach can be used for various surgical procedures, including nephroureterectomy,[8] pyeloplasty[9] and adrenalectomy.[10]

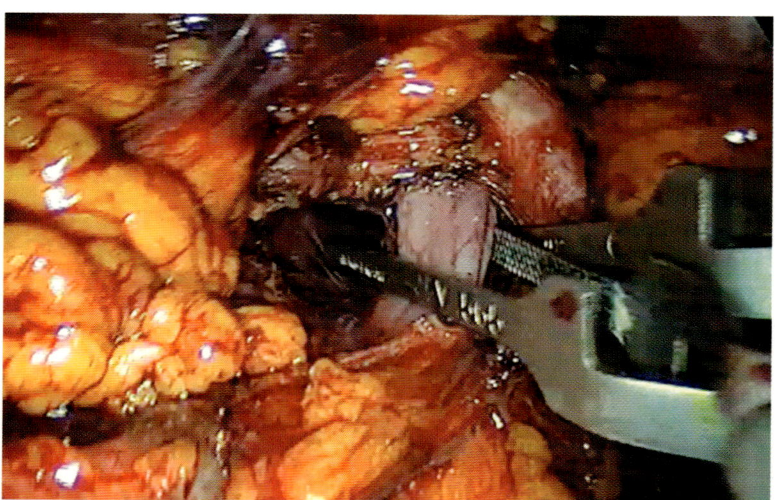

Fig. 19: Noncrushing vascular clamps are applied to the renal artery and vein

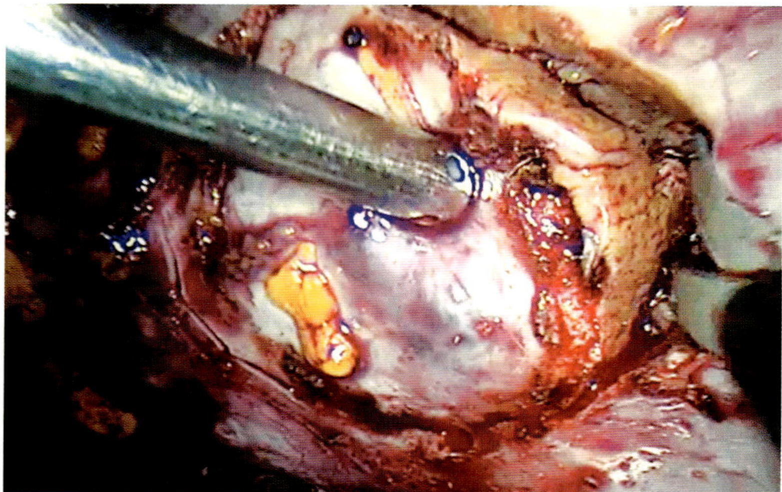

Fig. 20: Sharp scissor dissection along the premarked parenchymal margin

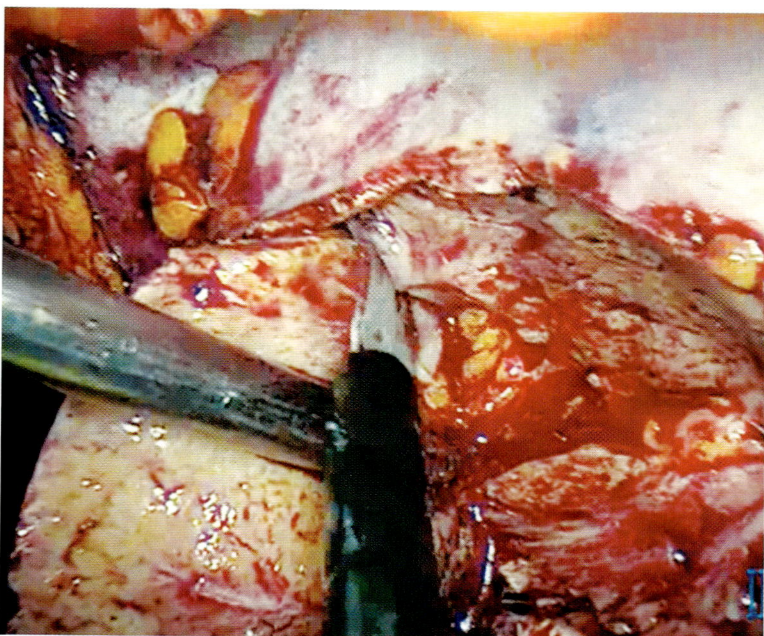

Fig. 21: The parenchyma is divided down to sinus fat

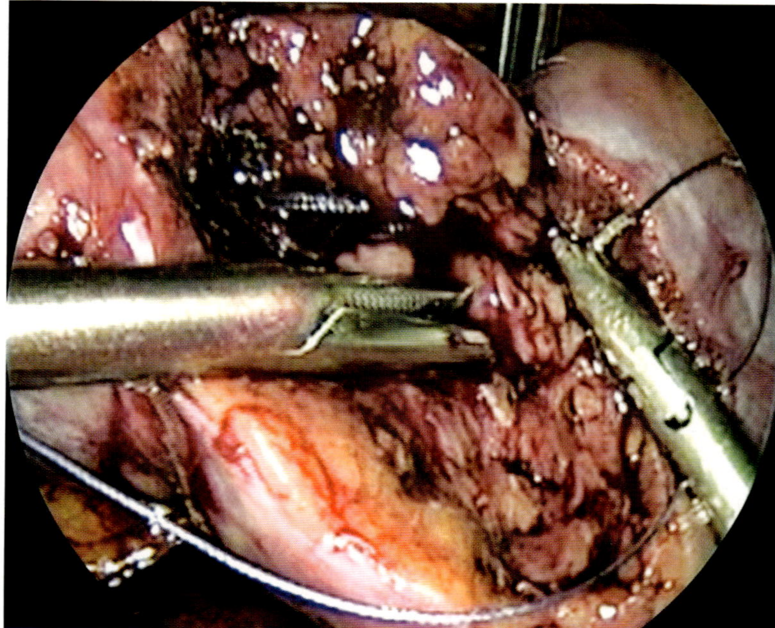

Fig. 22: Arterial perforators and venous sinus are suture ligated with absorbable suture

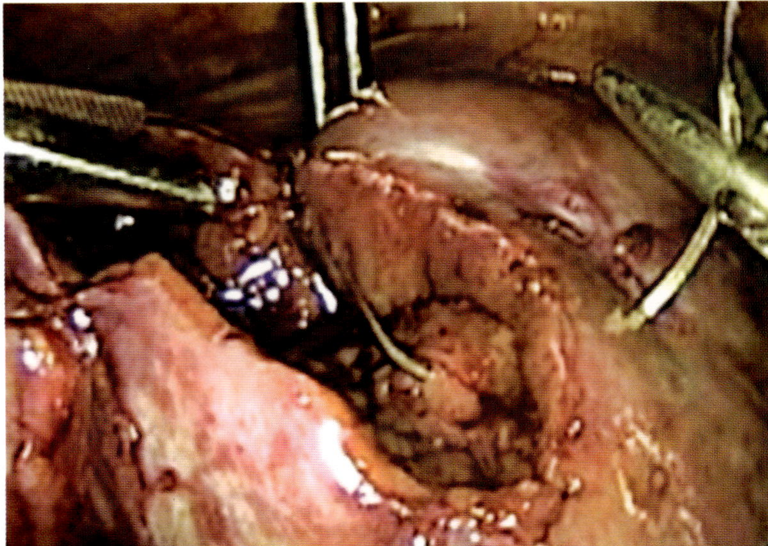

Fig. 23: Parenchymal resonstruction with preplaced 2-0 Vicryl stitches across the defect, through the capsule and superficial parenchyma

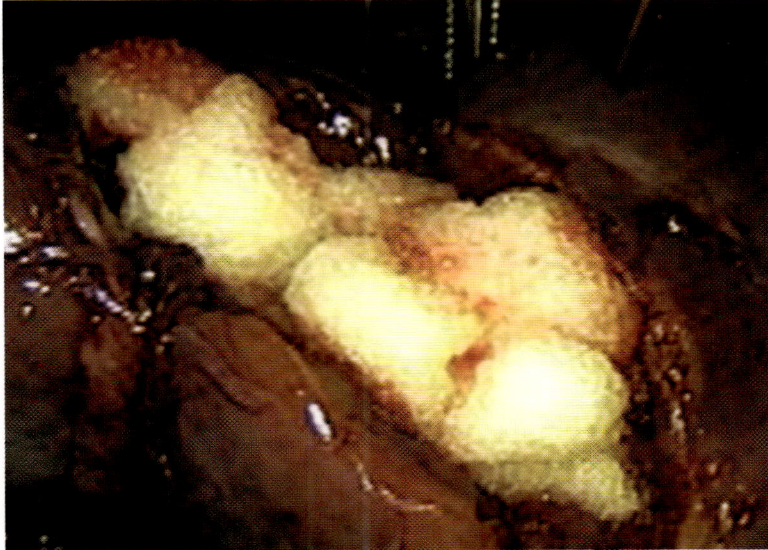

Fig. 24: Topical hemostatic agents are placed into the defect

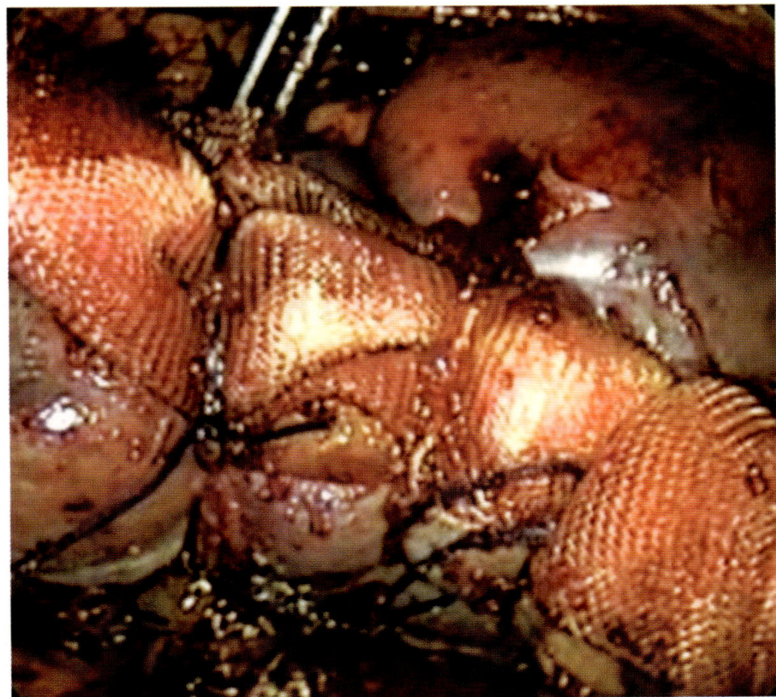

Fig. 25: The preplaced parenchymal reconstruction sutures are tied over an absorbable patch placed into the defect

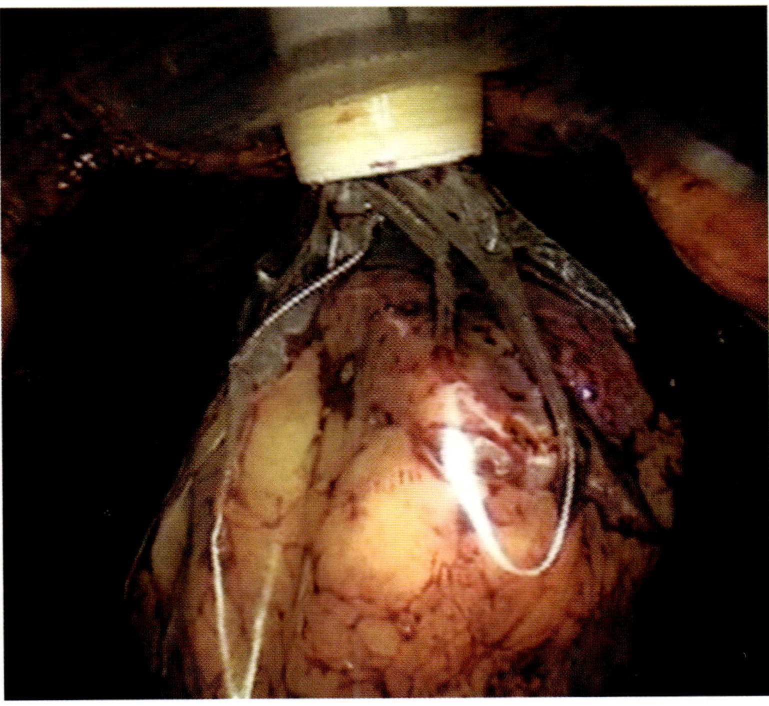

Fig. 26: The specimen is placed in a laparoscopic sac and removed through the middle port

REFERENCES

1. O'Malley RL, Godoy G, Kanofsky JA, et al. The necessity of adrenalectomy at the time of radical nephrectomy: a systematic review. J Urol. 2009;181(5):2009-17.
2. Hemal AK, Mishra S. Retroperitoneoscopic nephrectomy for pyonephrotic nonfunctioning kidney. Urology. 2010;75(3):585-8.
3. Kohei N, Kazuya O, Hirai T, et al. Retroperitoneoscopic living donor nephrectomy: experience of 425 cases at a single center. J Endourol. 2010;24(11):1783-7.
4. Pyo P, Chen A, Grasso M. Retroperitoneal laparoscopic partial nephrectomy: surgical experience and outcomes. J Urol. 2008;180(4): 1279-83.
5. Gill IS, Delworth MG, Munch LC. Laparoscopic retroperitoneal partial nephrectomy. J Urol. 1994;152(5 Pt 1):1539-42.
6. Gaur DD, Agarwal DK, Purohit KC. Retroperitoneal laparoscopic nephrectomy: initial case report. J Urol. 1993;149(1):103-5.
7. Gaur DD. Retroperitoneoscopy: the balloon technique. Ann R Coll Surg Engl. 1994;76(4):259-63.
8. Gill IS, Sung GT, Hobart MG, et al. Laparoscopic radical nephroureterectomy for upper tract transitional cell carcinoma: the Cleveland Clinic experience. J Urol. 2000;164(5):1513-22.
9. Moon DA, El-Shazly MA, Chang CM, et al. Laparoscopic pyeloplasty: evolution of a new gold standard. Urology. 2006;67(5):932-6.
10. Yuan Q, Li F. Laparoscopic adrenalectomy in pheochromocytoma: a retroperitoneal approach versus transperitoneal approach. J Endourol. 2010;24(9):1441-5.

5 Chapter

Hand-Assisted Laparoscopic Radical Nephrectomy

Shadi Al Ekish, Gyan Pareek

INTRODUCTION

Since its description by Robson in 1969, open radical nephrectomy has been the standard of care for the management of renal carcinomas.[1] In 1990, Clayman et al. performed the first laparoscopic nephrectomy, propelling this approach as an alternative to traditional open nephrectomy.[2] Because of the technical challenges and steep learning curve of a pure laparoscopic nephrectomy, widespread usage has been limited. In 1996, Bannenberg et al.[3] performed the first hand-assisted laparoscopic nephrectomy in a porcine model. In that report, operative times were shorter and maneuverability was easier with the hand-assisted approach when compared with a purely laparoscopic approach. One year later, Nakada and colleagues performed the first human hand-assisted laparoscopic nephrectomy for a chronically infected kidney. Since that time, many publications have reported the use of the hand-assisted techniques for performing radical nephrectomies, nephroureterectomies, partial nephrectomies, dismembered pyeloplasties and donor nephrectomies.[4-7]

There is a tremendous interest in the hand-assisted approach for many reasons. Specifically, the hand offers a tactile feedback and facilitates blunt dissection, palpation of lesions or blood vessels, organ retraction, hemorrhage control, and knot tying.[8-10] Ultimately, this approach is the most transferrable approach, while maintaining all the benefits of minimally invasive surgery. Proponents also emphasize that the hand-port utilized during the hand-assisted approach not only allows for excellent tactile feedback, but also serves as the necessary extraction site needed after radical kidney surgery. Herein, the authors report on the indications, preoperative evaluation, patient work-up and technique for performing a hand-assisted laparoscopic radical nephrectomy (HALRN) for carcinoma of the kidney.

INDICATIONS

Any condition that warrants an open nephrectomy may be considered an indication for HALRN. The most common indication to perform a HALRN is a renal mass, most commonly due to a renal cell carcinoma. The hand-assisted approach is also utilized to perform such procedures as a simple nephrectomy, live-donor nephrectomy and adrenalectomy in conjunction with removal of large renal tumors.

CONTRAINDICATIONS

Many factors and circumstances have to be taken into consideration during the preoperative planning phase of a HALRN. These circumstances include a history of peritonitis, bowel obstruction, abdominal wall infection, prior renal inflammation or surgery and tumor size (> 10 cm). Additionally, as is the case for other laparoscopic procedures, a patient with a history of cardiac or pulmonary disease may get an increased risk for complications from pneumoperitoneum, the latter resulting from reduced venous return and/or impairment of ventilation.

PATIENT EVALUATION AND PREPARATION

Prior to HALRN, a full metastatic evaluation should be obtained. This includes a complete blood count, serum creatinine, chest radiograph, serum liver function tests, serum calcium, and computed tomography of the abdomen and pelvis with and without intravenous contrast to assess the size and boundaries of the tumor. Additional information gleaned from the latter includes details such as possible lymph node enlargement, evidence of metastatic disease, venous invasion, and the ability to fully assess the renal vascular anatomy. A bone scan is advised for patients with elevated calcium, elevated alkaline phosphatase, or bone pain. A mechanical bowel preparation is prescribed. On the day prior to surgery, a clear liquid diet is started and a mechanical bowel preparation utilizing MiraLax® is taken by the patient. The patient is kept nil per os (NPO) or nothing by mouth after midnight. Prior to surgery, antibiotic therapy in the form of a second generation cephalosporin is administered. Prior to induction of general anesthesia and endotracheal intubation, pneumatic stockings are applied bilaterally. In the obese patient or in those with a history of deep venous thrombosis, 5,000 units of heparin are administered subcutaneously 1 hour prior to the procedure and continued every 12 hours postoperatively until the patient is ambulatory. Just prior to any skin incision, a nasogastric or orogastric tube and a Foley catheter are placed in order to decompress the stomach and bladder.

HAND-ASSISTED LAPAROSCOPIC PORT PLACEMENT

The surgeon's hand placement without the loss of the pneumoperitoneum is facilitated by the hand-access laparoscopy device. Currently, there are five different types of those devices with each having its pros and cons (Table 1). Selection of the type depends on the surgeon's preference, patient's body habitus and location of the hand

Table 1: Various hand-port devices
Hand-Port System (Smith & Nephew, Inc., London, England)
Lap Disc (Hakko Shoji, Tokyo, Japan)
Omni-Port (InterMed, Selling, Nevada, USA)
Gel-Port (Applied Medical Resources, Rancho Santa Margarita, CA, USA)
Dexterity Pneumo Sleeve device (Dexterity Inc., Roswell, GA)

incision. The operating room (OR) set up for HALRN is similar to that of most standard laparoscopic procedure (Figs 1A and B).

Table 2 outlines the most important equipment used in hand-assisted laparoscopic surgery.

PATIENT POSITIONING

The patient is positioned in a lateral decubitus position utilizing gel pads on the operative table to prevent sliding as well as to prevent pressure injuries. With the affected side up break at the level of the umbilicus, the patient is secured to the OR table with 3 inch wide cloth tape across the pelvis, and one application over the shoulder. These measures secure the patient and allows the physician to rotate the patient to the right and left. A padded arm rest is used to support the upper arm. The lower leg is flexed and the upper extended with pillows placed in between the upper aspect of each lower extremity. Careful padding of bony prominences and soft tissue is of paramount importance to avoid neurapraxia and pressure injury. The kidney rest is usually positioned in between the costal margin and the iliac crest and may be utilized for greater exposure (Fig. 2). This step is not always necessary as the internal space created by the pneumoperitoneum is normally sufficient for exposure. Upper and lower body warming blankets, in order to minimize hypothermia, are utilized throughout the procedure. The patient's entire abdomen and flank is then prepped and draped.

TROCARS AND HAND-PORT PLACEMENT

The initial step is the creation of the hand portal incision and inserting the hand access device. The size of the incision is calculated based on the surgeon's glove size.

LEFT HAND-ASSISTED LAPAROSCOPIC RADICAL NEPHRECTOMY

For a right-handed surgeon performing a left radical nephrectomy, a midline incision is placed just above or around the umbilicus. The hand-port is placed in the abdomen after the dissection carried

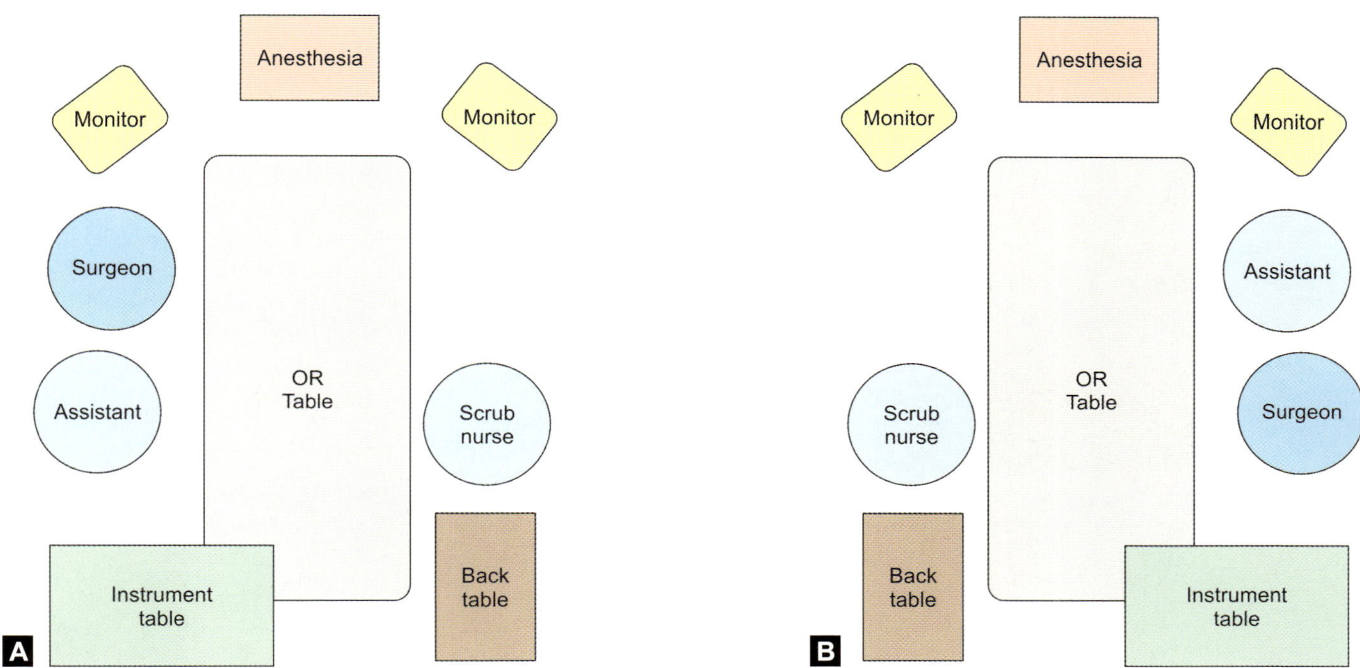

Figs 1A and B: Operating room set-up for a hand-assisted (A) Left; (B) Right laparoscopic nephrectomy

Table 2: HALRN Instrument List[11]

Nondisposable	Disposable
Two monitors, flat screen (Stryker)	Hand-access device (Gelport, Applied Medical)
5 mm or 10 mm (Stryker) 30° laparoscope	Nonbladed trocars, one 5 mm, two 10 mm (Visiport, Ethicon)
5 mm or 10 mm (Stryker) 0° laparoscope	Port reducers (Ethicon)
High-flow insufflator	LapSac (Cook)
Three-chip camera (Stryker)	Endo-GIA stapler, vascular load (10 mm) (Ethicon)
5 mm Maryland dissector	Sutures, 1-0 PDS for fascial closure of hand-port
5 mm Atraumatic grasper	0 Vicryl for 10 mm ports
5 mm scissors, curved and straight blades	4-0 Vicryl for skin closure
5 mm suction/irrigation system (Nehzat)	
Carter-Thomason closure device (Inlet Medical, Eden Prairie, MN)	
5 mm curved harmonic scalpel (Ethicon)	

through the midline into the abdomen. The hand-port device is placed and insufflation is carried out through the CO_2 tubing attached to the trocar. A 0 or 30-degree camera is placed through the trocar and full inspection is conducted (Fig. 3A). The remaining trocars are then placed and include a 12-mm trocar just above the hand-port for camera placement and a second 12-mm trocar in the left lower quadrant.

RIGHT HAND-ASSISTED LAPAROSCOPIC RADICAL NEPHRECTOMY

On the right side, the hand-assist incision is placed in the right lower quadrant, halfway between the umbilicus and the anterior superior iliac spine. After hand-port placement and insufflation as outlined above, the remaining ports are placed. A 5 mm port is placed in the midaxillary for placement of a liver retractor. Alternatively, a 5 mm port may be placed just below the xiphoid process through which a grasping device may be utilized to retract the liver in an upward fashion. The two remaining trocars are placed and include a 12-mm trocar in the midline just above the umbilicus and a 12-mm trocar in the midline one hand-breadth below the xiphoid process. The latter is utilized for camera placement (Fig. 3B).

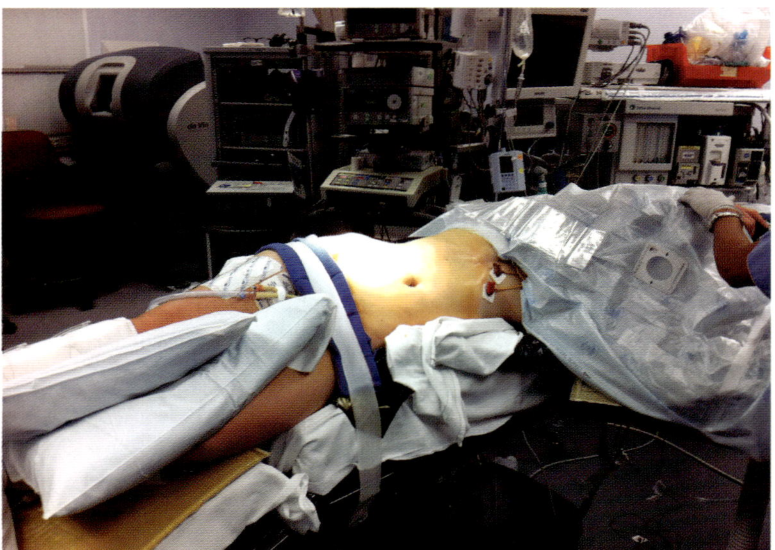

Fig. 2: The patient is placed in a lateral decubitus position with slight flexion of the operating table to extend the flank gently

STEPS OF THE PROCEDURE

Step 1: Colon Mobilization

Utilizing the harmonic scalpel, the colon is mobilized from lateral to medial along the white line of Toldt (Fig. 4). The utility of hand-assistance helps with medial traction of the colon and aids in the dissection carried out cephalad to the hepatic or splenic flexure and caudally to the iliac vessels. Additional maneuvers include medial rotation of colon, spleen and tail of pancreas. Care must be taken when mobilizing the tail of the pancreas on the left side to avoid bleeding from the splenic vessels that course along the lateral aspect of the pancreas.

On the right side, the liver is freed from the lateral attachment by incising the triangular ligament. The surgeon may encounter significant attachments between superior aspect of Gerota's fascia and the undersurface of the liver which must be released using the harmonic scalpel. The duodenum is mobilized medially by performing the Kocher maneuver with sharp and blunt dissection to reveal the inferior vena cava (IVC) and the right renal vein.

Step 2: Access to the Renal Hilum

Once the colon is retracted medially, a tissue plane is created between the large bowel mesentery and the anterior aspect of Gerota's fascia. This tissue plane is incised by the harmonic scalpel to gain access to the renal hilum. The superior and lateral attachments of the kidney are released while the posterior attachment is kept intact at this stage for better control of the kidney. The surgeon must make sure not to violate the Gerota's fascia when dissecting, adhering to all the surgical principles of a radical nephrectomy.

Step 3: Dissection of the Ureter

The ureter is identified upon reflection of the colon medially and is typically located along the medial border of the psoas muscle. Along

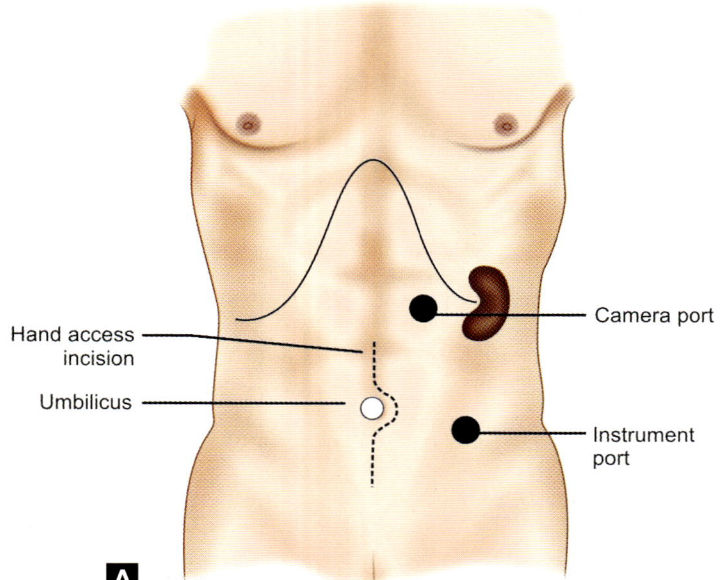

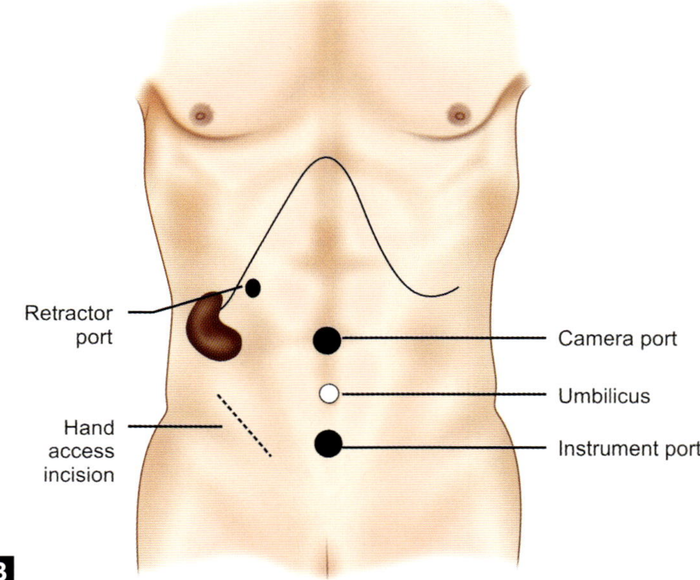

Figs 3A and B: Trocars and hand access incisions sites for hand-assisted (A) Left; (B) Right laparoscopic nephrectomy for right-handed surgeon

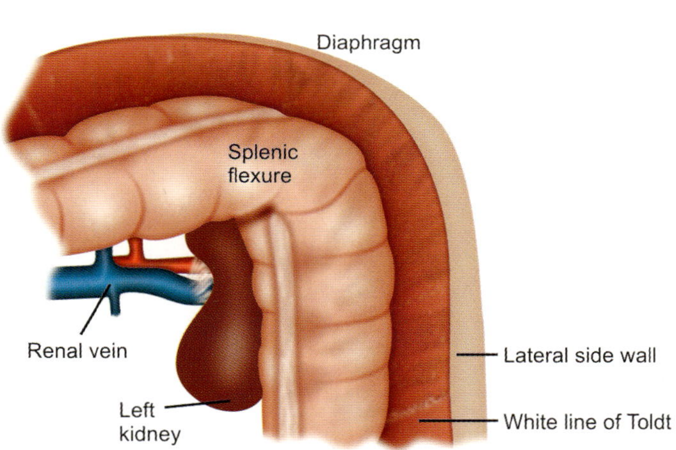

Fig. 4: Schematic drawing of the splenic flexure, left kidney and the white line of Toldt that attaches the colon to the lateral side wall

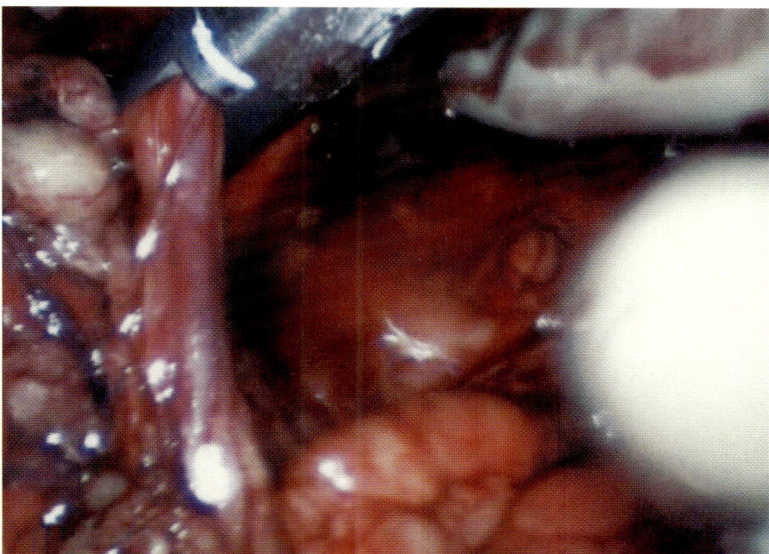

Fig. 5: Stapling of the ureter

with the gonadal vein, located in a superior and medial plane, the ureter leads the surgeon to the renal hilum. Once the lower pole of the kidney is identified, it is displaced laterally with the fingers while the thumb pushes the bowel medially. The ureter is divided between clips or with the vascular stapler and the proximal stump is used to retract the kidney in a cephalad manner (Fig. 5).

Step 4: Division of the Renal Blood Vessels

On the left side, the renal vein is found by following the gonadal vein cranially. The gonadal vein can be divided by using the harmonic scalpel or clipped and sharply divided (Fig. 6). Lumbar vein(s) and the adrenal vein need to be clipped and divided, facilitating the subsequent division of the renal vein. On the right side, Gerota's fascia is opened longitudinally just lateral to the IVC to identify the ureter and the gonadal vein. The gonadal vein can be clipped and divided as it enters the IVC to prevent traction injury and bleeding. The renal vein and artery should be dissected free and dissected off of the hilar fat for proper application of the endovascular stapler. Palpation of the hilum can help with identifying the artery. If difficulty arises at this step, the posterior attachments are divided, allowing medial retraction of the kidney. This latter maneuver is paramount in exposing the renal artery (Fig. 7). Next, the kidney is stretched superiorly by hand-assistance allowing maximum exposure of the artery and the vein. The renal artery is divided using the endovascular stapler followed by the vein (Fig. 8).

Step 5: Adrenal Sparing or Adrenalectomy

For adrenal-sparing nephrectomy, the plane between the adrenal gland and the upper pole of the kidney can be dissected by combined blunt and sharp dissection using the surgeon's fingers and the harmonic scalpel. In order to avoid injury to the adrenal vessels, dissection should be lateral and inferior to the gland. If the adrenal gland is to be removed with the left kidney, it should be done after division of the renal vessels. The tissue plane between the adrenal and the aorta is divided using harmonic scalpel and clips. Right adrenalectomy may be challenging. The right adrenal excision requires complete visualization of the vena cava to clearly clip and divide the adrenal vein. Additionally, the liver must be completely mobilized medially to the superior phrenic attachments, allowing for identification of the feeding vessels.

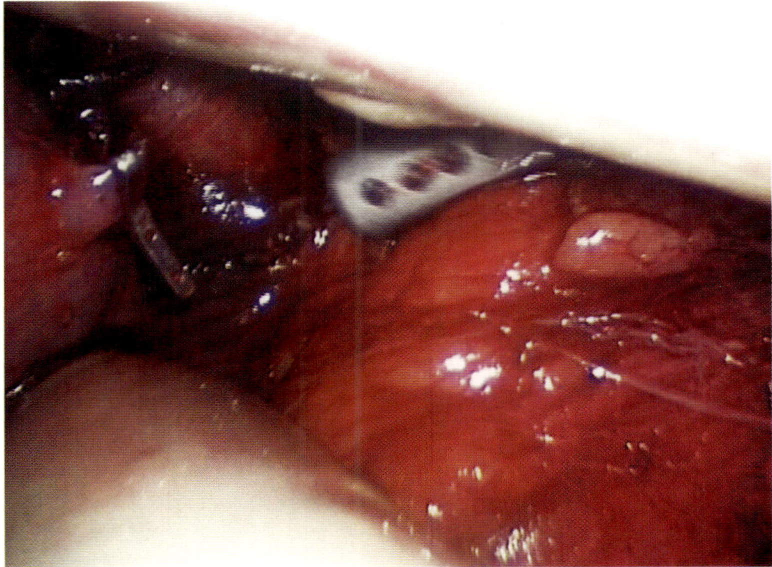

Fig. 6: Clipped and divided gonadal vein

Some venous bleeding might be undetected under the usual pressure of the pneumoperitonuem. Thus at the end of the procedure, lowering the pressure and surveying the area where clipping and ligation occurred may reveal small bleeding site that are identified at the time of the procedure, rather than in the postoperative setting.

Step 6: Specimen Extraction and Closure

Hand-port site metastasis of renal cell carcinoma following hand-assisted laparoscopic radical nephrectomy is rare, but has been reported.[12] All specimens may be placed in an extraction sac to protect the wound edges from potential tumor seeding. In addition, the sac may facilitate the extraction of large specimens through small wounds. A suture-passing device is utilized to close the 12-mm trocar site incisions; it can be visualized by inserting the laparoscope through the hand access device. The fascia in the hand-site incision is closed with a running 1-0 PDS suture. The skin is closed with a 4-0 monocryl suture in a subcuticular fashion.

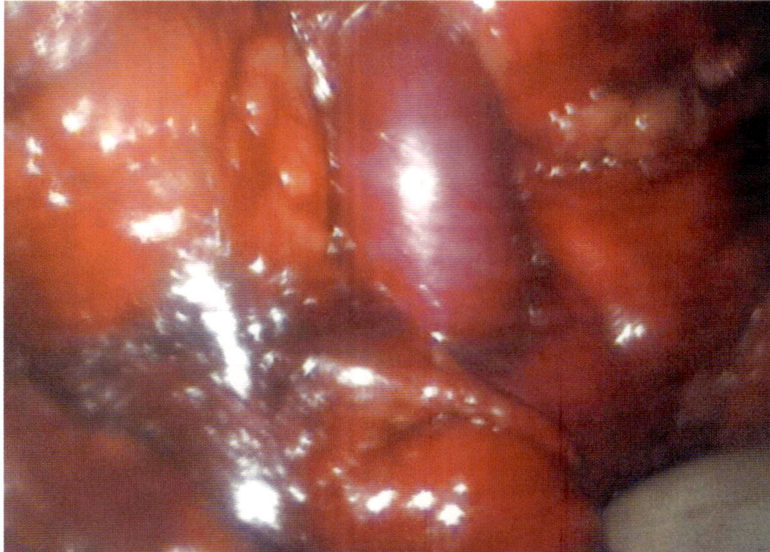

Fig. 7: Posterior approach maneuver to explore the renal artery

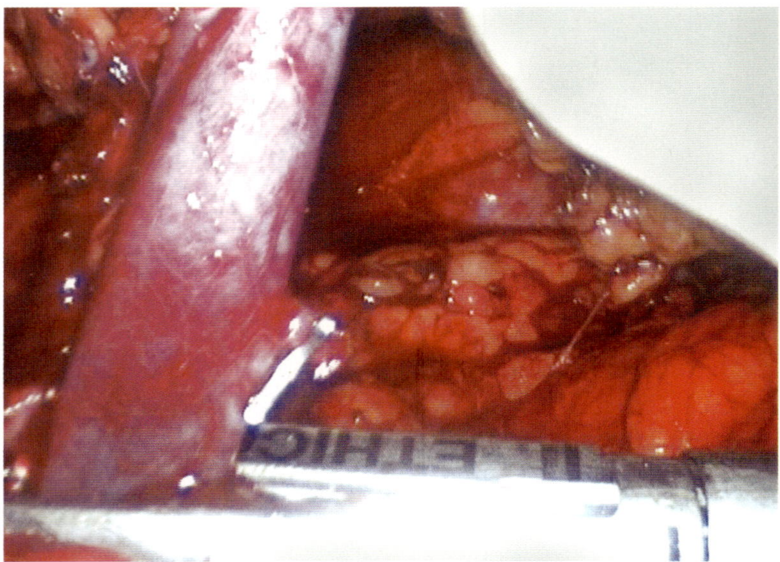

Fig. 8: Renal vein stapling

CONCLUSION

HALRN combines the advantages of open surgery and the postoperative benefits of laparoscopic surgery. It has clear advantages over traditional open techniques including less blood loss, hospital stay, narcotics requirements and recovery time. The technical skills necessary to perform a HALRN are paramount for the practicing urologist in order to provide the patient with a less morbid option for the management of their disease.

REFERENCES

1. Robson CJ. The results of radical nephrectomy for renal cell carcinoma. J Urol. 1969;101:297-301.
2. Clayman RV, Kavousi LR, Soper NJ, et al. Laparoscopic Nephrectomy; initial case report. J Urol. 1991;146:278-82.
3. Bannenberg JJ, Meijer DW, Bannenberg JH, et al. Hand-assisted laparoscopic nephrectomy in the pig: initial report. Min Invasive Ther Allied Technol. 1996;5:483-7.
4. Stifelman MD, Sosa RE, Andrade A, et al. Hand-assisted laparoscopic nephroureterectomy for the treatment of transitional cell carcinoma of the upper urinary tract. Urology 2000;56:741.
5. Wolf JS, Seifman BD, Montie JE. Nephron sparing surgery for suspected malignancy: open surgery compared to laparoscopy with selective use of hand assistance. J Urol. 2000;163:1659-64.
6. Wolf JS, Moon TD, Nakada SY. Hand-assisted laparoscopic nephrectomy: comparison to standard laparoscopic nephrectomy. J Urol. 1998;160:22.
7. Wolf JS, Tchetgen MB, Merion RM. Hand-assisted laparoscopic live donor nephrectomy. Urology. 1998;52:885.
8. Stifelman MD, Sosa RE, Nakada SY, et al. Hand-assisted laparoscopic partial nephrectomy. J Endourol. 2001;15:161.
9. Darzi A. Hand-assisted laparoscopic colorectal surgery. Surg Endosc. 2000;14:999-1004.
10. Cushieri A. Laparoscopic hand-assisted surgery for hepatic and pancreatic disease. Surg Endosc. 2000;14:991-6.
11. Lowry PS, Nakada SY. Hand-assisted laparoscopic nephrectomy. In: Caddedu JA (Ed). Laparoscopic Urologic Oncology. Totowa, NJ: Humana Press, 2004. p. 56.
12. Chen YT, Yang SS, Hsieh CH, et al. Hand port-site metastasis of renal-cell carcinoma following hand-assisted laparoscopic radical nephrectomy: case report. J Endourol. 2003;17:771-5.

Chapter 6

Robotic Radical Nephrectomy and Robotic Nephrectomy with Caval Thrombectomy

Praneeth Vemulapalli, Ronney Abaza

INTRODUCTION

Radical nephrectomy can be performed with standard laparoscopic techniques, but the addition of robotic instrumentation to the procedure allows additional visualization and control that may be of benefit to some surgeons, particularly for more complex nephrectomies. This chapter will describe techniques for performing robotic radical nephrectomy, including for complex scenarios such as very large tumors and vena caval tumor thrombi.

POSITIONING

Robotic radical nephrectomy is similar to standard laparoscopic nephrectomy in positioning in that a modified flank position allows ideal exposure to the kidney. Transperitoneal access is more often used given that the retroperitoneal space, while adequate for standard retroperitoneoscopic surgery, can be challenging for robotic surgery. This is due to the reduced working space with the retroperitoneal approach such that positioning of robotic ports requires experience to prevent and reduce collisions.

While the patient can be placed anywhere between 30° and 90° of laterality as with standard laparoscopy, the 90° flank position maximizes gravity retraction of bowels away from the anatomy of interest and minimizes reliance on a bedside assistant for retraction of bowels or other organs.

Positioning should be optimized to prevent injury but maintain patient stability on the table. Unlike with standard laparoscopy, once the robot is docked to the patient, the table position cannot be modified to compensate for inadequate exposure. Therefore, positioning should be optimized initially rather than compromised and later adjusted, which requires undocking and redocking of the robot. The authors prefer using a beanbag to secure the patient in 90° flank position with flexion only if necessary and strict avoidance of kidney rest elevation. Attention should be paid to arm positioning not only to avoid patient injury, but also to allow clearance of the robotic arms and adequate access at the bedside to the assistant port(s) if used.

INSTRUMENTS AND PORT PLACEMENT

With experience, simple robotic radical nephrectomies can be performed without an experienced bedside assistant such that a scrub nurse able to change instruments is adequate. In such cases, a robotic camera and two working instruments, allowing dissection and cutting, are all that is needed as well as the robotic clip applier for vascular control. For newer surgeons, a skilled bedside assistant is recommended to aid in progression of the procedure and for safety in the event of an intraoperative crisis, and the robotic fourth arm can also be used.

The authors' preference is to use the robotic cautery scissor and fenestrated Maryland bipolar for the entirety of the procedure, using the robotic Hem-o-Lok clips for the renal artery, renal vein, and ureter (and gonadal vein when appropriate). Other robotic energy instruments can be substituted, including hook cautery or other robotic bipolar energy instruments. Suction is typically not needed if hemostasis is maintained, but if no assistant port is being used and suction is needed, it can be accomplished through a robotic instrument port by temporarily removing the robotic instrument and applying the included reducer cap on the port valve.

Additionally, in a surgeon's early experience or for more complex procedures, additional ports are recommended until reliance on a bedside assistant is minimized, to better respond to unforeseen potential crises, or for portions of complex procedures where it is necessary, such as caval thrombectomy (Figs 1A and B). Retraction can be achieved with the robotic fourth arm and an instrument such as the robotic Prograsp or with one or more assistant ports for the bedside assistant to manipulate various instruments and the laparoscopic suction device when needed. A dedicated port can be placed for a liver retractor if desired but is not necessary in straightforward right nephrectomy with experience.

The authors prefer to place the camera port at the umbilicus and rarely deviate from this position, but other positions have been described including a lateral camera port to provide additional room for the bedside assistant. In extremely obese individuals, the umbilicus at the skin level will not correspond where the umbilicus meets the linea alba at the fascial level, such that the camera port should be moved laterally to meet the linea alba. This allows extraction of the specimen through the linea alba by extending the camera port incision (in both normal and obese patients) without any muscle splitting incisions.

With the camera port at the umbilical level through the midline, the working robotic instrument ports can then be placed in the lower and upper quadrants ipsilateral to the diseased kidney. Adjustments in the exact position of these ports can be made to match tumors with a predominantly upper pole position where instruments will need to reach high in the abdomen or vice versa, but any port placement should be planned to still allow access to the hilum (overly lateral port placement should be avoided). To prevent robotic arm clashes, the robot should be docked to the table at the angle best suited to the triangulation of the robotic ports once placed rather than always approaching the bedside with the robotic cart at 90° to the table.

Assistant ports can be placed depending on the intended use. A 5 mm port for suction or retraction can be placed in the right upper

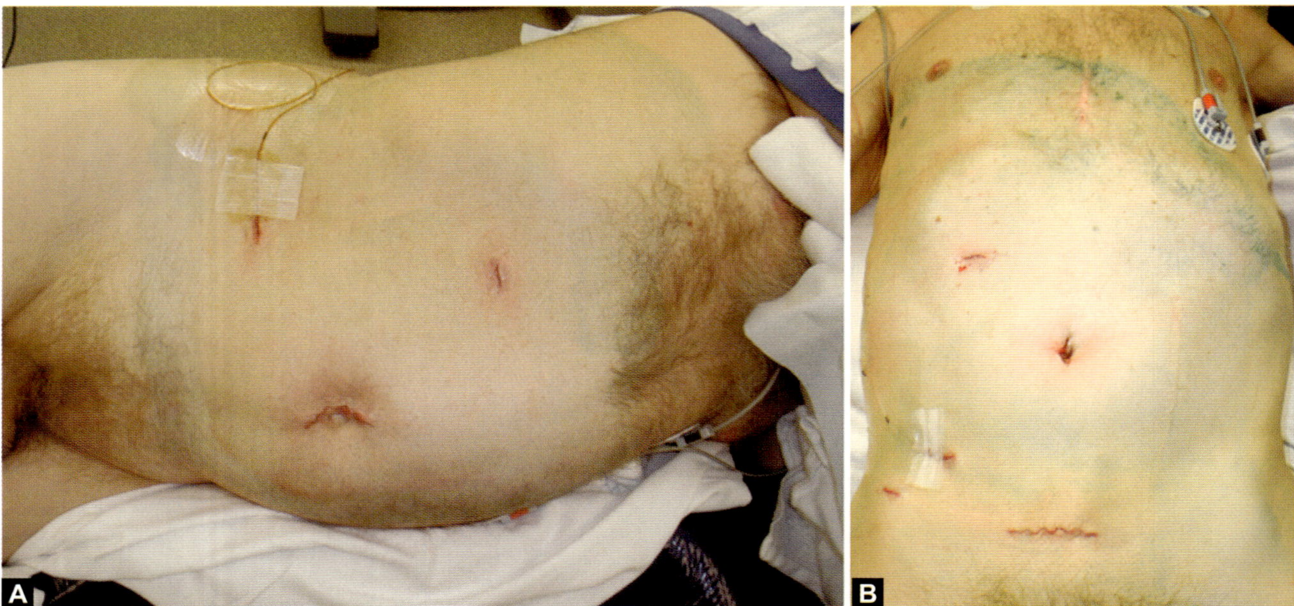

Figs 1A and B: (A) Robotic radical nephrectomy performed with three-port approach with extension of periumbilical camera port for specimen extraction (note patient in full flank position with catheter for continuous infusion of local anesthetic tunneled to extraction site); (B) Additional ports can be placed when needed as for tumors with IVC thrombus, and specimen extraction can be performed with a Pfannenstiel or midline incision

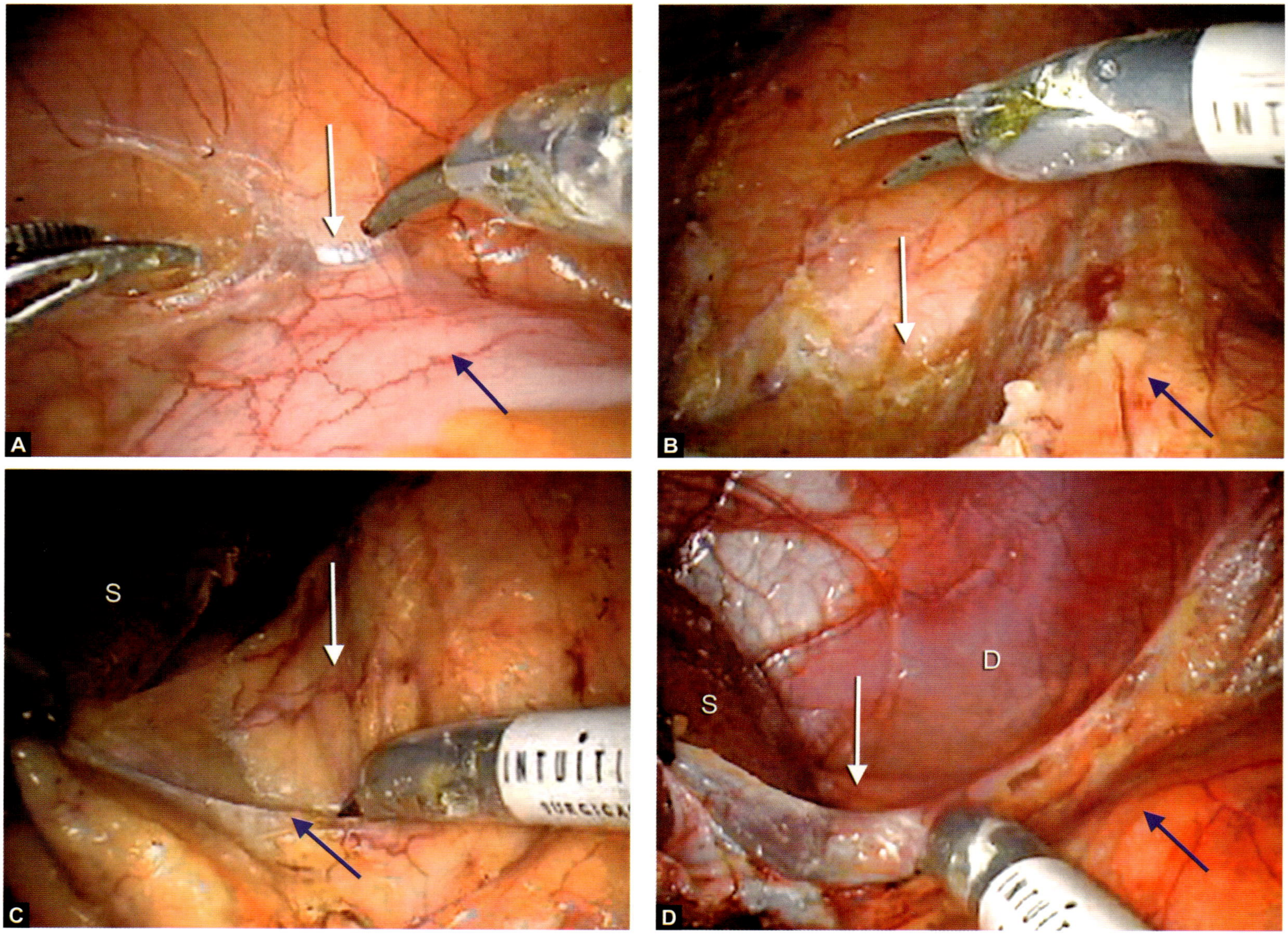

Figs 2A to D: Initial dissection of the left line of Toldt: (A) Blue arrow, colon; White arrow, colon attachment to the abdominal sidewall; (B) Blue arrow, colon fat; White arrow, boundary between colon fat and underlying Gerota's fascia; (C) Blue arrow, reflected margin of the colon; White arrow, Gerota's fascia; S, spleen; (D) Blue arrow, upper pole of kidney; White arrow, incision towards diaphragm; D, diaphragm; S, spleen

quadrant for liver retraction, for example, or in the lower quadrant for intended retraction of bowels if needed. If the surgeon prefers that the bedside assistant place clips or use a stapler to secure the renal vessels, a 12 mm port can be placed and should be optimized to allow access at the bedside for the assistant with adequate distance from robotic arms and with an angle of approach to allow adequate access to the vessels.

LEFT NEPHRECTOMY

Robotic left nephrectomy can be divided into four major segments. After achieving access and docking the robot, the initial step is to reflect the descending colon to gain access to the retroperitoneum (Figs 2A to D). The left hemicolon can be reflected without dividing the lateral attachments of the spleen more cephalad, but doing so will limit the ability to medially displace the colon because of the attachments between the splenic flexion of the colon and the spleen itself. Rather than trying to release the corner of the colon at the splenic flexure, reflecting the colon and spleen as one unit by continuing the incision of the peritoneal reflection lateral to the spleen will allow the colon and spleen to fall away from the retroperitoneum medially by gravity alone and remain out of the operative field for the remainder of the procedure without need for retraction by an assistant. Once complete, the second segment of the operation is lifting of the kidney within Gerota's fascia off of the underlying psoas muscle in approach to the hilum (Figs 3A to C). The third segment involves division of the renal vessels including adrenal sparing when possible (Figs 4A to D), and the operation is then completed by incising all remaining attachments between the abdominal wall and Gerota's fascia as well as ligation and division of the ureter (Figs 5A and B). A retroperitoneal lymph node dissection can then be performed when indicated (Figs 6A and B).

The left colon is reflected by incising the left line of Toldt and using gentle retraction to develop the natural plane between the colon and the underlying Gerota's fascia. Once the line of Toldt has been incised, the colon is further reflected by developing the retroperitoneal space between the colon and the left kidney within Gerota's fascia. Once the colon has been mobilized, the incision of the peritoneal reflection is continued lateral to the spleen in a cephalad direction beyond the upper pole towards the diaphragm to allow the colon and spleen to be reflected medially as one unit away from the underlying kidney without need for constant retraction.

Opening of a window between the posterior aspect of Gerota's fascia and the underlying psoas muscle allows elevation of the kidney. Dissection cephalad is continued until the renal hilum is reached, and the gonadal vein can be traced to the renal vein, if needed.

The left renal artery is clipped with the robotic clip applier and can be divided between clips or clipped once and then further cleared once the renal vein has been divided. The renal vein is divided between

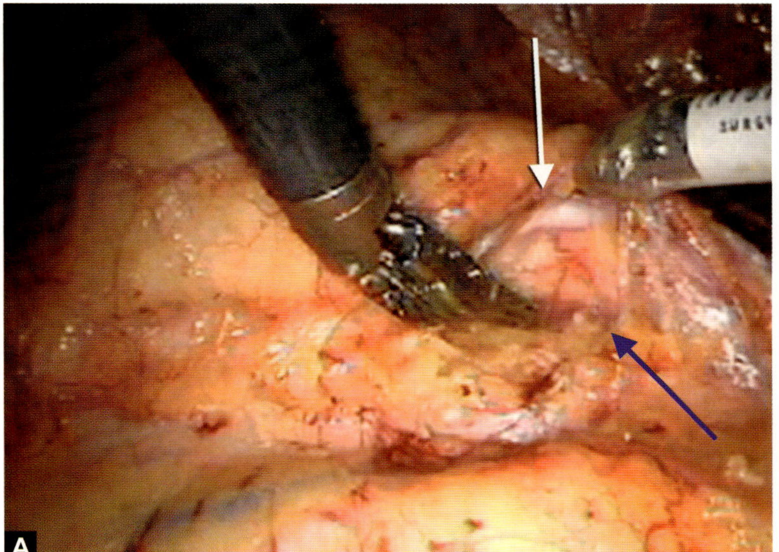

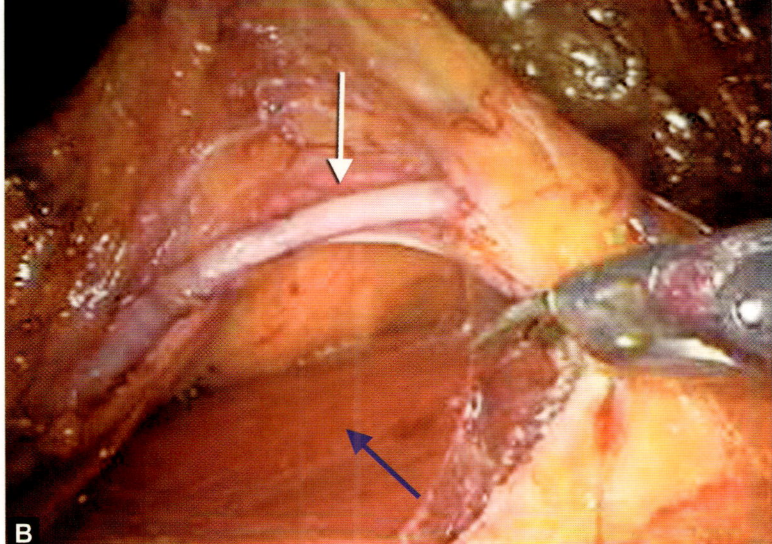

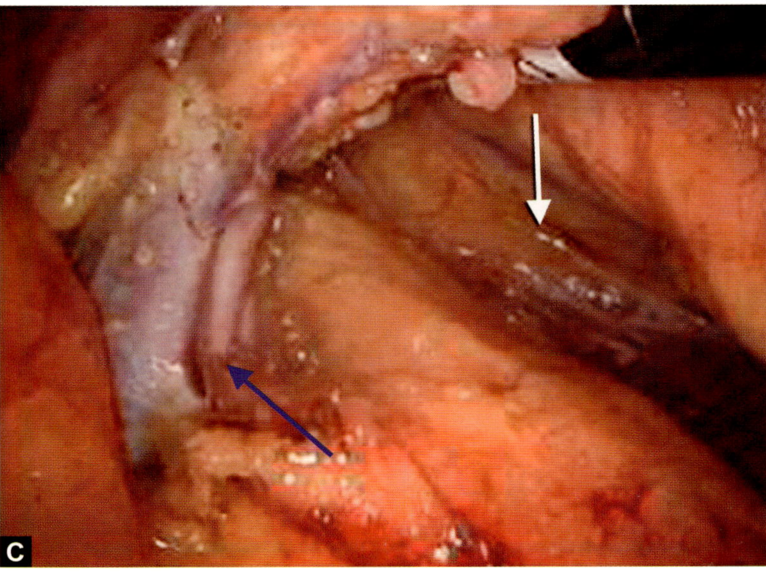

Figs 3A to C: Psoas window to elevate lower pole and identify the left renal vessels: (A) Blue arrow, initial identification of plane between posterior Gerota's and red of psoas muscle; White arrow, ureter within Gerota's fascia; (B) Blue arrow, further cleared psoas muscle, White arrow, ureter within elevated Gerota's fascia; (C) Blue arrow, renal vessels; White arrow, further development of space between elevated Gerota's contents and underlying psoas

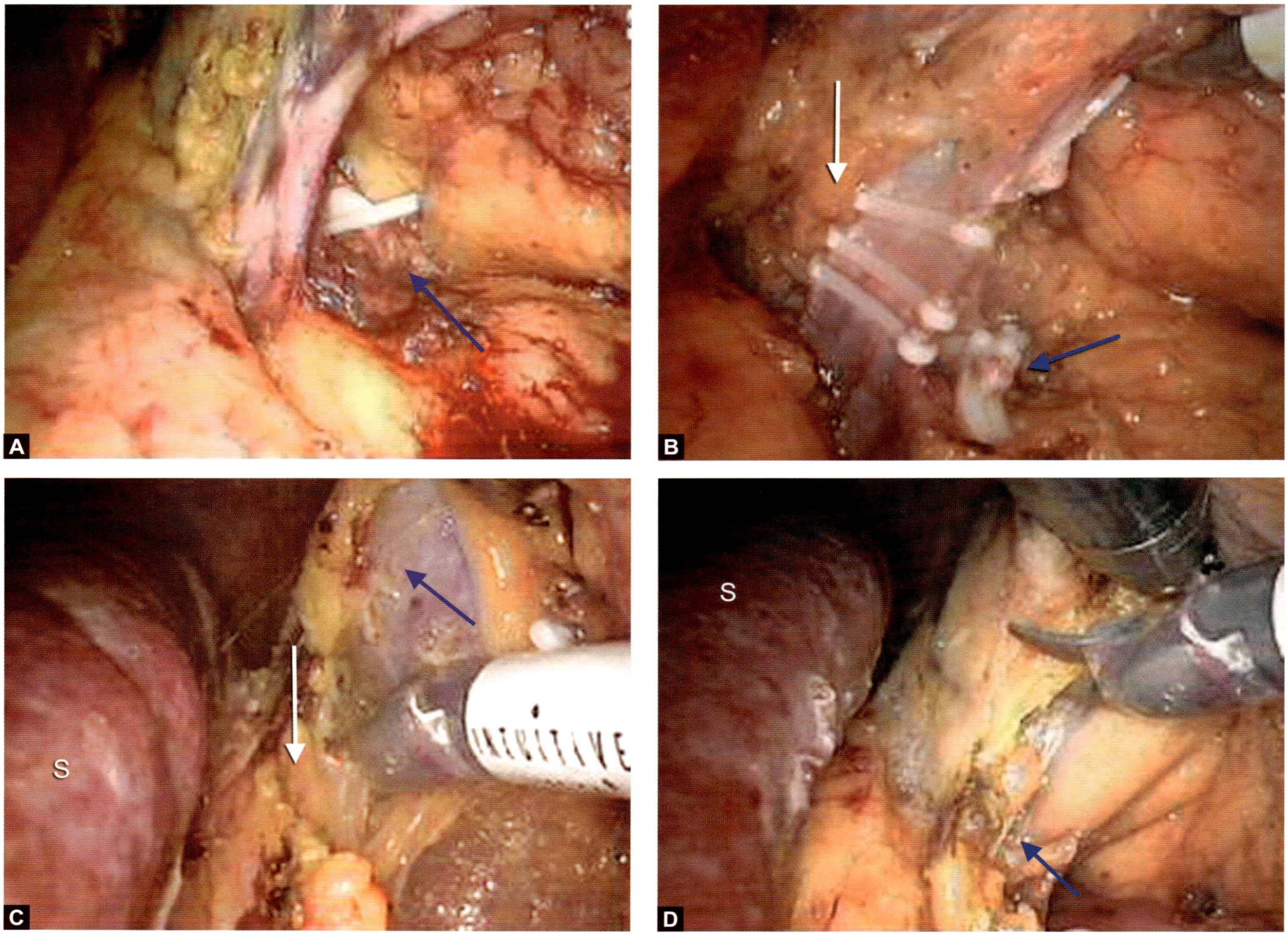

Figs 4A to D: Division of left renal vessels and upper pole dissection: (A) Blue arrow, clipped renal artery before division; (B) Blue arrow, divided renal artery; White arrow, clipped renal vein; (C) White arrow, plane between visualized edge of adrenal gland and kidney; Blue arrow, upper pole of kidney; S, spleen; (D) Blue arrow, plane between medial aspect of adrenal gland and peritoneal fat and spleen; S, spleen

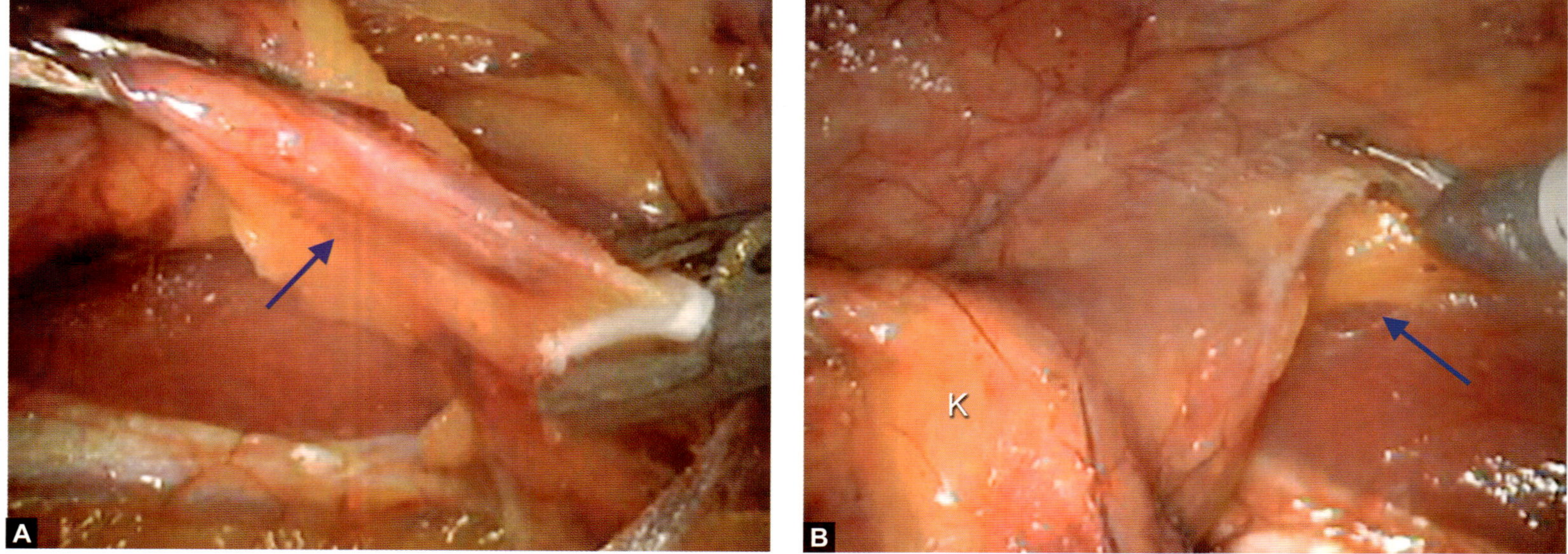

Figs 5A and B: Final steps: (A) Blue arrow, ureter; (B) Blue arrow, division of lateral attachments; K, kidney within Gerota's fascia

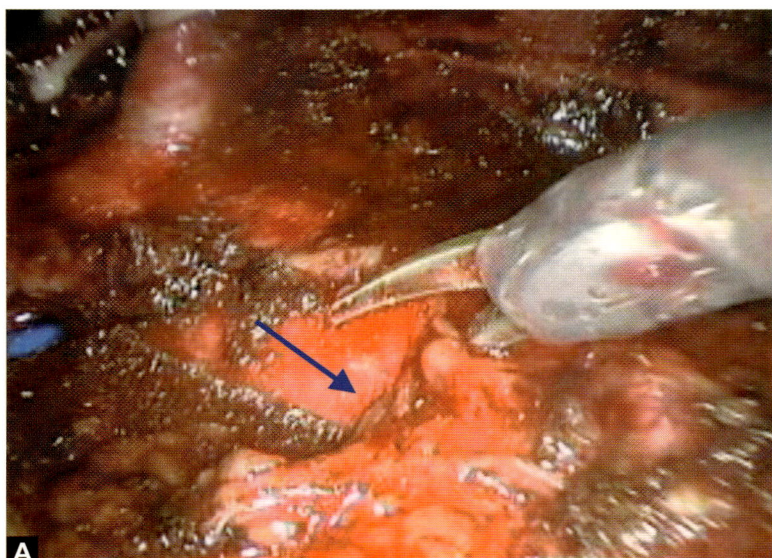

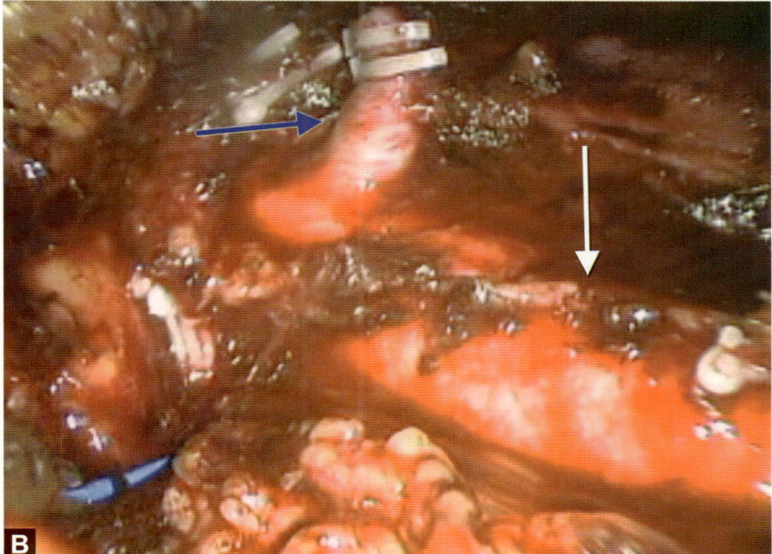

Figs 6A and B: Lymph node dissection: (A) Blue arrow, nodal packet peeled away from underlying aorta; (B) Blue arrow, stump of renal artery; White arrow, aorta after interaortocaval dissection

clips in similar fashion. In an adrenal-sparing procedure, the left adrenal gland is separated from the upper pole of the devascularized left kidney after entering Gerota's fascia and identifying the upper pole parenchymal surface (Fig. 4C). If the adrenal is to be excised, the upper pole is excised widely with the adrenal gland included with Gerota's fascia (Fig. 4D).

The ureter is clipped prior to transection. The kidney within Gerota's fascia is then dissected off of the lateral abdominal wall to complete the nephrectomy. The lateral attachments are divided last to prevent the kidney from falling medially and interfering with vascular and adrenal dissection (Figs 5A and B).

If indicated during left nephrectomy, a para-aortic lymphadenectomy can also be performed robotically (Figs 6A and B). The lymph node packet lateral to the aorta is dissected first, followed by the interaortocaval nodes.

RIGHT NEPHRECTOMY

Robotic right nephrectomy is similar to the left but has several distinguishing features. The colon is reflected in similar fashion as on the left side but typically with less difficulty achieving adequate medial retraction due to the absence of the splenocolic attachments. On the right, once the colon has been partially reflected, the duodenum will be seen overlying the vena cava and will require reflection along with the retroperitoneal surface of the mesentery of the colon to visualize the vena cava (Figs 7A to D). The underlying vena cava will make identification of the renal vein very simple in contrast to the left side, and lifting the kidney within Gerota's fascia off of the underlying psoas muscle as on the right will allow access to the renal artery, typically found posterior to the vein. The artery can also be accessed in the interaortocaval space when the presence of an exceedingly large renal tumor, short renal vein, or large vein or caval thrombus precludes dissection of the artery on the right side of the cava (Figs 8A to D). The vein is then ligated with clips, stapler, or other techniques (Figs 9A to D) with less length than the left renal vein but with less concern for the location of gonadal, adrenal, or lumbar veins as on the left. Thereafter, the remainder of the procedure is identical to the left side.

The right colon is reflected, in a similar fashion to the left, by incising the right line of Toldt and using gentle retraction to develop the natural plane between the right colon and the Gerota's fascia. Once the colon has been adequately reflected, the dissection is continued further into the retroperitoneum to the level of the duodenum. The attachments of the duodenum to the Gerota's fascia are incised in a standard Kocher maneuver to mobilize the duodenum medially.

Once the duodenum has been mobilized, the inferior vena cava (IVC) is visualized. The kidney is lifted within Gerota's fascia off of the underlying psoas just lateral to the edge of the IVC. This allows the vessels to be placed on stretch for dissection of the artery behind the vein. The artery can be clipped behind the vein or alternatively, the artery can be approached in the interaortocaval space when the renal vein is very short or when the artery branches early behind the IVC.

Once the right renal artery is controlled, the right renal vein is dissected. After circumferential dissection, it can be clipped with robotic clips and transected.

RIGHT NEPHRECTOMY WITH EXCISION OF VENA CAVAL THROMBUS

Robotic right nephrectomy can be performed even in the presence of tumor thrombus in the infrahepatic vena cava due to the readily achieved access to the cava achieved in the course of dissection. Extreme caution should be taken in performing such cases to prevent both bleeding from inadequate control of the vena cava prior to entering its lumen as well as embolism of the tumor thrombus during mobilization of the thrombus, which can be fatal. Major critical steps beyond those performed in standard right nephrectomy include identification of the extent of the thrombus in preparation for caval clamping (Figs 10A and B) and complete circumcaval mobilization along the entire length of the involved cava as well as for an adequate length above and below the thrombus to allow clamping (Figs 11A to D). This requires control of all lumbar veins with or without division by clips or energy ligation (e.g. bipolar cautery) and dissection of the left renal vein (Figs 12A and B). The renal artery is dissected and ligated as early in the procedure as possible to allow partial retraction and shrinkage of the thrombus but may not be readily accessed until the cava has been partially mobilized as typically necessary in particular when clipping the artery in the interaortocaval space (Figs 13A to D). Modified Rommel tourniquets allow clamping of the cava and left renal vein without concern for inadvertent dislodgement of bulldog clamps internally or Satinsky clamps externally by robotic arm movement. Internal space and visualization is also maximally conserved by use of such tourniquets, and the gentle application of the tourniquet on the cava above the thrombus will minimize the risk of

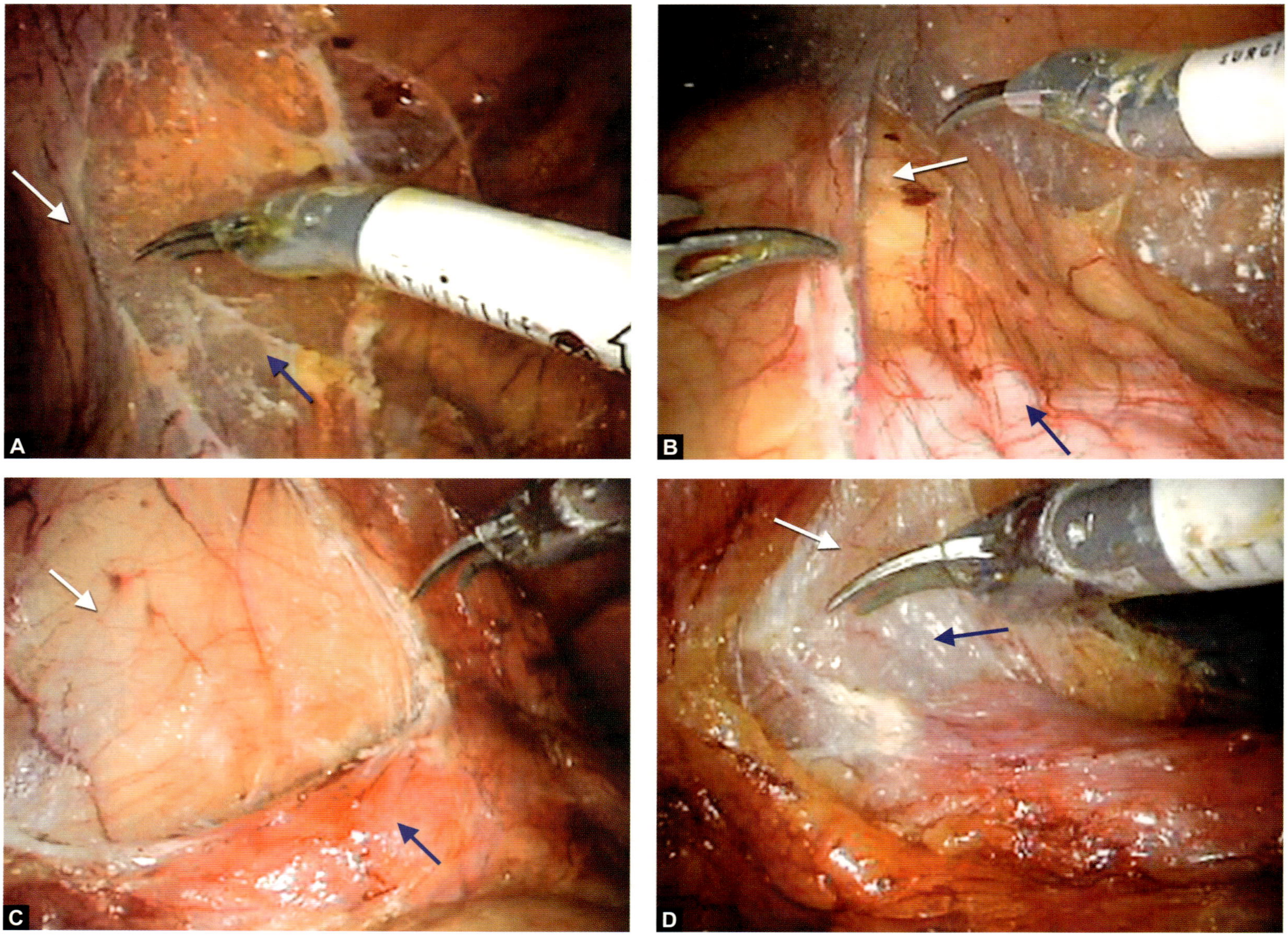

Figs 7A to D: Right colon reflection and Kocherization of duodenum: (A) Blue arrow, colon; White arrow, right line of Toldt; (B) Blue arrow, colon; White arrow, boundary between colon fat and underlying Gerota's fascia; (C) Blue arrow, duodenum; White arrow, Gerota's fascia; (D) Blue arrow, incision of the lateral duodenal attachments in Kocher maneuver; White arrow, Gerota's fascia

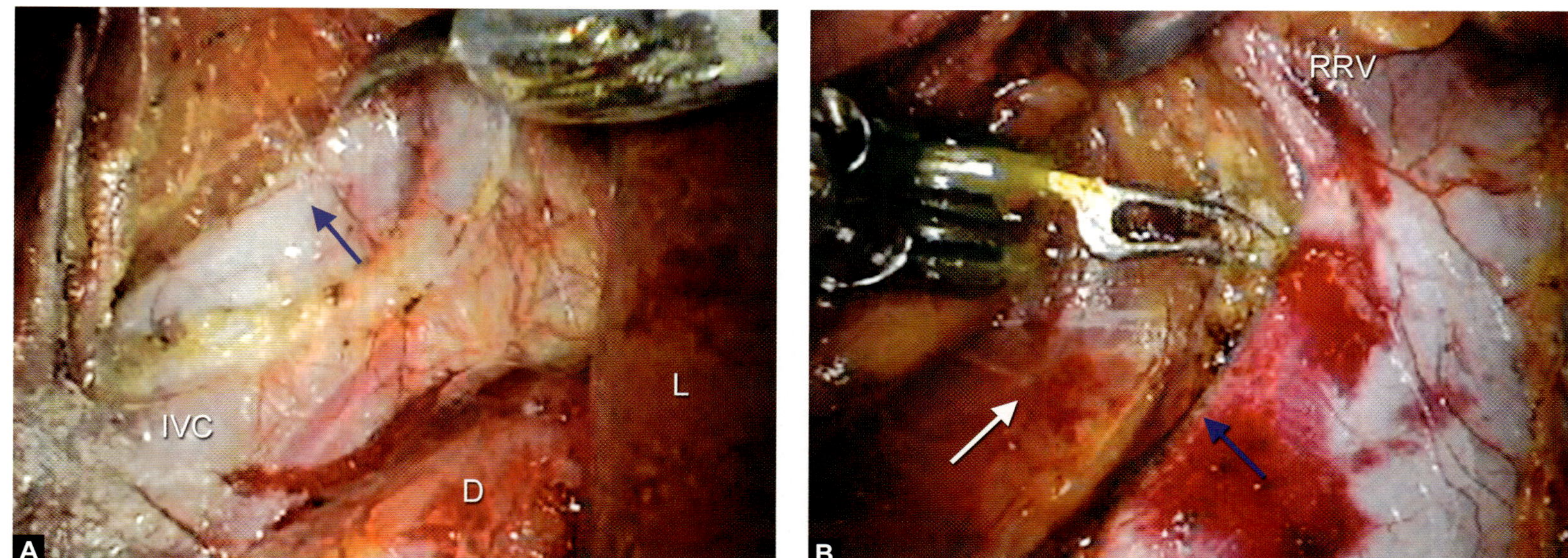

Figs 8A and B

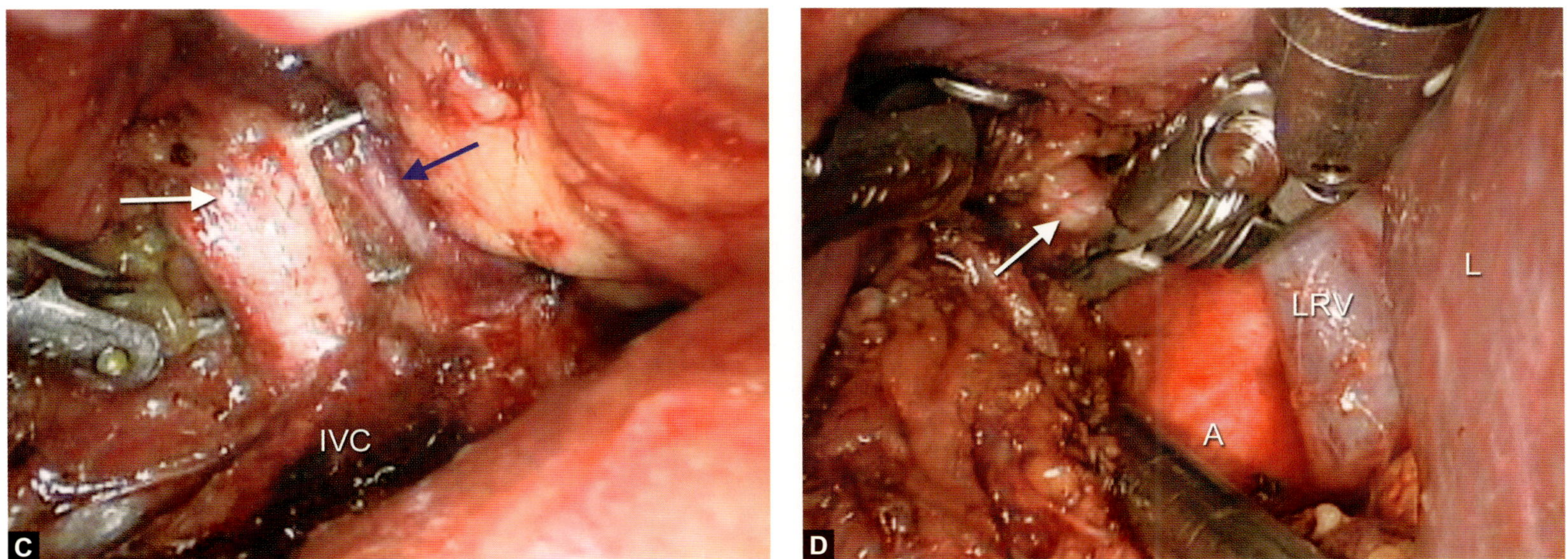

Figs 8A to D: Identification of renal hilum and renal artery ligation: (A) Blue arrow, lateral margin of inferior vena cava (IVC); L, liver, D, duodenum; (B) Blue arrow, lateral edge of IVC; White arrow, psoas muscle; RRV, right renal vein; (C) Blue arrow, inferior edge of renal vein; White arrow, renal artery; IVC, inferior vena cava; (D) White arrow, renal artery in interaortocaval space; A, aorta; L, liver; LRV, left renal vein; IVC, retracted inferior vena cava

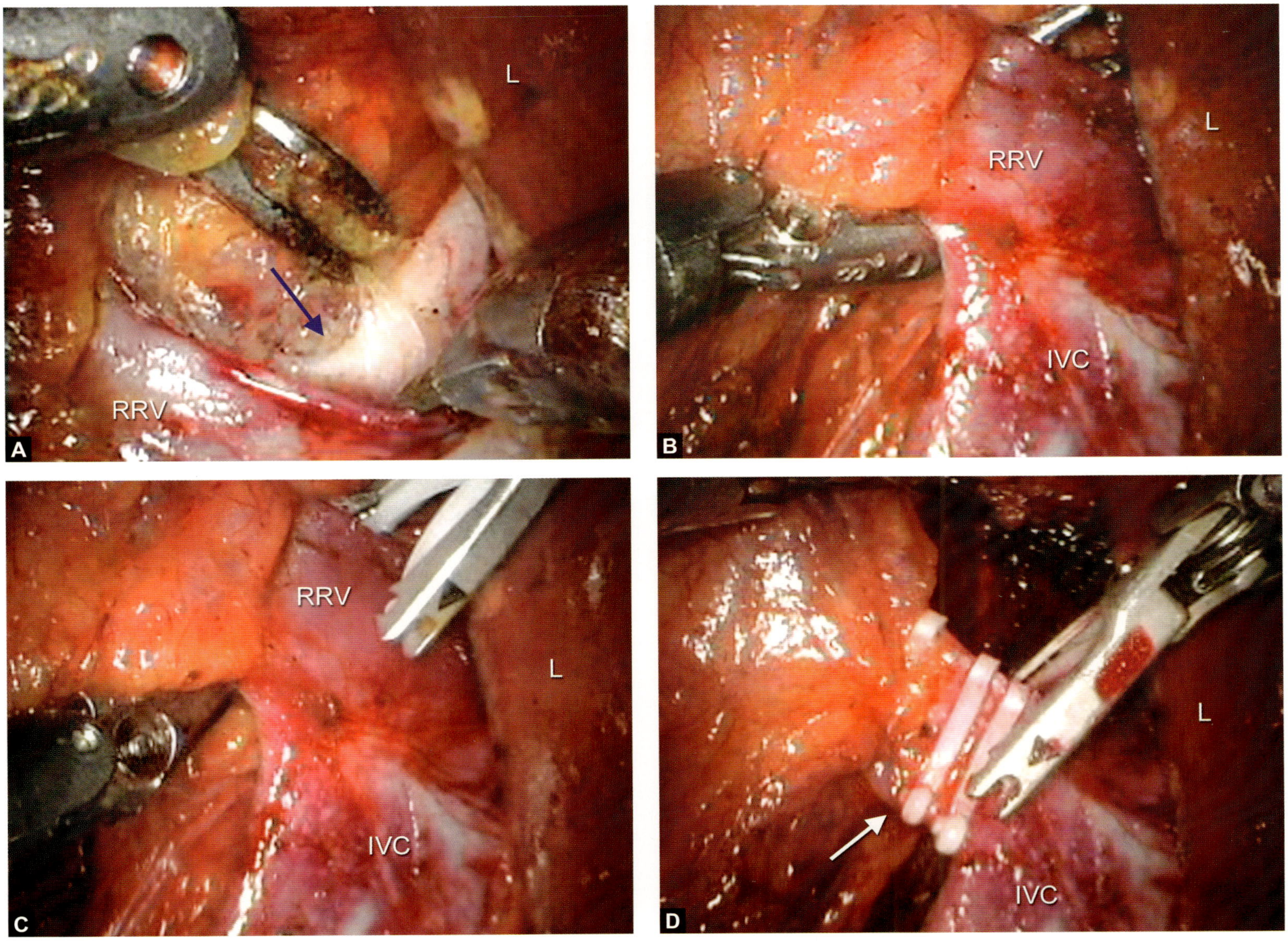

Figs 9A to D: Dissection and ligation of right renal vein (RRV): (A) Blue arrow, edge of inferior vena cava (IVC); RRV, right renal vein; L, liver; (B) RRV, right renal vein; IVC, inferior vena cava; L, liver; (C) RRV, right renal vein; IVC, inferior vena cava; L, liver; (D) White arrow, clipped right renal vein; IVC, inferior vena cava; L, liver

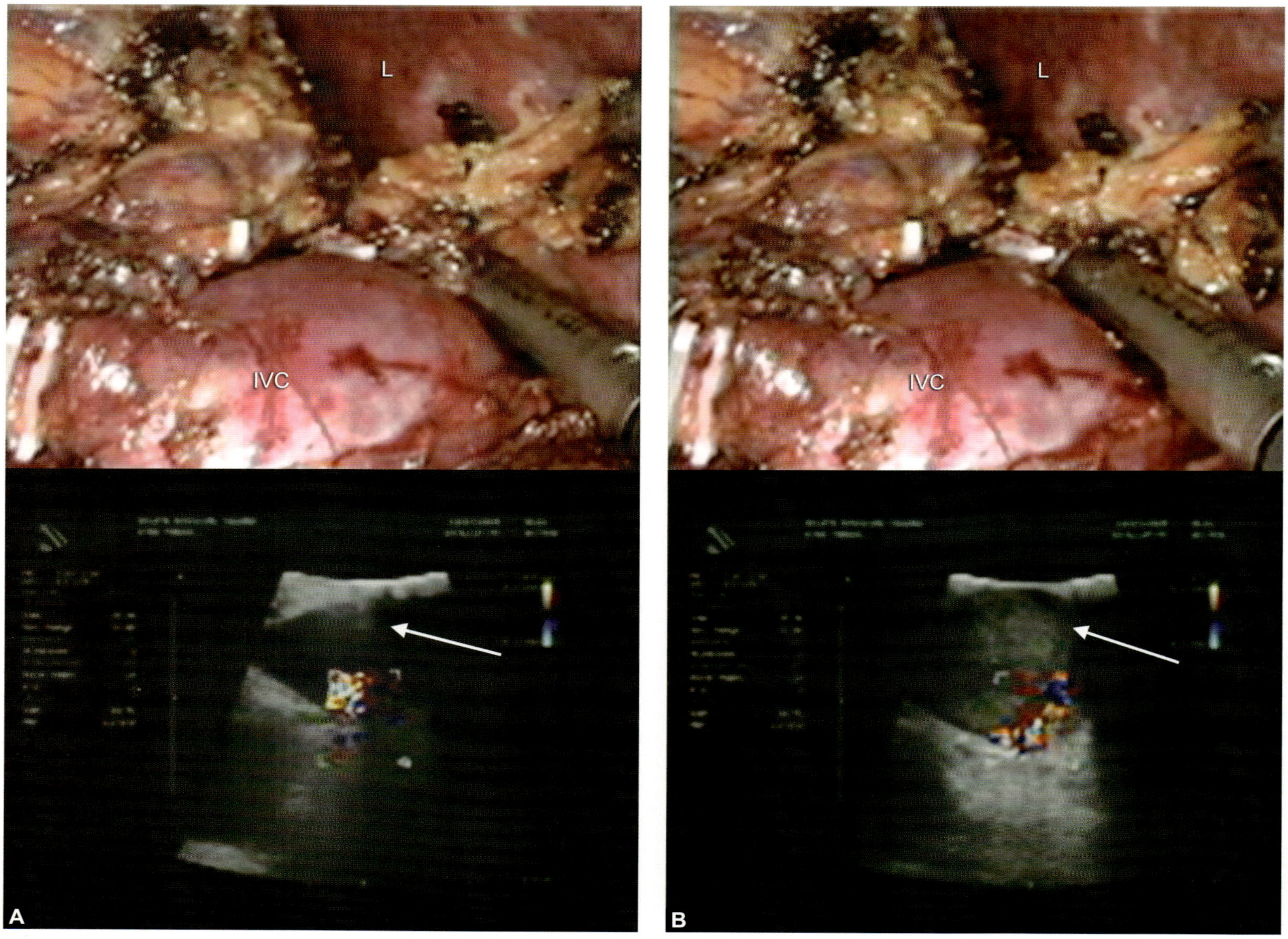

Figs 10A and B: Identification of caval thrombus with intracorporeal ultrasound: (A) White arrow, cranial tip of caval thrombus in patent vena cava; L, liver; IVC, inferior vena cava; (B) White arrow, body of caval thrombus; L, liver; IVC, inferior vena cava

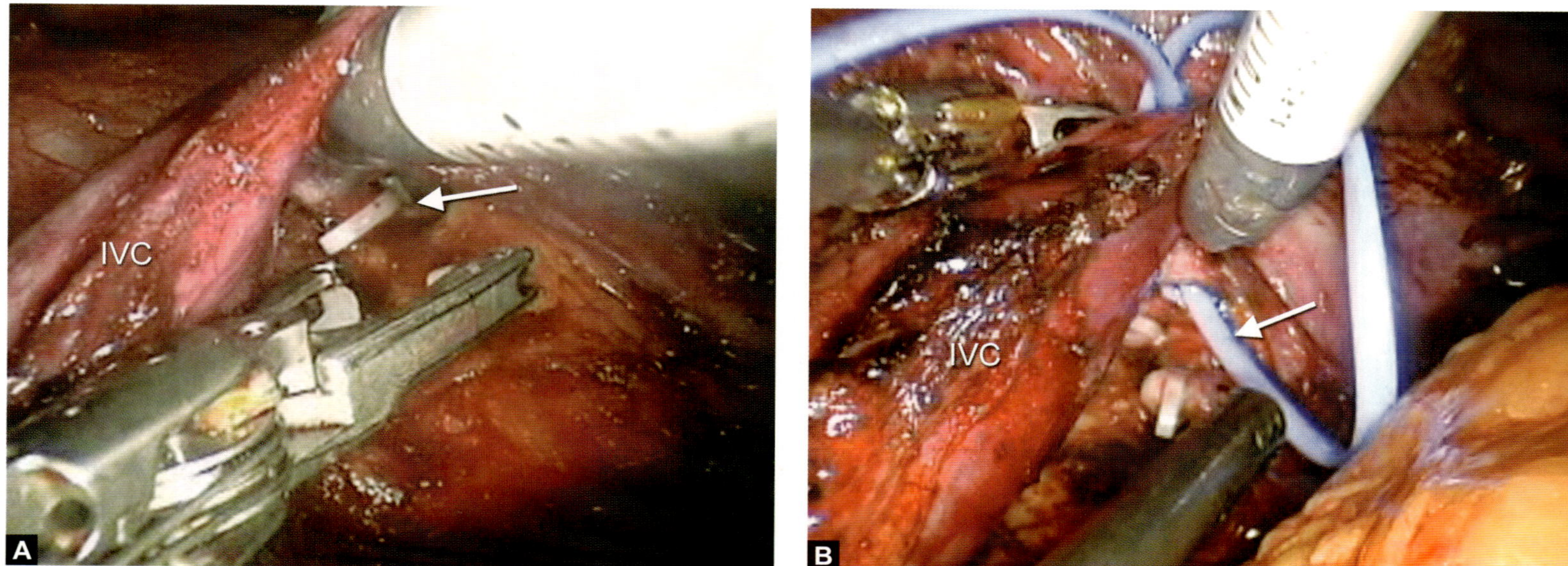

Figs 11A and B

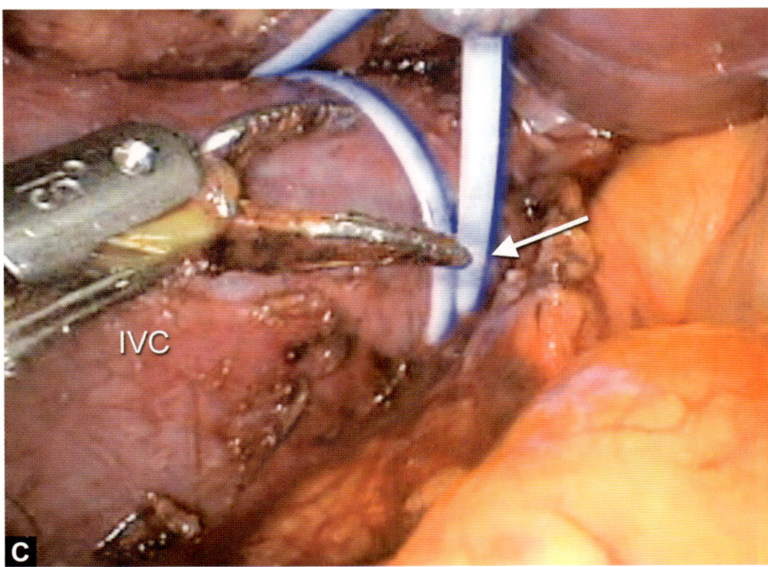

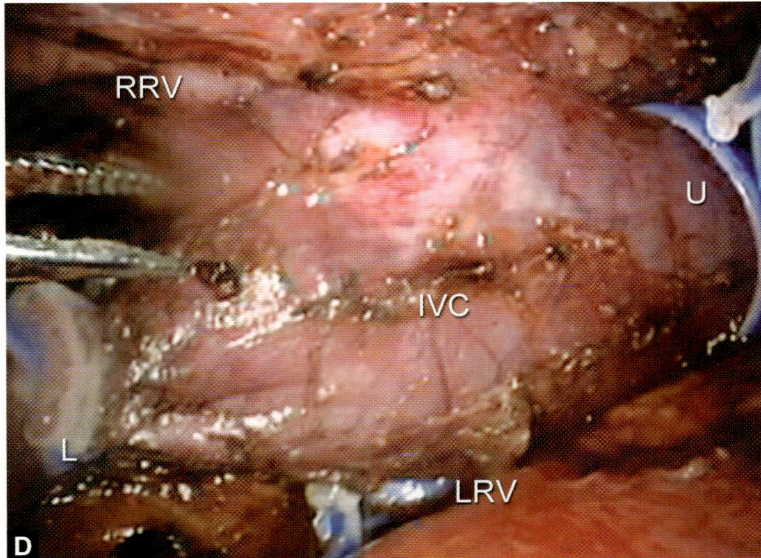

Figs 11A to D: Vascular control of the inferior vena cava: (A) White arrow, clipped lumbar vein; IVC, retracted inferior vena cava; (B) White arrow, vessel loop placed twice around cava; IVC, inferior vena cava; (C) White arrow, vessel loop placed around cava just below liver edge; IVC, inferior vena cava; (D) RRV, right renal vein with thrombus; IVC, inferior vena cava; L, lower cava with tightened Rommel; LRV, left renal vein with tightened Rommel; U, uppermost Rommel prior to tightening

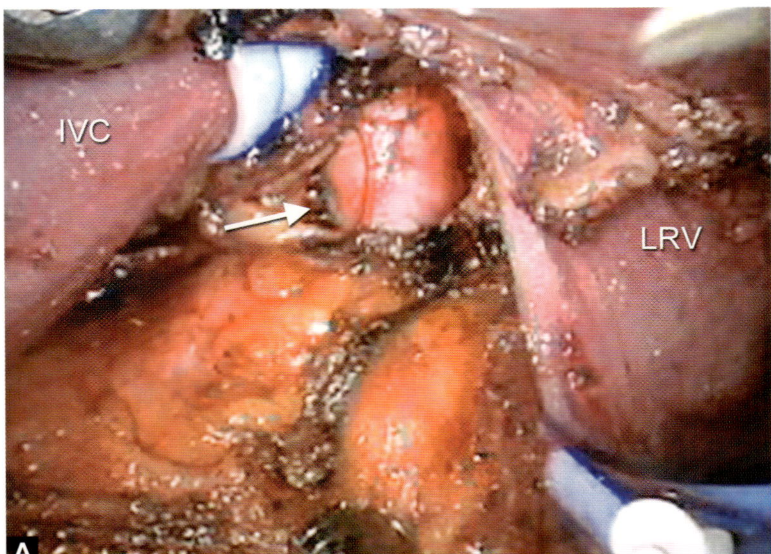

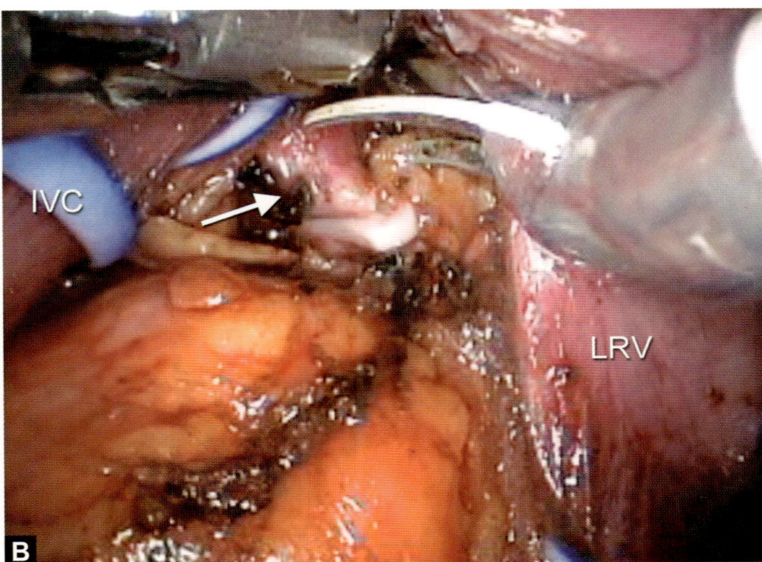

Figs 12A and B: Right renal artery dissection in the interaortocaval space: (A) White arrow, right renal artery; IVC, inferior vena cava with prepared Rommel tourniquet; LRV, left renal vein with prepared Rommel tourniquet; (B) White arrow, clipped right renal artery; IVC, inferior vena cava; LRV, left renal vein

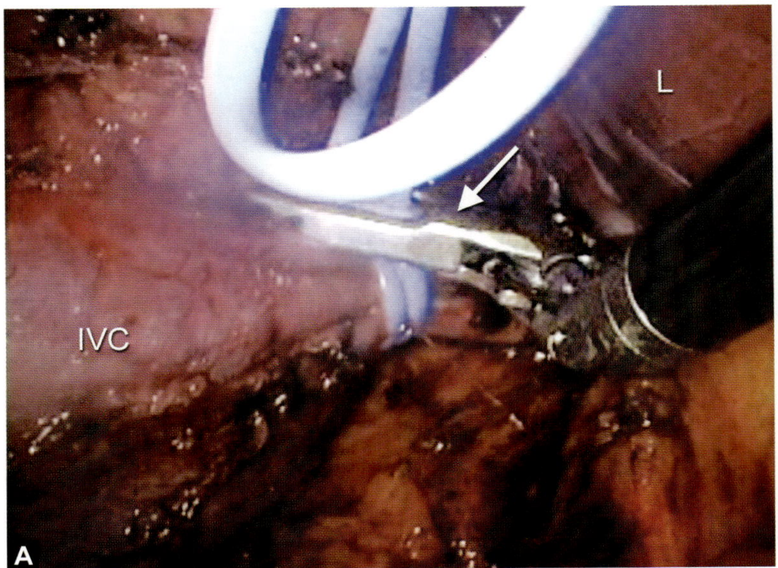

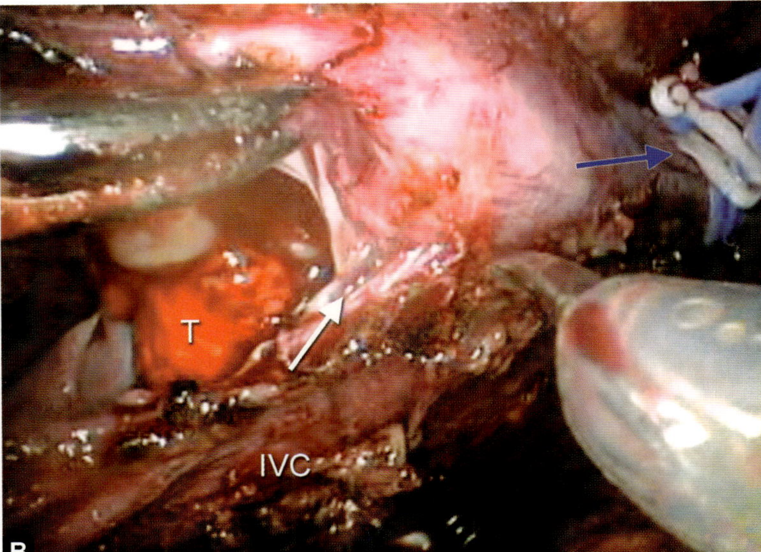

Figs 13A and B

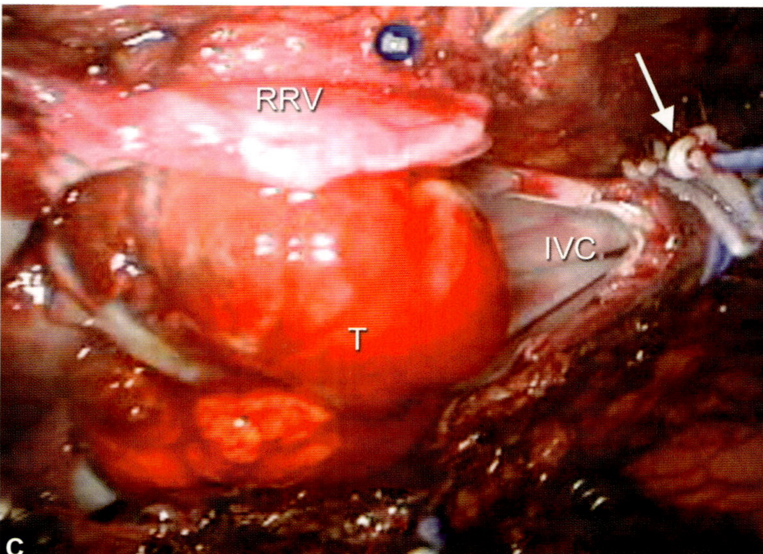

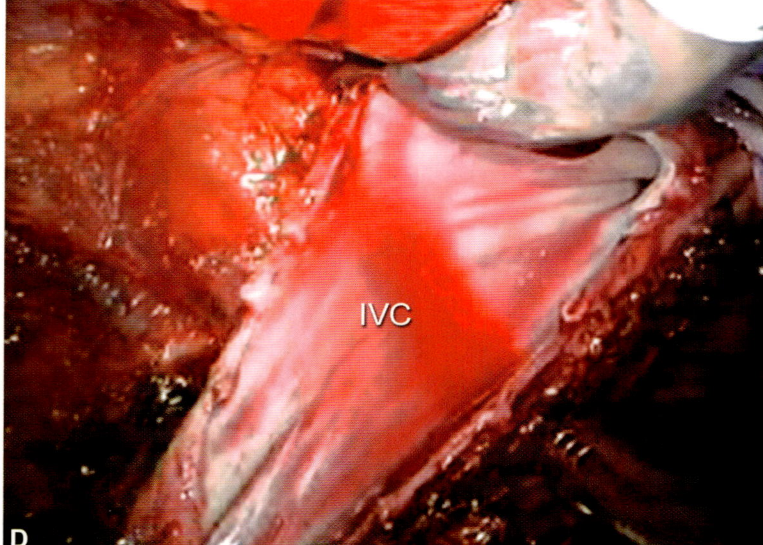

Figs 13A to D: Incision into vena cava and extraction of tumor thrombus: (A) White arrow, vessel looped is cinched and clip placed to secure; IVC, inferior vena cava; L, liver; (B) Blue arrow, cinched uppermost caval tourniquet; white arrow, incision into inferior vena cava; IVC, inferior vena cava; T, tumor thrombus; (C) White arrow, cinched proximal vena cava; IVC, inferior vena cava lumen; T, tumor thrombus; RRV, right renal vein edge; (D) IVC, exposed lumen of inferior vena cava after tumor thrombus extraction

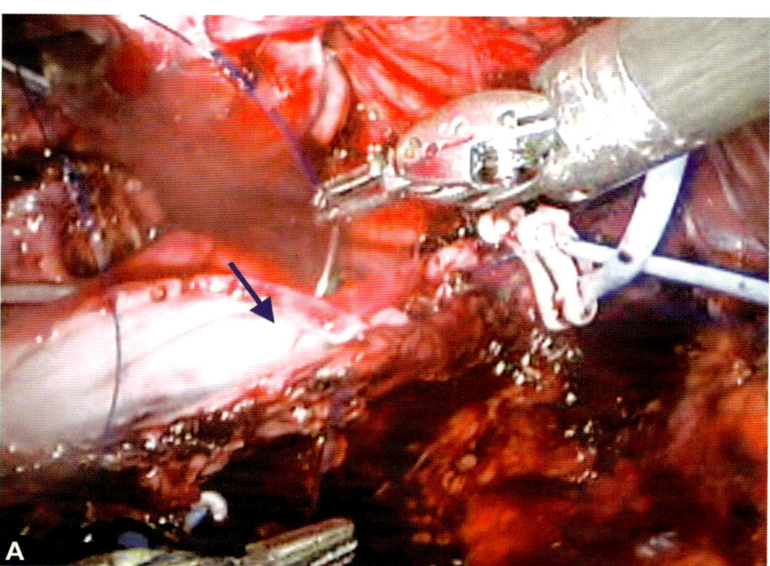

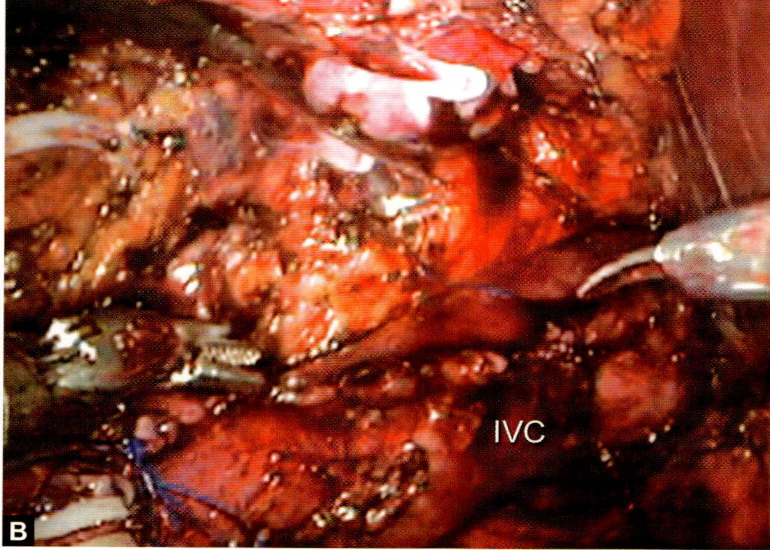

Figs 14A and B: Reconstruction of inferior vena cava: (A) Blue arrow, cavotomy closure with polypropylene suture; (B) IVC, reconstructed inferior vena cava after removal of vessel loop tourniquets

accidental thrombus fracture by a clamp if the extent of the thrombus is underestimated. Once the cava and left renal vein are controlled, complete hemostasis upon entering the cava should be tested with a small cavotomy that ceases to bleed once the cava is gently squeezed to extract all blood within; if continuous flow of bleeding is encountered, the cavotomy should be closed and the cava reassessed for a missed lumbar vein or inadequate tightness of the tourniquets. The cava can then be opened for tumor thrombus extraction in a bloodless field (Figs 13A to D), and the cava can then be sutured prior to loosening of the tourniquets to reestablish flow (Figs 14A and B).

Once the right colon has been reflected and the vena cava is identified, laparoscopic ultrasound is used to identify the location and extent of the tumor thrombus.

The vena cava is dissected circumferentially. All lumbar veins must be controlled, using robotic clips to ligate larger lumbar vessels and bipolar cautery for smaller veins (lumbar veins need not be divided once ligated). Cross clamping of the vena cava is achieved with modified Rommel tourniquets by placing vessel loops twice around the inferior vena cava (IVC) above and below the thrombus as well as around the left renal vein.

The right renal artery is dissected and clipped in the inter-aortocaval space as the thrombus in the renal vein will limit access to the artery behind the vein on the right side of the IVC. The artery can be dissected and clipped as early as possible (and need not be divided yet) to allow partial retraction of the thrombus upon devascularization of the kidney.

Once the right renal artery has been ligated and Rommel tourniquets have been placed, the vessel loops are pulled tightly to cinch down before placing a robotic clip. The vena cava can then be incised in a dry field, allowing for extraction of the tumor thrombus. Prior to closure, the IVC is inspected to confirm that the entire thrombus has been removed.

The vena cava is closed with permanent suture after tumor thrombus extraction and flushed with heparinized saline. Once the cavotomy is closed, the vessel loops are released to test the repair and then removed.

Chapter 7 Laparoscopic Partial Nephrectomy

Reza Ghavamian

INTRODUCTION

Partial nephrectomy (PN) is now considered the gold standard treatment for the solid renal cortical neoplasms amenable to nephron-sparing surgery (NSS). The enthusiasm and necessity for the performance of PN is the higher incidence of long-term renal insufficiency associated with radical nephrectomy (RN).[1] RN is also associated with increased long-term morbidity including cardiovascular disease and mortality.[2] The guidelines document for the management of small renal cortical neoplasms published by the American Urological Association lists PN as the preferred treatment option for these lesions.[3] Open NSS has now been established as the gold standard treatment option in the management of the solid renal mass up to 7 cm even in the presence of a normal contralateral kidney.[4] In the last 7 years, laparoscopic partial nephrectomy (LPN) has emerged as a minimally invasive alternative to open PN.[5] Several studies have demonstrated equivalent perioperative, renal functional and oncologic outcomes to open PN for the same indications and for lesions with the same size characteristics.[6] These include complex scenarios including endophytic central tumors, hilar tumors, solitary kidneys and heminephrectomies.[7-10] LPN provides equivalent oncologic efficacy to open PN in larger tumors up to 7 cm as well.[11] However it remains a technically challenging operation that requires advanced laparoscopic expertise and surgical skill set for the operating surgeon. This chapter provides a step by step procedure guide for LPN. As different tumor characteristics mandate different surgical considerations and hence dictate different surgical maneuvers, select unique clinical scenarios are additionally depicted.

INSTRUMENTATION

The basic instrumentation for laparoscopic partial nephrecotomy is provided in Table 1.

Table 1: Core instrumentation for laparoscopic partial nephrectomy
Atraumatic bowel graspers
Laparoscopic right angle clamps
Laparoscopic bipolar graspers
Laparoscopic needle holders
Laparoscopic bulldog clamps (large, small, curved and straight)
Dissection and energy device (laparoscopic scissors, ultrasonic shears or LigaSure®)
Laparoscopic ultrasound machine and probe
Hemostatic agents (Fibrin glue, Surgicel®, Gelfoam®, Floseal®)
Laparoscopic specimen extraction bag
Hem-o-lok® (Weck) and Lapra-Ty® clips

PREPARATION, POSITIONING AND PORT PLACEMENT

General endotracheal anesthesia is instituted. The patient is placed in a lateral decubitus position. All pressure points are padded and the patient is securely taped to the operating table. An axillary roll is placed and the ipsilateral arm is supported by an armrest. The video tower and all instrumentation are placed behind the patient and the main video screen is positioned directly in front of the surgeon. A secondary video tower is placed behind the surgeon for the assistants as needed. A 4-port approach is utilized and their positions are marked (Fig. 1). The right and left dissecting trocars are placed in the midclavicular line a fingerbreadth below the costal margin and 2–3 fingerbreadths below the umbilical line. The camera trocar is placed in the anterior clavicular line at or just above the umbilicus. Insufflation is carried out at the infracostal trocar level or at the level of the 4th trocar just medial to the anterior superior iliac spine. A Fast Clamp retractor is placed through this trocar later for optimal liver retraction on the right (Fig. 2). The anesthesiologist is instructed to keep the patient well hydrated throughout the procedure as is done in donor nephrectomy cases to perfuse the kidney and optimized postoperative renal function.

TECHNIQUE OF RIGHT-SIDED LAPAROSCOPIC PARTIAL NEPHRECTOMY

To demonstrate the technique of right-sided LPN, a case of an intraparenchymal predominantly posterior tumor is presented (Figs 3A and B).

The key points to the safe performance of a right-sided LPN are adequate mobilization and retraction of the liver and identification

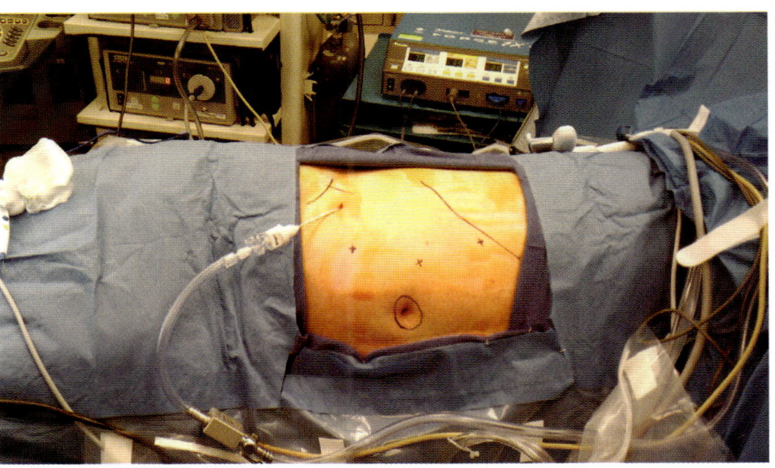

Fig. 1: Right-sided port placement

and kocherization of the duodenum. This allows for safe and clear visualization of the vena cava and the renal hilum for optimal control. The liver can be retracted with a Fast Clamp retractor (Fig. 4A) or alternatively with a locking laparoscopic forceps through an alternatively placed upper and medial port (Fig. 4B).

The line of Toldt is divided, and the ascending colon is retracted medially. The plane between Gerota's fascia and the mesentery of the colon is identified, and the lower pole of the kidney enveloped by Gerota's fascia is identified. The gonadal vein and the ureter are identified and retracted laterally with the left-handed bowel grasping forceps exposing the psoas muscle and the lateral edge of the vena cava and duodenum (Fig. 5A). An ultrasonic shear is used to kocherize and mobilize the duodenum (Fig. 5B).

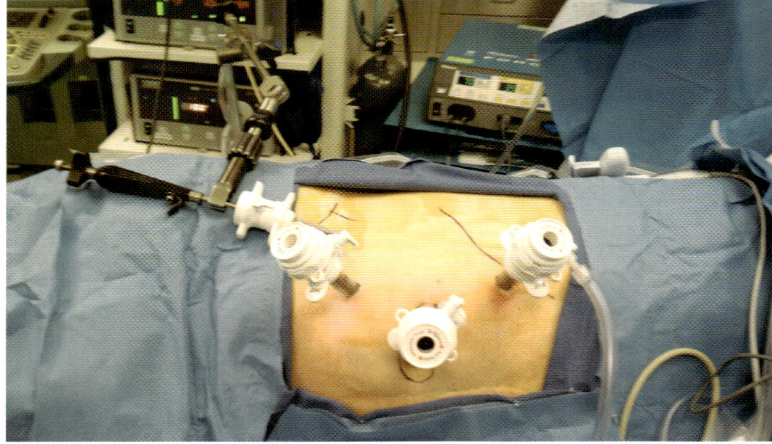

Fig. 2: A liver retractor is applied and secured to the table

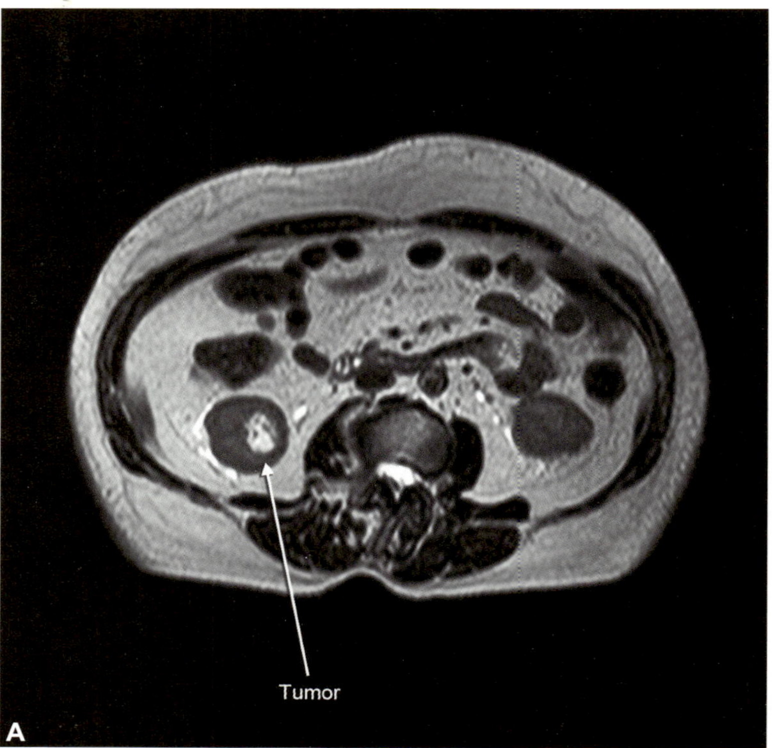

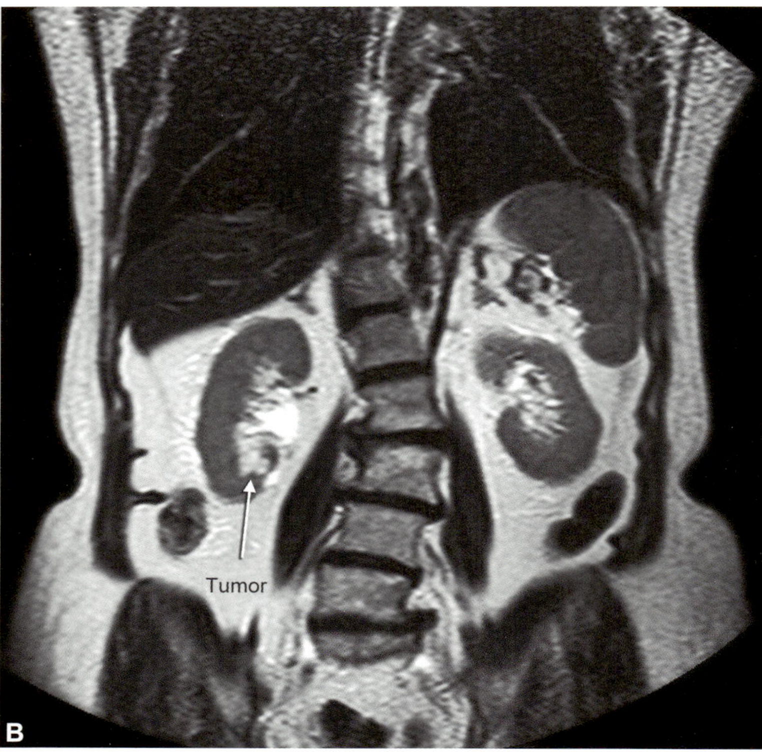

Figs 3A and B: (A) Transverse and (B) Coronal magnetic resonance images of a cystic Bosniak 4 lesion with intramural solid nodules encroaching the collecting system

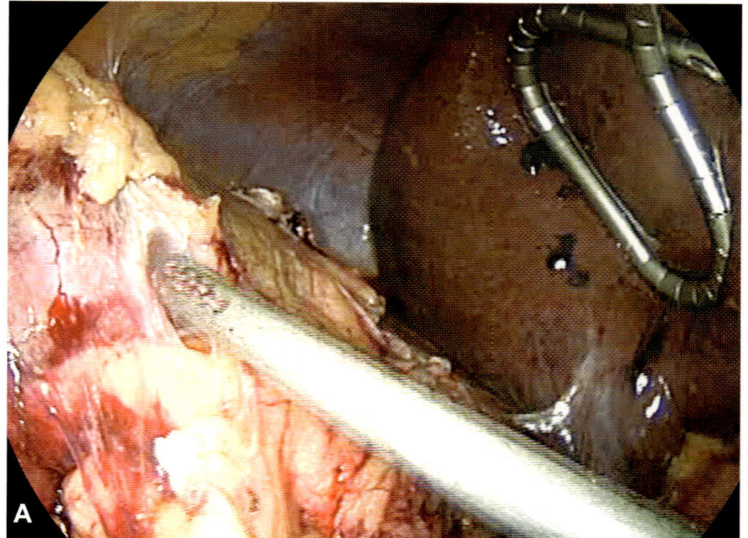

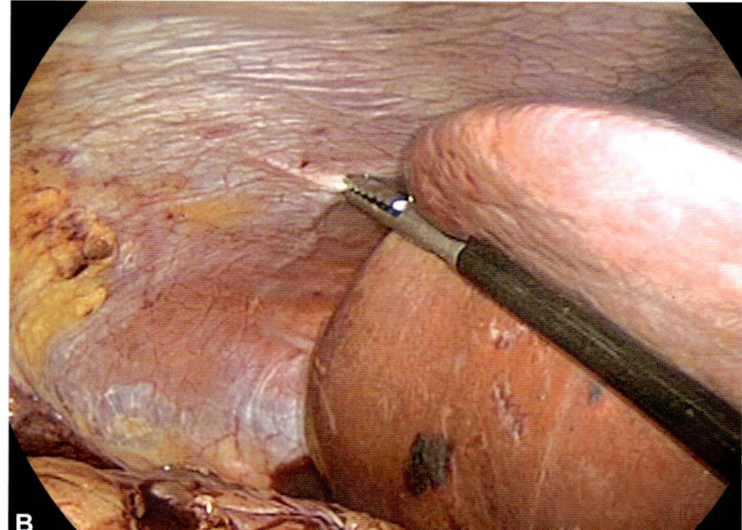

Figs 4A and B: (A) Fast Clamp retractor on the liver and (B) A Davis and Geck laparoscopic forceps retracting the liver

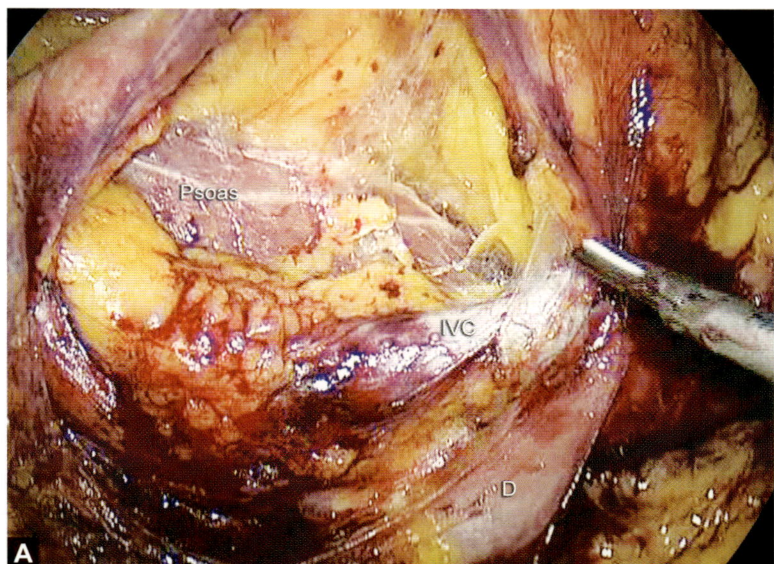

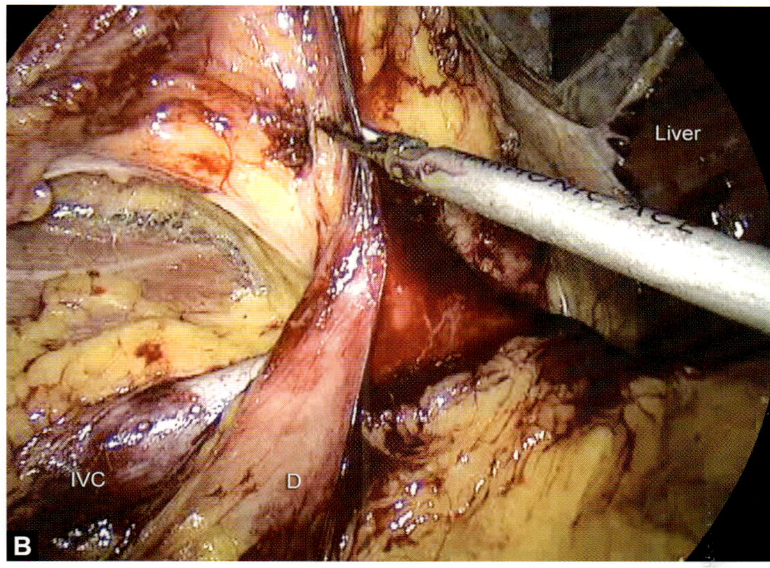

Figs 5A and B: (A) The inferior vena cava (IVC) is identified and (B) The duodenum 'D' is kocherized

The renal hilum is exposed. Along the dissection the retracting left-armed instrument is advanced cephalad along the medial border of the kidney, providing gentle lateral exaggerated retraction for optimal exposure and dissection with the dissecting right arm (Fig. 6).

The right kidney is mobilized and defatted circumferentially to expose and inspect the full cortical surface of the kidney. In this particular case, the kidney is fully mobilized using the ultrasonic shears to expose the lower pole medial and partially posterior tumor (Fig. 7). The ureter is identified and dissected carefully off the tumor to prevent injury during resection and is medially rotated (flipped) to expose the posterior surface of the lower pole for adequate tumor resection (Fig. 8). At this point, 12.5 g of mannitol is administered intravenously to promote diuresis and decrease the chance for postoperative acute tubular necrosis (ATN). During the infusion of mannitol, laparoscopic intraoperative ultrasonography is performed to delineate the renal parenchymal and deep resection margins for adequate resection (Fig. 9).

Prior to clamping, it should be made sure that all sutures necessary for reconstruction are available and loaded to decrease warm ischemia time. A hemostatic bolster is introduced into the field for future use for parenchymal reconstruction. After 7–10 minutes following the infusion of mannitol, the kidney is rotated back to its anatomical position and the renal hilum is then controlled with laparoscopic bulldog clamps to allow for bloodless resection (Fig. 10). Alternatively, the renal artery and vein could be controlled with separate bulldogs. The renal vein could be left unclamped to allow for retrograde renal perfusion. However the merits of this maneuver and its true advantage are debatable.

The tumor is then circumscribed with laparoscopic scissors. The parenchymal resection is then carried out in sequential depths with cold scissors paying particular attention not to abrogate the tumor psuedocapsule (Fig. 11). Collecting system entries are noted for subsequent repair. No cautery is used for the tumor resection. A laparoscopic scalpel blade is a valuable adjunct to help complete tumor resections, when a parallel resection line in the deep tumor crater is needed. The tumor is then entrapped in a specimen entrapment sac (Figs 12A and B).

The tumor crater is inspected for any signs of collecting system entry, large segmental vessels that need to be closed and the optimal method of parenchymal closure allowing for less tension on approximation. The collecting system is closed with 3-0 polyglactin

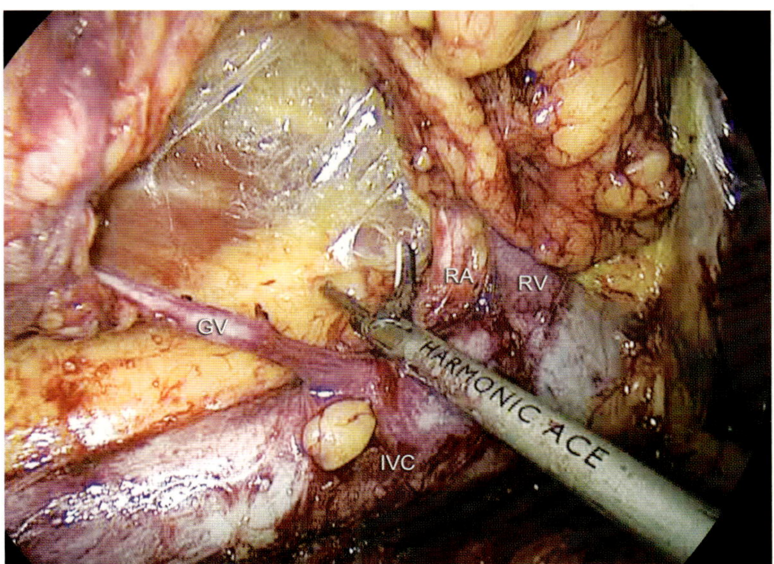

Fig. 6: The right renal artery (RA) and renal vein (RV). Note inferior vena cava (IVC) and gonadal vein (GV)

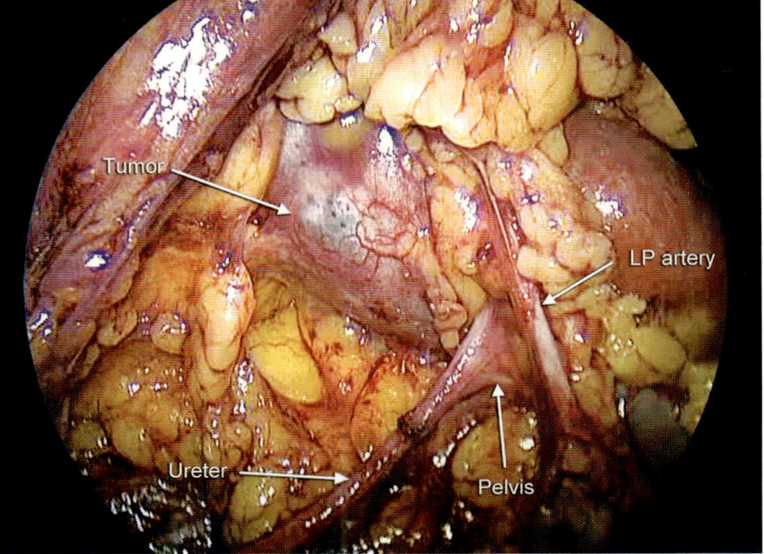

Fig. 7: Anterior view of endophytic medial, partially cystic and predominantly posterior lower pole tumor. Note lower pole (LP) arterial branch crossing anterior to the renal pelvis

suture with absorbable Lapra-Ty® clips to decrease freehand suturing and decrease warm ischemia time (Figs 13A and B).

In cases where large resections are performed or if there is any doubt of violation of the tumor pseudocapsule, frozen sections from the tumor crater can be sent for pathologic evaluation. The hemostatic bolster is placed in the tumor crater and the Floseal® is applied. The renal parenchymal edges are approximated with 2-0 polyglactin sutures with freehand suturing technique (Figs 14A and B). The first knot is a triple surgeon's knot to lay down the suture without slipping. With optimal resection angles of the tumor, it can be ensured that the parenchymal edges can be closely approximated with the parenchymal sutures with no tension or risk of parenchymal fracture. At this point, the hilar clamp is removed. In cases where separate clamps are used for the artery and the vein, the venous clamp is removed first followed by the arterial clamp(s). Another 12.5 g of mannitol is administered intravenously followed by 10 mg of furosemide to promote diuresis and decrease the incidence of ATN. The remaining Floseal is placed over the repair with a Surgicel® blanket (Fig. 15). The recommended warm ischemia time for PN is generally considered to be 30 minutes.[12] A recent comprehensive

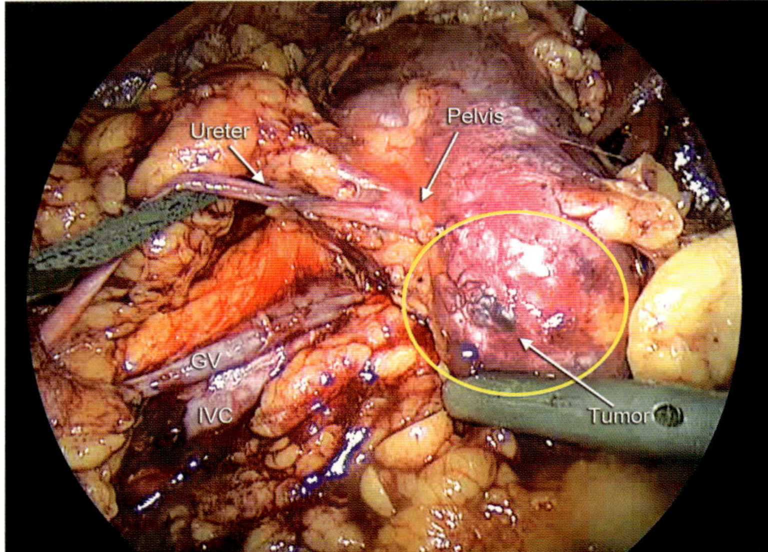

Fig. 8: The kidney is rotated medially (flipped) and the tumor is visualized for resection

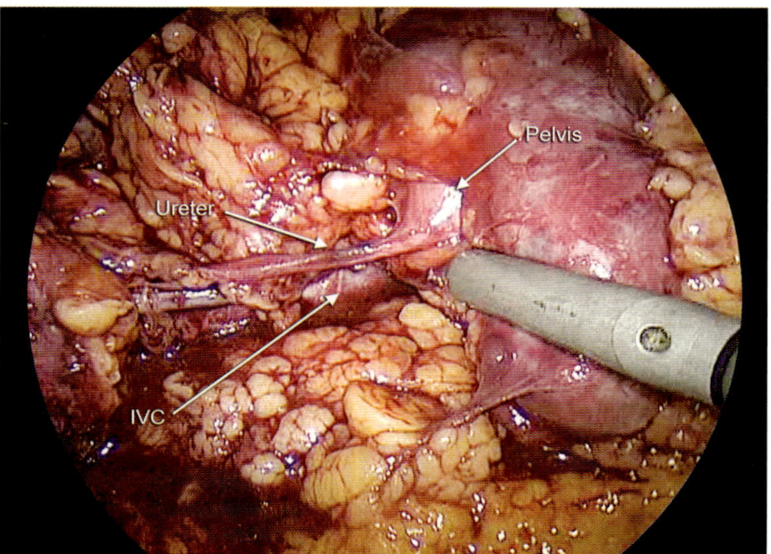

Fig. 9: Intraoperative ultrasonography is performed (Abbreviation: IVC—inferior vena cava)

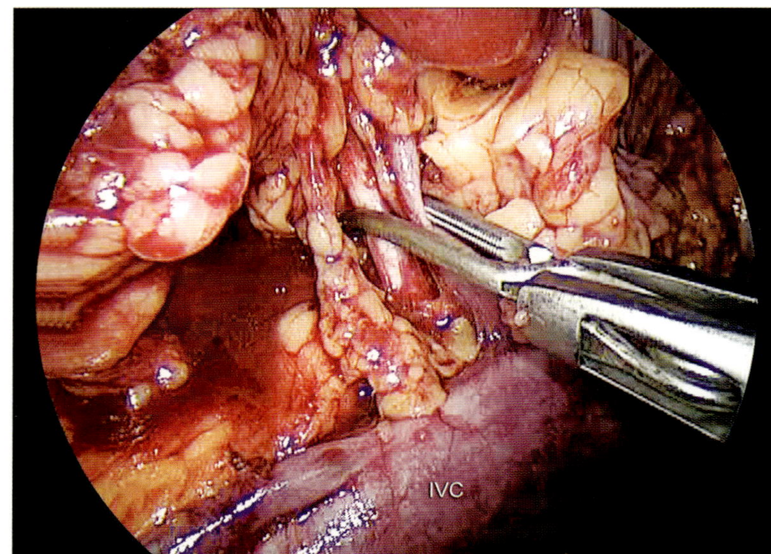

Fig. 10: The renal hilum is controlled en bloc

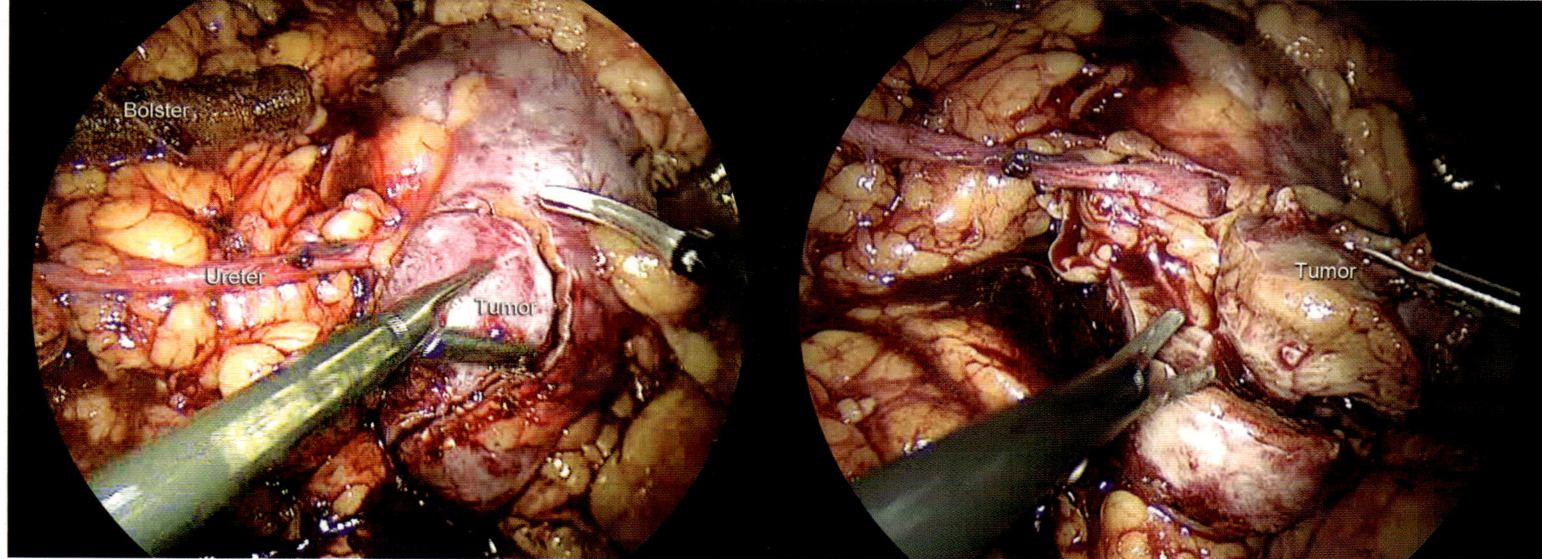

Fig. 11: Tumor resection with cold scissors

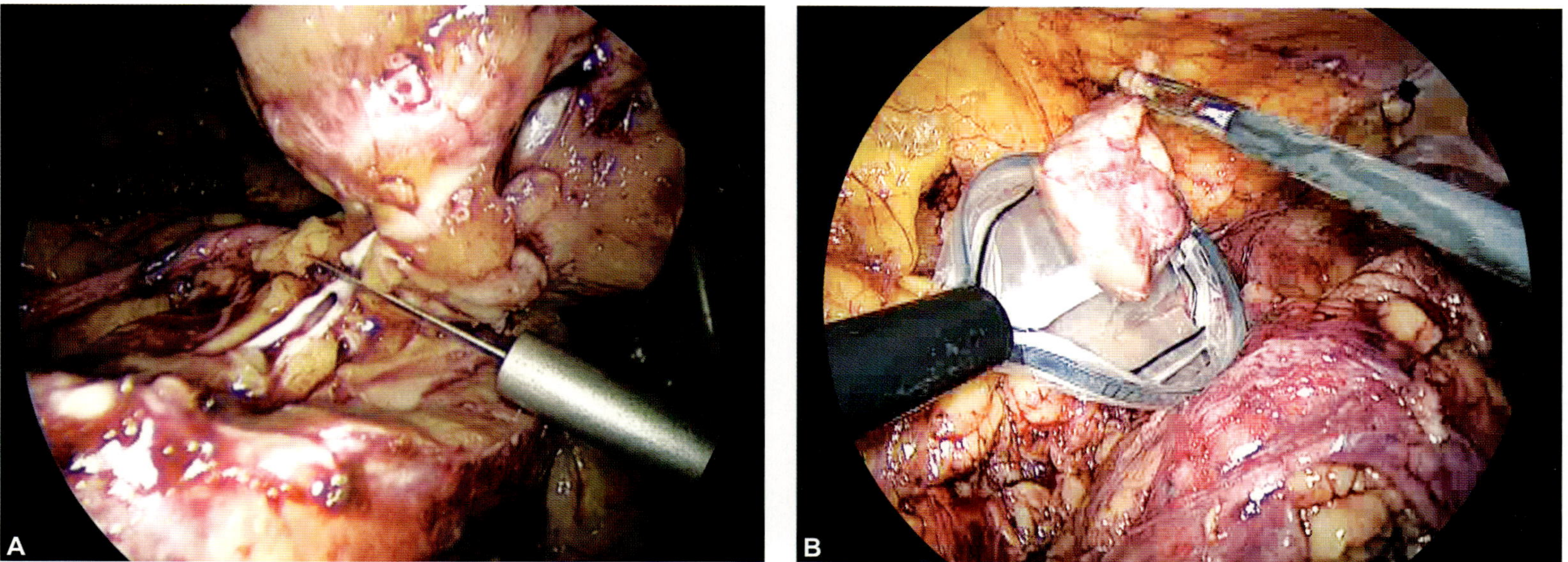

Figs 12A and B: (A) Collecting system entry and the use of laparoscopic scalpel blade for a clean resection line and (B) Tumor entrapment

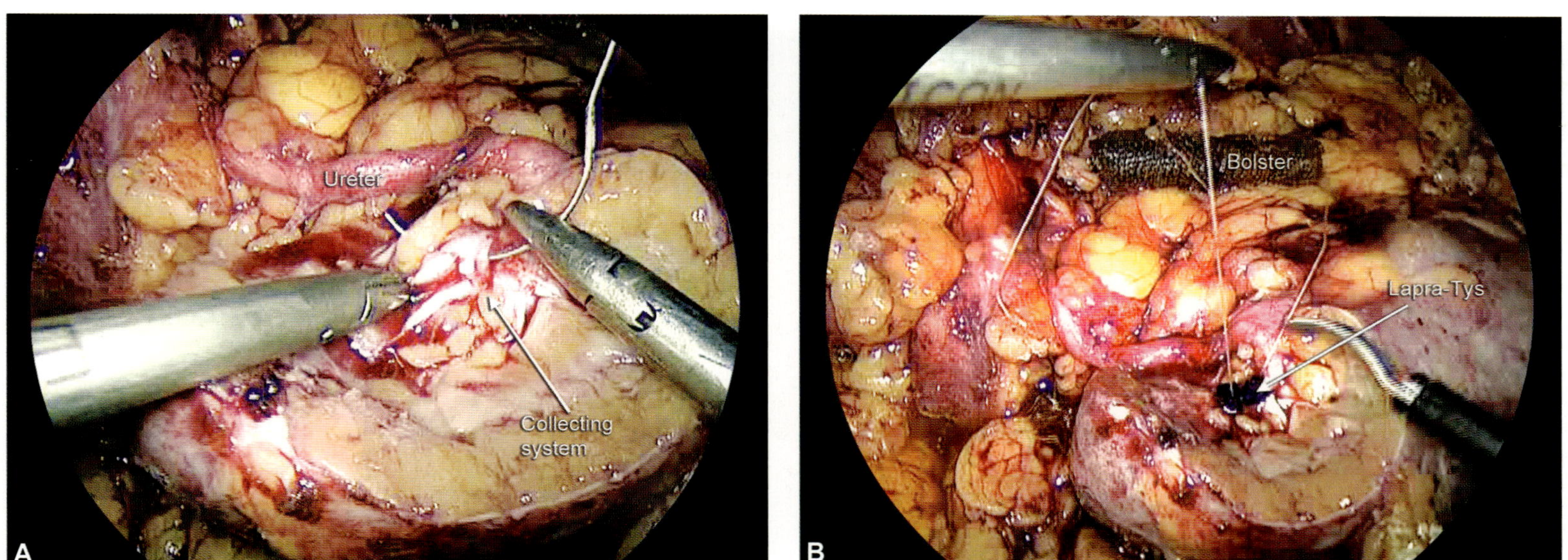

Figs 13A and B: (A) Collecting system closure and (B) Lapra-Tys are used to secure the suture. Note the hemostatic bolster in the background

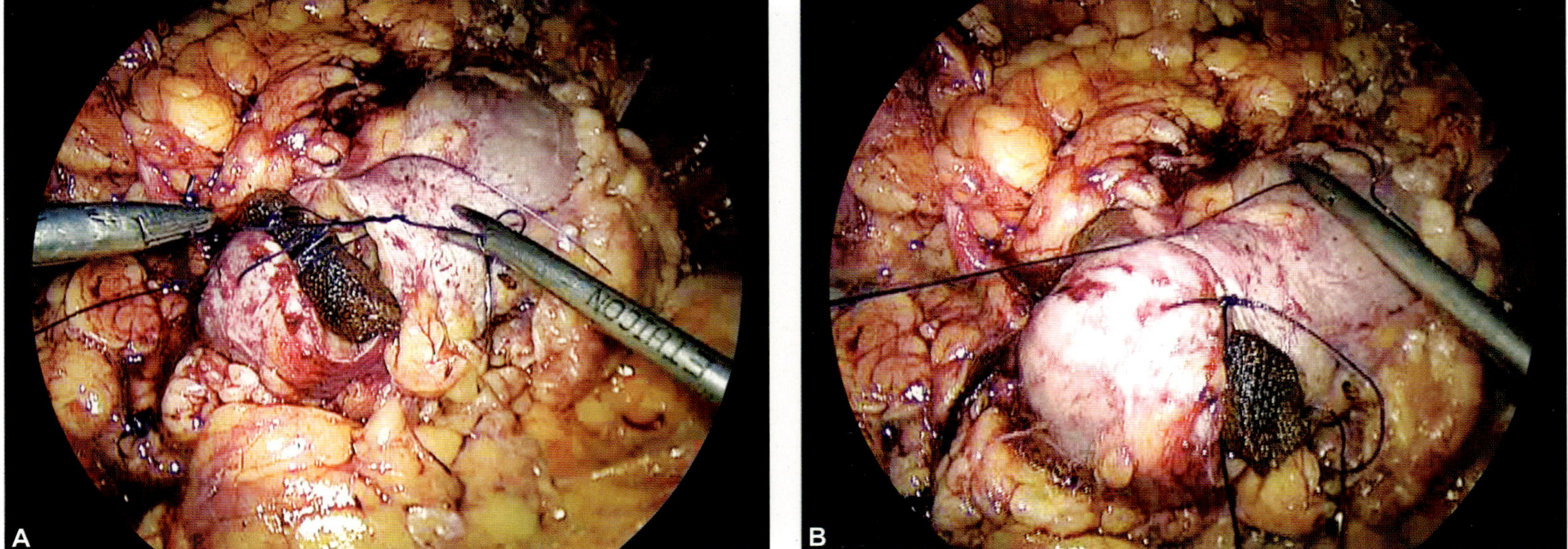

Figs 14A and B: (A) Parenchymal sutures are placed and (B) Excellent parenchymal edge approximation under no tension can be achieved

study advocates a maximum warm ischemia time of 20 minutes.[13] Therefore, every attempt should be made to expedite the operation and keep ischemia times at a minimum.

Postoperative computerized tomography scans, 6 months postoperatively, demonstrate excellent repair and renal function (Fig. 16).

TECHNIQUE OF LEFT-SIDED LAPAROSCOPIC PARTIAL NEPHRECTOMY

The nuances of a left-sided LPN include considerations for the mobilization of the descending colon, the tail of the pancreas and the spleen. The operation for the most part mirrors the right-sided operation as far as renal mobilization and tumor resection and reconstruction.

The images for the index patient demonstrated are shown in Figure 17. A large renal mass is demonstrated in the mid pole of the right kidney encroaching the renal sinus.

The line of Toldt is mobilized and the plane between the kidney and the colon is identified (Figs 18A and B).

The renal hilum is identified and dissected ready for clamping (Figs 19A and B). At this point, 12.5 g of mannitol is administered intravenously. The clear margins of the tumor are defined, by peeling off the Gerota's fat and intraoperative ultrasonography is performed delineating the parenchymal margins and the depth of the tumor. The renal hilum is now clamped and tumor resection is commenced (Figs 20A and B).

The parenchyma is scored with electrocautery and cold scissors are used to resect the tumor. Entry into the collecting system is noted (Fig. 21). The collecting system is closed with a figure of eight

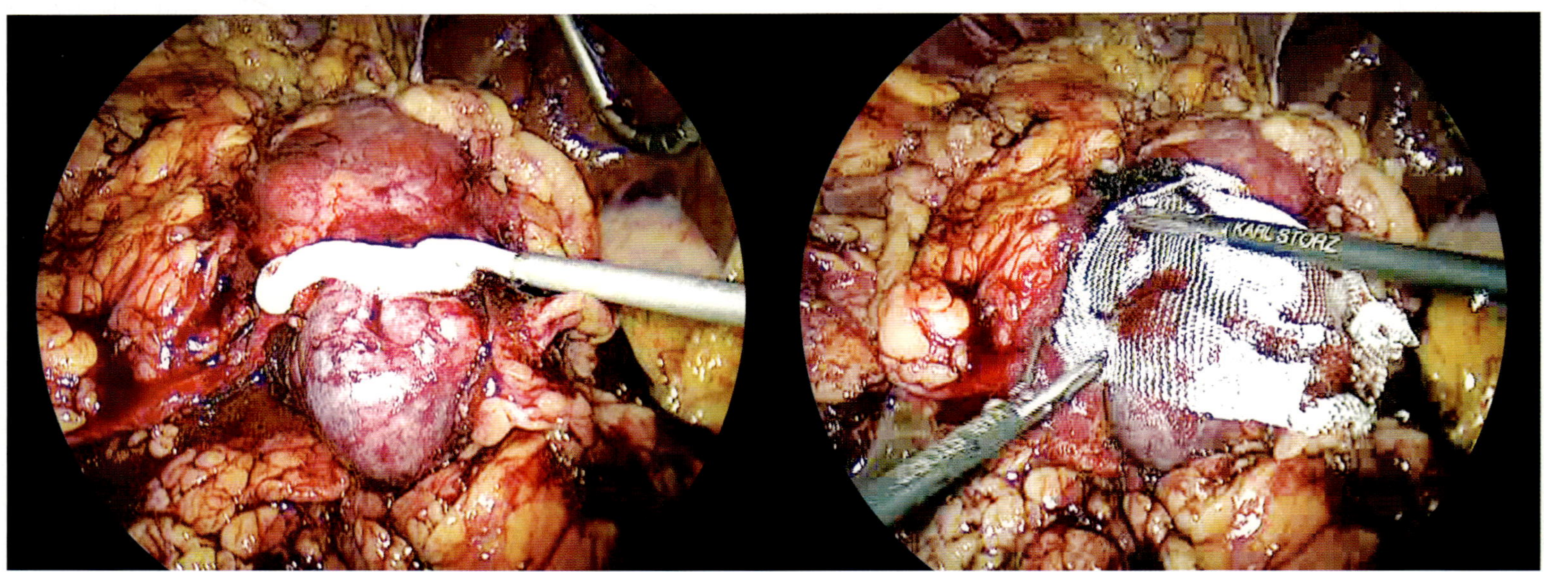

Fig. 15: Completed repair with additional hemostatic agent and Surgicel® blanket

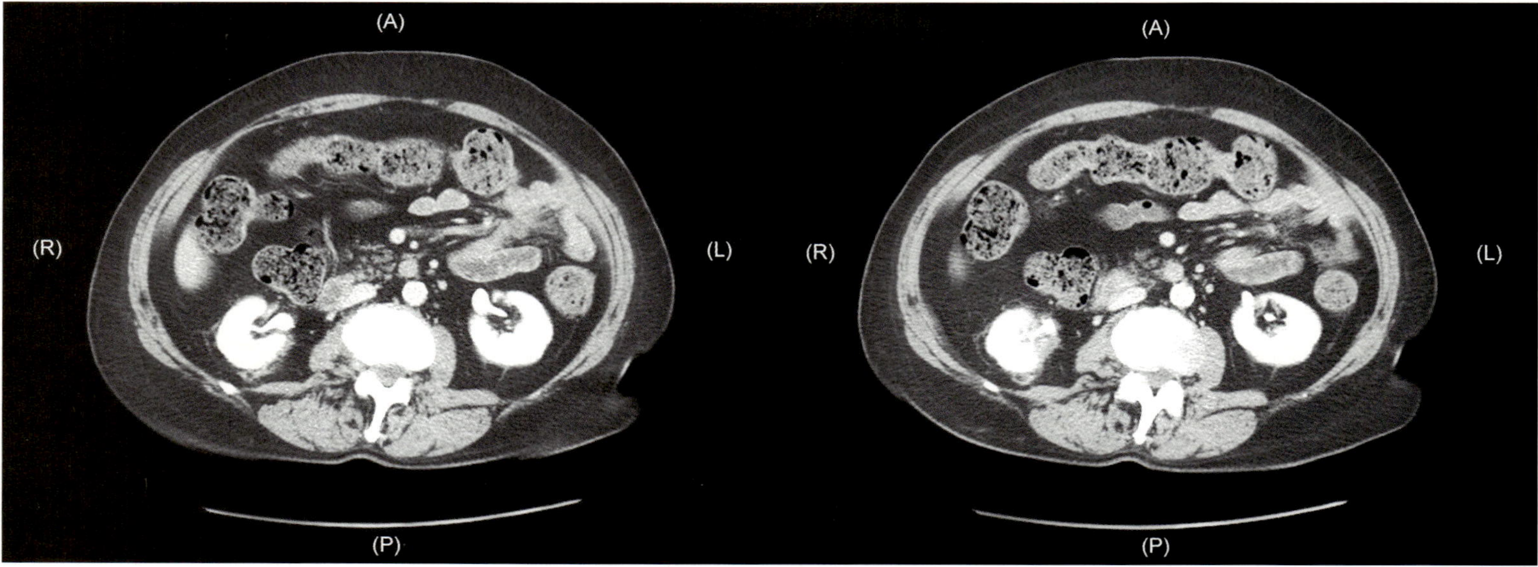

Fig. 16: Six-months postoperative CT scan demonstrate excellent healing and function

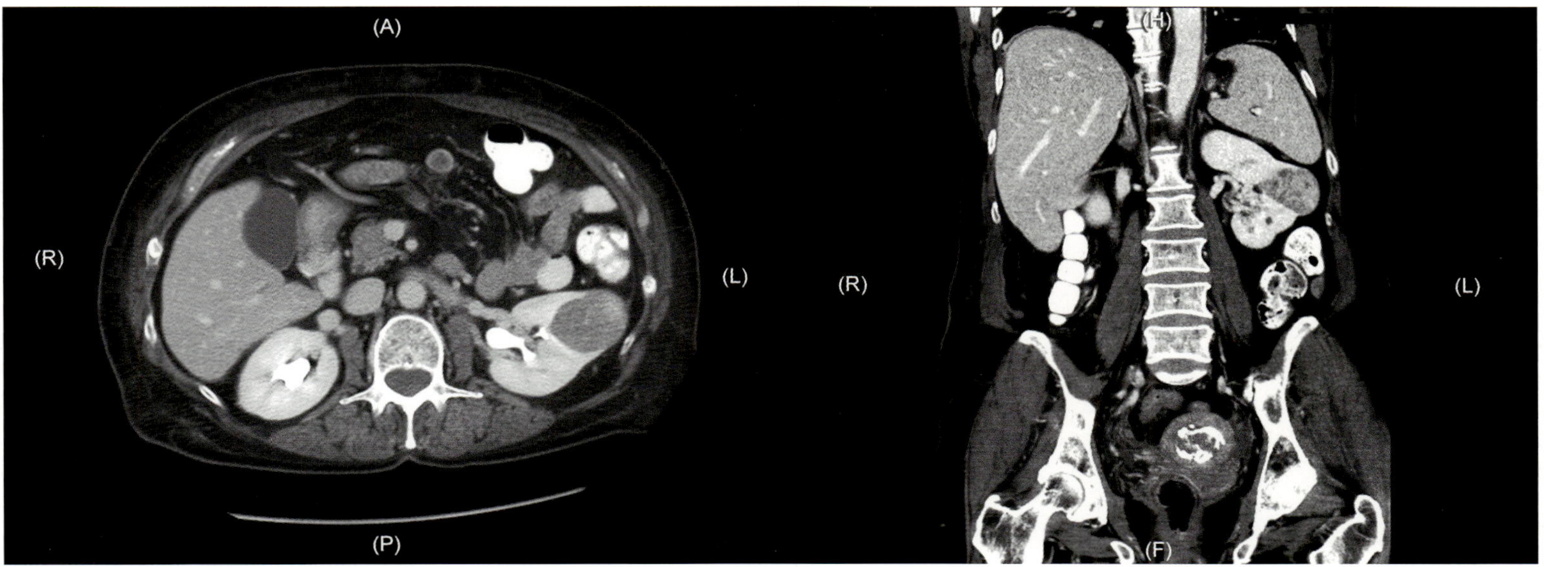

Fig. 17: CT scan demonstrating a 5 cm interpolar solid renal mass

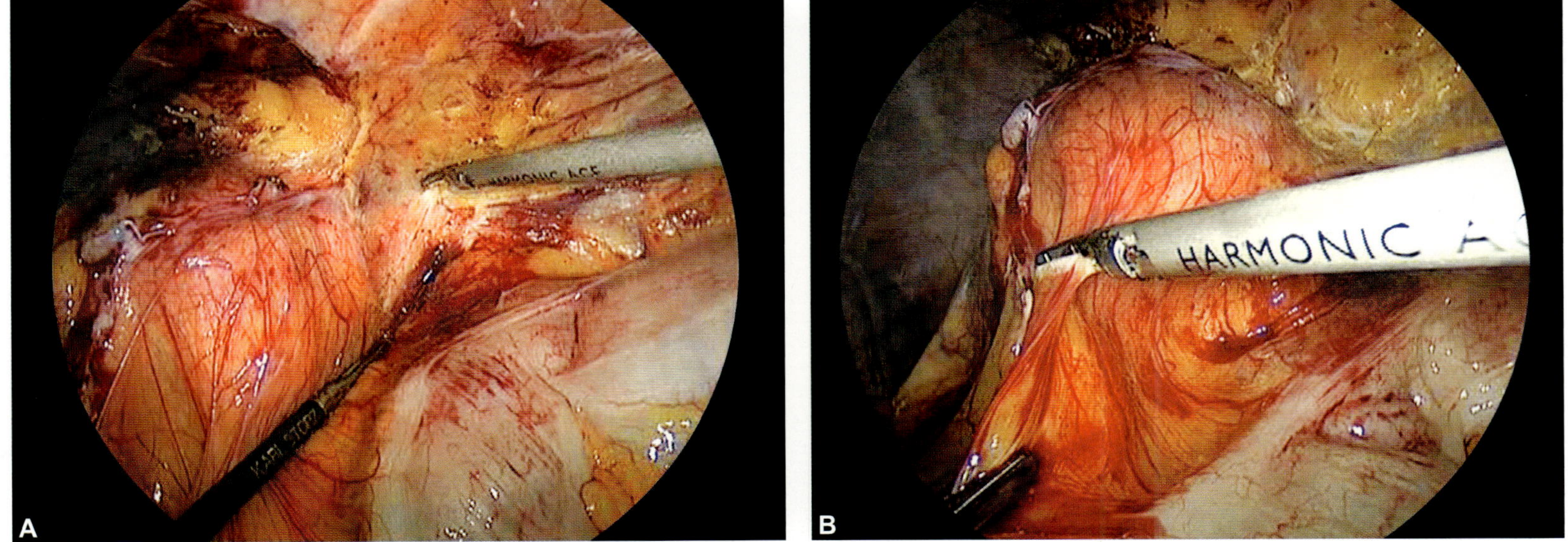

Figs 18A and B: (A) Mobilization of the kidney and (B) Note tumor in background

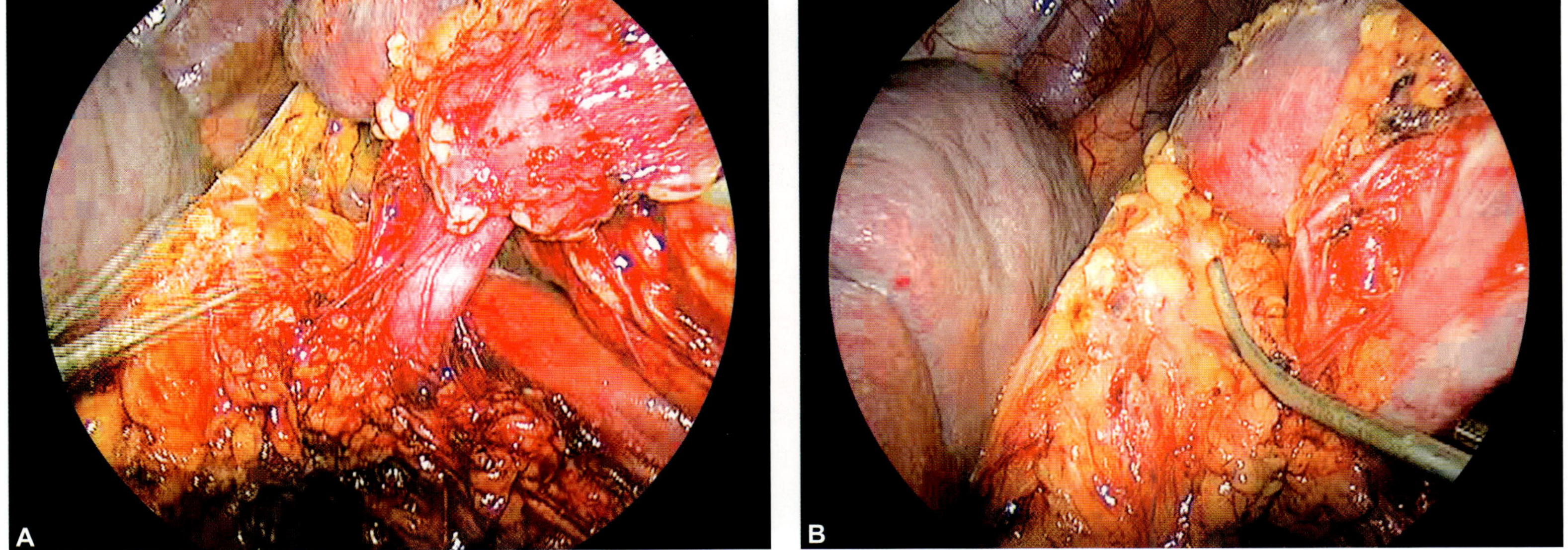

Figs 19A and B: (A) Dissected renal hilum and (B) En bloc hilar clamping

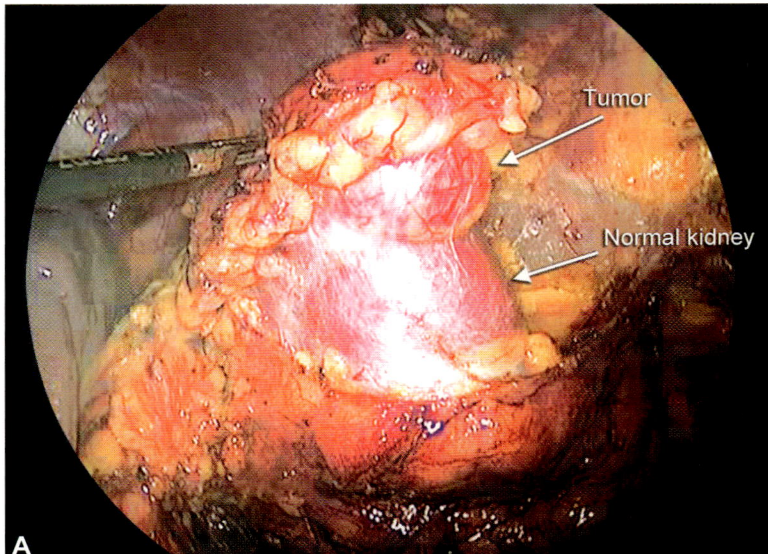

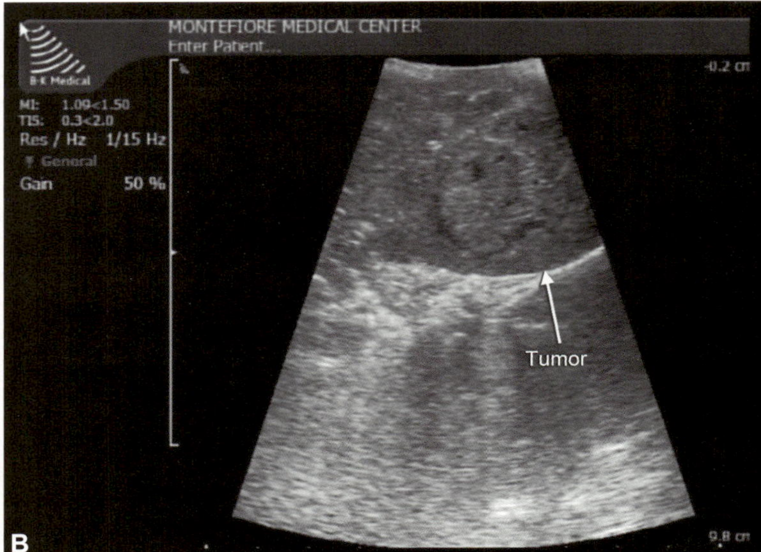

Figs 20A and B: (A) Dissection of tumor and (B) Ultrasonography

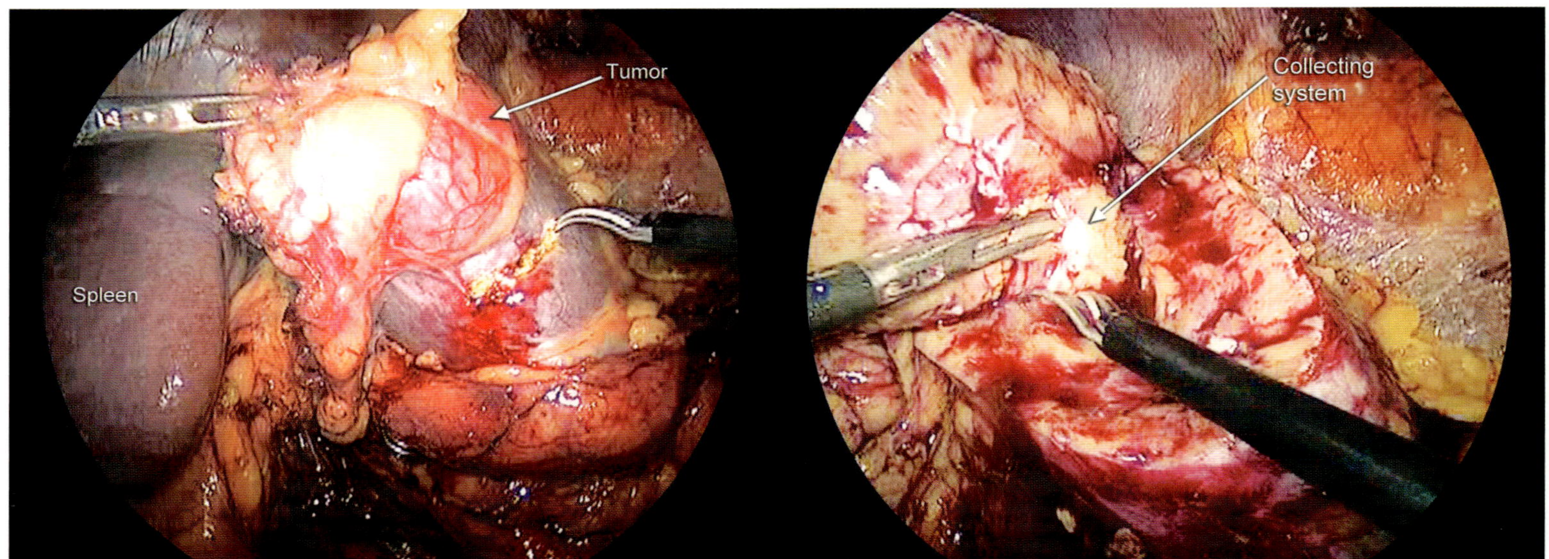

Fig. 21: Tumor resection

3-0 polyglactin suture in this instance. A second suture line is run in the tumor crater with 3-0 polyglactin secured by Lapra-Ty® at each end for hemostasis. The absorbable hemostatic bolster is placed in the tumor crater and Floseal® is applied (Fig. 22).

The parenchymal closure is then performed with 2-0 polyglactin sutures with freehand suturing. Freehand suturing provides excellent approximation of the parenchymal edges for the adept laparoscopic surgeon (Fig. 23).

At this point, the hilar clamps are removed. Another 12.5 g of mannitol and 10 mg of furosemide are administered intravenously. As needed, hemostatic Surgicel® blanket and fibrin glue are applied and a drain is placed laterally (Fig. 24).

At 6 months postoperatively cross-sectional imaging reveal excellent healing and function of the renal remnant (Fig. 25).

LAPAROSCOPIC PARTIAL NEPHRECTOMY FOR LARGE TUMORS

Large polar and interpolar tumors can be approached laparoscopically utilizing the same techniques as in open PN. The techniques for laparoscopic mobilization, preparation, resection and repair are the same as outlined (Figs 26A and B).

In these large tumor resections, often large segmental vessels can be identified and separately controlled with Hem-o-lok® clips during the resection (Fig. 27). In cases where deep entry into renal sinus and multiple entries into the collecting system are contemplated, retrograde infusion of diluted indigo-carmine or methylene blue through a previously cystoscopically placed ureteral catheter allows for accurate identification and closure of all points of collecting

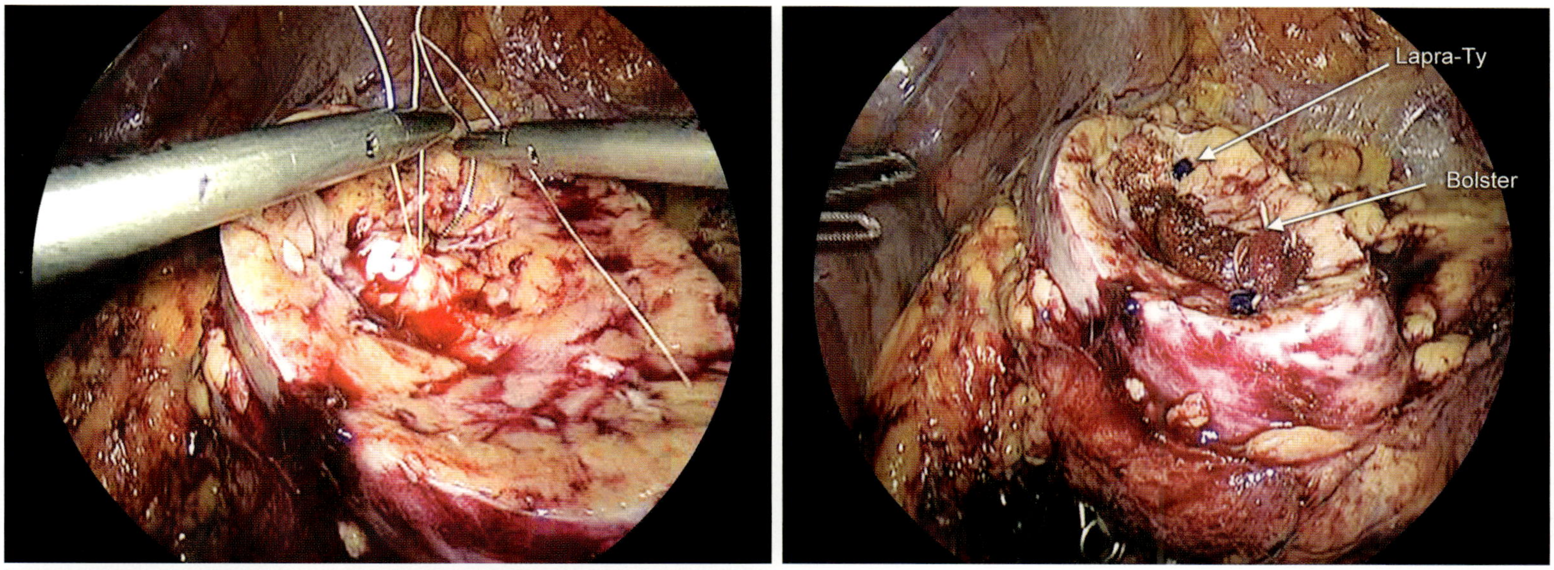

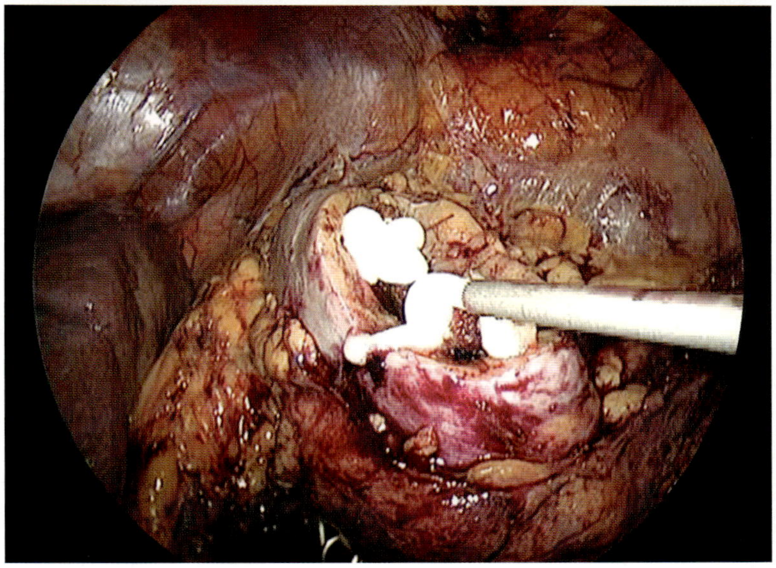

Fig. 22: Closure of collecting system and preparation of the tumor crater

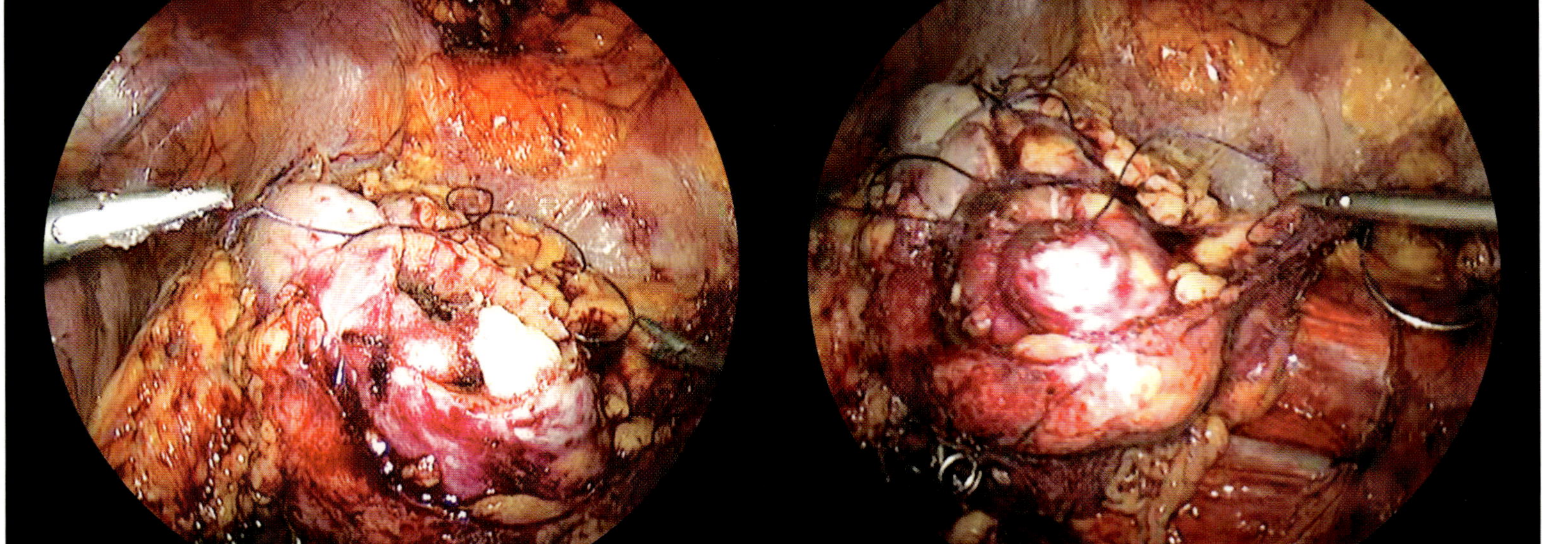

Fig. 23: Parenchymal closure

system entry in the large resection crater (Fig. 28). The collecting system is then closed over a bolster in the manner described above resulting in a functioning and substantial renal remnant (Fig. 29).

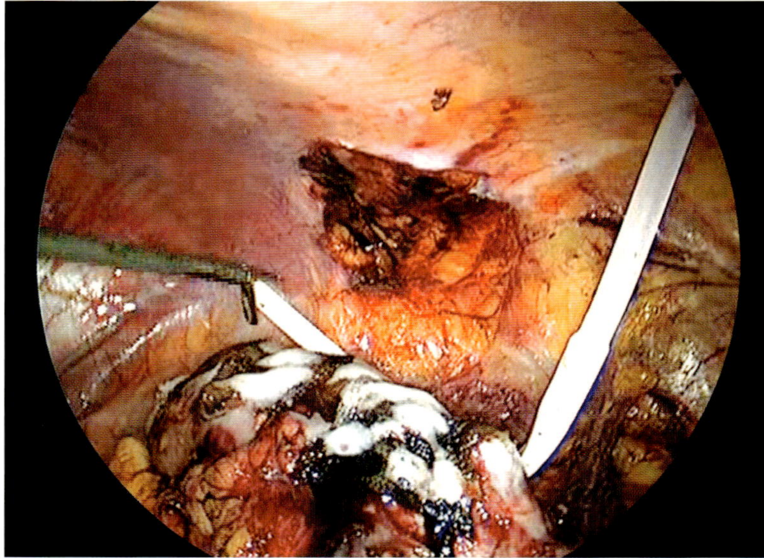

Fig. 24: Final repair with drain placement

Large polar resections can also be accomplished utilizing the technique of guillotine heminephrectomy (Figs 30A and B). The upper pole of the kidney is resected straight across and multiple collecting system entries are repaired. The renal parenchymal edges are approximated in the standard fashion described above (Fig. 31).

Occasionally with large polar tumors close to the hilum, individual segmental vessels can be identified on preoperative imaging and can be ligated intraoperatively prior to parenchymal resection (Figs 32 and 33A and B). In these tumors that encroach the hilum care is taken to fully dissect the ureter and always keep it in site to decrease the risk of ureteral injury or transection.

SLIDING CLIP RENORRHAPHY

In order to facilitate renal parenchymal closure and in an effort to decrease warm ischemia time, the technique of sliding clip renorrhaphy could be employed.[14] With this maneuver, a 2-0 polyglactin suture is used with a Hem-o-lok® and Lapra-Ty® at the end. After passage through the defect, the suture is further anchored again with Hem-o-lok® and Lapra-Ty® as it is tightened (Fig. 34).

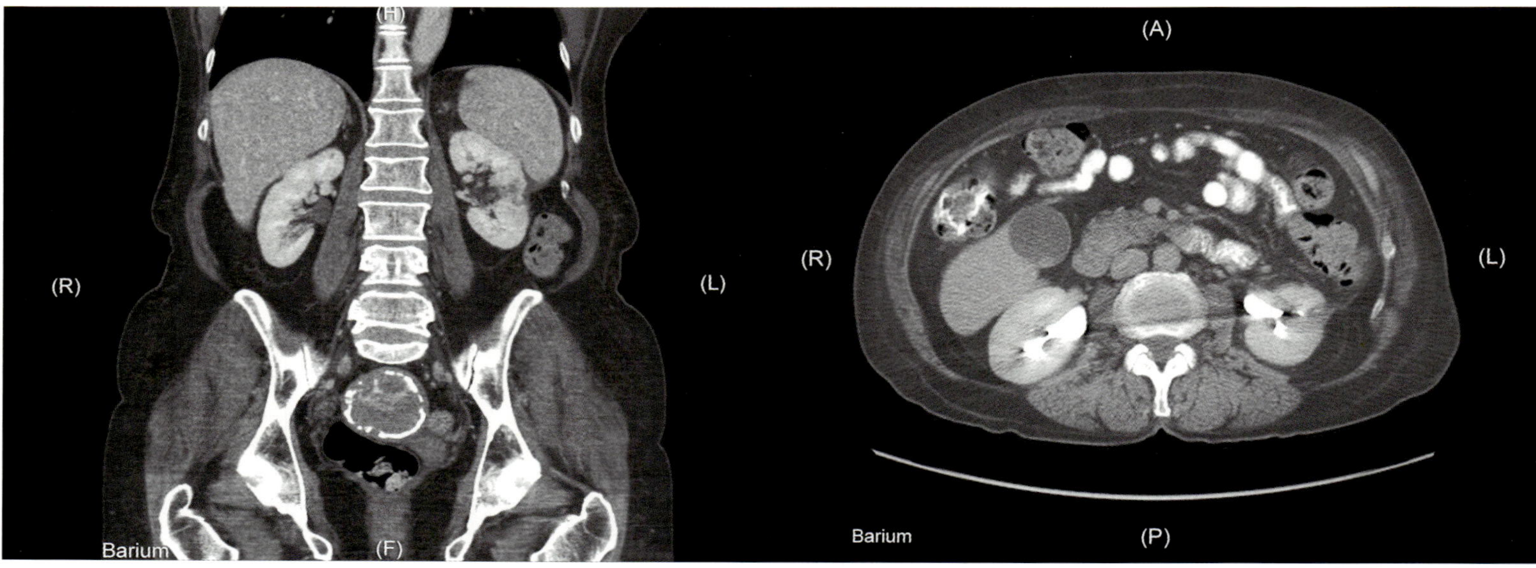

Fig. 25: CT scan at 6 months postoperative visit

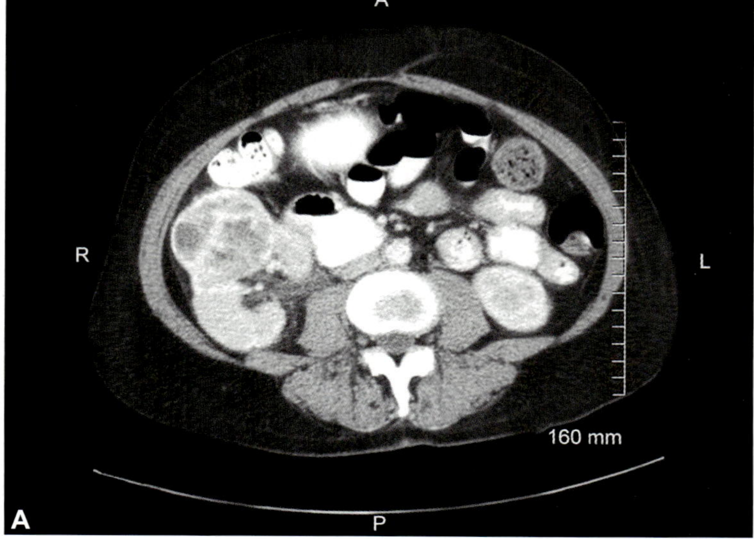

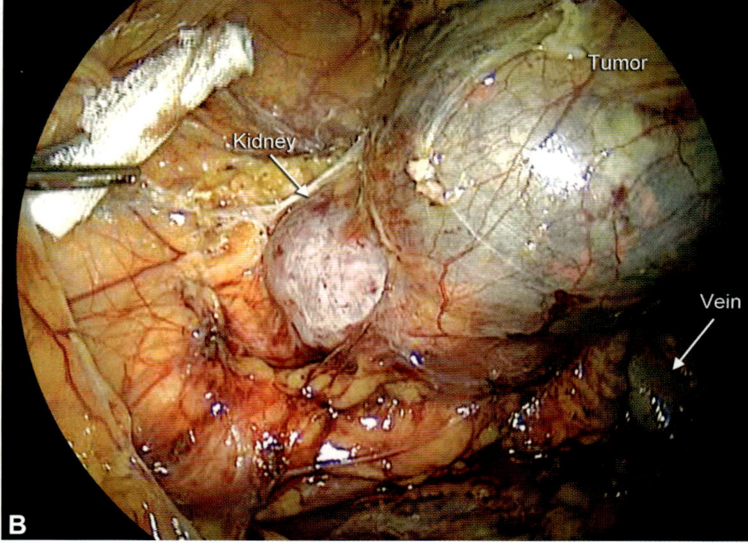

Figs 26A and B: (A) CT scan demonstrating a large (7 cm) interpolar tumor and (B) Intraoperative view

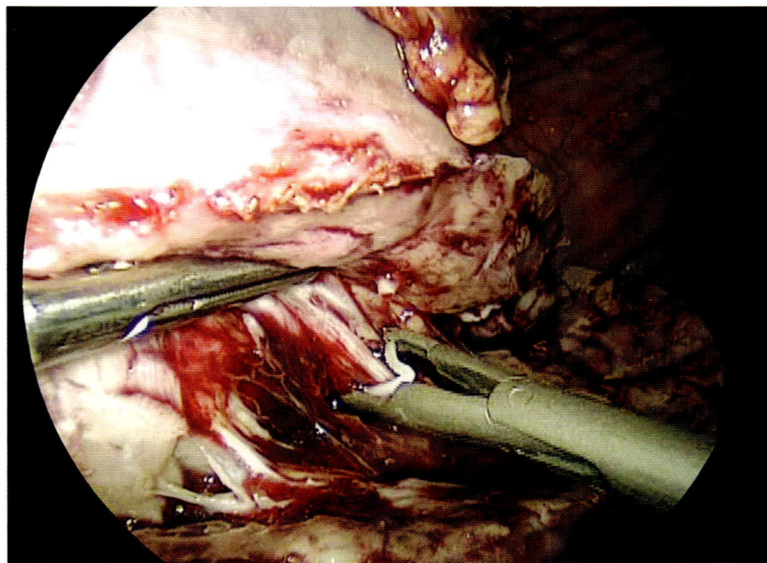

Fig. 27: Control of segmental arterial branches

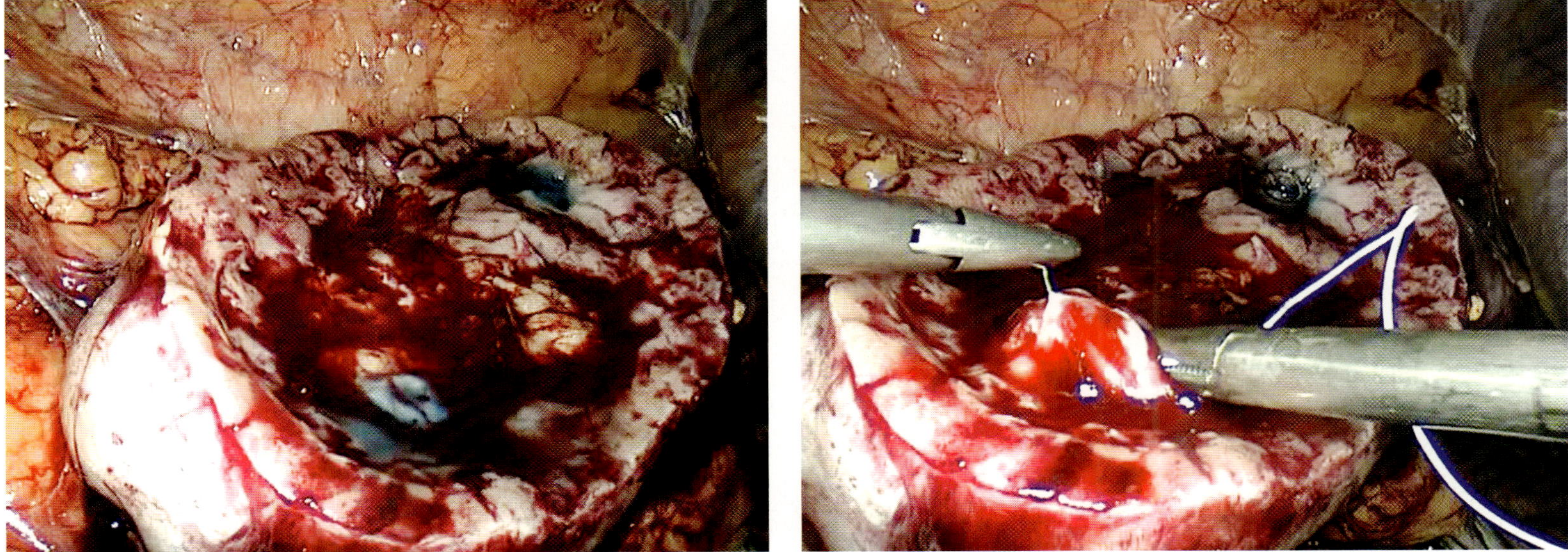

Fig. 28: Retrograde infusion of diluted indigo-carmine solution and collecting system closure

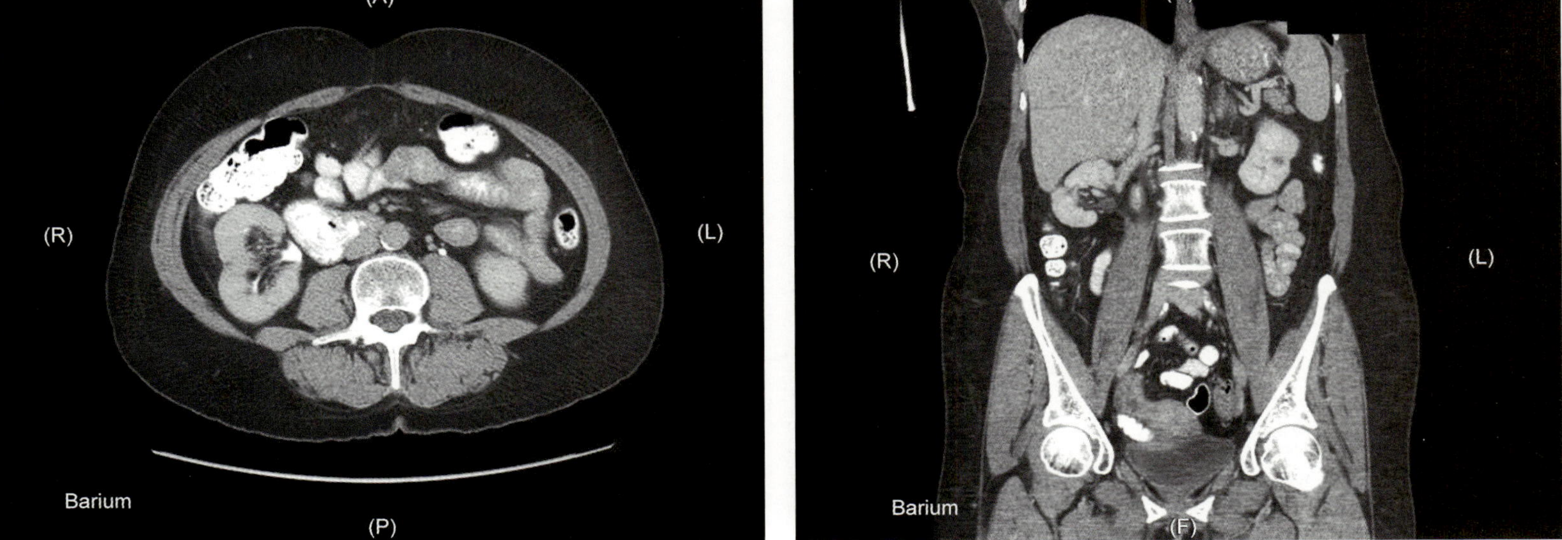

Fig. 29: Postoperative image 6 months after partial nephrectomy

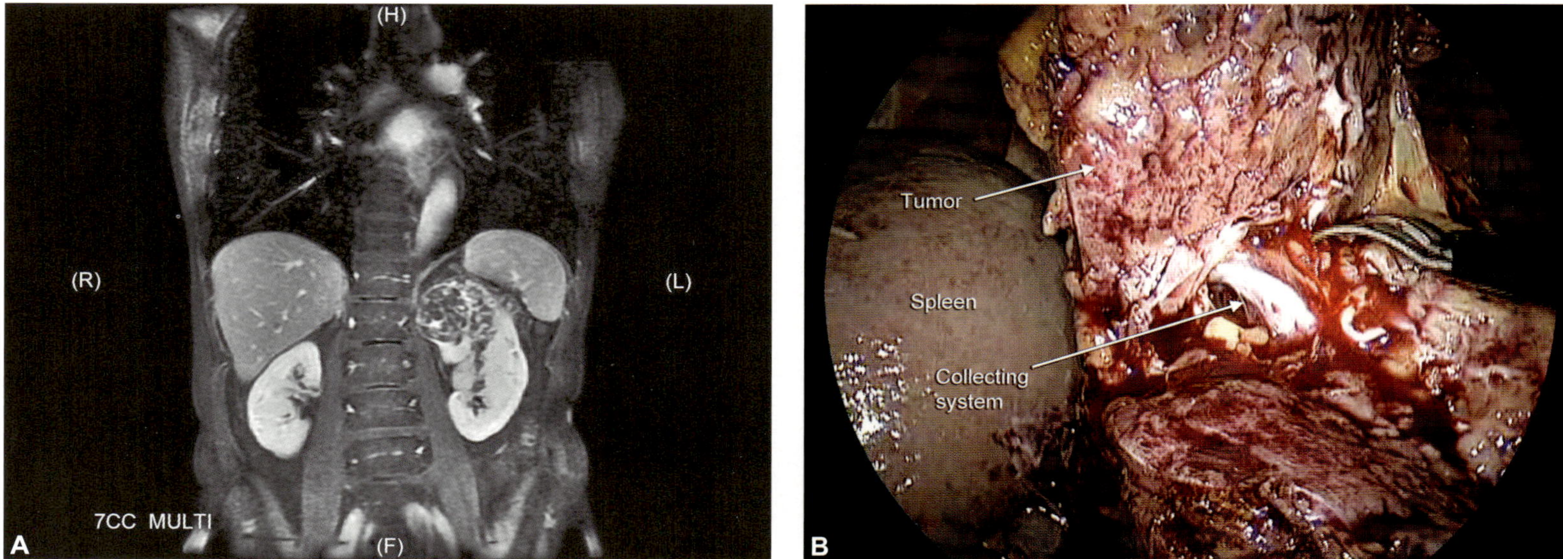

Figs 30A and B: (A) Large upper pole tumor and (B) Upper pole tumor resection

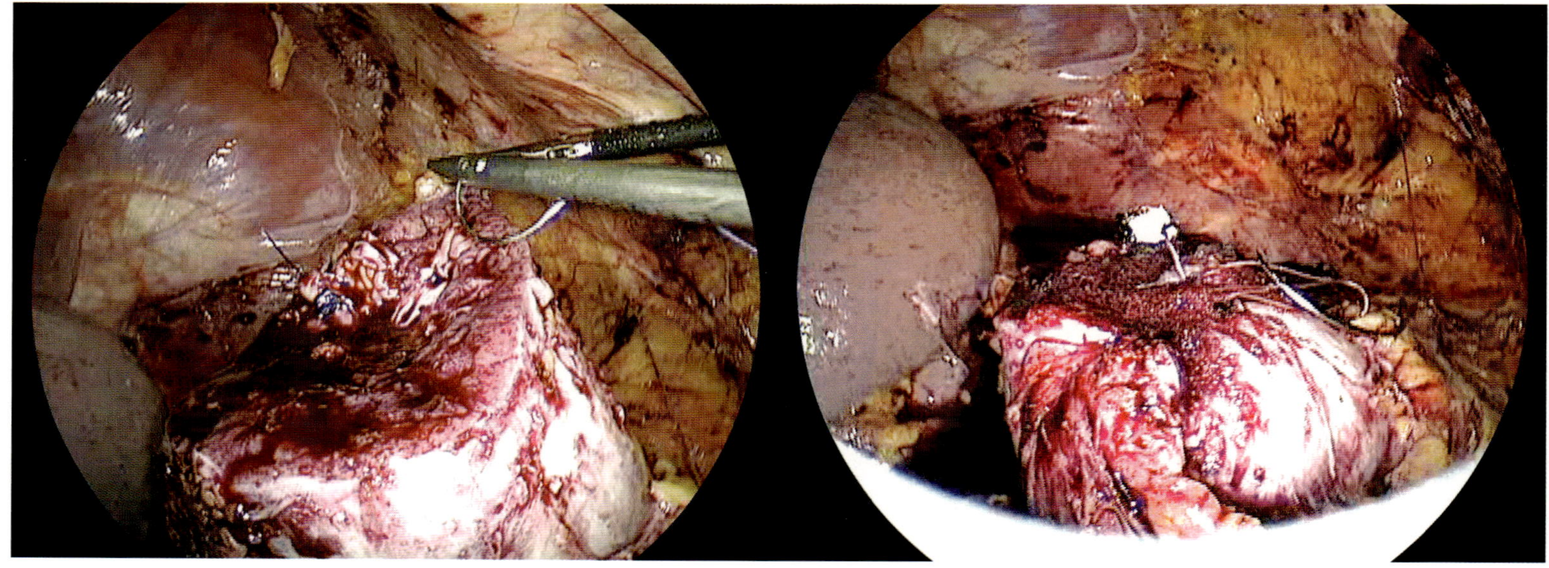

Fig. 31: Large tumor crater and resulting closure of the defect

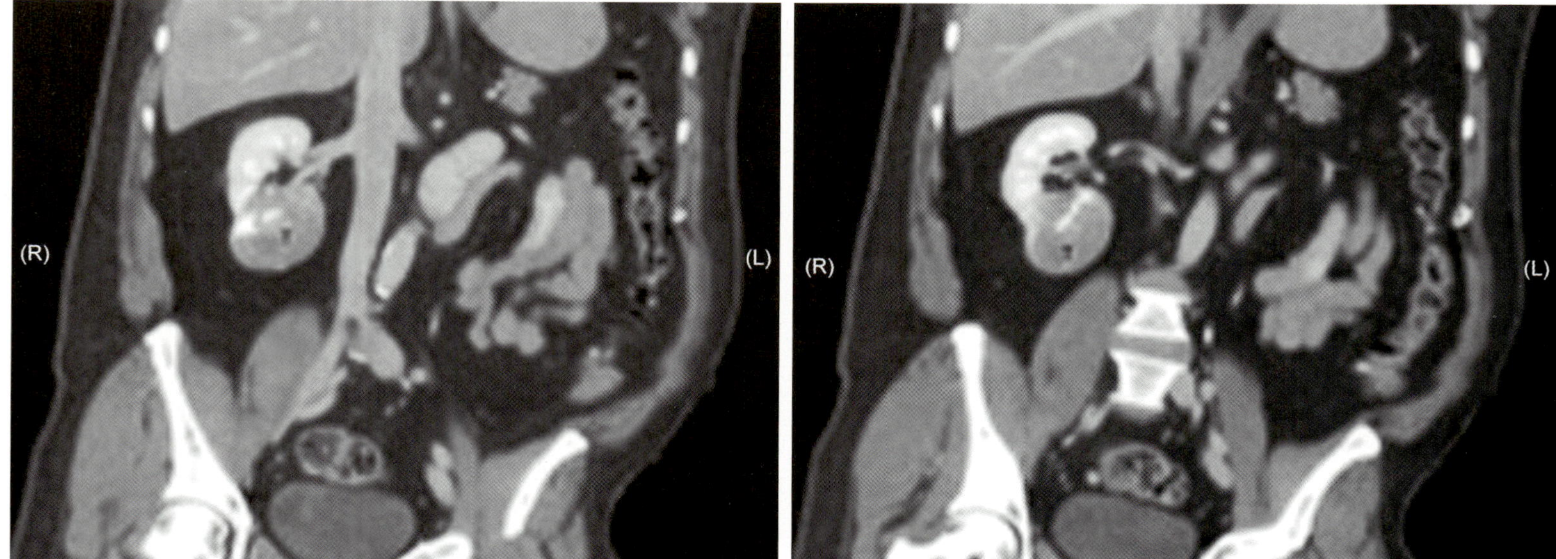

Fig. 32: CT scan of large lower pole, hilar tumor with feeding venous and arterial vessels (Abbreviation: T—tumor)

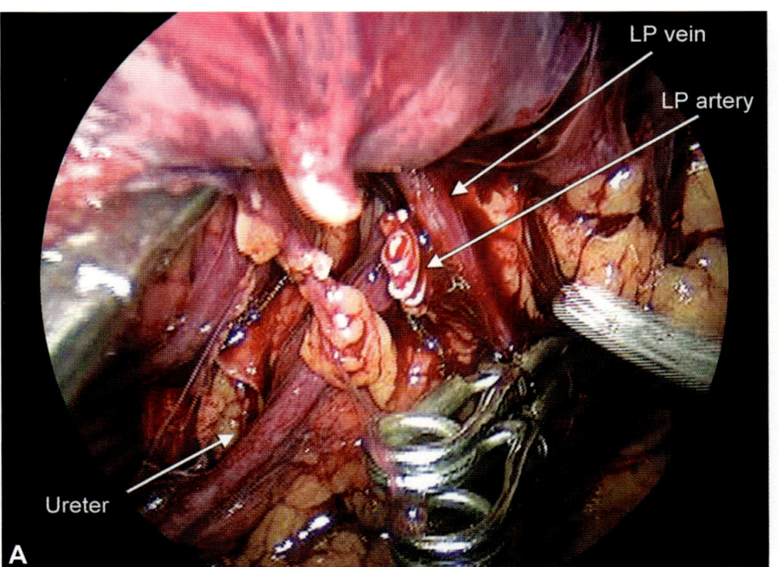

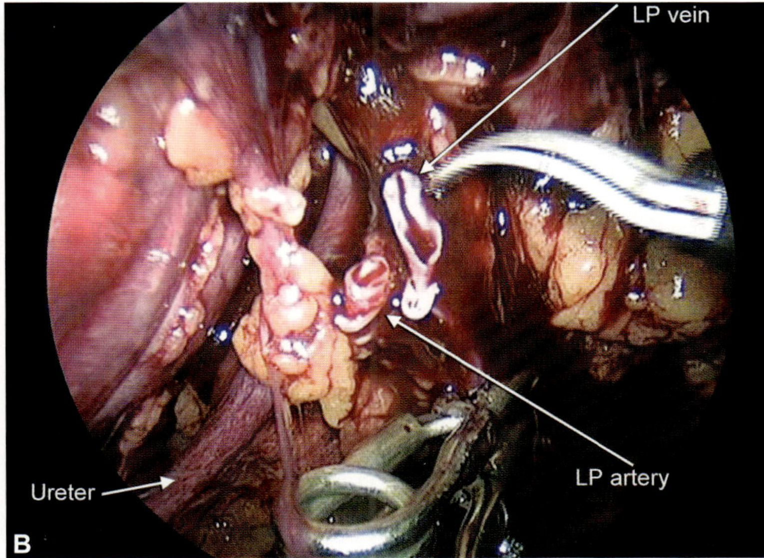

Figs 33A and B: (A and B) Renal hilar clamp is applied and lower pole (LP) artery and vein are isolated and divided. Note ureter in the background

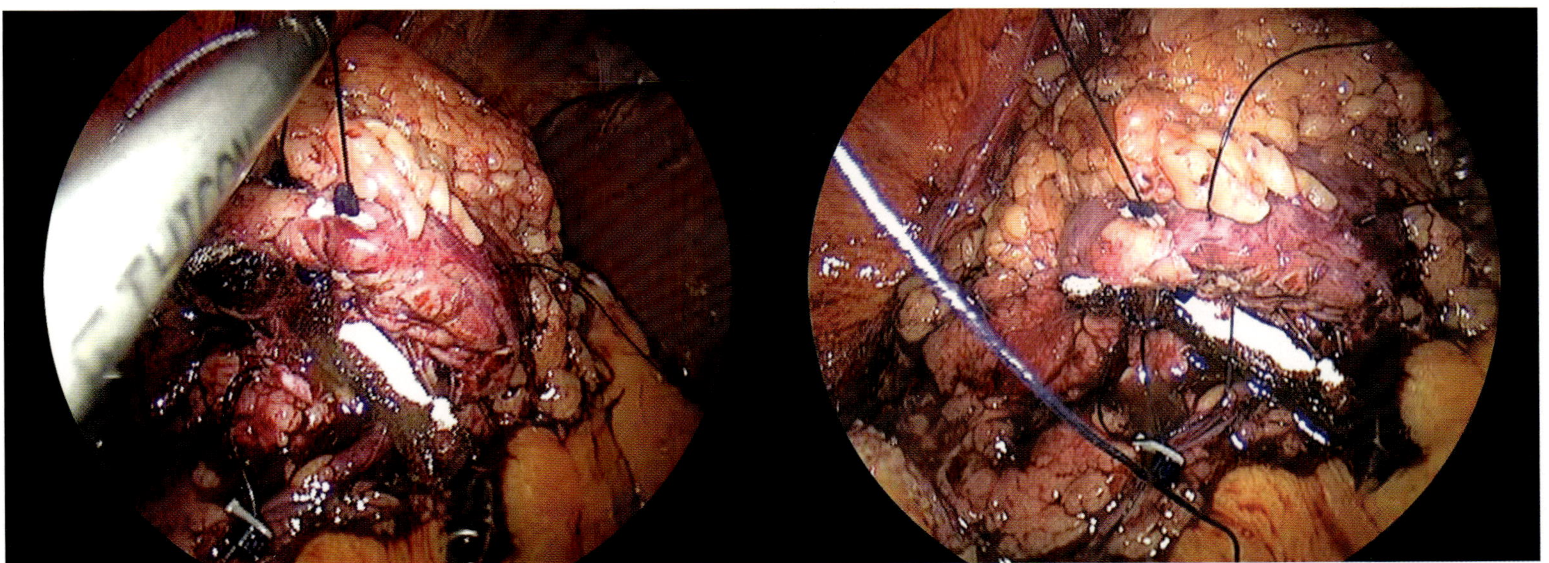

Fig. 34: Sliding clip renorrhaphy for closure of a right lower pole heminephrectomy

REFERENCES

1. Huang WC, Levey AS, Serio AM, et al. Chronic kidney disease after nephrectomy in patients with renal cortical tumours: a retrospective cohort study. Lancet Oncol. 2006;7:735-40.
2. Weight CJ, Larson BT, Fergany AF, et al. Nephrectomy induced chronic renal insufficiency is associated with increased risk of cardiovascular death and death from any cause in patients with localized cT1b renal masses. J Urol. 2010;183:1317-23.
3. Campbell SC, Novick AC, Belldegrun A, et al. Guideline for management of the clinical T1 renal mass. J Urol. 2009;182:1271-9.
4. Leibovich BC, Blute ML, Cheville JC, et al. Nephron sparing surgery for appropriately selected renal cell carcinoma between 4 and 7 cm results in outcome similar to radical nephrectomy. J Urol. 2004;171:1066-70.
5. Lane BR, Novick AC, Babineau D, et al. Comparison of laparoscopic and open partial nephrectomy for tumor in a solitary kidney. J Urol. 2008;179:847-52.
6. Eisenberg MS, Brandina R, Gill IS. Current status of laparoscopic partial nephrectomy. Curr Opin Urol. 2010;20:365-70.
7. Nadu A, Kleinmann N, Laufer M, et al. Laparoscopic partial nephrectomy for central tumors: analysis of perioperative outcomes and complications. J Urol. 2009;181:42-7.
8. Richstone L, Montag S, Ost M, et al. Laparoscopic partial nephrectomy for hilar tumors: evaluation of short-term oncologic outcome. Urology. 2008;71:36-40.
9. Gill IS, Kamoi K, Aron M, et al. 800 laparoscopic partial nephrectomies: a single surgeon series. J Urol. 2010;183:34-42.
10. Finelli A, Gill IS, Desai MM, et al. Laparoscopic heminephrectomy for tumor. Urology. 2005;65(3):473-8.
11. Simmons MN, Weight CJ, Gill IS. Laparoscopic radical versus partial nephrectomy for tumors > 4 cm: intermediate-term oncologic and functional outcomes. Urology. 2009;73:1077-82.
12. Simmons MN, Schreiber MJ, Gill IS. Surgical renal ischemia: a contemporary overview. J Urol. 2008;180(1):19-30.
13. Becker F, Van Poppel H, Hakenberg OW, et al. Assessing the impact of ischaemia time during partial nephrectomy. Eur Urol. 2009;56:625-34.
14. Benway BM, Cabello JM, Figenshau RS, et al. Sliding-clip renorrhaphy provides superior closing tension during robot-assisted partial nephrectomy. J Endourol. 2010;24(4):605-8.

8

Chapter

Robotic Partial Nephrectomy

Aron Bruhn, Michael Stifelman

INTRODUCTION

The incidental detection of renal tumors has increased over the past decades—significantly contributing to a downward size and stage migration of renal masses.[1,2] Nephron sparing partial nephrectomy is rapidly becoming the treatment of choice for renal masses less than 4 cm and up to 7 cm as it offers decreased risk of chronic renal insufficiency with equivalent oncologic outcomes.[3] Advances in robotics and minimally invasive techniques allow the surgeon to perform a partial nephrectomy on more complex renal masses as well as allowing for shorter warm ischemia and therefore potentially less impact on renal function. Furthermore, robotics may allow the surgeon to perform a partial nephrectomy through a minimally invasive approach, in what would have otherwise required an open procedure. Urologists already familiar with robotic surgery by from their experience with robotic prostatectomy will have a strong robotic skill set that can be easily applied to robotic partial nephrectomy, even with minimal experience in laparoscopic partial nephrectomy. A strong knowledge of anatomy, as well as the ability to follow the steps outlined in this chapter on how to best utilize the robot and define the anatomy will add greatly to the proficiency of the surgeon. The equipment used in the surgery is mentioned in Table 1.

PROCEDURAL STEPS

The steps of the surgery are (Figs 1 to 39):

In our institution, the camera port is placed via the Hassan technique halfway between the umbilicus and the sternum. The Nathanson retractor is used to elevate the liver prior to placement of the right robotic arm port. This allows for the most cephalad placement of the superior port without collision with the liver.

Table 1: Selection of preferred equipment
Robotic needle drivers
Maryland grasper
Bowel grasper
Endoshears
Doppler probe
Laparoscopic Ultrasound probe
V-loc™ sutures
Bull dog clamps

Fig. 1: A proper setup will allow for access to the whole operative field and avoid external collisions. The left and right arm ports, as well as the camera port are placed as high as possible to void external collision with the fourth arm, which is placed in the lower quadrant

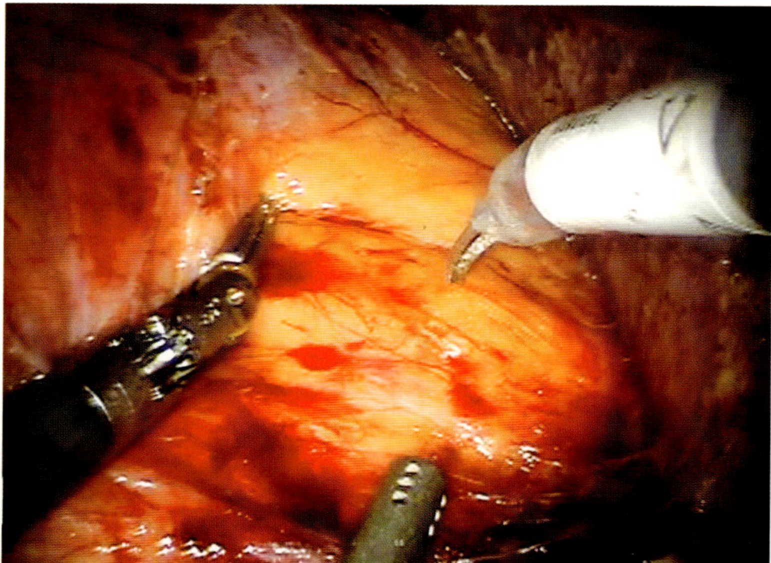

Fig. 2: Reflect the liver and put it on stretch. Once the adrenal gland can be visualized (under the scissors), the most cephalad portion of the dissection has been achieved. This becomes important during the dissection of the renal hilum in order to be able to achieve full control of the hilum if necessary

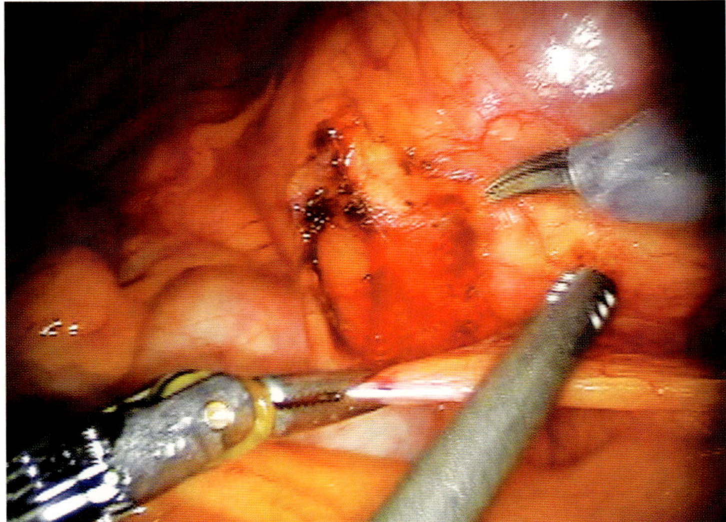

Fig. 3: The dissection begins on the lower medial pole just lateral to the colon. Incise the peritoneum and identify the anterior layer of Gerota's fascia. Develop the avascular plain between the peritoneum and Gerota's fascia and carry this dissection out like a hockey stick below the lower pole and to the sidewall. This will begin reflecting the colon medially

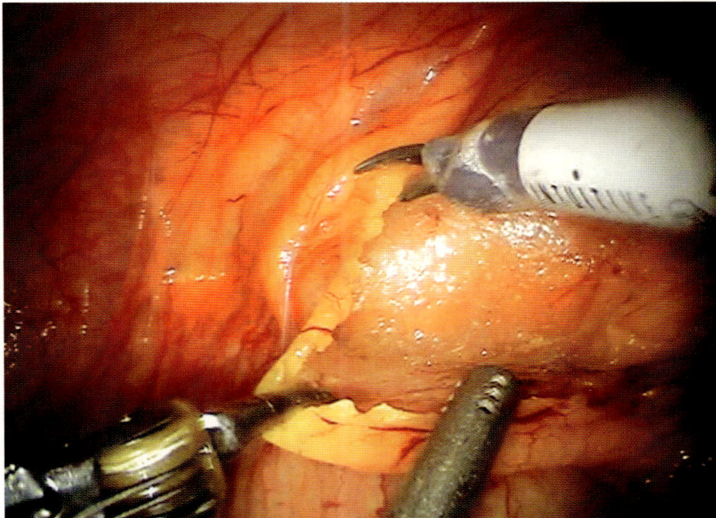

Fig. 4: Continue dropping the colon off the sidewall, allowing the pneumoperitoneum to guide the dissection while using good stretch with your left hand

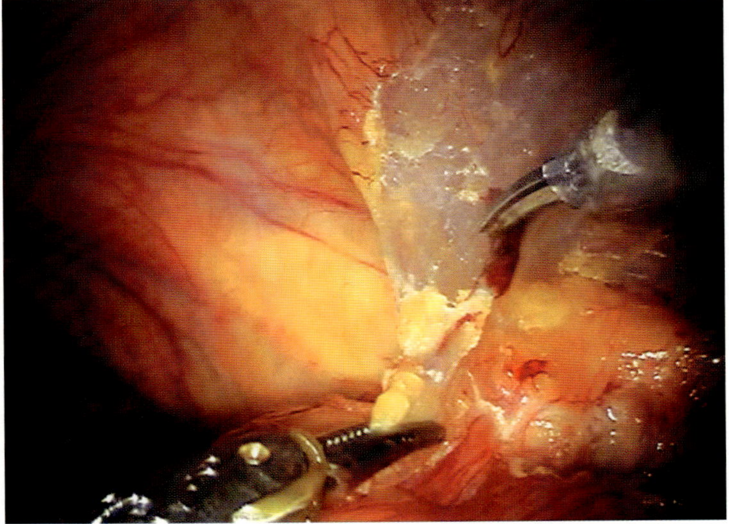

Fig. 5: Continue to release the colon all the way down to the iliac vessels to allow for maximal exposure

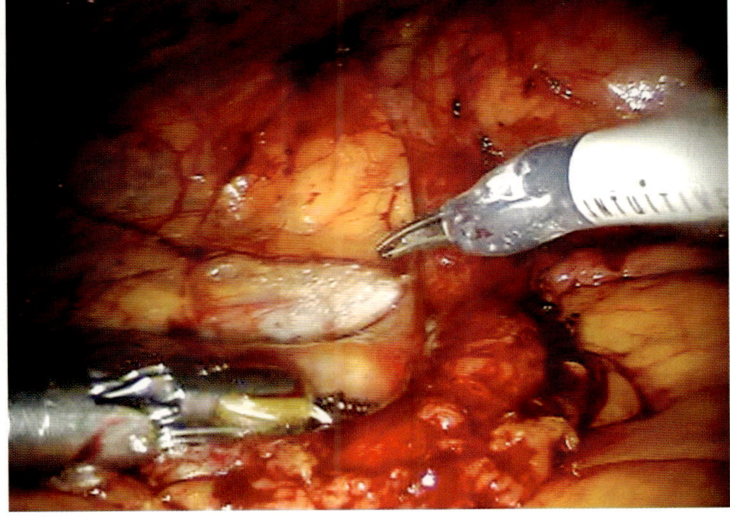

Fig. 6: Continue reflecting the colon until the vena cava is exposed inferior to lower pole

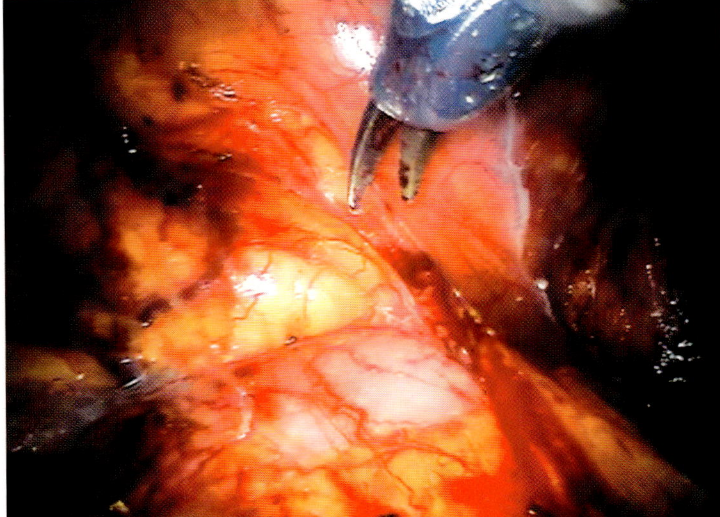

Fig. 7: Continue the dissection superiorly. The duodenum will often be encountered medial to the kidney. Kocherize the duodenum so that the vena cava at the level of the kidney can continue to be skeletonized anteriorly. Avoid using any cautery near the duodenum

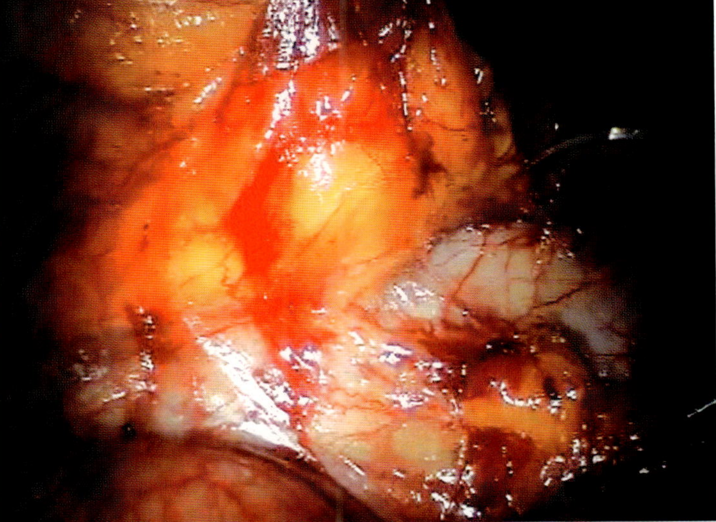

Fig. 8: Continue to take down the duodenum until the vena cava is exposed from the level of the adrenal vein to the lower pole of kidney to maximize exposure

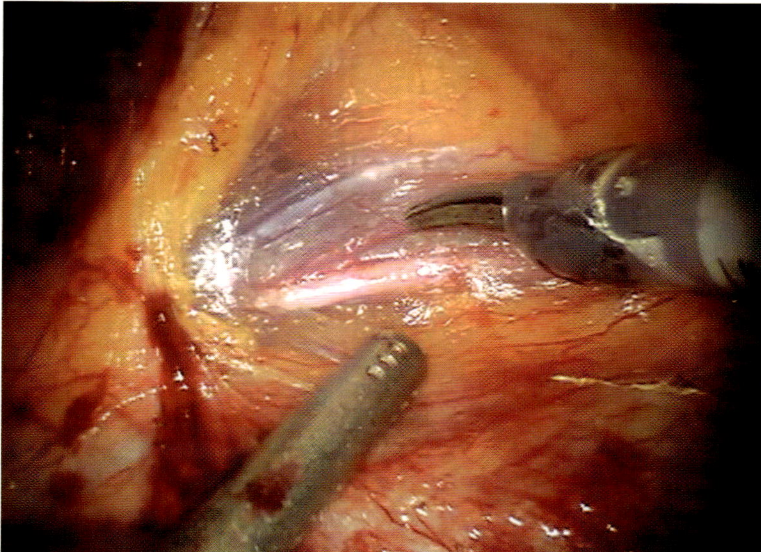

Fig. 9: Once the vena cava is exposed, the gonadal vein and the ureter can be identified inferior to kidney. Incidentally, this view is the same for both the right and left kidney

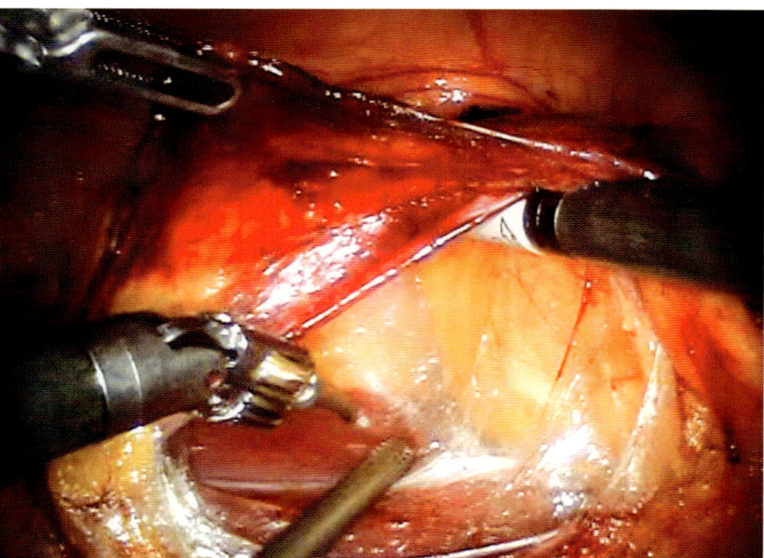

Fig. 10: Medialize the gonadal vein and elevate the ureter and lift the kidney off of the psoas. This creates a triangle with anterior side ureter, posterior side gonadal and superior side lower pole kidney

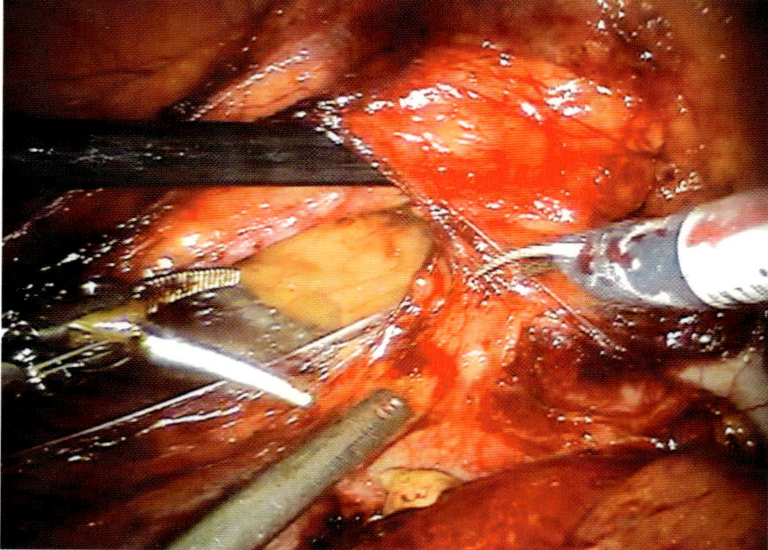

Fig. 11: Only now should the fourth arm be brought into the field. The fourth arm is used to elevate the kidney by placing it under the ureter after bluntly dissecting the posterior aspect of the kidney off of the psoas fascia. The kidney should be mobilized off the psoas all the way to the superior pole of the kidney. This maneuver will maximize the exposure of the hilum by placing the kidney on stretch. Only once the kidney has been placed on stretch should the renal hilum be dissected

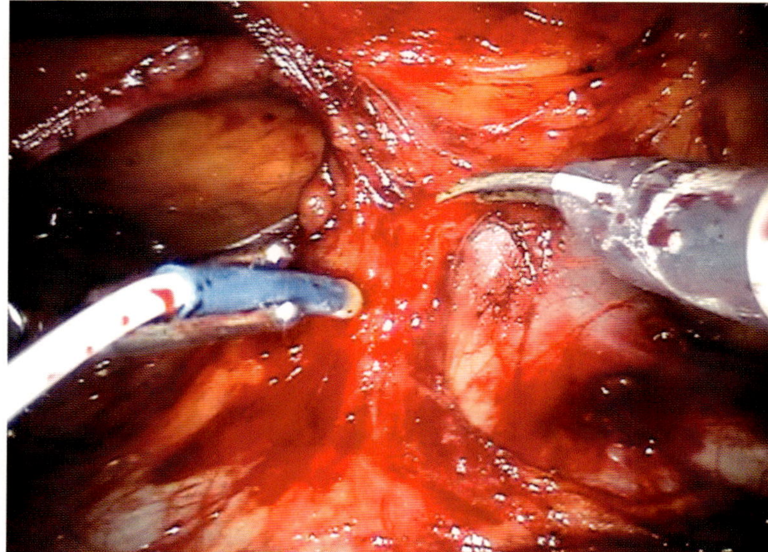

Fig. 12: The fourth arm should then extend posteriorly beyond the hilum to ensure maximal stretch and exposure. At this point, a Doppler probe, which is controlled by the surgeon, can be introduced to efficiently identify major vessels and allow the division of surrounding tissue with no signal, with impunity

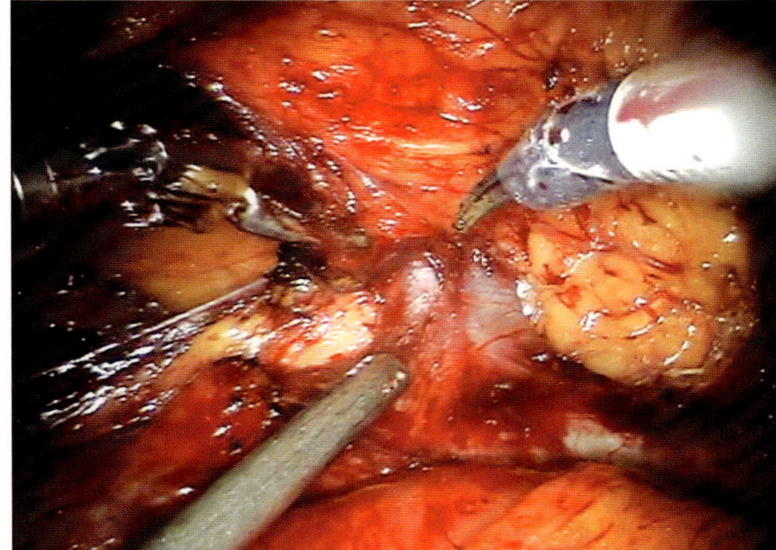

Fig. 13: Prior to dissecting the hilum of the kidney, ensure you have the correct exposure and anatomy by identifying the angle formed on the inferior aspect of the renal vein where it inserts into the vena cava. This will ensure you identify the renal artery as medially as possible

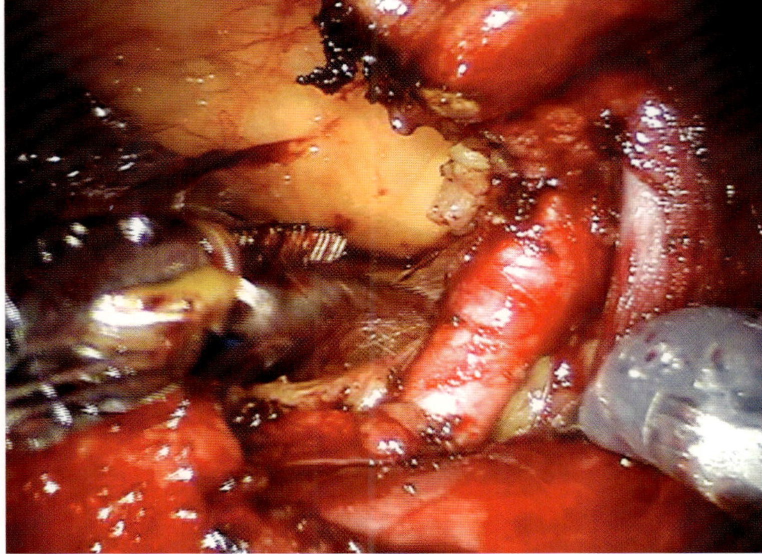

Fig. 14: Fully dissect the renal artery and expose it close to the aorta to avoid missing any early branches. By skeletonizing the renal artery, the bulldog clamps can achieve greater occlusion pressure. The Doppler probe is utilized again to confirm no early branches or accessory arteries have been missed

For left-sided procedures, a similar dissection can be carried out with the same principle that a wide dissection allows for increased safety and ease during the critical portions of the case.

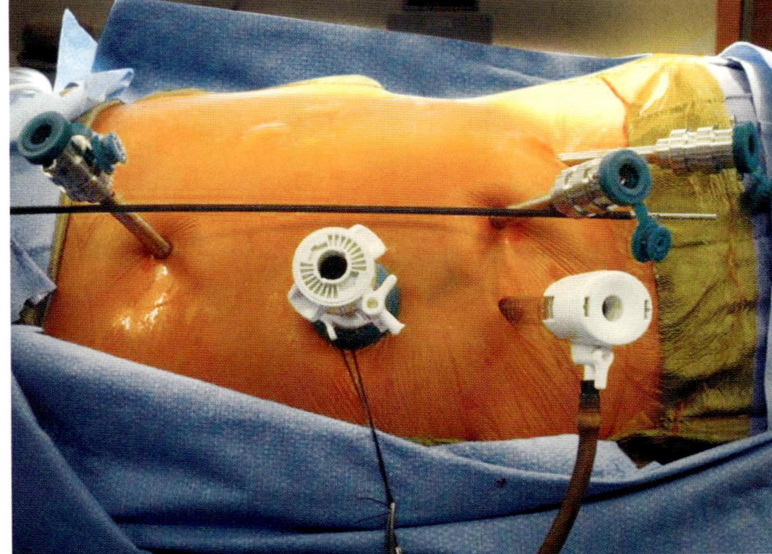

Fig. 15: The left-sided port placement follows a similar principle of moving the four main ports as far cephalad as possible to allow the fourth arm to be placed in the lower quadrant

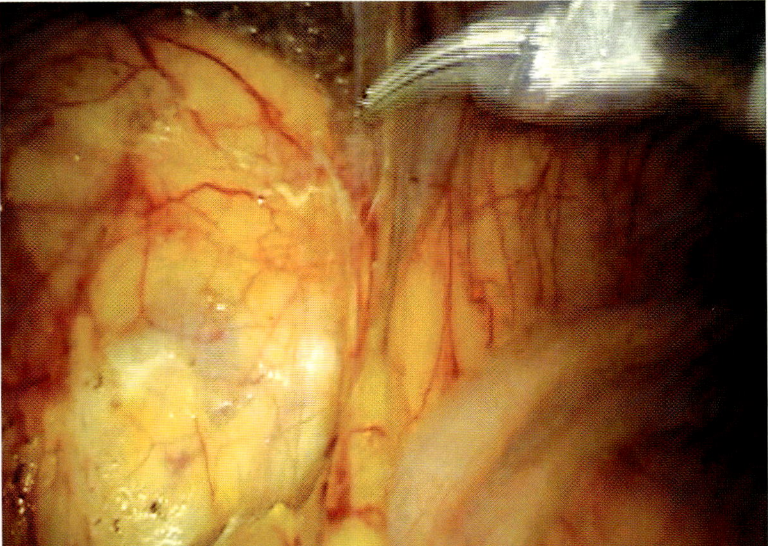

Fig. 16: Begin by medializing the colon by incising the peritoneum as it drapes over the anterior surface of the kidney at the level of the mid to lower pole of the kidney. Once Gerota's fascia is identified as a pearly, shiny covering over kidney, create an avascular plane that separates the peritoneum from Gerota's fascia. Continue this dissection to the iliacs as described previously

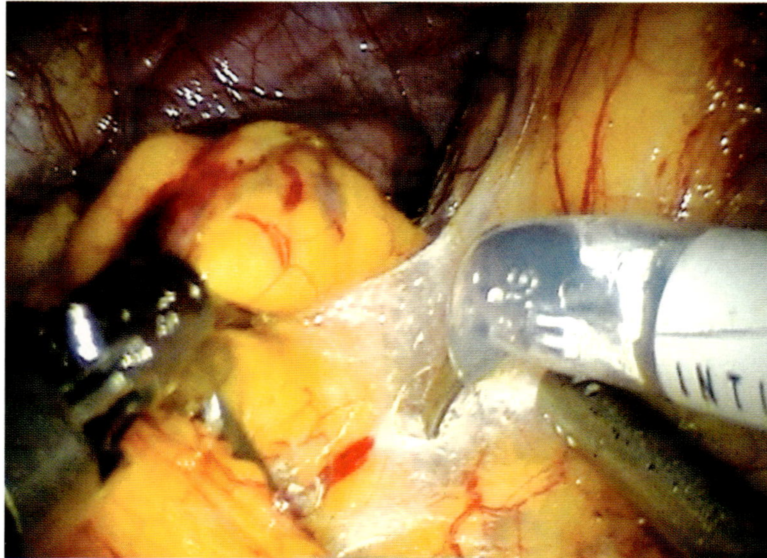

Fig. 17: Once the colon is dropped to the iliacs, work more cephalad and over the upper pole of the kidney. As you reach the upper pole, angle your dissection laterally toward the lateral splenic attachments. Continue releasing these attachments as superiorly as possible. The shaft of the left robotic instrument is used to place traction on spleen and pancreas superiorly and medially while the assistant places traction on upper pole inferiorly to open up the plane of dissection

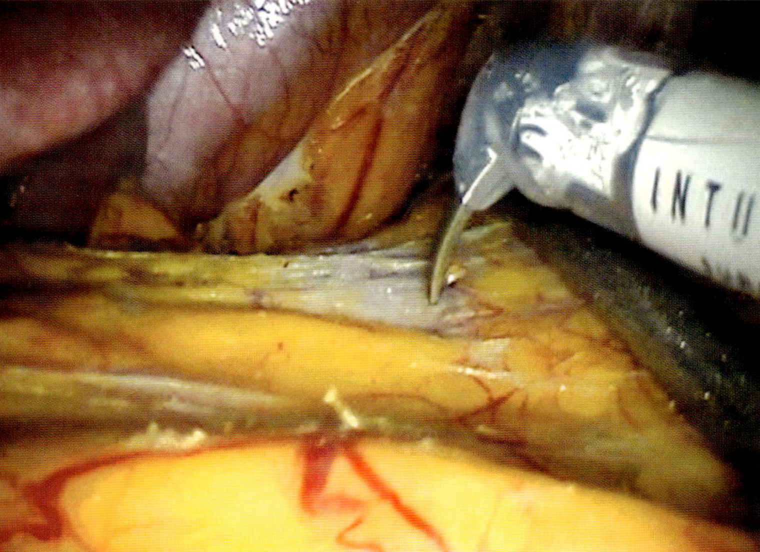

Fig. 18: Continue the dissection of the upper pole until the spleen can be flipped medially and superiorly away from its normal lie. This allows for greater release of the colon and pancreas for optimal exposure of the renal hilum. Care should be taken to avoid the stomach, which should be decompressed with a nasogastric tube (NGT). Similar to the right side, the left adrenal should be visualized without the need for significant traction from the assistant. This ensures optimal exposure

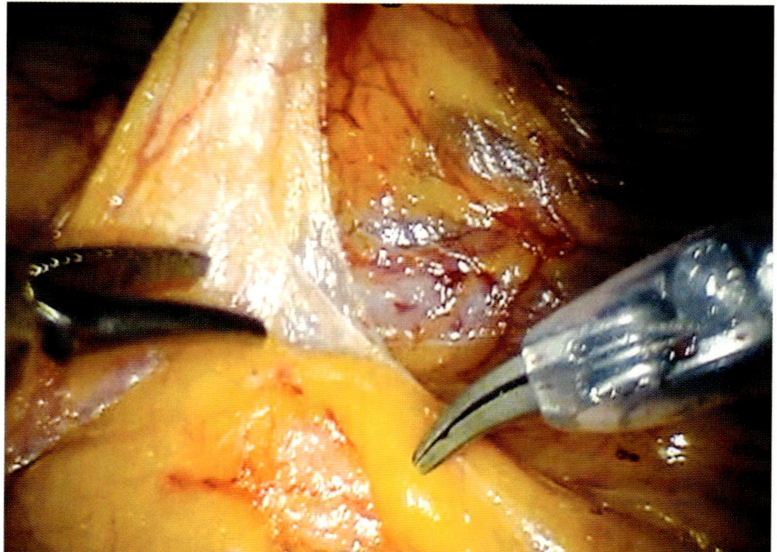

Fig. 19: Caudal to the kidney, continue the dissection of the colon in the avascular plane until the gonadal vein is identified. At this point, the fourth arm can be introduced to help with countertraction to best allow dissection of the gonadal vein anteriorly all the way to the renal vein

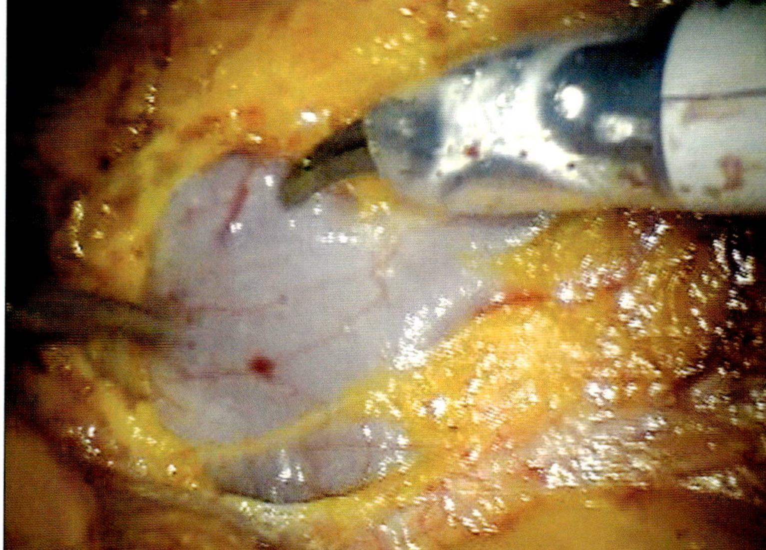

Fig. 20: Dissecting the anterior surface of the gonadal vein cephalad will expose the anterior surface of the renal vein

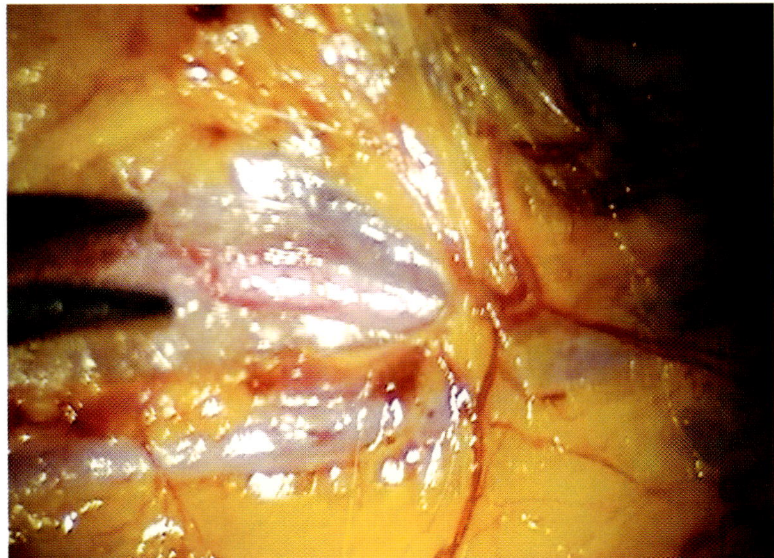

Fig. 21: The gonadal vein can then be medialized to expose the ureter, which is anterior to the gonadal vein. Like the right side, the gonadal vein is dropped and the ureter is then elevated

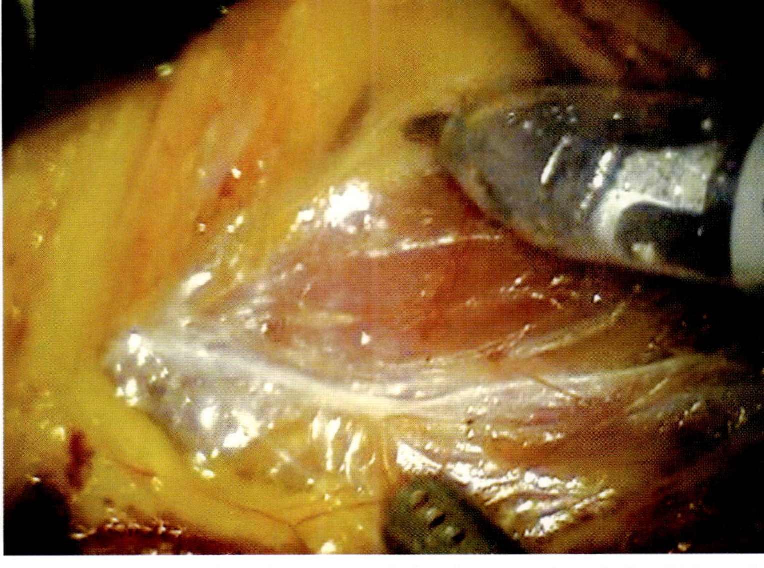

Fig. 22: Continue the dissection of the lower pole of the kidney by elevating the ureter and entering the avascular plane between the kidney and psoas, keeping the psoas fascia on the psoas muscle. Sweep under the kidney to elevate the kidney, moving towards the hilum

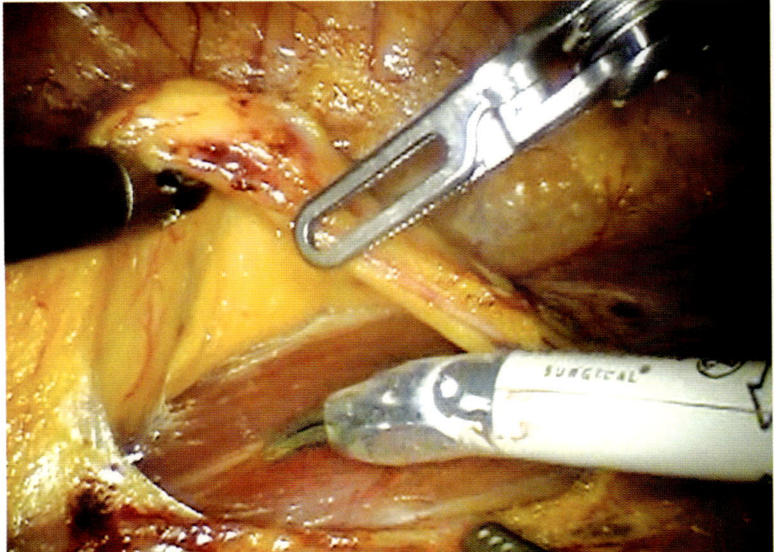

Fig. 23: Use the fourth arm to continue to elevate the kidney, marching towards the hilum

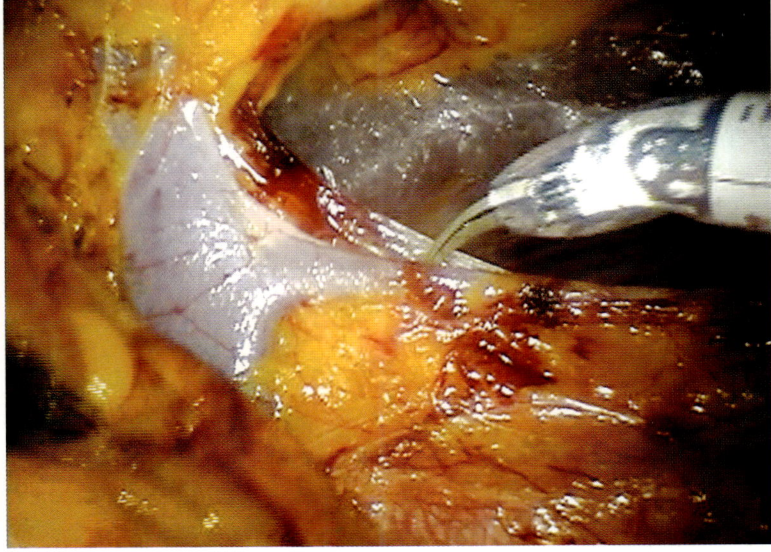

Fig. 24: Ensure that the kidney is freed posteriorly to the upper pole so that the fourth arm can be placed superior to the hilum for maximal stretch. The gonadal vein can then be divided and used as a landmark to find the artery, which is usually just medial and superior to the divided vein. Care should be taken to identify any lumbar veins, which also may insert here. At this point, a Doppler probe, which is controlled by the surgeon, can be introduced to efficiently identify major vessels and allow the division of surrounding tissue with no signal, with impunity

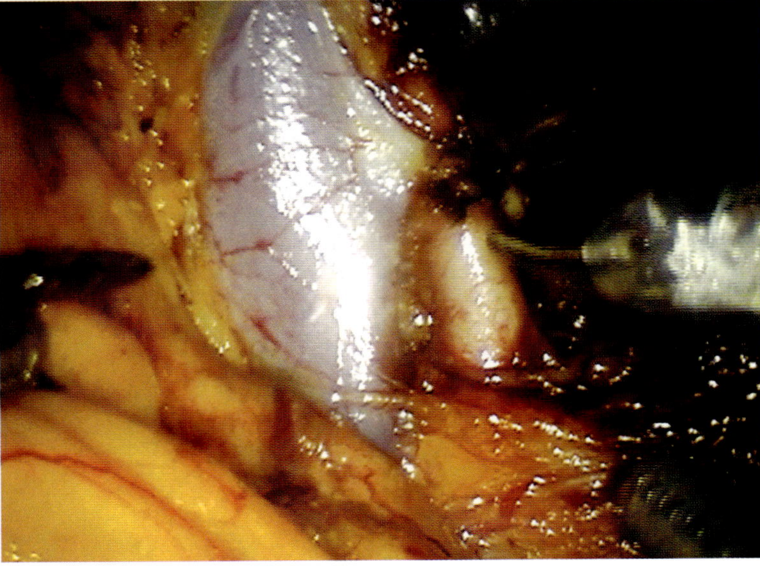

Fig. 25: Fully dissect the renal artery and expose it close to the aorta to avoid missing any early branches. By skeletonizing the renal artery, the bulldog clamps can achieve greater occlusion pressure. The Doppler probe is utilized again to confirm no early branches or accessory arteries have been missed

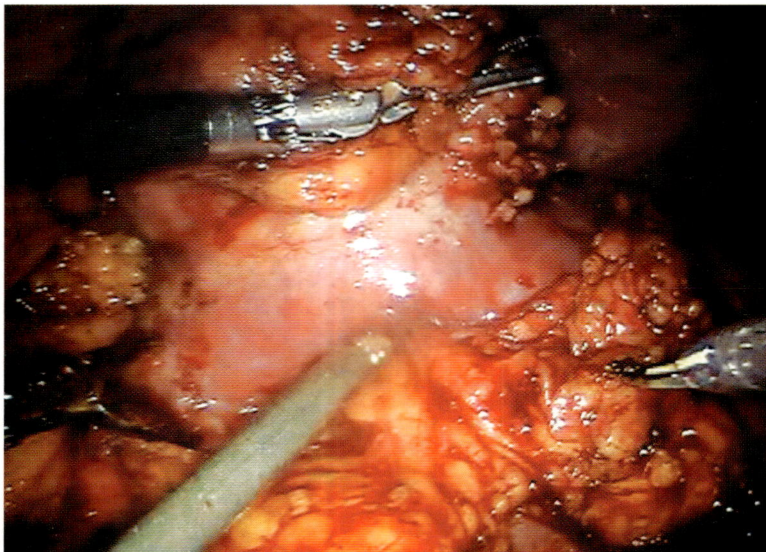

Fig. 26: With ureter, artery and vein dissected and isolated attention is paid to identifying location tumor and preparing kidney for tumor excision. Depending on the location of the tumor, the kidney may need to be mobilized to access the mass. In addition, intraoperative ultrasound (US) may be required to locate the tumor if endophytic or there is significant overlying fat. The kidney should be sufficiently mobilized such that the kidney can be rotated or flipped so that the tumor is in an optimal position, facing toward the camera. Gerota's fascia is divided circumferentially around the tumor and dissected down to expose normal kidney capsule approximately 1 cm from the renal tumor. US may be necessary for this step should "toxic fat," or fat that is adherent to the capsule of the kidney be encountered. Note, we believe this fat is best divided and removed from the capsule sharply with scissors

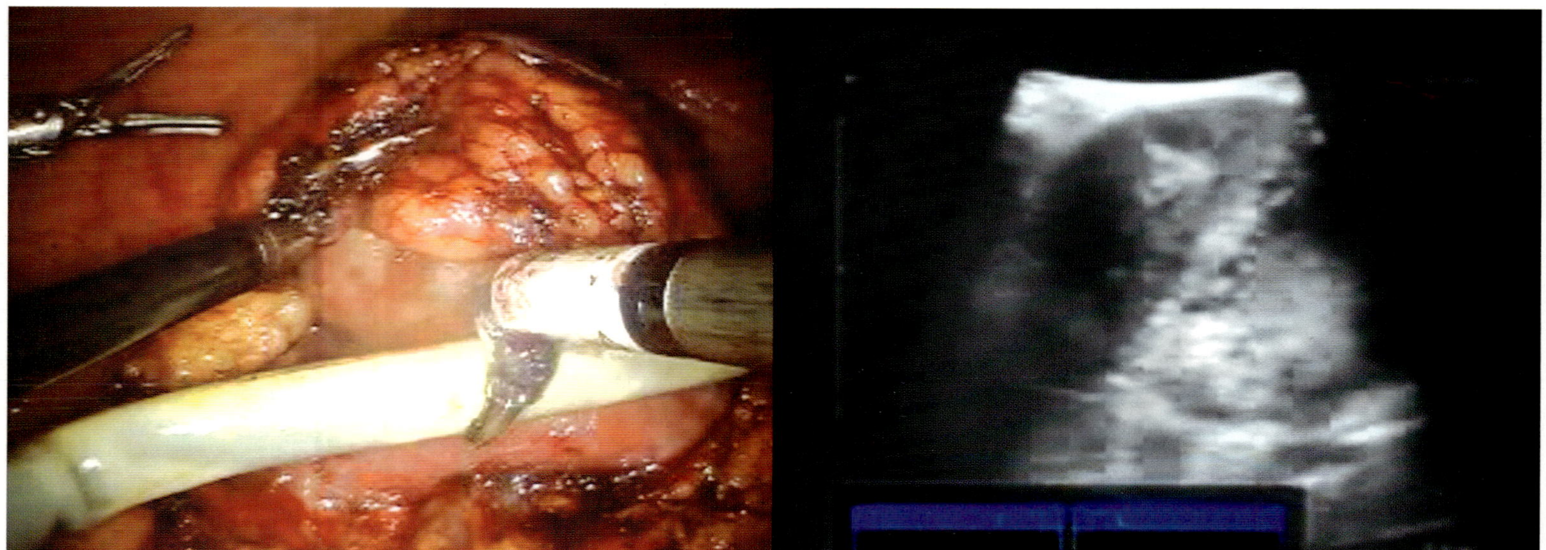

Fig. 27: Use the fourth arm to either help create traction/countertraction and to manipulate the kidney to allow for an ideal view of the segment of the kidney which is involved with tumor

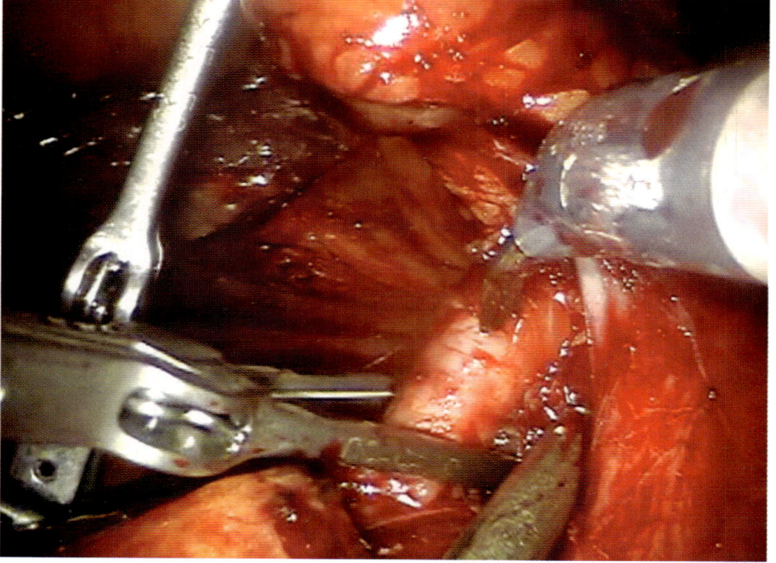

Fig. 28: After the kidney capsule has been exposed circumferentially around the tumor, the use of an ultrasound (US) is used to identify the borders circumferentially and to define the endophytic portion of the tumor. The probe is introduced by the assistant and manipulated such that the crystal is flush and perpendicular to the kidney and the tumor. Beginning on the tumor, the US is then swept off of the tumor, towards normal kidney to define where the lateral margins of the tumor end. The capsule is then scored with cautery to mark the border of the excision. This is repeated circumferentially around the tumor, until the capsule is scored over the entire course of the planned resection

Prior to going on clamp, we perform a checklist to ensure everything is ready to facilitate a short warm ischemia time. See Table 2 for our checklist.

Table 2: Preclamp checklist
Anesthesia
• Did you give mannitol?
• How much fluids have the patient received?
Circulator
• Do you have at least 4 bars of CO_2
• Is the Tissuelinke set at 70 coag and the saline primed and open
Surgical Technology
• Do you have 10 ml of Floseal® on the field
• Do you have a Satinsky clamp on the field
• Has the number of uses been checked on the needle drivers preoperatively?
• Do you have the sutures prepared?
– Six of the 2-0 V-locs, v-20 at 6 inches with a know, small weck, and large weck closest to the needle
– Prepare Three 3-0 vicryl RB-1 cut at 6 inches
• What bulldog clamp is loaded?
– Do you have the other three available?
– Which clamp would the surgeon like to clamp the second vessel with?

Whenever possible, we use selective ischemia to eliminate warm ischemia time for healthy parenchyma while still providing the vascular control and visualization of the traditional clamping techniques.

If, good ischemia is not achieved with selective clamping, the kidney can be placed back on stretch using the fourth arm and apply the bulldog clamps. Robotic controlled bulldogs allow for greater control by the surgeon. Clamps should be placed in the field and clipped to the fat before the artery is clamped to decrease the warm ischemia time.

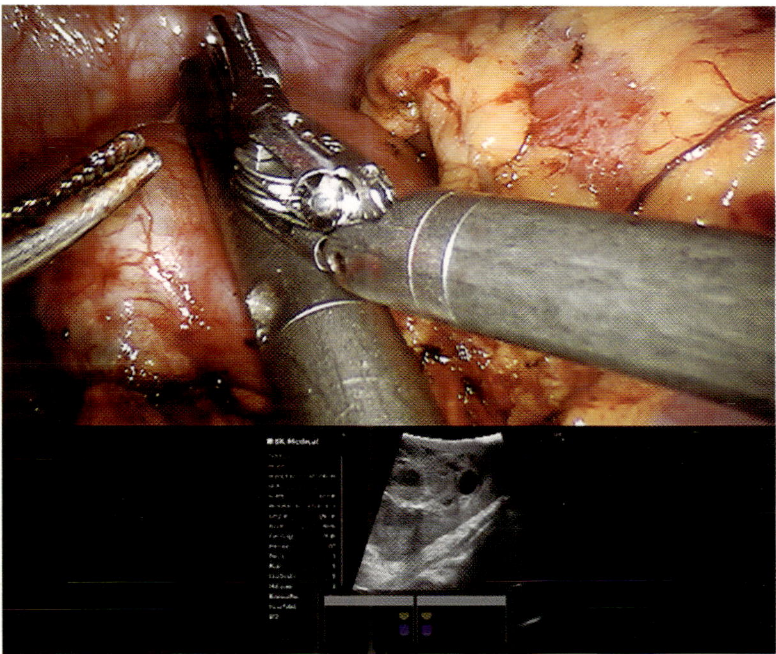

Fig. 29: In this case, the renal lesion is demonstrated by a drop-in ultrasound probe which allows the robotic surgeon to control the orientation of the probe. The borders of the lesion thus defined

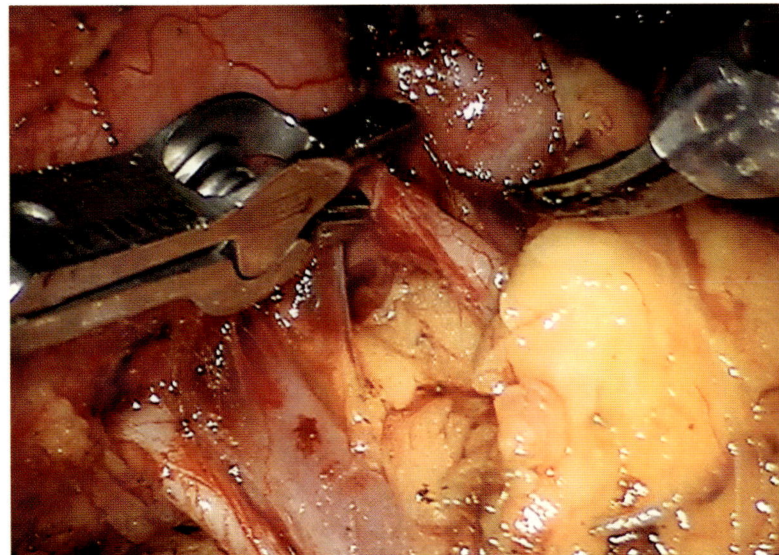

Fig. 30: A selective dissection of the renal hilum is then performed to define the secondary and tertiary branches of the renal artery. Using micro-bulldog clamps, the vessels feeding the lesion is clamped

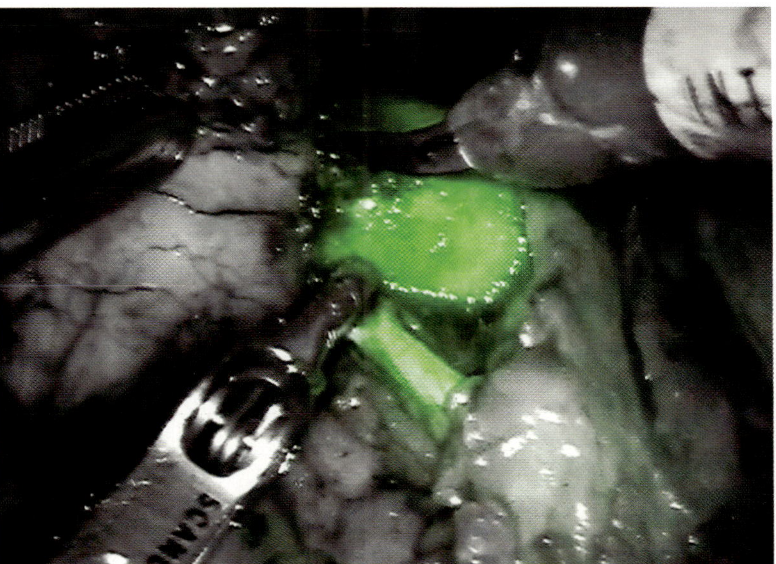

Fig. 31: After the branching artery is clamped, we then utilized the robotic infrared camera and inject intravascular Indocyanine Green. In this case, the tumor is black while the normal parenchyma is green, clearly demonstrating excellent ischemia of the renal lesion while preserving blood flow to the rest of the kidney

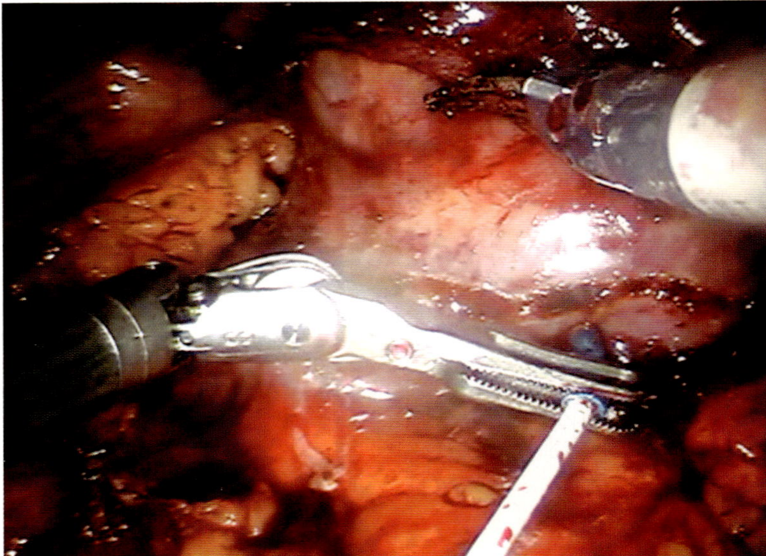

Fig. 32: The Doppler probe is then used to verify that there is no blood flow to the kidney

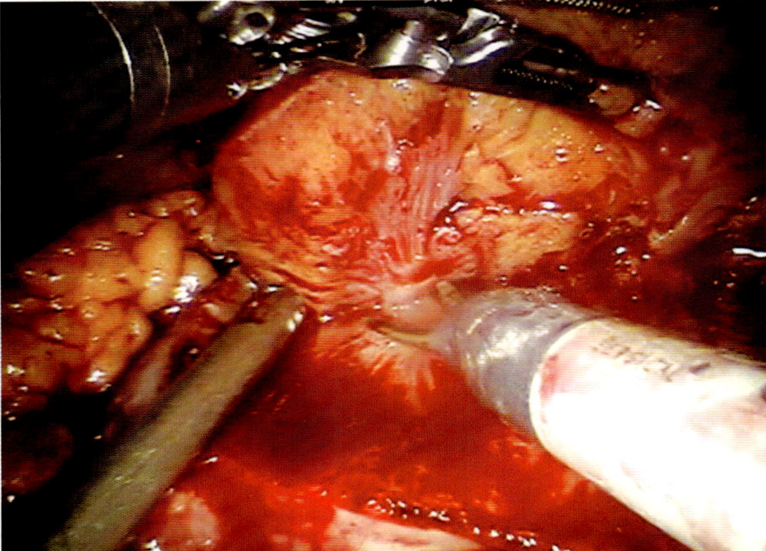

Fig. 33: Using the left hand to gently retract the tumor away from kidney, the assistant uses the sucker to gently apply counter downward traction and intermittent suction to expose the plane of dissection. It is important to cut broadly to avoid working in a hole

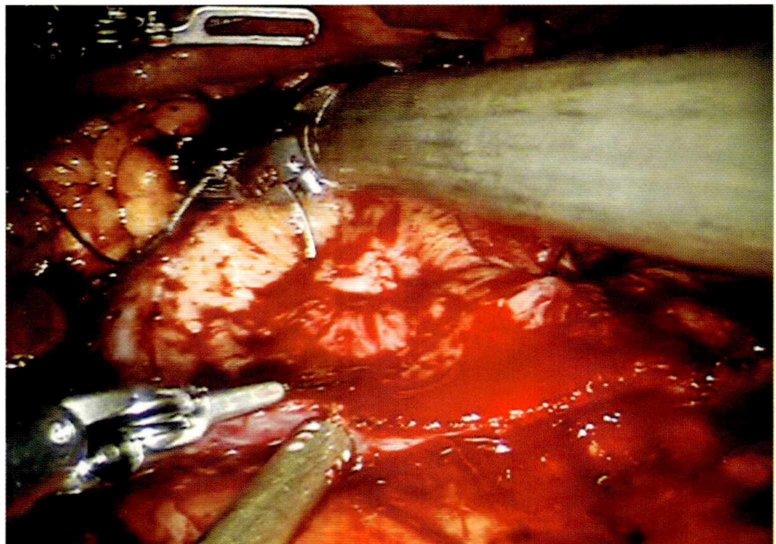

Fig. 34: Once the tumor is removed, any open vessels and collecting system can be over sown individually with a vicryl RB. Alternatively, as seen here, a 6–8 inch barbed suture with a preplaced Weck clip can be anchored outside the defect on the capsule, then run across the defect, compressing any small vessels and closing deep portions of the defect. A Weck clip can again be placed to secure the barbed suture outside the defect and against the collecting system. A hemostatic device such as tissue link, cautery or argon can be used on the cortex once the major defects are closed. Be carful not to cauterize the collecting system as this may prevent proper healing

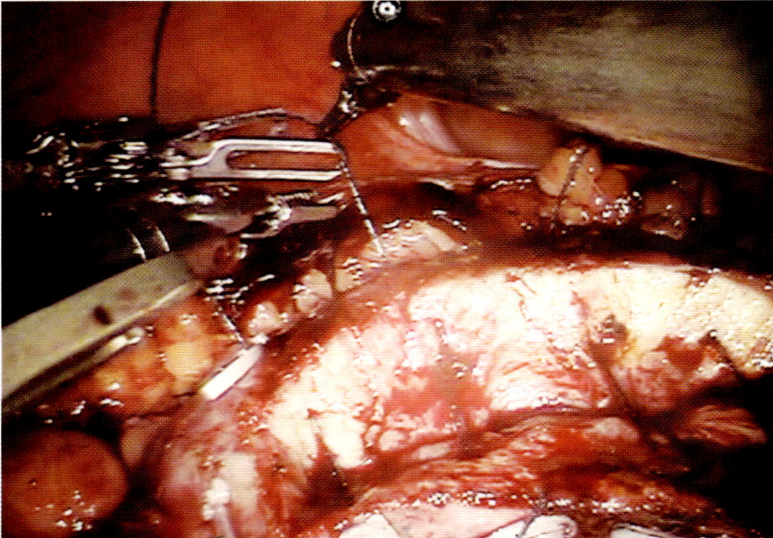

Fig. 35: Additional barbed sutures with preplaced weck clips are used across the defect. These sutures also enter and exit outside the defect and are secured against the capsule of the kidney with weck clips. These should be placed across the span of the defect approximately 1 cm apart. Place the sutures toward you to ensure easier exposure and angles during tightening

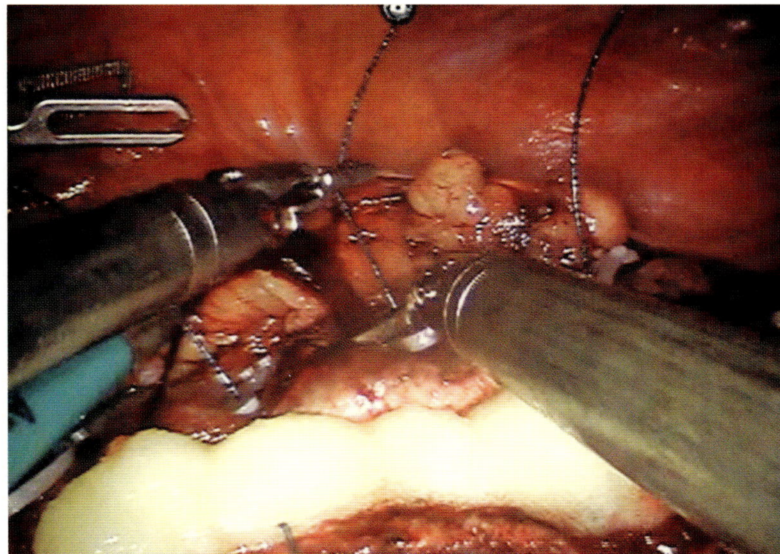

Fig. 36: We apply a hemostatic agent (Floseal®, Baxter) and tighten each of these sutures sequentially by sliding the weck clip down on the suture. To avoid ripping through the edge of the defect when tightening the suture, retract with the left hand in the direction the suture exits the parenchyma and slide the clip down with the right

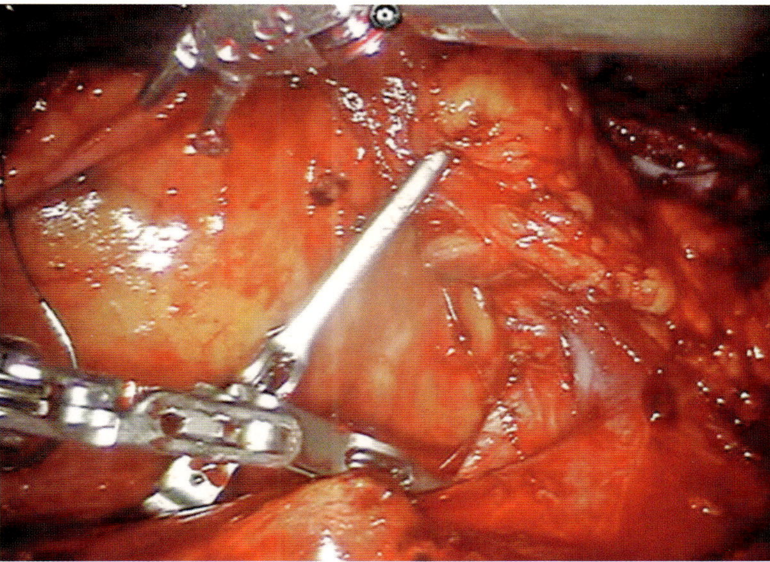

Fig. 37: Unclamp the vein followed by the artery and reaccess the defect for any bleeding. Any bleeding can be controlled by additional bolstering sutures or by tightening the existing sutures

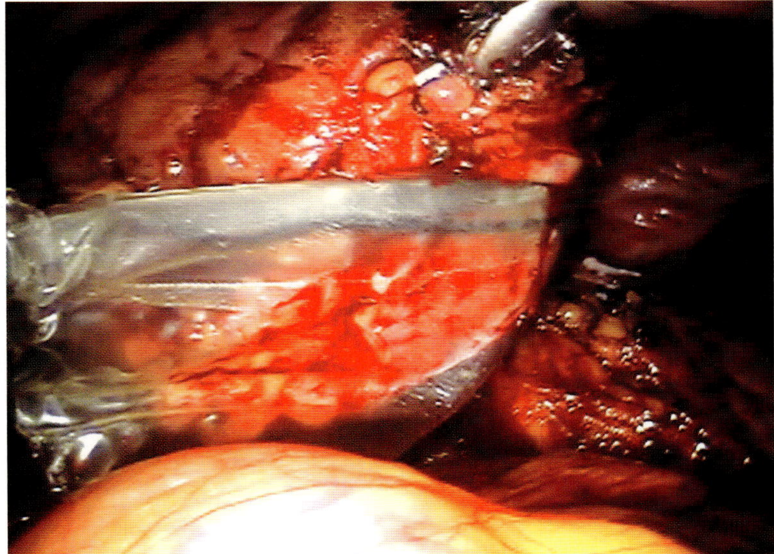

Fig. 38: Use an Endocatch™ bag to remove the tumor

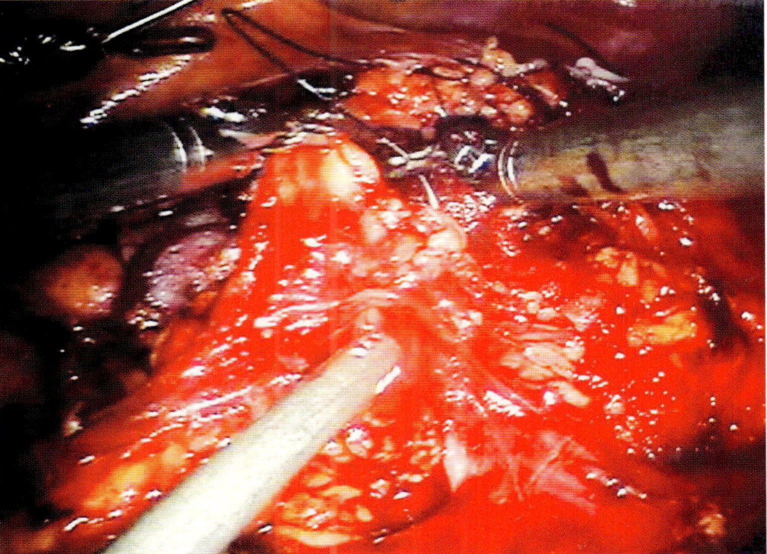

Fig. 39: Close Gerota's fat around the defect to help prevent adhesions on the defect and to restore normal anatomy. Fix the kidney to the sidewall if the kidney is sufficiently mobilized such that the kidney could rotate. Place a JP drain through the fourth arm port and, if the Hassan technique was utilized, remove the specimen from that port and close the fascia in the standard manner

REFERENCES

1. Chow WH, Devesa SS, Warren JL, et al. Rising incidence of renal cell cancer in the United States. JAMA. 1999;281(17):1628-31.
2. O'Connor SD, Pickhardt PJ, Kim DH, et al. Incidental finding of renal masses at unenhanced CT: prevalence and analysis of features for guiding management. AJR Am J Roentgenol. 2011;197(1):139-45.
3. Maclennan S, Imamura M, Lapitan MC, et al. Systematic review of oncological outcomes following surgical management of localised renal cancer. Eur Urol. 2012;61(5):972-93.

9

Chapter

Laparoendoscopic Single-Site (LESS) Live Donor Nephrectomy and Renal Surgery

Michael B Marean, James S Rosoff, Joseph J Del Pizzo

INTRODUCTION

Since the advent of laparoscopic surgery, there has been a dramatic shift towards the minimally invasive approach for management of many urologic conditions. Laparoscopic surgery has been shown to minimize morbidity and shorten recovery time, while maintaining comparable surgical outcomes. This trend has extended into the realm of live donor nephrectomy and, as such, the laparoscopic approach has become the standard of care at most major academic centers. This procedure typically requires three to four small incisions for trocar access and a small extraction incision for removing the specimen. Long-term studies have confirmed that allograft outcomes and complication rates after laparoscopic donor nephrectomy (LDN) are equivalent to those of the open approach.[1,2]

Laparoendoscopic single-site (LESS) surgery is a new advancement in minimally invasive technology that attempts to further minimize morbidity, decrease convalescence and improve cosmesis. This procedure is performed through a single small skin incision, most often at the umbilicus (although some centers have used a Pfannenstiel incision). LESS donor nephrectomy (LESS-DN) has been shown to have equivalent postoperative outcomes to standard LDN in terms of allograft function and overall 30-day complication rates.[3] Although measures of in-house morbidity between the two groups appear to be equivalent, there is some evidence that following discharge from the hospital, patients undergoing LESS-DN have decreased pain medication requirements, return to work sooner and have faster resolution of physical symptoms than patients undergoing LDN.[4] Although overall complication rates are equivalent, trocar site morbidity is a factor in LDN, including port-site hernia, pain and bleeding from epigastric vessel injury.[5]

In addition to minimizing morbidity, LESS-DN seems to provide improved cosmesis, an important factor in a young, otherwise healthy donor population. Placement of a single small incision at the umbilicus allows for a well-concealed scar.

Overall, the benefits of minimally invasive surgery have decreased barriers to kidney donation and LESS-DN may further minimize disincentives to live organ donation.[6] Donor kidneys are in short supply and increasing the population of organ donors is a potentially significant benefit of LESS-DN.

Although this chapter focuses on LESS-DN, single-site surgery is not limited to living donor nephrectomy. LESS surgery is a feasible technique for performing simple nephrectomy, radical nephrectomy, partial nephrectomy, or pyeloplasty in the hands of an experienced laparoscopic surgeon.[7]

Technical limitations do exist with LESS surgery. These include decreased working space and lack of instrument triangulation.

The use of a specialized multichannel port, such as the GelPOINT device, helps to decrease instrument clashing by providing increased space for triangulation. It also enables the surgeon to easily modify port configuration throughout the procedure to assist in retraction and dissection. Using a bariatric laparoscope with a parallel light cord in place of a traditional laparoscope serves to further minimize instrument collision and space restrictions. Articulating instruments are being developed that will help to further reduce these technical limitations.

Patient-specific challenges also exist with LESS-DN, such as BMI > 30, accessory renal arteries and right-sided donation. These patient factors make LESS-DN more difficult than LDN. However, they do not exclude this patient population from single-site surgery. LESS-DN has been shown to be feasible and safe in these patients in the hands of an experienced laparoscopic surgeon.[8-10]

PROCEDURE

The procedure is mentioned below in steps (Figs 1 to 19).

1. Position patient in 45° flank position on the operating table with adequate padding for the brachial plexus, dependent hip, knees and ankles. The lower leg is flexed while the upper leg is gently extended with a pillow placed between them. The table is then gently flexed to open either the right or left flank.
2. Once the patient is prepped and draped a 5 cm periumbilical incision is made with the skin on stretch, through which the GelPOINT Advanced Access Platform is placed. Two 5 mm trocars and one 15 mm trocar are then passed through the GelPOINT platform into the peritoneal space. A fourth trocar may be necessary for right-sided nephrectomy to assist with liver retraction.

Right Side

3. In a right-sided case, the right triangular ligament is incised while the liver is retracted medially and anteriorly. The coronary ligament is then opened in a lateral-to-medial direction.
4. The ascending colon is mobilized medially by incising the line of Toldt caudally to the bifurcation of the iliac vessels.
5. The hepatic flexure is gently lifted to identify the plane between Gerota's fascia and the mesocolon. A Diamond-Flex retractor can be used through a fourth trocar to provide continued retraction of the liver. Division of colorenal attachments improves mobilization of the ascending colon and provides access to the retroperitoneum.
6. The duodenum is identified and kocherized to expose the inferior vena cava (IVC). The adventitia surrounding the IVC is lifted with a Maryland dissector and incised, providing better exposure of the vena cava and the renal vein.

Left Side

7. In a left-sided case, the dissection begins by incising the line of Toldt from the level of the upper sigmoid colon to the splenic flexure. This dissection can be carried further medially by dividing the phrenicocolic and splenorenal ligaments.
8. The descending colon is gently lifted, thereby identifying the plane between Gerota's fascia and the mesocolon. Any colorenal attachments are sharply divided.
9. The pancreas is gently dissected off Gerota's fascia medially.
10. The operating room table is rotated in order to place the patient in lateral decubitus position at 90°. This helps to mobilize the spleen, pancreas and descending colon medially and expose the renal hilum.
11. The investing tissues over the renal hilum are lifted and incised to expose the renal vein. Maryland and right-angle dissectors are used to dissect the tissues off the renal vein and to isolate the adrenal and gonadal veins.
12. Both the adrenal and gonadal veins are clipped and divided flush with the renal vein.
13. The renal artery is identified posterior to the renal vein and dissected free of surrounding tissues close to the vena cava or aorta. This can be done with a Maryland or right-angle dissector.
14. Attention is turned towards identifying the ureter in the retroperitoneal fat, medial to the psoas muscle and lateral and posterior to the gonadal vein. The ureter and gonadal vein are dissected en bloc to maintain periureteral attachments and preserve the ureteral blood supply. The dissection is continued proximally to the renal hilum and distally to the iliac vessels or pelvic brim. On the right side, the gonadal vein is ligated at its confluence with the vena cava.
15. The psoas muscle is exposed laterally and posteriorly while dissecting cephalad from the lower pole of the kidney towards the upper pole, dividing any inferior and posterior side-wall attachments.
16. The adrenal gland is dissected off the superior medial aspect of the kidney with a harmonic scalpel. Any identified adrenal veins are cauterized and ligated.
17. The ureter and gonadal vein are divided together with a 10 mm Endo GIA™ stapler at the level of the iliac vessels. Prior to using the Endo GIA™ stapler, one of the 5 mm trocars is replaced with a 12 mm trocar.
18. The renal artery is divided with an Endo GIA™ vascular stapler, flush with the aorta on the left side. The renal vein is then similarly divided, flush with the vena cava on the right side.
19. A 15 mm Endo Catch™ is positioned behind the kidney and opened. The kidney is gently placed within the bag and delivered intact through the periumbilical incision.
20. The operative field is carefully inspected to ensure adequate hemostasis. The periumbilical incision is closed in standard fashion.

Tips and Tricks

1. Using the bariatric laparoscope with the right-angle attachment reduces interference between the camera and the laparoscopic instruments.
2. Placement of an occlusive barrier (e.g. Tegaderm transparent film dressing) on the GelPOINT prior to insertion of trocars reduces air leaks.
3. The GelPOINT device allows the surgeon to adjust the position of trocars as necessary to aid in dissection. For right-sided cases, the liver retractor can be placed through the GelPOINT as well.
4. Use the nondominant hand to provide traction in a 12 o'clock to 6 o'clock direction (as opposed to the 3 o'clock to 9 o'clock retraction used in traditional laparoscopy).
5. Most cases will require the extended-length Maryland dissector and extended-length harmonic scalpel in order to reach the limits of dissection.

INSTRUMENTS

- GelPOINT Advanced Access Platform
- 5 mm, 12 mm and 15 mm trocars
- Bariatric 10 mm rigid 30° laparoscope with right angle attachment for light cord
- Maryland dissector
- Right angle dissector
- Laparoscopic scissor
- Harmonic scalpel
- Endo TA™ vascular stapler
- Endo GIA™ vascular stapler (10 mm)
- Endo Catch specimen bag (15 mm)
- Diamond-Flex retractor
- Titanium clips
- Tegaderm transparent film dressing (large)

Fig. 1: A 5 cm incision is marked out with the skin stretched

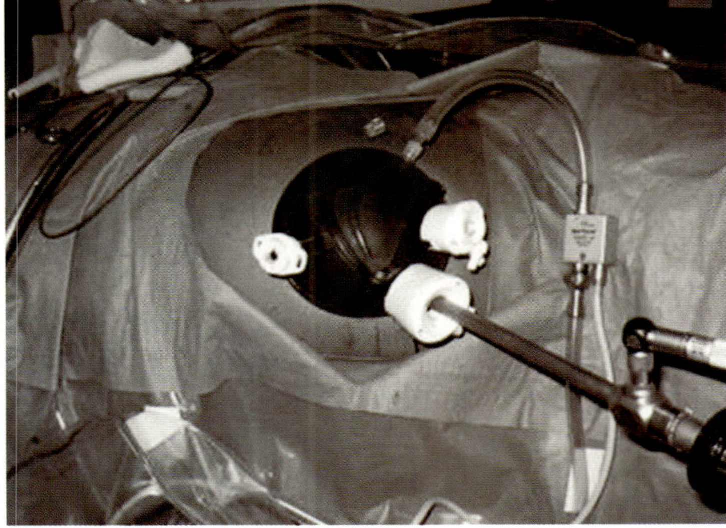

Fig. 2: The single port device is inserted; trocar placement for left-sided nephrectomy

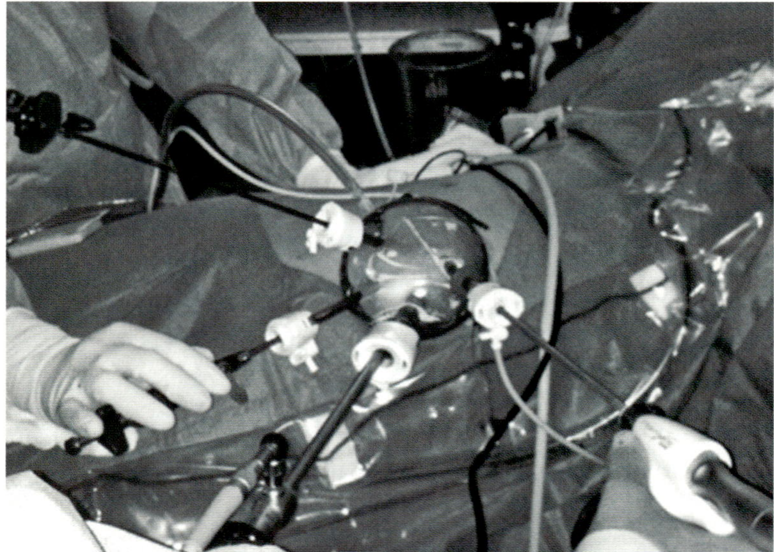

Fig. 3: Trocar placement for right-sided nephrectomy

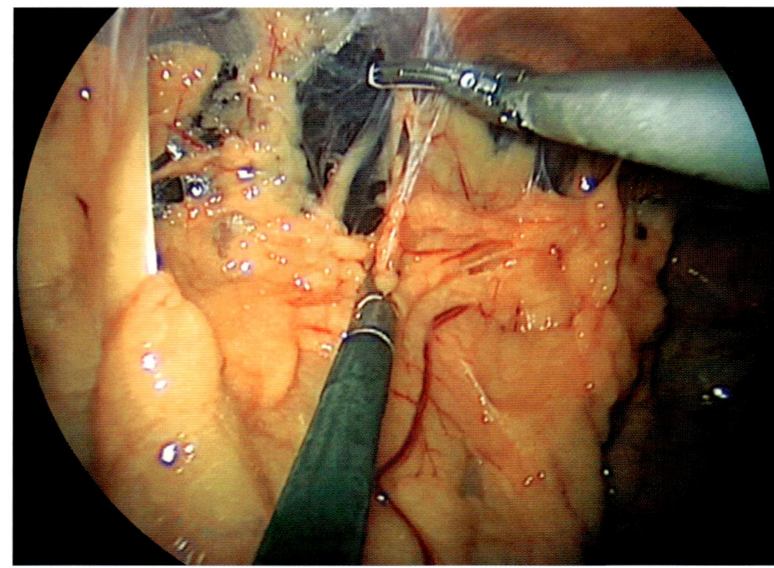

Fig. 4: Omental and bowel adhesions are lysed with the harmonic scalpel

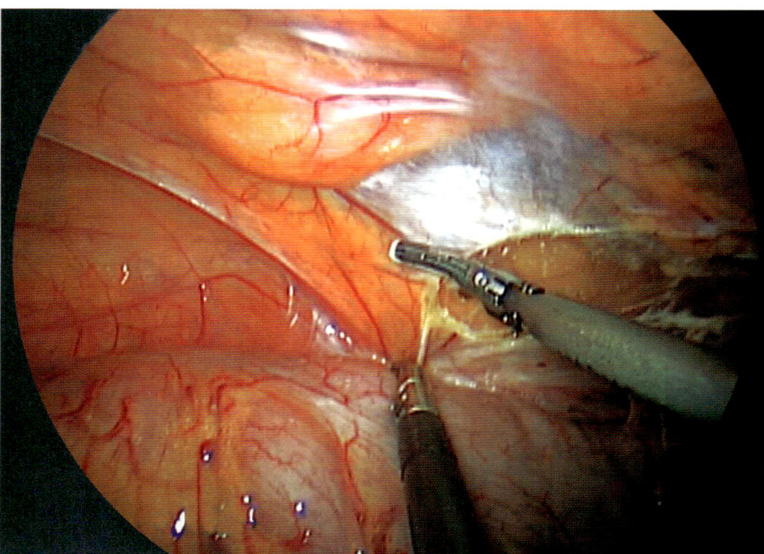

Fig. 5: The white line of Toldt is incised

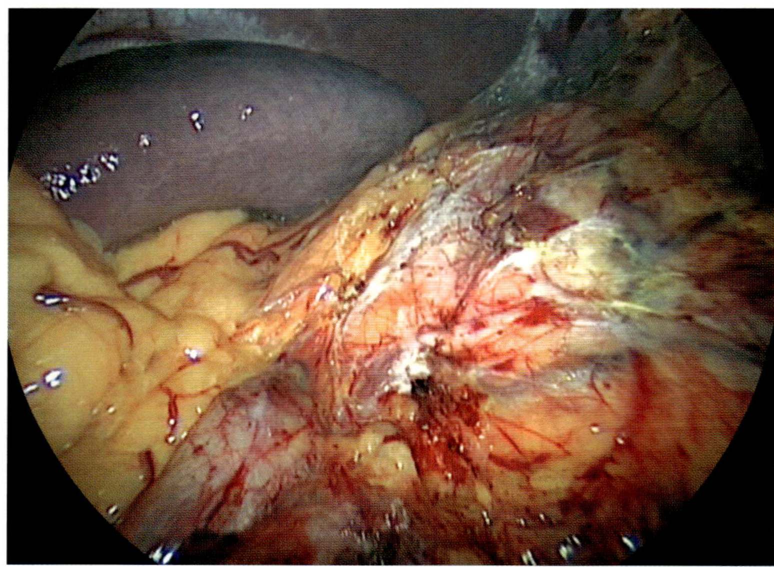

Fig. 6: The colon is swept medially

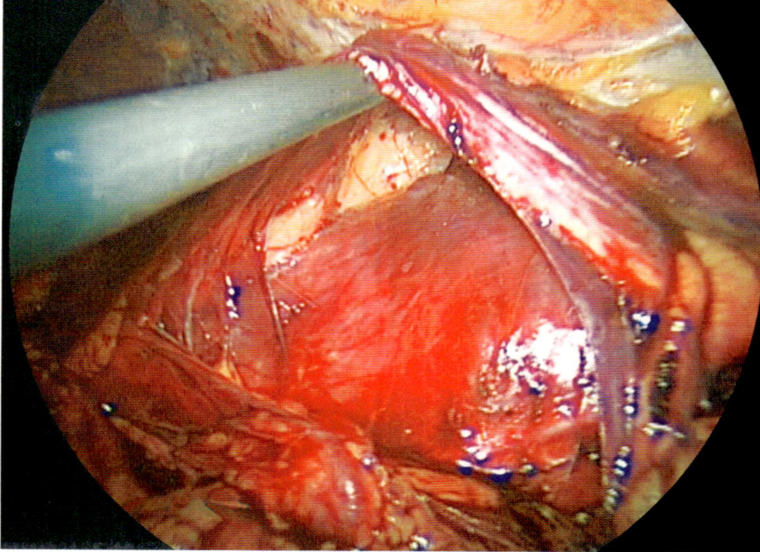

Fig. 7: The gonadal vein and ureter are identified and isolated

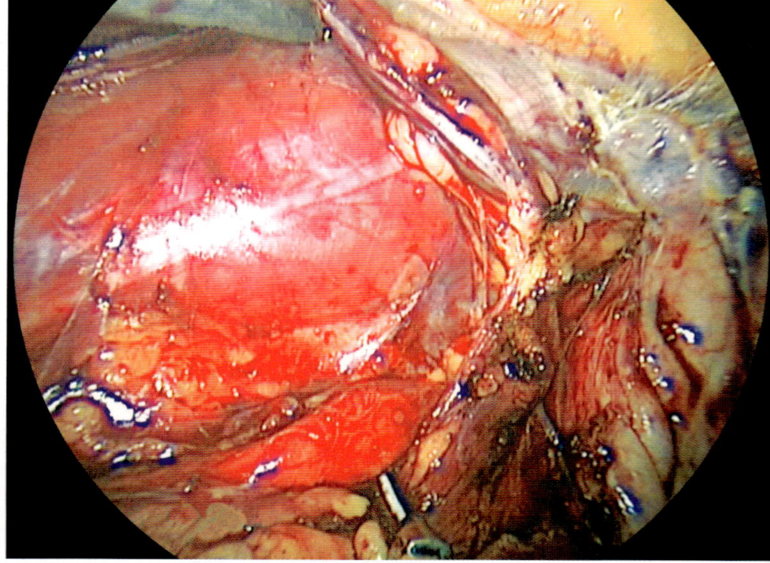

Fig. 8: Attachments to the gonadal vein and ureter are divided caudally to isolate this packet

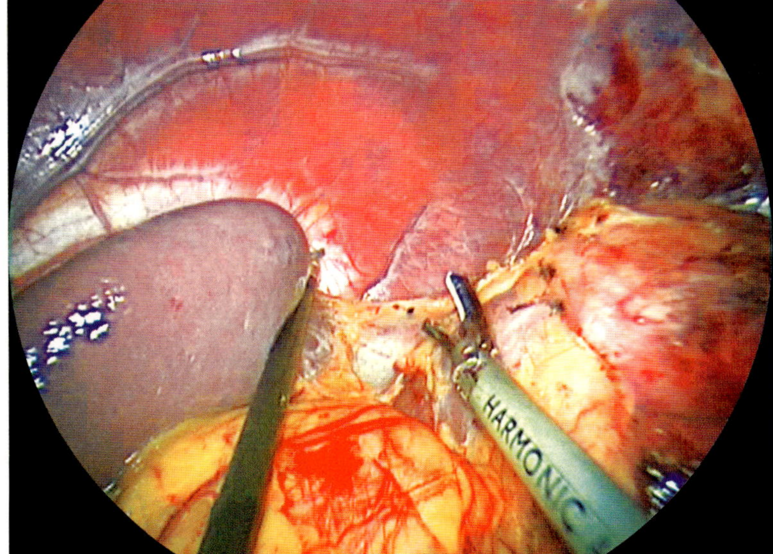

Fig. 9: Splenorenal attachments are divided

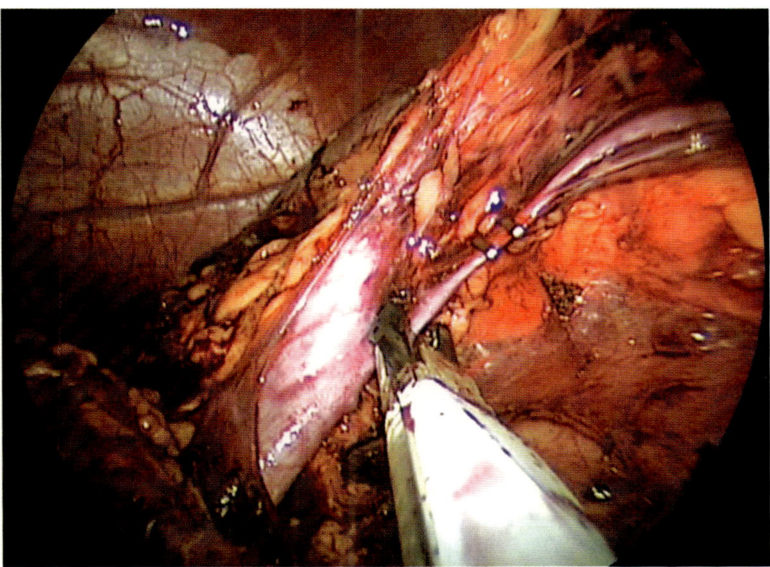

Fig. 10: The gonadal vein is clipped and divided

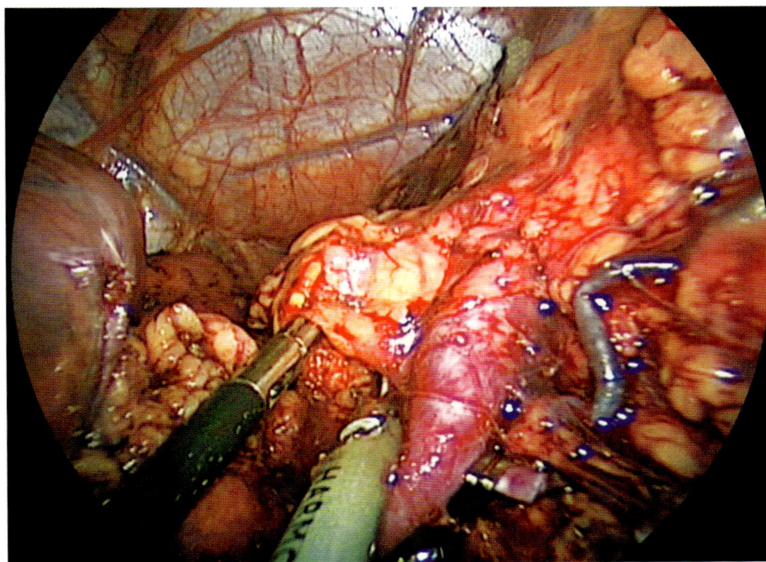

Fig. 11: The adrenal gland is separated off the upper pole of the kidney (after the adrenal vein is identified and divided)

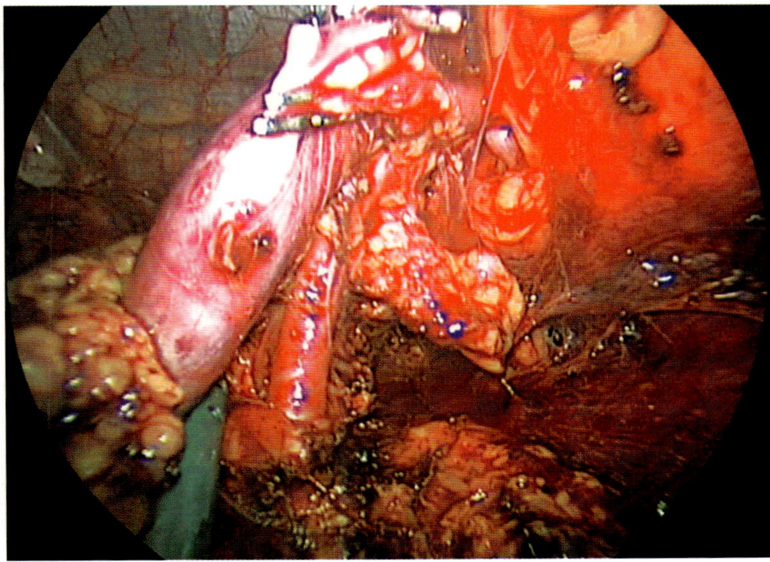

Fig. 12: The renal artery is identified and dissected free of surrounding tissues

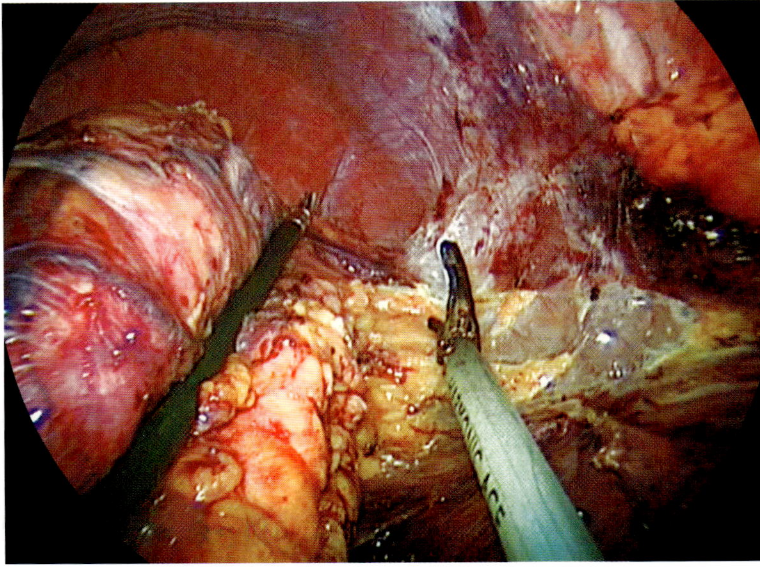

Fig. 13: The posterior and lateral attachments to the kidney are divided

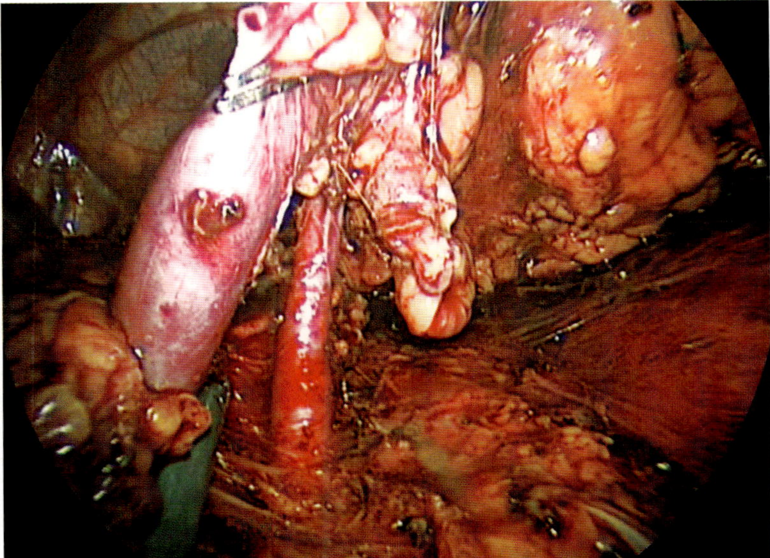

Fig. 14: The renal artery is cleaned off down to its origin at the aorta

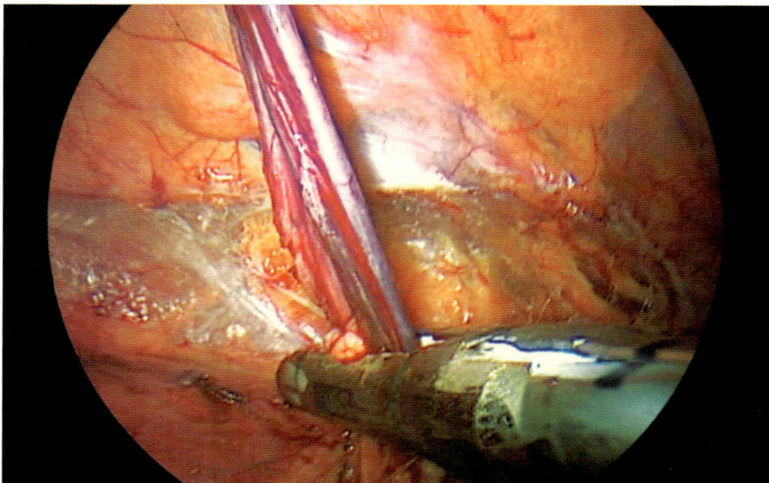

Fig. 15: The gonadal vein/ureter packet is divided with the Endo GIA™ vascular stapler, just above the bifurcation of the iliac vessels

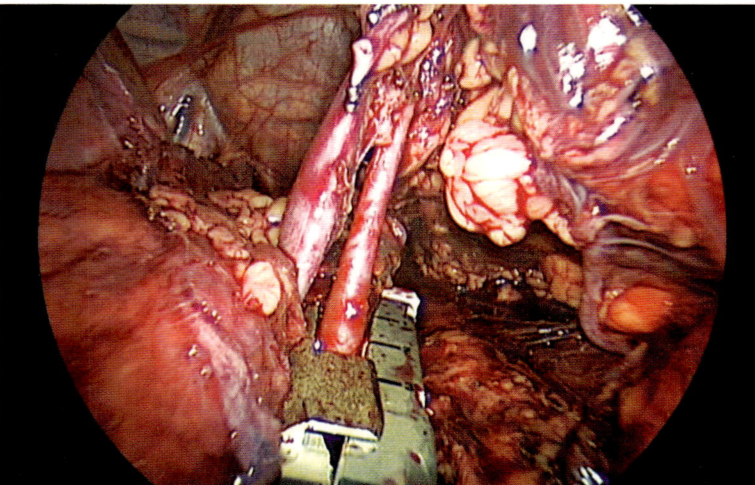

Fig. 16: The gonadal vein/ureter packet is divided with the Endo GIA™ vascular stapler, just above the bifurcation of the iliac vessels

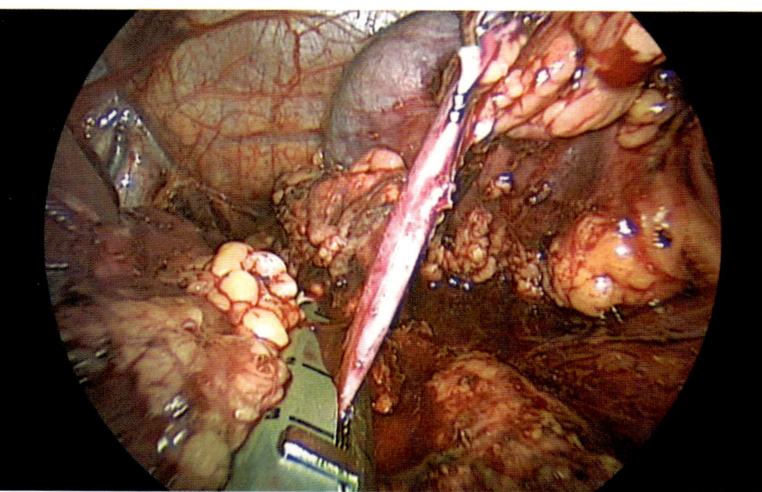

Fig. 17: The renal vein is divided with the Endo GIA™ stapler

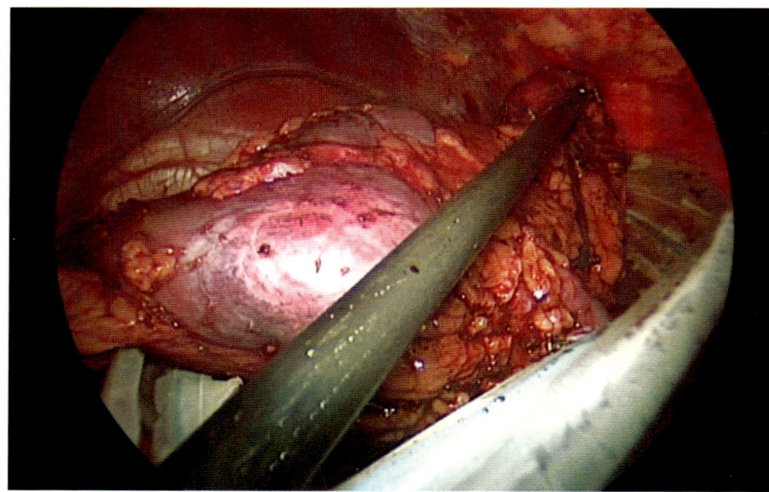

Fig. 18: The specimen is placed in a 15 mm Endo Catch™ bag

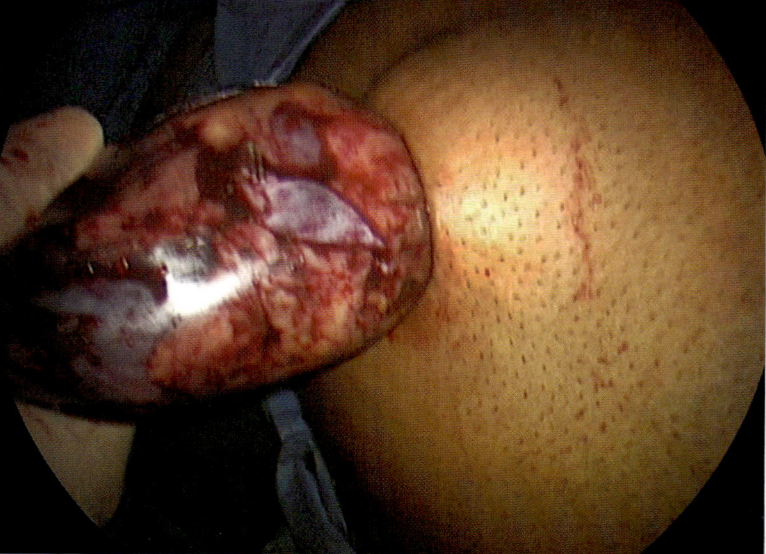

Fig. 19: The single port device and wound protector are removed, the specimen is removed through the perumbilical incision

REFERENCES

1. Skrekas G, Papalois VE, Mitsis M, et al. Laparoscopic live donor nephrectomy: a step forward in kidney transplantation? JSLS. 2003;7:197-206.
2. Eng M. The role of laparoscopic donor nephrectomy in renal transplantation. Am Surg. 2010;76:349-53.
3. Ramasamy R, Afaneh C, Katz M, et al. Comparison of complications of laparoscopic versus laparoendoscopic single site donor nephrectomy using the modified Clavien grading system. J Urol. 2011;186:1386-90.
4. Canes D, Berger A, Aron M, et al. Laparo-endoscopic single site (LESS) versus standard laparoscopic left donor nephrectomy: matched-pair comparison. Eur Urol. 2010;57:95-101.
5. Siqueira TM, Paterson RF, Kuo RL, et al. The use of blunt-tipped 12 mm trocars without fascial closure in laparoscopic live donor nephrectomy. JSLS. 2004;8:47-50.
6. Rodrigue JR, Cross NJ, Newman RC, et al. Patient-reported outcomes for open versus laparoscopic living donor nephrectomy. Prog Transplant. 2006;16:162-9.
7. Rais-Bahrami S, Montag S, Atalla MA, et al. Laparoendoscopic single-site surgery of the kidney with no accessory trocars: an initial experience. J Endourol. 2009;23:1319-24.
8. Gimenez E, Leeser DB, Wysock JS, et al. Laparoendoscopic single site live donor nephrectomy: initial experience. J Urol. 2010;184:2049-53.
9. Afaneh C, Ramasamy R, Leeser DB et al. Is right-sided laparoendoscopic single-site donor nephrectomy feasible? J Urol. 2011;186:1386-90.
10. Afaneh C, Sheth S, Aull M, et al. Laparoendoscopic single site nephrectomy in obese living renal donors. Endourology 2011 [in press].

10

Chapter

Robotic Nephroureterectomy with Resection of Distal Bladder Cuff

Jan Colli, Benjamin R Lee

INTRODUCTION AND INDICATIONS

Indications for nephroureterectomy include organ-confined urothelial carcinoma involving the renal pelvis or middle to upper ureter. Additional indications include end-stage upper tract disease due to ureterolithiasis or recurrent infections resulting in chronic pyelonephroureteritis and leading to a nonfunctioning kidney with lower tract calculus. Indications for robotic nephroureterectomy are the same as for open nephroureterectomy. This chapter focuses on oncological principles of robotic nephroureterectomy.

In 2011, an estimated 2,270 new cases of upper tract urothelial carcinoma were diagnosed in the United States, and approximately 790 patients died of this disease.[1] Oncologic principles for treatment involve en bloc removal of the kidney, ureter and an ipsilateral bladder cuff. Open radical nephroureterectomy has been the gold standard for patients with normal contralateral kidney.[2] Laparoscopic nephrectomy techniques were first described by Clayman[3] in 1991. The technique evolved to laparoscopic nephroureterectomy in 2002 by McNeill.[4] Robotic nephroureterectomy was first described by Authors in 2006.[5-7] They describe and outline their technique for robotic nephroureterectomy.

TECHNIQUE

Equipment and Patient Positioning

Equipment and sutures for robotic nephroureterectomy are listed in Table 1. After general anesthesia is administered to the patient, an orogastric tube and Foley catheter are inserted and secured. Initially, the patient is placed in a modified lateral position with a gel bolster and pressure points padded.

Trocar Placement

In a paramedian location, a Veress needle is used to insufflate the abdomen. Once the abdominal pressure reaches 15 mm Hg, a 12 mm port is placed lateral and slightly cephalic to the umbilicus. Next, under direct vision, the two 8 mm robotic arm ports are placed. The cephalic port is placed 8 cm cephalic to the camera port, in a longitudinal pararectus line. The caudal robot port is placed 8 cm lateral to the camera port, creating a V-pattern aligned toward the focus of the kidney. A 12 mm working port is placed caudal and medial to the lower robotic port. Figure 1 illustrates port sites and trocar placement.

Nephrectomy Procedure

The nephrectomy part of the nephroureterectomy is performed identical to a standard laparoscopic radical nephrectomy. The lateral peritoneum is incised along the white line of Toldt, and the colon is reflected medially. The splenic or hepatic flexure is incised. Next, the anterior surface of Gerota's fascia is exposed by incising the thin colorenal attachments (Fig. 2). On the right side, the duodenum is gently mobilized medially with sharp, cold dissection.

Once the colon is mobilized, the lower pole is elevated and the ureter and gonadal vein are identified. A clip is placed on the ureter to prevent the risk of malignant cells migrating distally during the manipulation of the kidney (Fig. 3).

Next, dissection toward the renal hilum continues with the lower pole of the kidney elevated along with ureter to help expose the renal hilum (Fig. 4).

The Maryland dissector is used to help divide adventitial attachments and isolate the renal vein (Fig. 5).

The renal artery is identified and attachments released such that a gastrointestinal anastomosis (GIA) can pass freely around the vessel (Fig. 6). A plane is developed above the hilum, caudal to the adrenal gland. The attachments between the adrenal gland and the upper pole of the kidney are divided with bipolar cauterization. Care should be taken to identify the adrenal vein. The renal artery is ligated with

Table 1: Select equipment and sutures for robotic laparoscopic renal surgery
Monopolar cautery curved endoshears (Intuitive)
Maryland bipolar cautery dissector (Intuitive)
Large needle drivers (Robotic, Intuitive)
8 mm robotic trocar/port (x 2) (Intuitive)
12 mm and 5 mm bladed and dilating trocars/ports (Ethicon)
Titanium clips, 5 mm or 10 mm automatic applier (Ethicon)
Lapra-Ty absorbable clips and applier (Ethicon)
Weck Hem-o-loc clips and laparoscopic clip applier (Weck)
5 mm endoshears (Ethicon)
5 mm locking graspers (Ethicon)
5 mm blunt Kitners (Ethicon)
5 mm laparoscopic needle drivers (Ethicon)
Suction-Irrigator (5 mm and 10 mm) (Stryke-Flow)
Laparoscopic vascular bulldog clamps (applier and remover) (Ethicon)
Endocatch bags (10 mm and 15 mm) (Aesculap)
Carter-Thomason needlepoint passer (Medical CloSure System)
Surgicel (Johnson and Johnson)
Vessel loops (red, blue)
3-0 Vicryl, SH needle, 2-0 Vicryl, CT-1 and CT-2 needles (Ethicon)
Rigid cystocope and resectoscope with Collins knife
Jackson-Pratt drain and Foley catheter

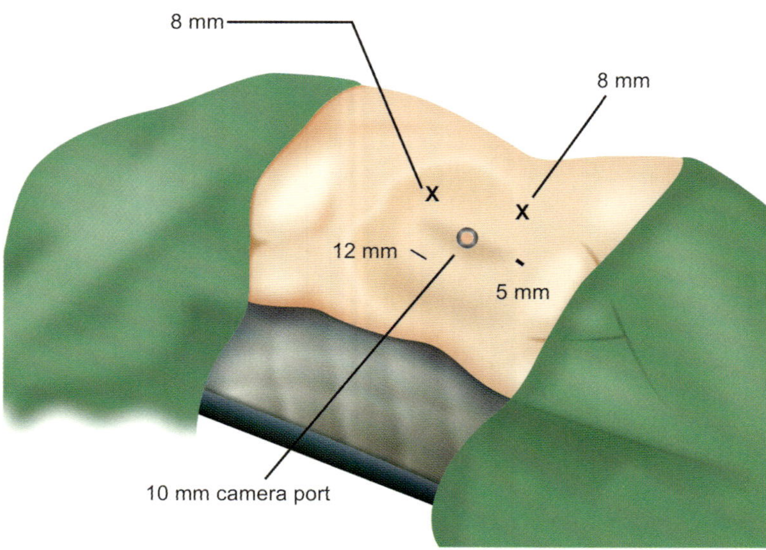

Fig. 1: Port sites and trocar placement

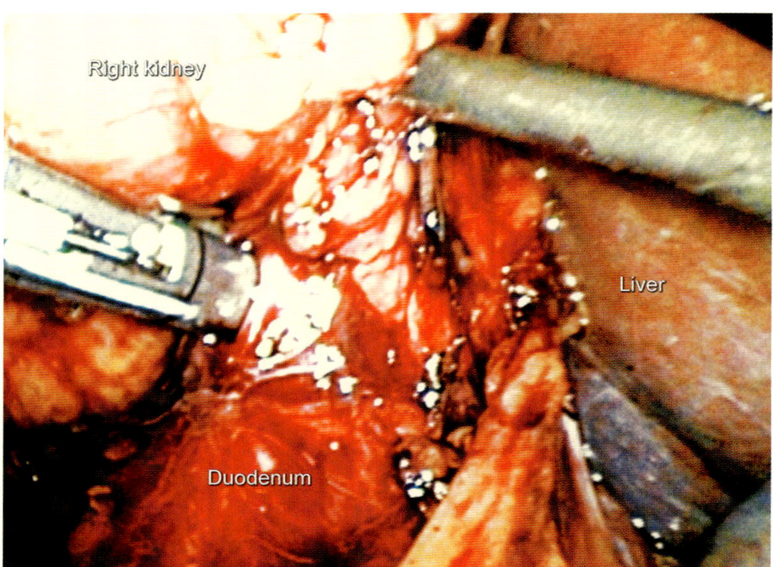

Fig. 2: Isolation of kidney with separation of intestinal attachments

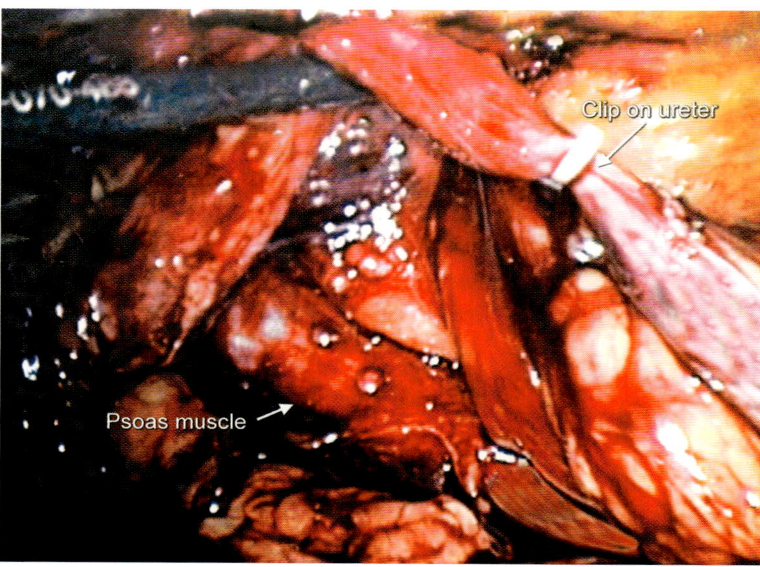

Fig. 3: Isolation of ureter, with early placement of clip on ureter, to prevent distal migration of malignant cells

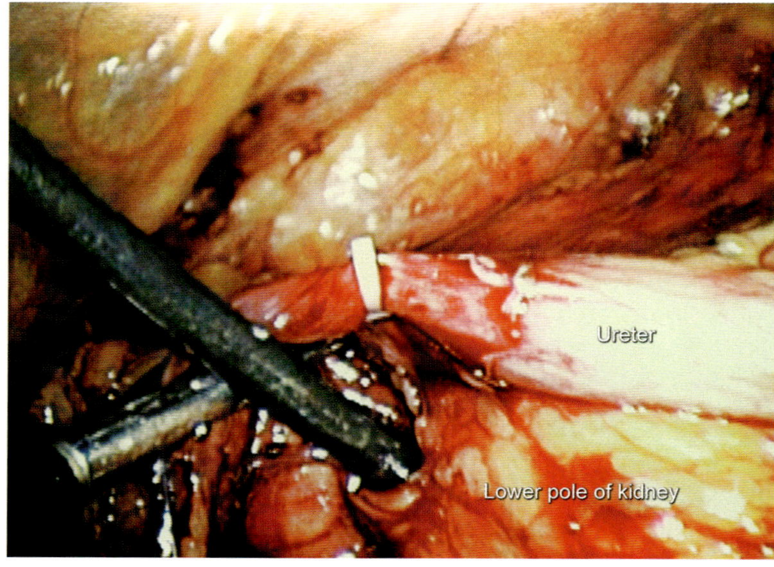

Fig. 4: Ureter placed on traction and dissection of lower edge of renal hilum

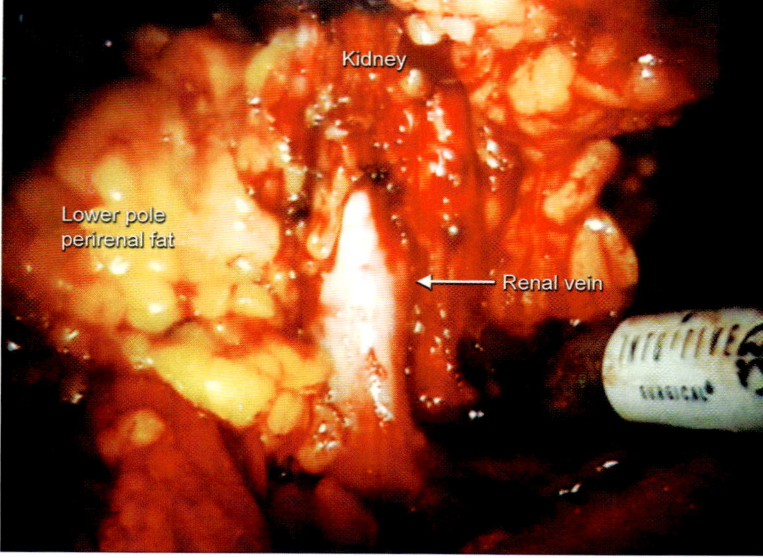

Fig. 5: Renal vein isolation

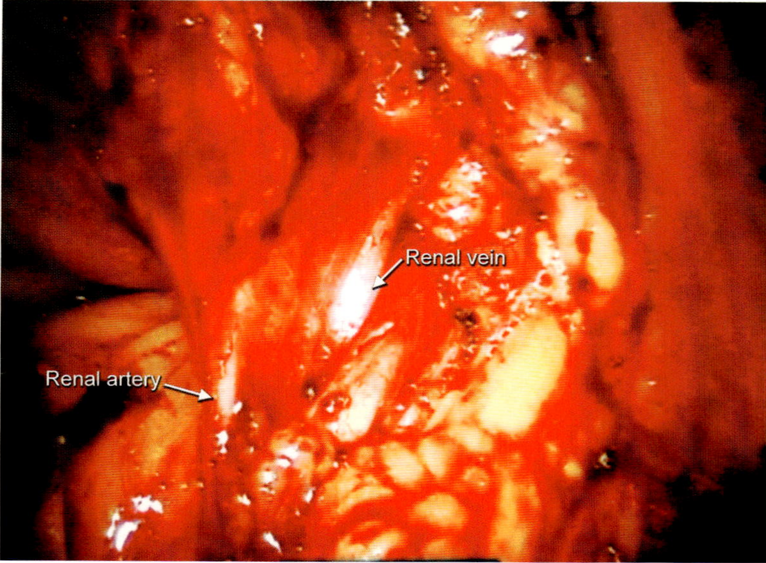

Fig. 6: Renal hilar dissection

the endovascular stapler. Once the renal artery is divided, the vein can likewise be divided with the endoscopic vascular stapler. Next, attachments to the upper pole of the kidney are mobilized.

As the final step in the nephrectomy portion, the lateral attachments to the kidney are isolated and divided. The ureter is isolated from surrounding retroperitoneal tissue distally to the iliac brim.

Dilemma of the Distal Ureter

A variety of techniques have been described to secure the distal ureter in a minimal invasive manner.[8-16] However, there has been concern about the oncologic control of urothelial carcinoma with minimal invasive techniques.[17]

The first technique described in the literature, involves transurethral resection of the ureteral orifice—'pluck' technique.[9] In this method, the patient is placed in the lithotomy position and endoscopic resection of the intramural ureteral orifice is performed until perivesical fat is visualized and the ureter is completely detached from the bladder, allowing for it to be 'plucked' during the laparoscopic dissection.[9] There is great concern regarding 'tumor spillage' into the peritoneal cavity and authors therefore adapted a modification which involves early ligation of the ureter.[10-14] Another minimal invasive technique involves intussusception 'stripping' technique.[14] During this method, a ureteral catheter is inserted at the start of the procedure, and during the nephrectomy portion of the operation, the ureter is dissected as distally as possible and ligated. The ureteral catheter is secured to the transected ureter. The patient is repositioned in the lithotomy position, and by using traction on the ureteral catheter, the distal ureter is intussuscepted into the bladder. A resectoscope is used to release the distal ureter. Another technique, described by Gill et al.,[15] involves a transvesical laparoscopic approach, using two transvesical 2 mm suprapubic trocars to secure the ureteral orifice with a loop ligature placed around the ureteral stent creating a closed system, and a Collins knife is then used to excise the ureteral orifice.

Distal Ureterectomy and Bladder Cuff Procedure

Our technique includes a combination of cystoscopic and robotic techniques. The ureter had undergone early ligation (at the time of the nephrectomy) to prevent distal tumor migration followed by a coalescent of cystoscopic and then robotic transperitoneal circumferential excision of bladder cuff. The patient is repositioned into dorsal lithotomy position and a resectosope is introduced into the bladder. A 2 cm margin around the distal ureter is circumscribed with the Collins knife through all the bladder layers (Fig. 7), until perirenal fat is encountered.

Next, the robot is redocked, and the remaining ports are adjusted to position the camera port now periumbilical and a robotic arm is placed on the contralateral side, 8 cm from the robotic camera port. The ureter is isolated from the iliac vessels (Fig. 8) and followed all the way down to the intramural portion at the ureterovesical junction.

The ureter is retracted cephalad and dissected down to its insertion into the bladder (Fig. 9).

The overlying detrusor fibers are dissected exposing the intramural ureter. A bladder cuff is circumferentially incised 2 cm around the distal ureter (Fig. 10).

The dissection is carried down to the cystotomy previously made by the Collins knife. The bladder is entered as the bladder cuff is transected en bloc with the distal ureter (Fig. 11).

The bladder cuff, ureter and kidney are placed in an endocatch bag taking precautions to ensure no tumor spillage. The cystotomy is closed, mucosa to mucosa, watertight and tension-free with a two-layer closure of absorbable suture (Figs 12 and 13).

The midline ports are connected and the specimen is extracted within the endocatch bag. A Jackson-Pratt drain is passed through the lateral port and positioned in proximity to the bladder closure. A urethral catheter is left in place for a minimal of 5 days. Although removal of the distal ureter via this technique requires moving the patient to lithotomy position after the nephrectomy portion, doctors feel this method offers superb oncological advantage compared to the other methods of minimal invasive distal ureterectomy. Overall, prior studies have found similar long-term oncological results when comparing open nephroureterectomy to minimal invasive nephroureterectomy.[16,18] While at the same time, laparoscopic and robotic techniques have less morbidity than open surgery and offer distinct advantages for the patient with upper tract urothelial carcinoma.

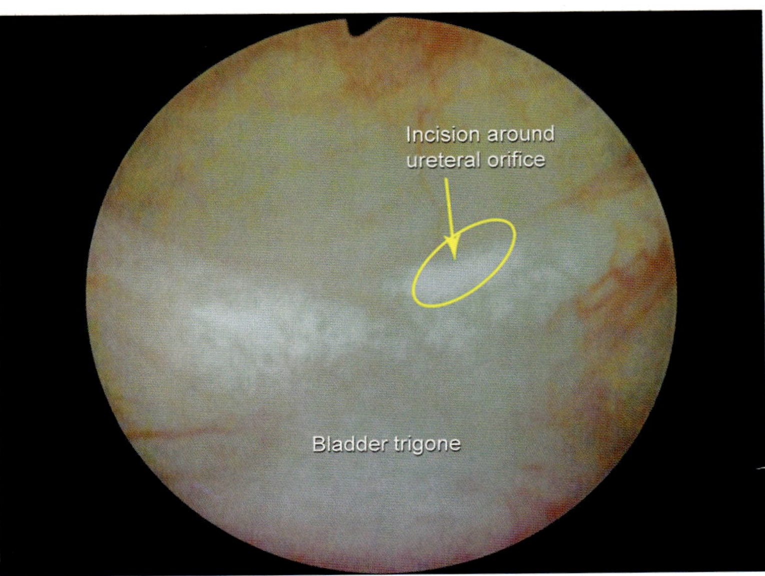

Fig. 7: Transurethral resection of ureteral orifice

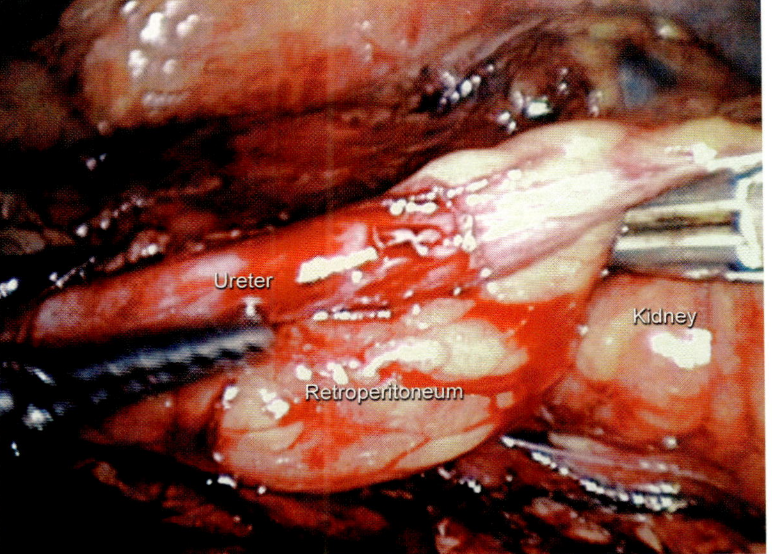

Fig. 8: Separation of ureter from retroperitoneal tissue

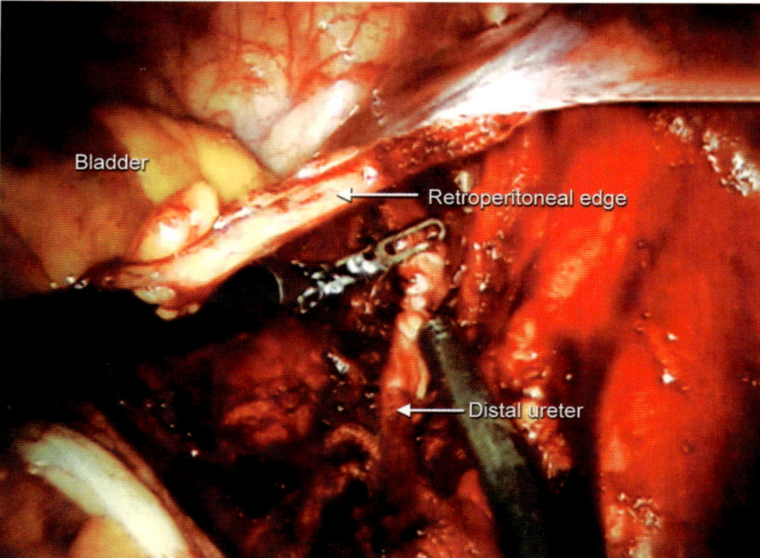

Fig. 9: Isolation of ureter, down to bladder

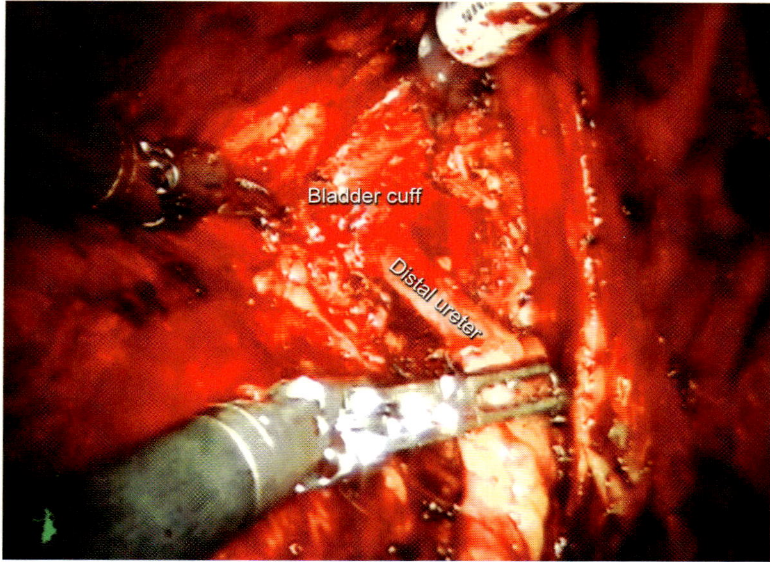

Fig. 10: Incision of bladder cuff around distal ureter

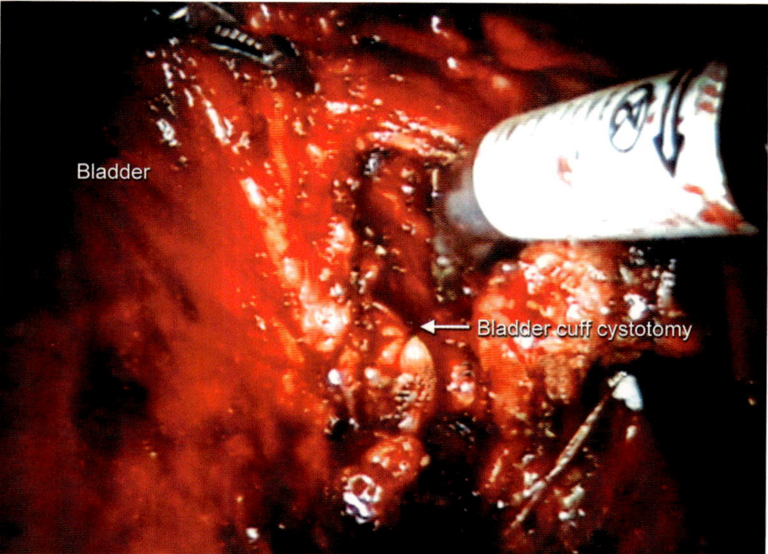

Fig. 11: Bladder cuff transected, and distal ureter and bladder cuff removed en bloc with kidney

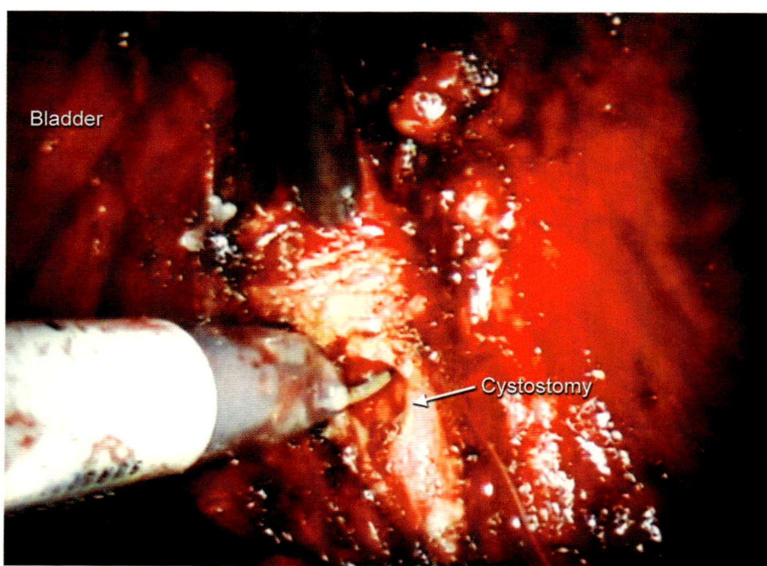

Fig. 12: First layer closure of cystotomy

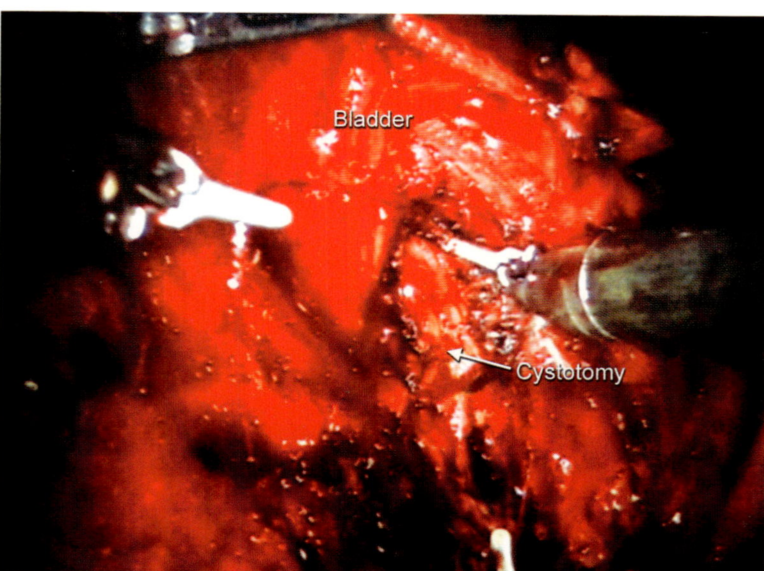

Fig. 13: Second layer closure of cystotomy

REFERENCES

1. American Cancer Society, Facts and Figures 2010, Atlanta, GA: American Cancer Society; 2010.
2. Sagalowsky A et al. Management of urothelial tumors of the renal pelvis and ureter. In: Wein A, et al. (Eds). Campbell-Walsh Urology, 9th edition. Philadelphia: WB Saunders; 2007. pp. 1653-87.
3. Clayman R, Kavoussi L, Albala D. Laparoscopic nephrectomy: initial case report. J Urol. 1991;146(2):278-82.
4. McNeill S, Tolley D. Laparoscopic nephroureterectomy for upper tract transitional cell carcinoma. Arch Esp Urol. 2002;55(6):595-601.
5. Hu J, Silletti J, Williams S. Initial experience with robot-assisted minimally-invasive nephroureterectomy. J Endourol. 2008;22(4): 699-704.
6. Park SY, Jeong W, Ham WS, et al. Initial experience of robotic nephroureterectomy: a hybrid-port technique. BJU Int. 2009;104(11): 1718-21.
7. Nanigian DK, Smith W, Ellison LM. Robot-assisted laparoscopic nephroureterectomy. J Endourol. 2006;20:463-5.
8. Steinberg J, Matin S. Laparoscopic radical nephroureterectomy: dilemma of the distal ureter. Curr Opin Urol. 2004;14:61-5.

9. Jones DR, Moisey CU. A cautionary tale of the modified pluck' nephroureterectomy. Br J Urol. 1993;71: 486.
10. Wong C, Leveillee RJ. Hand-assisted laparoscopic nephroureterectomy with cystoscopic en bloc excision of the distal ureter and bladder cuff. J Endourol. 2002;16:329-32.
11. Kurzer E, Leveillee RJ, Bird VG. Combining hand-assisted laparoscopic nephroureterectomy with cystoscopic circumferential excision of the distal ureter without primary closure of the bladder cuff—is it safe? J Urol. 2006;175:63-7.
12. Gonzalez CM, Batler RA, Schoor RA, et al. A novel endoscopic approach towards resection of the distal ureter with surrounding bladder cuff during hand assisted laparoscopic nephroureterectomy. J Urol. 2001;165:483-5.
13. Stifelman MD, Sosa RE, Andrade A, et al. Hand-assisted laparoscopic nephroureterectomy for the treatment of transitional cell carcinoma of the upper urinary tract. Urology. 2000;56:741-7.
14. Giovansili B, Peyromaure M, Saïghi D, et al. Stripping technique for endoscopic management of distal ureter during nephroureterectomy: experience of 32 procedures. Urology. 2004;64:448-52.
15. Gill IS, Soble JJ, Miller SD, et al. A novel technique for management of the en bloc bladder cuff and distal ureter during laparoscopic nephroureterectomy. J Urol. 1999;161:430-4.
16. Tan BJ, Ost M, Lee BR. Laparoscopic nephroureterectomy with resection of bladder-cuff resection: techniques and outcomes. J Endourol. 2005;19(6):664-76.
17. Hetherington JW, Ewing R, Philp NH. Modified nephroureterectomy: a risk of tumour implantation. Br J Urol. 1986;58:368-70.
18. Waldert M, Remzi M, Klingler HC, et al. The oncological results of laparoscopic nephroureterectomy for upper tract transitional cell cancer are equal to those of open nephroureterectomy. BJU Int. 2009;103(1):66-70.

11

Chapter

Laparoscopic and Robot-Assisted Adrenalectomy

Jennifer K Yates, Samay Jain, Ravi Munver

INTRODUCTION

Adrenalectomy and partial adrenalectomy (PA) are indicated for the management of benign and malignant conditions, including functional tumors, masses with radiographic findings suspicious for malignancy, solitary metastatic lesions and nonfunctioning symptomatic lesions. Laparoscopic adrenalectomy (LA) was first described in 1992, and has gained popularity for the management of benign adrenal tumors. In many cases, malignant adrenal masses—including metastatic disease to the adrenal gland—can also be managed with LA. Compared with open adrenalectomy, LA has been associated with a decrease in postoperative pain, shorter hospital stay and improved cosmetic results.[1-4] Relative contraindications for LA include extensive adhesions from prior surgery, morbid obesity, uncorrected coagulopathy and cardiopulmonary disease that preclude hypercapnea that is associated with pneumoperitoneum. These cases must be evaluated on an individual basis, and the surgeon's experience and comfort level must be taken into consideration. While LA may be a feasible approach for many adrenal masses, a low threshold to convert to open surgery should be maintained. The robotic platform can also be utilized for adrenalectomy and PA, with indications similar to that of LA.

Preoperative patient evaluation includes a thorough history and physical examination, metabolic evaluation to determine whether the lesion is functional, and radiographic imaging. In this chapter, the surgical approaches to laparoscopic and robot-assisted laparoscopic adrenalectomy (RALA) and PA will be discussed.

LEFT TRANSPERITONEAL LAPAROSCOPIC ADRENALECTOMY

Left LA can be performed via a transperitoneal or retroperitoneal approach. The focus of this section will be on the transperitoneal approach, with a comment on modifications for retroperitoneal LA later in the chapter.

1. *Position:* The patient is placed in the right lateral decubitus position. The table can be flexed to increase the intra-abdominal working area. A bean bag or gel rolls are used to support the patient in the lateral decubitus position. An axillary roll is placed two fingerbreadths below the axilla. The lower arm is positioned on a well-padded armboard. The upper arm is supported either with a commercially available device or in another fashion such that it is parallel to the lower arm. The lower leg is bent and the upper leg remains straight, with adequate pillows and padding. Once all of the areas prone to pressure are well-padded, the patient is secured using 3-inch tape. Patient position is shown in Figure 1. A foley catheter and orogastric tube should be placed before starting the procedure.
2. *Trocar Placement:* A skin incision is made 2 cm superior to the umbilicus and left of the midline. Insufflation with a Veress needle to 15 mm Hg or a Hassan technique is used to obtain pneumoperitoneum. A 5 mm or 12 mm trocar is placed at this site and a laparoscope is used to inspect the abdominal contents (Table 1). A 5 mm or 12 mm trocar is placed 2 cm below the xiphoid process to the left of the midline, and is used for a 30-degree laparoscope lens. A 12 mm trocar is placed 2 cm above the umbilicus in the midclavicular line (MCL). An accessory 5 mm trocar can be placed below the costal margin at the anterior axillary line (AAL) to assist in retraction of the kidney and other maneuvers. The periumbilical and MCL trocars are used for instrument passage, starting with atraumatic grasping forceps at the periumbilical trocar, and ultrasonic shears or alternative energy device in the MCL trocar. Figure 2 demonstrates two options for trocar placement during left transperitoneal LA.
3. The descending colon is mobilized along the white line of Toldt (Fig. 3), avoiding entry into Gerota's fascia. The spleen is mobilized extensively to allow visualization of the upper pole of the kidney and adrenal gland.
4. Dissection and exposure of the adrenal gland can begin either at the inferomedial aspect or the superomedial aspect. Initial dissection of the inferomedial aspect of the adrenal gland is performed in order to identify the renal hilum.
5. The renal hilum—usually the renal vein—is identified and used as a landmark to identify the adrenal vein. A right-angle clamp

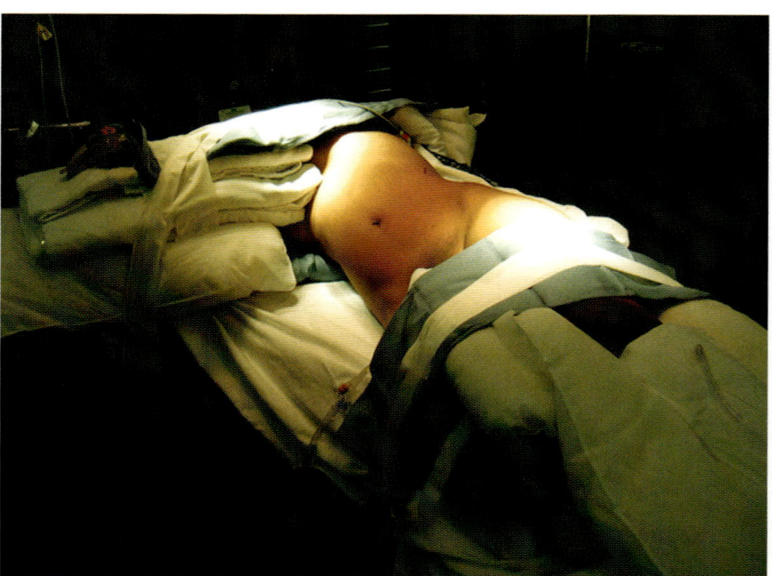

Fig. 1: Patient positioning for left transperitoneal laparoscopic adrenalectomy

Table 1: Instrumentation for laparoscopic adrenalectomy
Veress needle
5 mm or 10 mm laparoscope with 0 and 30-degree lenses
12 mm trocars
5 mm trocars
Laparoscopic atraumatic grasping forceps
Laparoscopic right angle
Ultrasonic shears
Laparoscopic liver retractor and holder
Bipolar vessel-sealing device
Laparoscopic Kittner
Laparoscopic suction/irrigator
Laparoscopic ultrasound probe
Laparoscopic stapling device
Laparoscopic retrieval bag
Polymer or titanium hemostatic clips (5 mm or 10 mm)
Oxidized cellulose polymer
Other hemostatic agents (optional)
Fascial closure device

is used to dissect the adrenal vein (Fig. 4). Once completely free from surrounding structures, the left adrenal vein can be divided between hemostatic polymer clips or with a bipolar vessel-sealing device. Figure 5 demonstrates use of a bipolar vessel-sealing device to ligate the vein. If a bipolar vessel-sealing device is used, the tissue should be sealed in several areas before transecting the vein in the middle of the sealed tissue.

6. After division of the adrenal vein, the adrenal gland can be gently retracted medially. The parenchyma of the kidney is identified as seen in Figure 6, and the lateral attachments of the adrenal are divided. Any remaining medial attachments are also divided. The ultrasonic shears or bipolar vessel-sealing device can be used as the adrenal attachments are often highly vascular. Small arterial branches from the inferior phrenic or renal arteries can be encountered, and should be carefully divided with clips or the bipolar vessel-sealing device. Any additional superior attachments of the adrenal are divided. Figure 7 shows division of the remaining adrenal attachments using the bipolar vessel-sealing device.
7. The specimen is placed in a laparoscopic retrieval bag (Fig. 8). The pneumoperitoneum is decreased to 5 mm Hg and the adrenal bed is inspected for bleeding. Hemostatic maneuvers, such as the use of oxidized cellulose polymer, can be used based on surgeon preference. Oxidized cellulose polymer can be used in the setting of minor bleeding. If indicated, a hemostatic matrix such as Floseal™ can be used as well.
8. The specimen can be extracted from any of the trocar sites. A 12 mm trocar site will typically accommodate the specimen better than a 5 mm trocar site. Often, the trocar site incision will require enlargement in order to accommodate the specimen. After specimen extraction, all trocar sites larger than 10 mm are closed under direct vision using a fascial closure device. Inspection of the trocar sites after removal of the trocars should be performed to confirm the absence of bleeding. Skin incisions are closed using subcuticular sutures or skin staples.

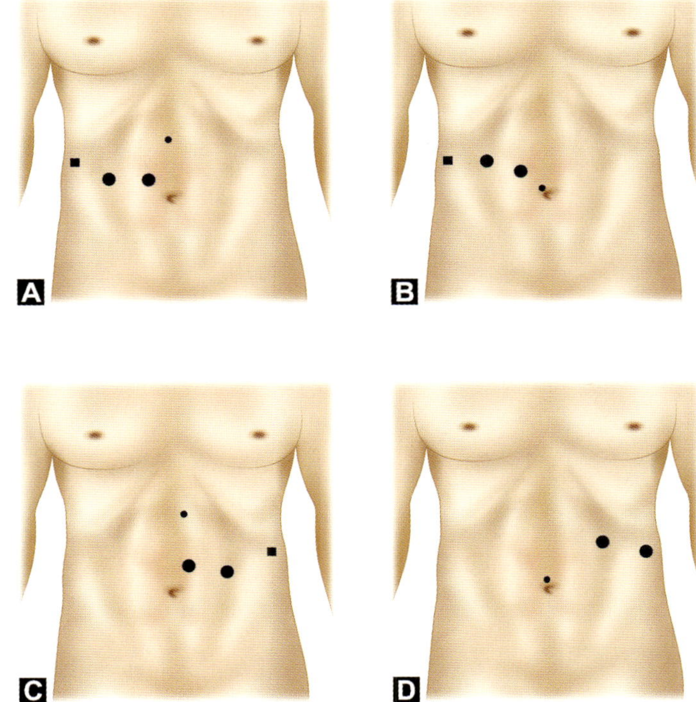

Figs 2A to D: (A and B) Right transperitoneal laparoscopic adrenalectomy trocar placement; (C and D) Trocar placement for left transperitoneal laparoscopic adrenalectomy

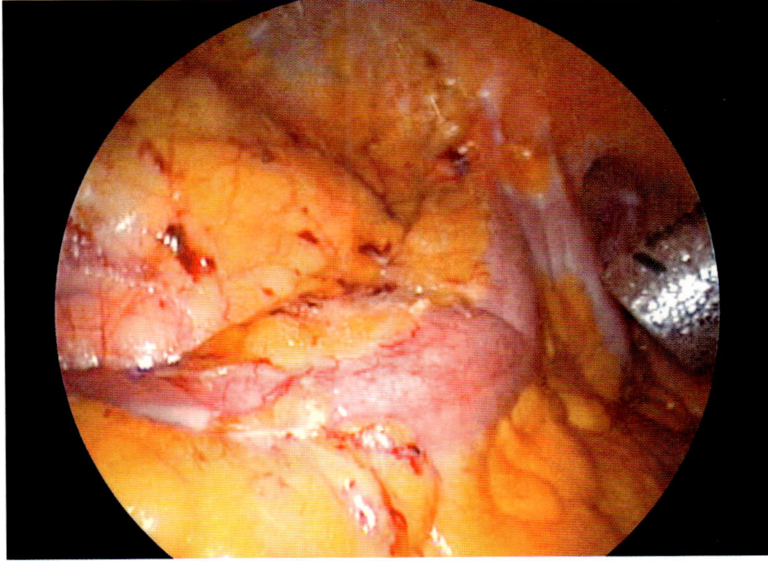

Fig. 3: The colon has been mobilized along the white line of Toldt to expose the kidney and left adrenal gland

RIGHT TRANSPERITONEAL LAPAROSCOPIC ADRENALECTOMY

1. *Position:* The patient is placed in the left lateral decubitus position. The table can be flexed to increase the intra-abdominal working area. A bean bag or gel rolls are used to support the patient in the lateral decubitus position. An axillary roll is placed two

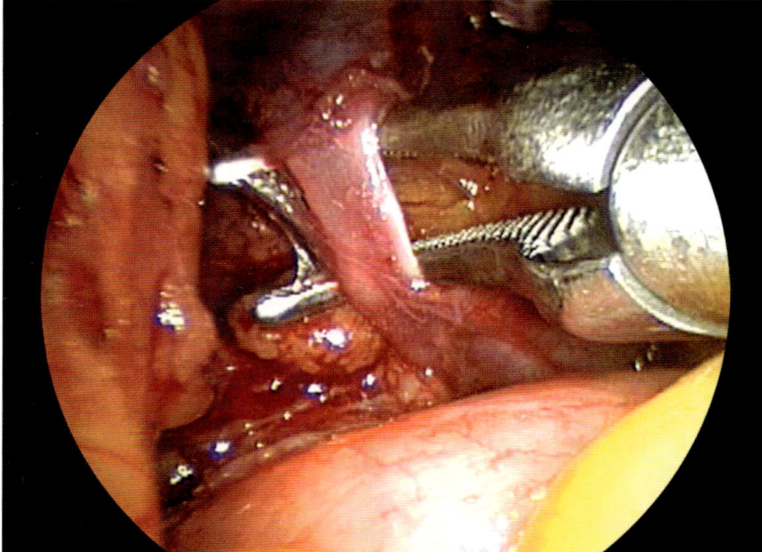

Fig. 4: A laparoscopic right-angle clamp is used to isolate the adrenal vein

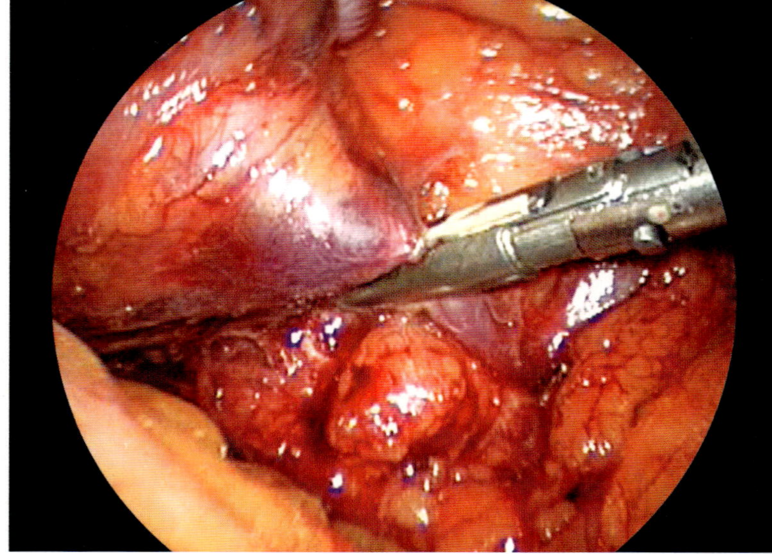

Fig. 5: The bipolar sealing device is used to seal the adrenal vein in several places before dividing the vein

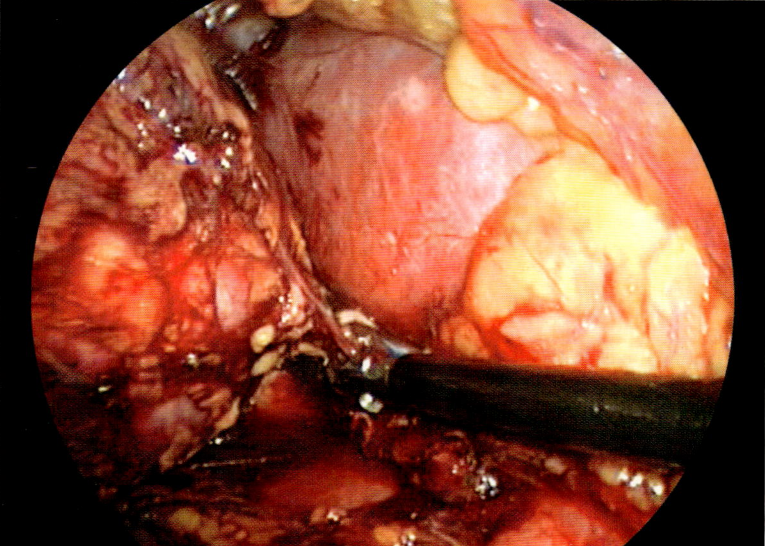

Fig. 6: After the adrenal vein is divided, the adrenal can be retracted medially to expose the kidney parenchyma and attachments of the adrenal gland

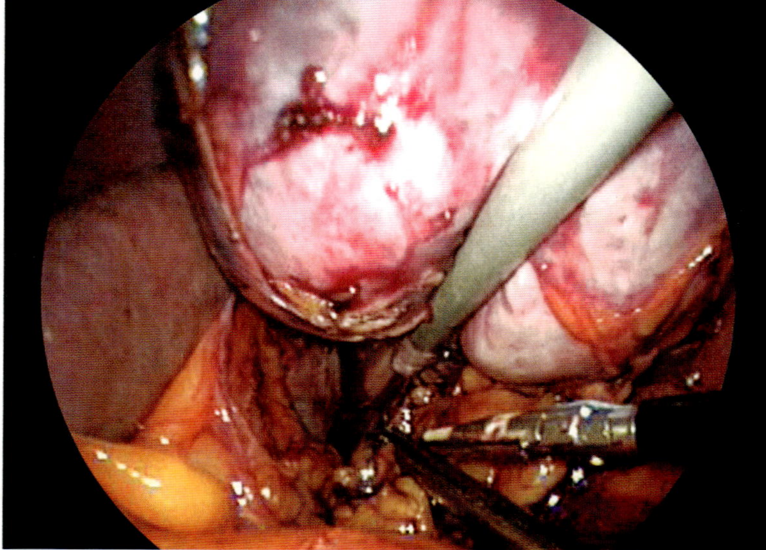

Fig. 7: The remaining medial attachments of the adrenal are divided. The adrenal mass can be seen at the top of the image

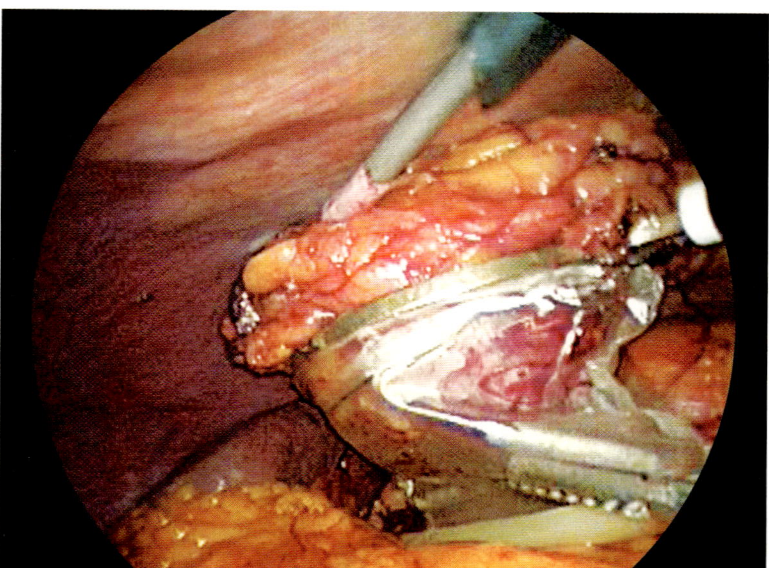

Fig. 8: The adrenal gland is placed in a laparoscopic retrieval bag

fingerbreadths below the axilla. The lower arm is positioned on a well-padded armboard. The upper arm is supported either with a commercially available device or in another fashion such that it is parallel to the lower arm. The lower leg is bent and the upper leg remains straight, with adequate pillows and padding. Once all of the areas prone to pressure are well-padded, the patient is secured using 3-inch tape. A foley catheter and orogastric tube should be placed before starting the procedure.

2. *Trocar Placement:* An incision is made to the right of the midline, 2 cm above and 2 cm lateral to the umbilicus. A Veress needle is introduced into the abdominal cavity through the incision, or alternatively, a Hassan technique is used, and the abdomen is insufflated to 15 mm Hg. A 12 mm trocar is placed at this site, and a laparoscope is used to inspect the abdominal contents. A 5 mm or 12 mm trocar is placed 2 cm below the xiphoid process to the right of the midline, and is used for a 30-degree laparoscope lens. A 5 mm or 12 mm trocar is placed 2 cm above the umbilicus in the MCL. An accessory 5 mm trocar is placed below the costal margin at the AAL. The instruments are advanced through the

trocars, including ultrasonic shears or alternative energy device through the periumbilical trocar, and atraumatic grasping forceps through the MCL trocar. The 5 mm accessory trocar is used for a liver retractor. The trocar configuration is shown in Figure 2.

3. The liver is first mobilized to expose the adrenal gland, starting with incision of the right triangular ligament. The posterior peritoneum is divided near the liver edge from the inferior vena cava to the abdominal side wall (Fig. 9). The liver must be mobilized extensively to provide adequate exposure to the inferior vena cava and the adrenal gland. A commercially available liver retractor is often useful to keep the liver out of the operative field, as shown in Figure 10. A Kocher maneuver is performed in order to expose the inferior vena cava. The medial aspect of the inferior vena cava can then be traced cephalad to identify the adrenal vein.
4. To localize the adrenal gland, the superior border of the kidney is identified and Gerota's fascia is entered (Fig. 11). The ultrasonic shears can be used for this maneuver, with a bipolar vessel-sealing device that can be used for more vascular tissue. The adrenal gland is identified along the superior-medial portion of the kidney.
5. Dissection is initiated lateral to the inferior vena cava, along the superomedial aspect of the adrenal gland. Branches of the renal artery and vein can be encountered here, and cautious dissection is warranted to avoid injury to these structures. The adrenal gland can be retracted laterally to expose the medial tissue with the assistance of a laparoscopic Kittner or a suction-irrigator device.
6. The right adrenal vein is identified and either clipped with hemostatic polymer clips and divided, or sealed and divided with a bipolar vessel-sealing device. Figure 12 demonstrates placement of a hemostatic polymer clip on the adrenal vein. The right adrenal vein is short in length, and care must be taken when manipulating and dividing the vein to avoid injury to the vein or inferior vena cava.
7. After division of the adrenal vein, the adrenal is dissected from the upper pole of the kidney and the surrounding structures. Ultrasonic shears or a bipolar vessel-sealing device is useful for the dissection of the adrenal tissue as this tissue often contains small perforating blood vessels. During dissection of the medial and lateral attachments of the adrenal, the renal artery and vein,

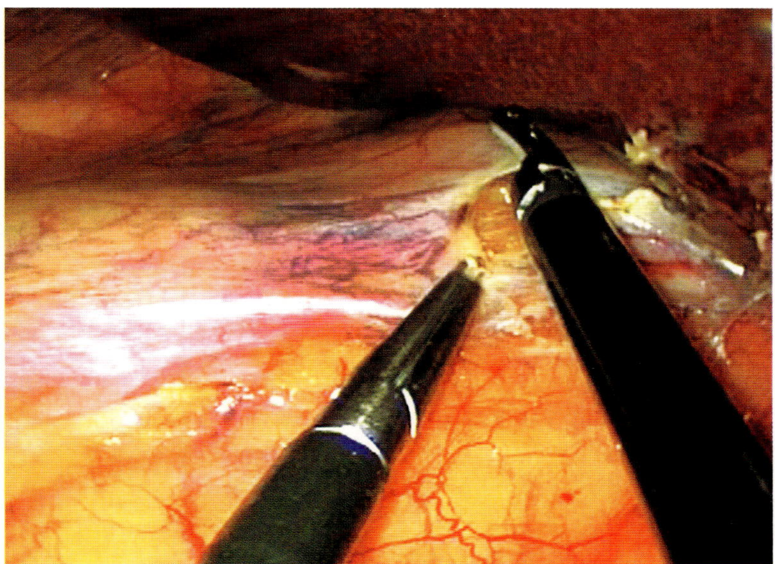

Fig. 9: Incision of the peritoneum overlying the kidney and adrenal gland to begin mobilization of the liver

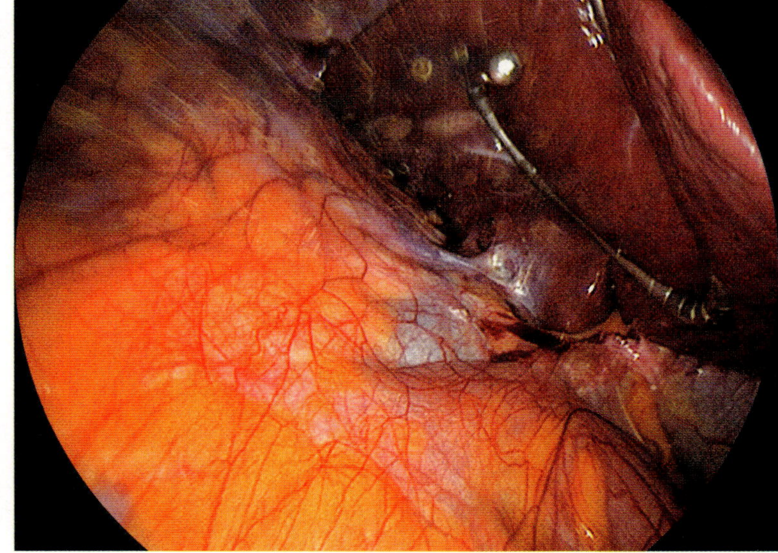

Fig. 10: A commercially available liver retractor can be used to provide exposure to the right adrenal gland

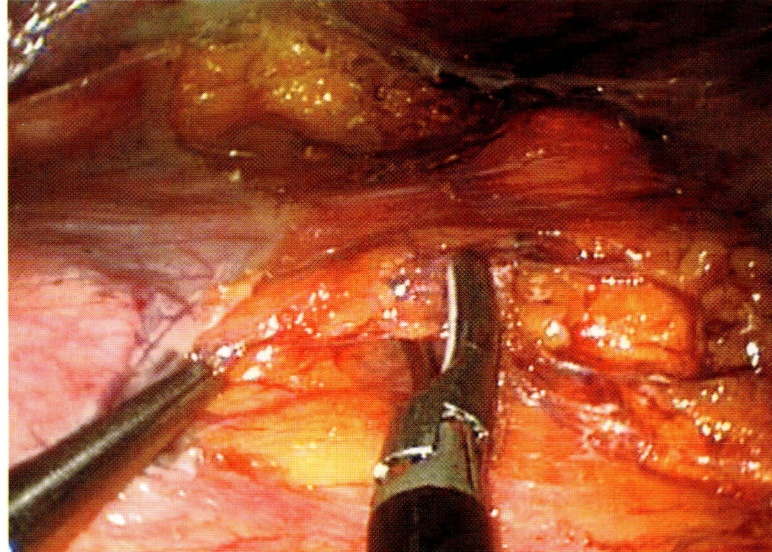

Fig. 11: Entry into Gerota's fascia using the bipolar sealing device to locate the adrenal gland

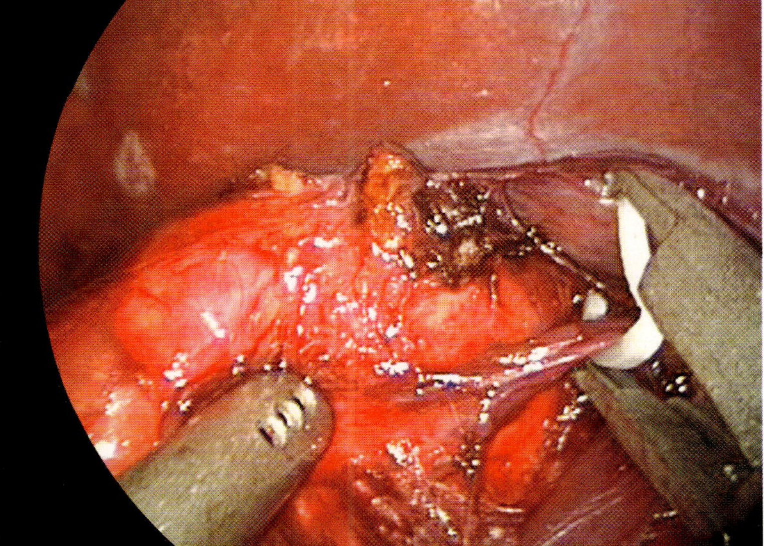

Fig. 12: Placement of a hemostatic polymer clip on the right adrenal vein. Note the short length and tangential course of the adrenal vein

including branches of the renal artery, can be seen and should be preserved. The bipolar vessel-sealing device is used in Figure 13 to divide adrenal attachments to the liver and psoas muscle.

8. The lateral attachments of the adrenal gland are divided last. Once the adrenal gland has been completely dissected from the surrounding structures it is placed into a laparoscopic retrieval bag. The pneumoperitoneum is lowered to 5 mm Hg and the area is inspected for bleeding. Hemostatic maneuvers, including the use of oxidized polymer matrix, can be used as needed, as shown in Figure 14. The specimen is removed through one of the 12 mm trocar sites, which can be enlarged as necessary. The trocars are removed under direct vision to confirm the absence of bleeding. Trocar sites 10 mm or larger are closed with a fascial closure device, and the skin incisions are closed with subcuticular sutures or skin staples.

RETROPERITONEAL LAPAROSCOPIC ADRENALECTOMY

Right Retroperitoneal Laparoscopic Adrenalectomy

A skin incision is made 2 cm below the costal margin in the midaxillary line and the underlying muscles are bluntly divided to gain access to the retroperitoneum. The peritoneum is gently retracted medially to provide room for the access device. A commercially available dissecting balloon is inserted into the incision, directed laterally and posterior to Gerota's fascia, and the balloon is inflated. A 30-degree lens can be placed through the balloon to assist in developing the retroperitoneal space. Once the retroperitoneal space is developed, a 10 mm or 12 mm trocar is placed and the retroperitoneal space is insufflated to 15 mm Hg. A 30-degree laparoscope lens is placed through the trocar, and additional trocars are placed under direct vision. While a variety of trocar configurations can be used, a common configuration involves placement of two additional trocars (5 mm and 12 mm) 3–4 cm cephalad to the initial trocar in the anterior and posterior axillary lines. If desired, an additional 5 mm trocar may be placed for additional retraction or suction. For proper orientation, the psoas muscle should be identified posteriorly, and the kidney should be displaced anteriorly and medially.

The first step of the retroperitoneal approach is medial reflection of the peritoneum, which in turn reflects the liver and ascending colon. The renal hilum is located medial to the psoas muscle. The adrenal vein is identified and controlled before manipulation of the adrenal gland.

Right retroperitoneal LA is initiated with identification of the inferior vena cava and the psoas muscle. The main adrenal vein is identified on the posterolateral aspect of the vena cava. The vein is isolated and divided, along with other anomalous vessels encountered during the dissection. Using ultrasonic shears, dissecting forceps, or a bipolar vessel-sealing device, the medial and inferior surfaces of the adrenal gland are dissected off the renal vein and vena cava. Small vessels, including branches from the inferior phrenic artery, are identified, clipped, and cut. The inferior surface of the adrenal gland is dissected off of the upper pole of the kidney. Finally, the lateral surface of the kidney is dissected free, and the specimen is placed in a laparoscopic retrieval bag. The pneumoperitoneum is lowered to 5 mm Hg and the adrenal bed is inspected for bleeding. The 12 mm trocar site can be enlarged for specimen removal, and trocar sites 10 mm and larger are closed with a fascial closure device. The skin is closed with subcuticular sutures or skin staples.

Left Retroperitoneal Laparoscopic Adrenalectomy

The configuration for left retroperitoneal LA is the mirror image of that used for the right side. Adrenalectomy begins with identification of the renal hilum. The renal artery is retracted caudally and blunt dissection helps to identify the left adrenal vein. The vein is then carefully dissected, isolated and divided. Next, the superior aspect of the adrenal is dissected from the diaphragm, and inferior phrenic vessels, if encountered, are divided. The lateral surface of the adrenal gland is dissected from the kidney. Cephalad retraction of the adrenal gland assists in dissection of the inferior surface from the kidney. Finally, the lateral surface of the adrenal gland is dissected free. The specimen is completely freed from its surrounding tissues and placed in a laparoscopic retrieval bag. The pneumoperitoneum is lowered to 5 mm Hg and the adrenal bed is inspected for bleeding. The 12 mm trocar site can be enlarged to allow specimen removal, and trocar sites 10 mm and larger are closed with a fascial closure device. Skin incisions are closed with subcuticular sutures or skin staples.

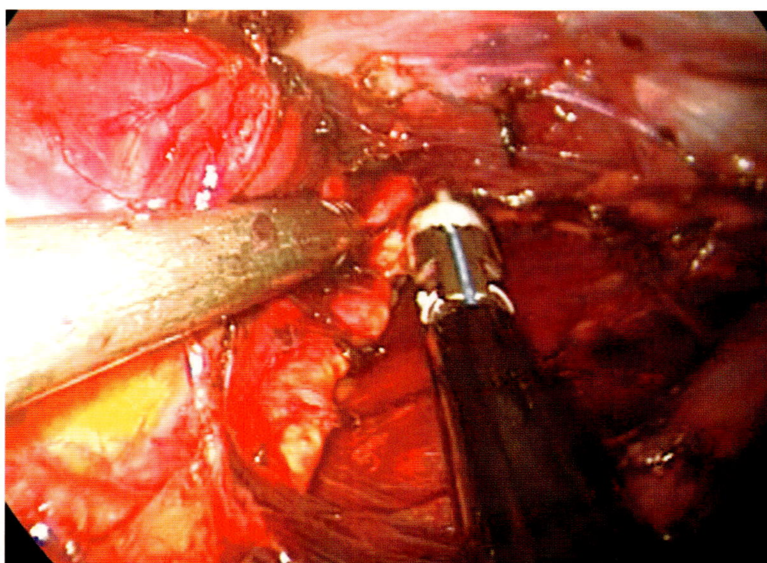

Fig. 13: After division of the adrenal vein, the adrenal gland is gently retracted away from the liver to allow division of the attachments to the liver and underlying psoas muscle. The bipolar sealing device is used to divide these attachments

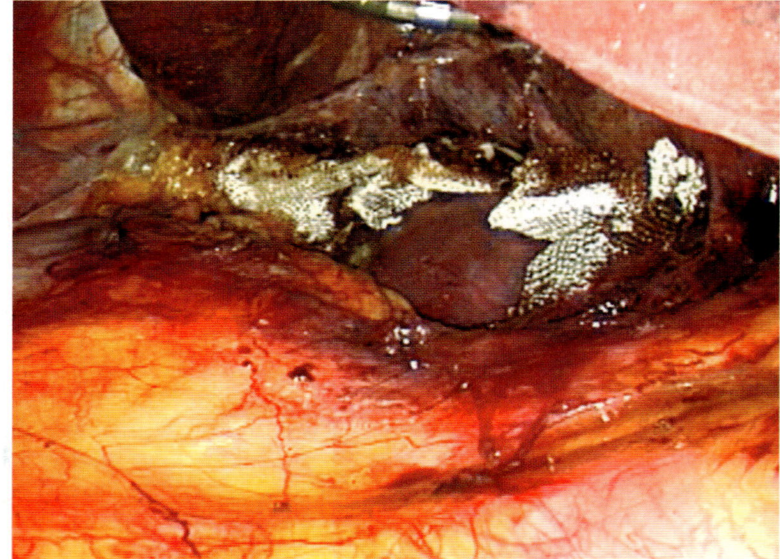

Fig. 14: After the adrenal gland has been placed in the laparoscopic specimen retrieval bag, the adrenal bed is inspected for any bleeding. Oxidized cellulose matrix can be placed in the adrenal bed to aid in hemostasis

ROBOT-ASSISTED LAPAROSCOPIC ADRENALECTOMY

1. Robot-assisted laparoscopic adrenalectomy requires several modifications to the standard transperitoneal LA. A three-arm approach, with rotation of the bed (the foot of the bed tilted away from the side of the surgery) is employed to facilitate docking of the robot. Trocar placement begins with placement of a 12 mm trocar lateral to the umbilicus, toward the side of the lesion. A 12 mm smooth, nonbladed trocar is placed in this location. The exact location varies depending on the body habitus of the patient. This trocar can be placed more lateral in larger patients to optimize visualization. Once the robotic laparoscope trocar is placed, two 8 mm robotic trocars are placed under direct vision in a triangulated fashion with a minimum distance of 8 cm between trocars to avoid robotic arm collision. A 12 mm assistant trocar is placed, usually caudad to the camera trocar, with 8 cm distance between the trocars. For right-sided procedures, a 5 mm trocar can be placed in the AAL for placement of a liver retractor. Trocar placement for left RALA is shown in Figure 15.
2. Recommended instrumentation for RALA is shown in Table 2. The fenestrated bipolar forceps are an ideal tool for both robot-assisted laparoscopic (RAL) kidney and adrenal surgery. The broad surface area of the instrument and rounded tip are idea for gentle dissection and bipolar cautery when working with vascular tissue. A fenestrated bipolar forceps in used for the left robotic arm and a monopolar scissors for the right arm. Alternatively, a Maryland bipolar forceps can be used for the left arm.
3. The steps for colon reflection and splenic mobilization (left side), liver and duodenal mobilization (right side), and identification of the adrenal vein are similar to those described above for laparoscopic transperitoneal adrenalectomy. When dissecting the adrenal vein, the assistant can advance a 10 mm laparoscopic right-angle dissector through the 12 mm assistant trocar. The assistant can also place hemostatic polymer clips on the adrenal vein as shown in Figure 16. Alternatively, the bipolar sealing device can be advanced through the assistant trocar to divide the vein.
4. Once the adrenal vein is divided, dissection of the adrenal gland from the surrounding tissue can be approached with several techniques. First, the fenestrated bipolar forceps are useful for hemostasis when working with vascular tissue, and can be used in combination with the monopolar scissors. Second, the assistant can utilize a bipolar vessel-sealing device through the 12 mm assistant trocar as shown in Figure 17. The remainder of the adrenalectomy proceeds as described in the previous sections, with the assistant trocar used to pass the bipolar sealing device and other instruments as indicated.

LAPAROSCOPIC AND ROBOT-ASSISTED LAPAROSCOPIC PARTIAL ADRENALECTOMY

1. Laparoscopic and RAL partial adrenalectomy is performed with the same configuration of trocars as used during laparoscopic and RAL total adrenalectomy.

Table 2: Instrumentation for robot-assisted total or partial adrenalectomy
Veress needle
12 mm robotic laparoscope with 0 and 30-degree lenses
5 mm or 10 mm laparoscope with 0 and 30-degree lenses (optional)
5 mm trocar
12 mm trocar
8 mm robotic trocars
Robotic fenestrated bipolar forceps
Robotic Maryland bipolar forceps
Robotic curved monopolar scissor
Laparoscopic suction/irrigator
Laparoscopic liver retractor and holder
Bipolar sealing device
Laparoscopic right angle
Laparoscopic Kittner
Laparoscopic ultrasound probe
Laparoscopic retrieval bag
Polymer or titanium hemostatic clips (5 mm or 10 mm)
Oxidized cellulose polymer
Other hemostatic agents (optional)
Fascial closure device

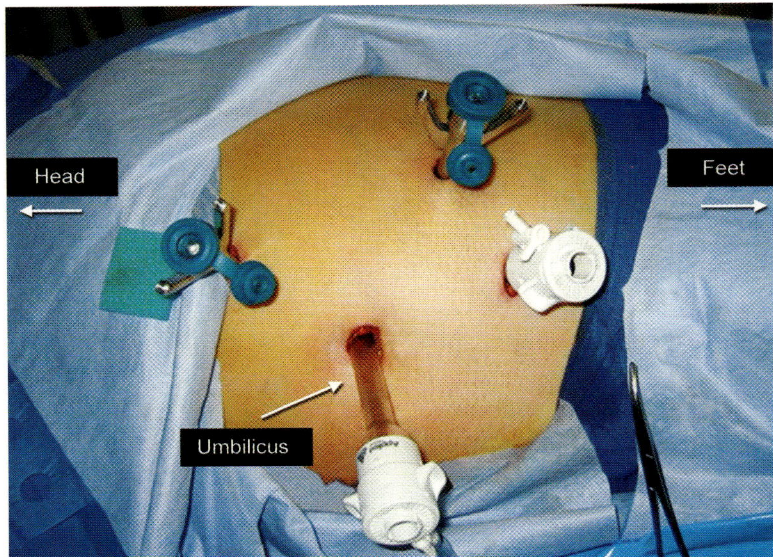

Fig. 15: Trocar placement for left robot-assisted laparoscopic adrenalectomy and partial adrenalectomy

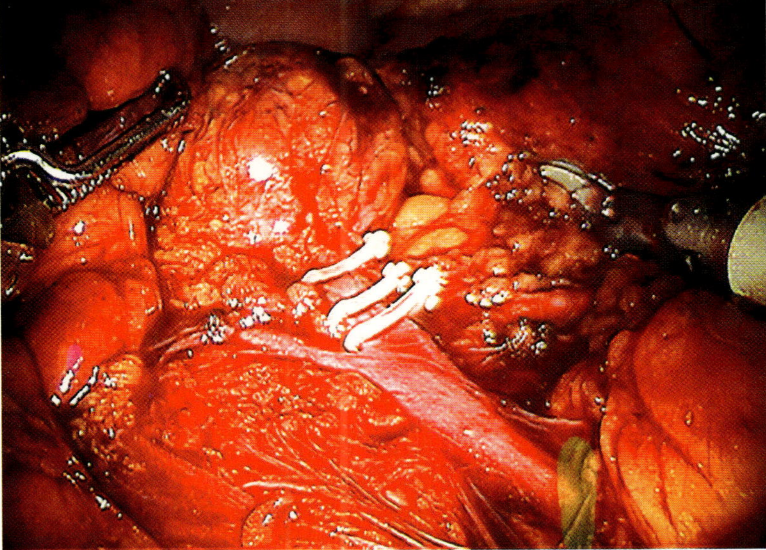

Fig. 16: The assistant has placed hemostatic polymer clips on the adrenal vein. The adrenal adenoma is seen beyond the third clip

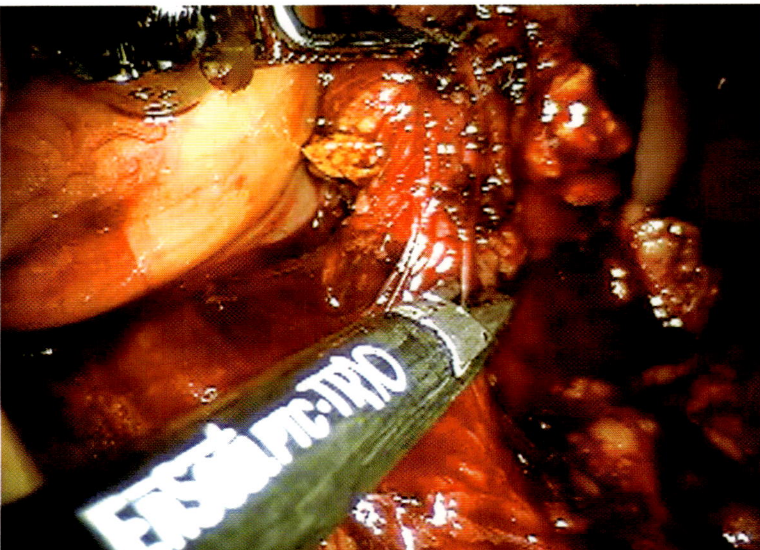

Fig. 17: The assistant can use the bipolar sealing device through the assistant trocar to divide the vascular tissue around the adrenal gland

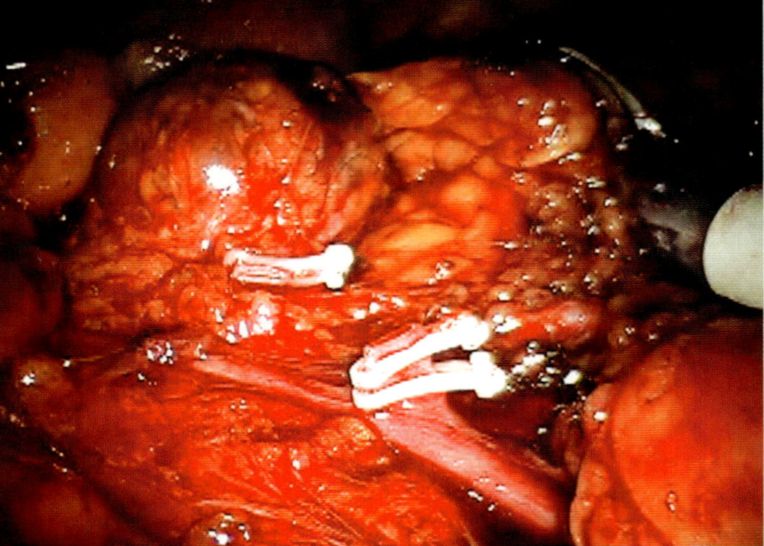

Fig. 18: The branch of the adrenal vein draining the adrenal mass is selectively divided, while the branch draining the normal adrenal is left intact

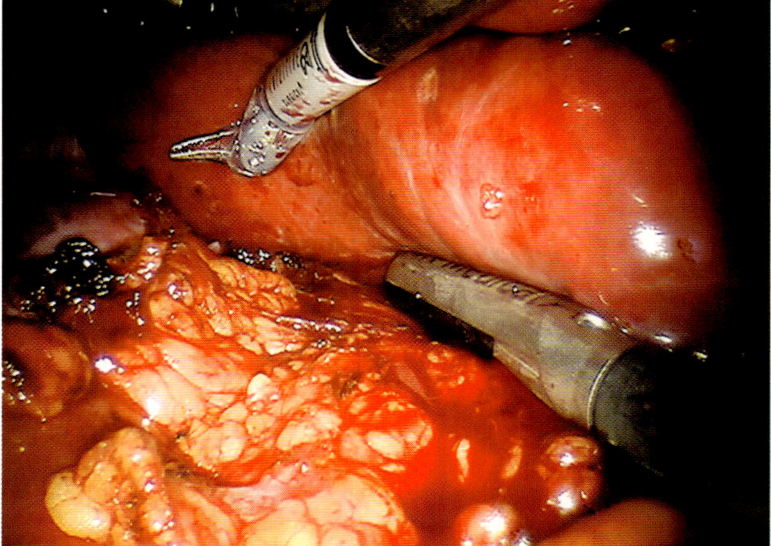

Fig. 19: Use of the ultrasound to identify the adrenal mass

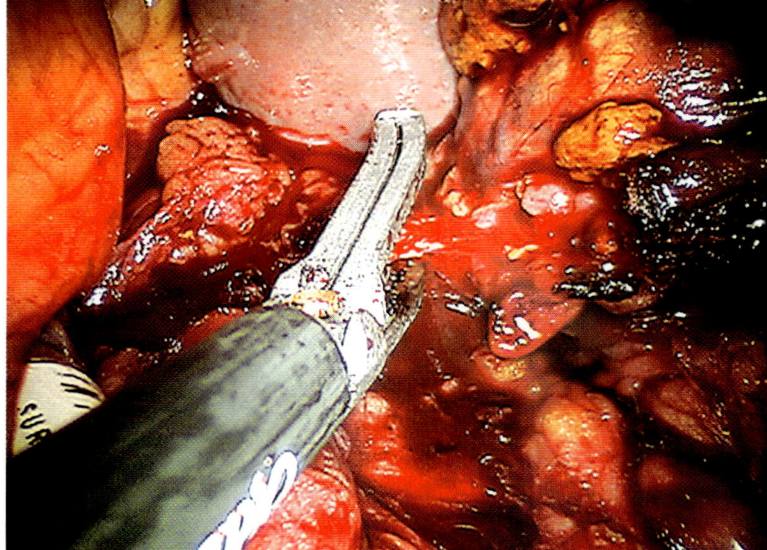

Fig. 20: The bipolar sealing device is used to excise the adenoma from the normal tissue

2. The decision to divide the adrenal vein is based on the vein's proximity to the adrenal mass. The vein can be left intact if the surgeon feels that the adrenal mass can safely be dissected from the normal adrenal tissue without damage to the vein. In some cases, a branch of the adrenal vein that drains the adenoma can be selectively divided, leaving the remainder of the vein intact, as shown in Figure 18.
3. Intraoperative ultrasound can be useful to help identify the adrenal mass, especially when there is a significant amount of perirenal fat. Use of the ultrasound device to localize the adrenal mass is shown in Figure 19.
4. Once the adrenal mass is identified, the bipolar vessel-sealing device—shown in Figure 20—can be used to excise the adenoma from the remainder of the adrenal gland. The bipolar vessel-sealing device provides excellent hemostasis when dividing the vascular adrenal tissue. Alternatively, an endovascular stapling device, bipolar forceps, hemostatic polymer clips or ultrasonic scalpel can be used to divide the adenoma from the uninvolved adrenal tissue.

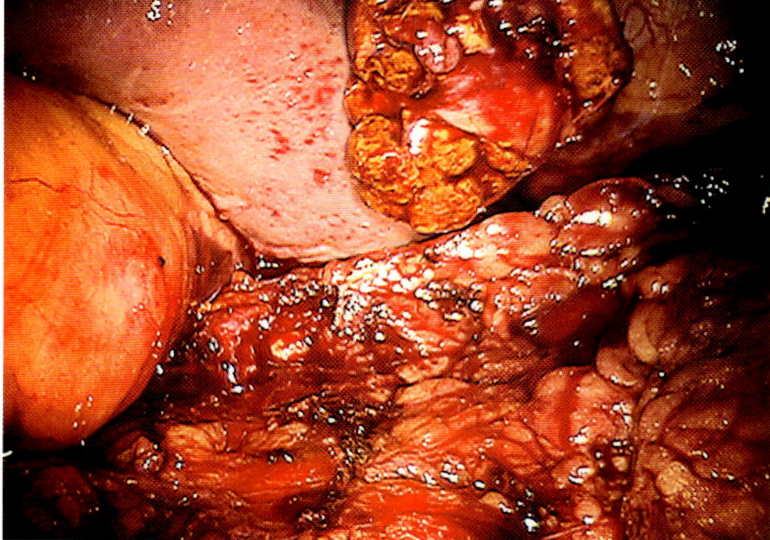

Fig. 21: The adrenal mass has been excised and is seen at the top of the image. The remaining adrenal tissue is inspected for bleeding

5. The remaining adrenal tissue is inspected for bleeding (Fig. 21) with the pneumoperitoneum decreased to 5 mm Hg. As discussed earlier, hemostatic agents such as oxidized cellulose polymer or other hemostatic matrices such as Floseal™ can be used.
6. The specimen is placed in a laparoscopic retrieval bag and removed through one of the 12 mm trocar sites. All trocar sites larger than 10 mm are closed with a fascial closure device, and the trocars are removed under direct vision. The skin is closed with subcuticular sutures or skin staples.

REFERENCES

1. Gagner M, Lacroix A, Bolte E. Laparoscopic adrenalectomy in Cushing's syndrome and pheochromocytoma. N Engl J Med. 1992;327:1033.
2. Prinze R. A comparison of laparoscopic and open adrenalectomies. Arch Surg. 1995;130:489-92.
3. Smith C, Weber C, Amerson J. Laparoscopic adrenalectomy: a new gold standard. World J Surg. 1999;23:389-96.
4. Gill I. The case for laparoscopic adrenalectomy. J Urol. 2001;166: 429-36.

SECTION

3

Lower Tract Surgery

12

Chapter

Transperitoneal Robotic Radical Prostatectomy

Abhishek Srivastava, Nishant Mishra, Prasanna Sooriakumaran, Ashutosh K Tewari

INTRODUCTION

Robotic-assisted radical prostatectomy using the da Vinci® surgical platform has become very popular in recent years, accounting for over 70% of all radical prostatectomies performed in the United States in 2008. Its postulated advantages over the conventional open approach include better intraoperative dexterity and visualization of periprostatic tissue architecture with up to 12-fold optical magnification for the surgeon, while patients experience less intraoperative blood loss, less painful recovery and shorter hospital stays. However, despite innovations in surgical techniques, surgeons are still faced with the daily dilemma of balancing complete cancer clearance while striving for potency preservation during surgery. In several series, 20–50% of patients still remain impotent at one year following nerve-sparing radical prostatectomy.

Over the past few years, the authors' group has made several advances in mapping out a trizonal approach to the complex periprostatic neural architecture through cadaveric and real-time operative dissections. The authors' subsequent appreciation of the course of the trizonal lattice of nerves around the prostate in different fascial planes enveloping the prostatic capsule led us to adopt a risk-stratified approach to nerve preservation while maintaining adequate clearance of cancer. Herein, surgeons describe current technique of athermal nerve-sparing robotic prostatectomy.

SURGICAL INSTRUMENTS

Table 1 represents the surgical instruments and surgical steps.

Table 1: Surgical instruments

Surgical step	Lens	Right robotic instrument	Left robotic instrument	Fourth robotic arm
Dropping the bladder	Zero	Monopolar Curved Scissors	Bipolar Maryland Forceps	N/A
Incising endopelvic fascia	Zero	Monopolar Curved Scissors	Bipolar Maryland Forceps	N/A
Bladder Neck Dissection	Zero	Monopolar Curved Scissors	Bipolar Maryland Forceps	N/A
Vas and seminal vesicle dissection	Zero	Monopolar Curved Scissors	Bipolar Maryland Forceps	N/A
Posterior Dissection (Risk-stratified approach)	Zero	Monopolar Curved Scissors	Bipolar Maryland Forceps	N/A
Posterior urethral transection (via retro-apical approach)	30° upward	Monopolar Curved Scissors	Bipolar Maryland Forceps	N/A
Anterior urethral transection	Zero	Monopolar Curved Scissors	Bipolar Maryland Forceps	N/A
DVC control and transection	Zero	Monopolar Curved Scissors	Bipolar Maryland Forceps	N/A
Anatomic reconstruction of bladder neck	Zero	Monopolar Curved Scissors	Bipolar Maryland Forceps	N/A
Posterior reconstruction	Zero	Needle Driver	Bipolar Maryland Forceps	N/A
Vesicourethral anastomosis	Zero	Needle Driver	Bipolar Maryland Forceps	N/A
Anterior reconstruction	Zero	Needle Driver	Bipolar Maryland Forceps	N/A

Accessory Instruments

- BairHugger: Lithotomy under body
- Bard (Bardex I.C. Complete Care Foley Tray)
- Da Vinci® 8 mm Bladeless Obturator
- Endo Catch Gold (10 mm)
- Endo Shears (5 mm)
- Endopath OneSeal Reducer Cap
- High Flow Insufflation Tubing (with Filter)
- Indermil Tissue Adhesive
- Intuitive Camera Arm Drape (X2)
- Intuitive da Vinci® single Use Seal (X2)
- Tip Cover Accessory
- Aircast VF DSP Calf Cuff
- Versaport Plus V2 w/ Fixation Cannula (Long)
- Versaport V2 (5 mm) (X2)
- Ethicon Endo-Surgery Endopath 512 DA (12 mm)
- Instrumental arm cannula (X2)

Laparoscopic Instruments and Trocars

- 5 mm laparoscopic suction
- 5 mm laparoscopic locking grasper
- 5 mm laparoscopic scissors
- 5 mm laparoscopic needle driver

- 10 mm laparoscopic Hem-o-lok clip applier
- 10 mm laparoscopic Endocatch Gold bag

Robotic Instruments

- Monopolar Curved Scissors
- Bipolar Maryland Scissors
- Large Needle Driver x2

Sutures

- DVC Stitch: 6-inch 3-0 V-Loc 180 barbed sutures
- Posterior reconstruction Stitch: 6-inch 3-0 V-Loc 180 barbed sutures
- Anastomosis Stitch: 6-inch 3-0 V-Loc 180 barbed sutures
- Endoclose: O Polysorb GS-21
- Drain stitch: 2-O Sofsilk C-15
- Fascia: O Maxon GS-24 (peri-Umbilical Incision)
- Subcutaneous: 3-O Chromic V-20
- Skin: 4-O Biosyn P-12
- Skin: Indermil Adhesive Tissue

TIPS AND TRICKS

Optimizing Erectogenic Outcomes

- Using a risk-stratified approach prior to surgery, determine the balance needed regarding extent of aggressiveness of nerve preservation and risk of extraprostatic extension of cancer
- Incise endopelvic fascia near to prostatic capsule
- Dissect the seminal vesicles beginning from the midline laterally outward to avoid injury to the proximal neurovascular plate that sits in close proximity to the tips of the seminal vesicles
- Avoid use of cautery after the seminal vesicles are dissected free-control potential bleeders using Hem-o-Lok® clips
- Commence posterior dissection in the appropriate fascial plane, beginning from the midline groove and working laterally outwards

Reducing Apical Margin Positivity

- Use a retroapical approach with a 30° upward lens to visualize the exact intersection between the prostatic apex and membranous urethra
- Divide the membranous urethra 1 mm from the apex posteriorly using sharp scissors
- Do not perform DVC control and transection until after urethral transection has been completed—this facilitates better visualization of the prostatic apex and reduces risk of causing inadvertent divots

Optimizing Anastomotic Healing and Early Continence

- Preserve the puboprostatic ligaments and arcus tendineus (collectively known as the puboprostatic collar)
- Optimize urethral stump length using a synchronous approach to urethral transection
- Reinforce Denonvilliers' musculofascial plate by suturing the posterior bladder neck close to the urethral stump—this significantly relieves tension off the anastomosis
- Complete the anastomosis with a continuous running pre-tied double suture
- Hitch bladder up to the puboprostatic collar—this relieves downward stress on the healing anastomosis during micturition

TECHNIQUE OF TRIZONAL ATHERMAL ROBOTIC PROSTATECTOMY

Anterior Dissection and Dropping the Bladder

After port placement, we develop the extraperitoneal space to expose the space of Retzius until the prostate and the prostatovesical junction are seen (Figs 1 and 2).

Incising Endopelvic Fascia

After clearing the fat, the endopelvic fascia is exposed and incised with scissors just medial to the white line sparing its most distal part, which is in continuity with the puboprostatic ligaments (Fig. 3). The arcus tendineus is dissected out on both sides and preserved (Fig. 4). These structures collectively form what we term the 'puboprostatic collar', which serves as a fibrotendinous scaffold for subsequent anterior reconstruction of the bladder neck after the prostate is removed.

Bladder Neck Dissection

The 'bimanual robotic pinch', together with simultaneous retraction of the indwelling catheter balloon against the bladder neck, helps the surgeon accurately identify the prostatovesical junction (Fig. 5).

The anterior bladder neck is then incised and the incision extended posteriorly taking care not to injure the ureteral orifices (Figs 6 and 7). This allows entry into the retrotrigonal fibromuscular layer, a musculofascial plane behind the posterior wall of the bladder neck (Figs 8 and 9).

Dividing the retrotrigonal layer exposes the vasa deferentia (VD) and the seminal vesicles (SVs). Electrocautery is avoided from this point onwards (Fig. 10).

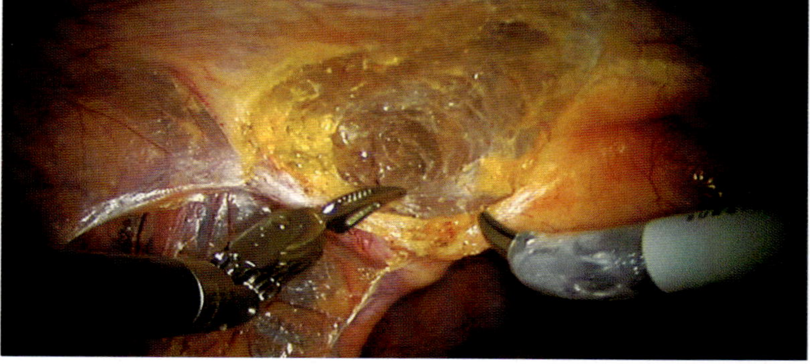

Fig. 1: Anterior dissection and dropping the bladder on the left side

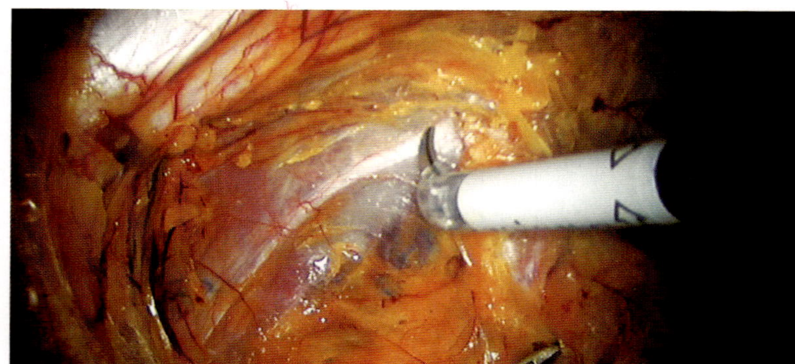

Fig. 2: The space of Retzius exposed on the left side until the prostate and the prostatovesical junction are seen

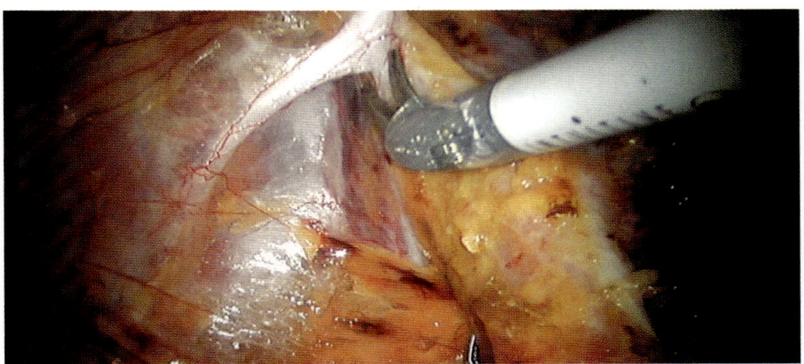

Fig. 3: The endopelvic fascia is exposed and incised with scissors just medial to the white line sparing its most distal part

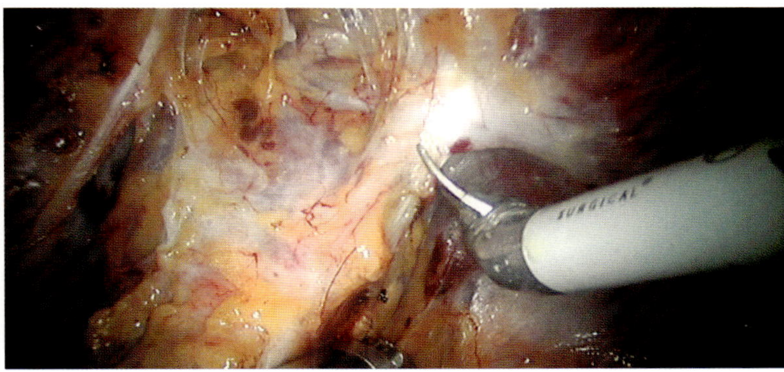

Fig. 4: The arcus tendineus is dissected out on both sides and preserved

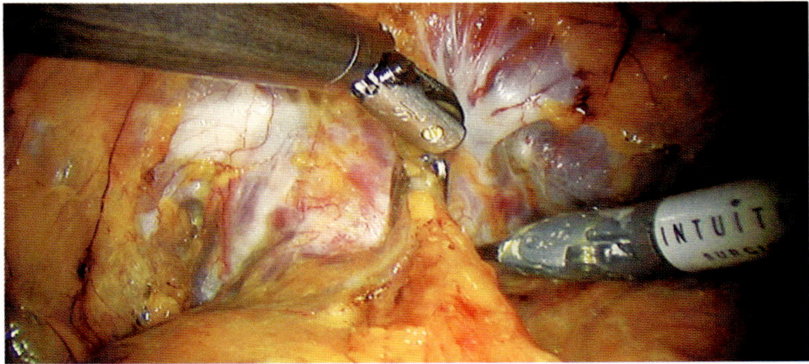

Fig. 5: Bimanual robotic pinch to identify the prostatovesical junction

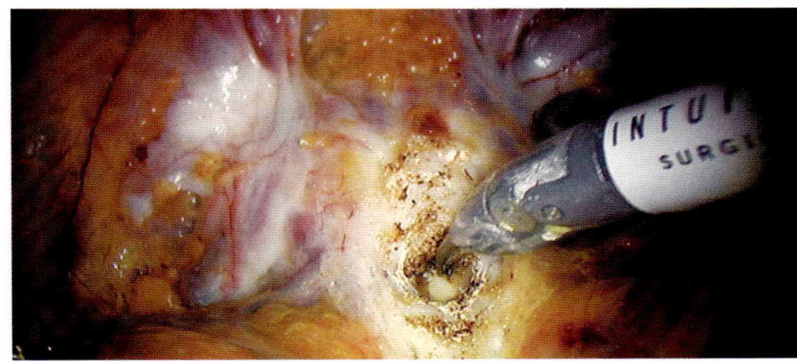

Fig. 6: Incision of the anterior bladder neck

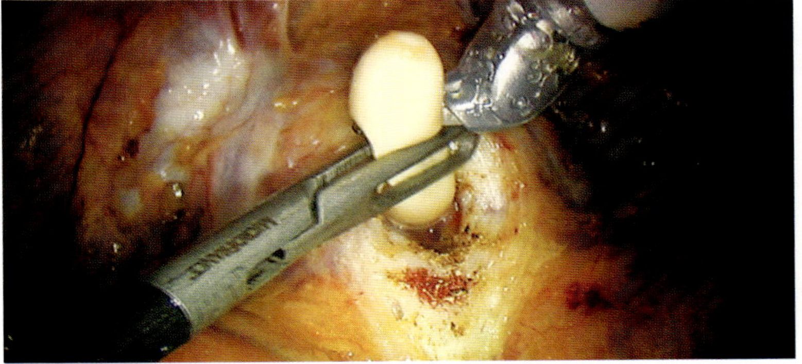

Fig. 7: Incision is widened and Foley catheter is withdrawn at the prostate-vesical junction

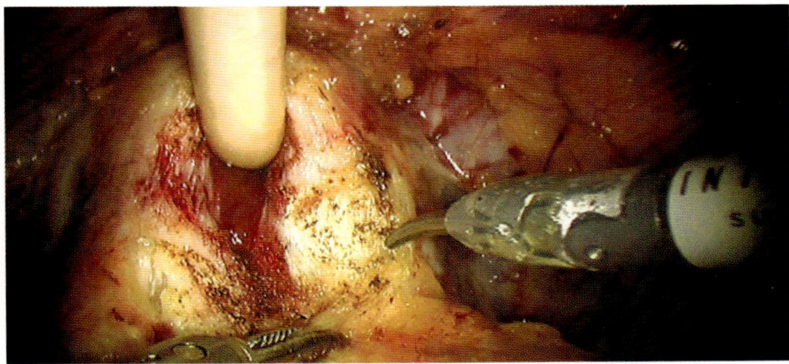

Fig. 8: The incision is extended posteriorly taking care not to injure the ureteral orifices

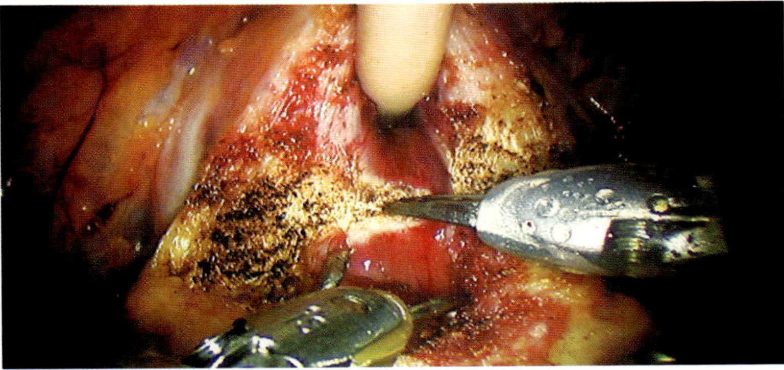

Fig. 9: Incision in the retrotrigonal fibromuscular layer

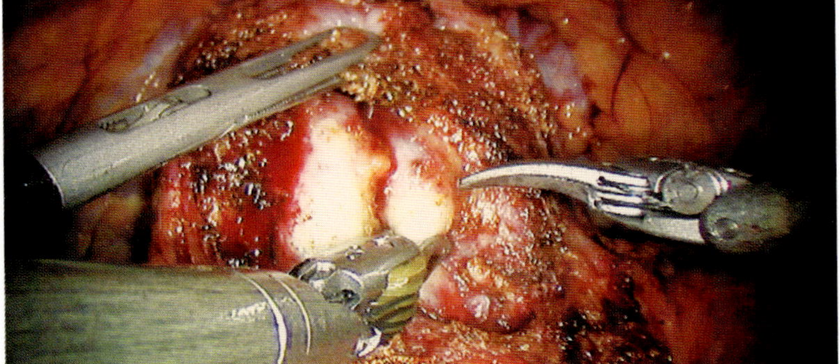

Fig. 10: The retrotrigonal layer is divided to expose the vasa deferentia (VD) and the seminal vesicles (SVs)

Dissection of the VD and SVs

The VD and SVs are identified behind the retrotrigonal layer. Each SV has its own compartment and most of the blood supply enters near its tip and anterolateral aspect. Lateral to this compartment and near the tip lies the proximal neurovascular plate. This spatial relationship has profound implications for our nerve-sparing technique because the crucial neural tissue can be damaged (or avulsed) by heat, crushing and the torque of pulling during seminal vesicle dissection. We then mobilize the VD and clip the proximal end behind the trigone (Figs 11 to 13).

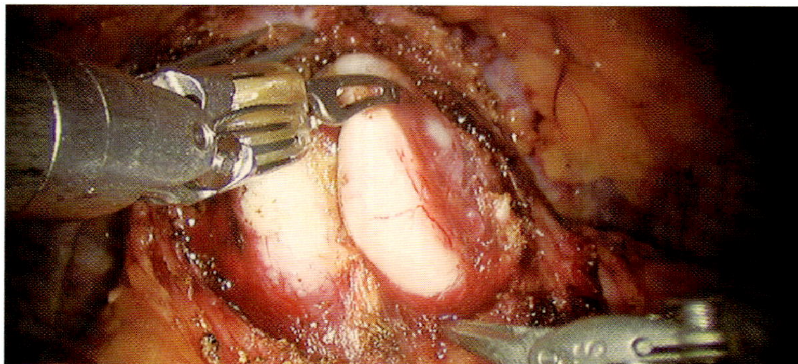

Fig. 11: The Vas Deferens is mobilized athermally

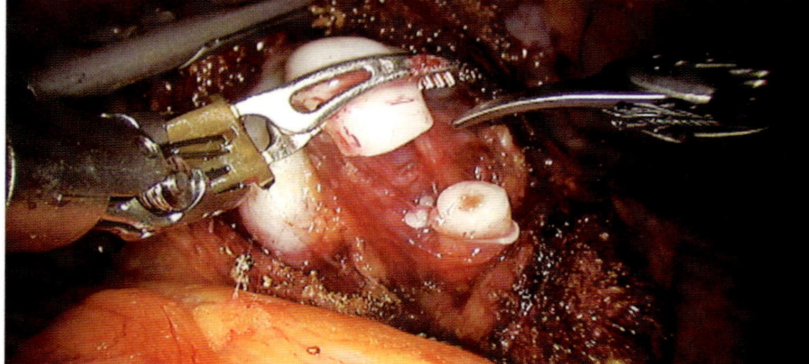

Fig. 12: The proximal end is clipped and divided

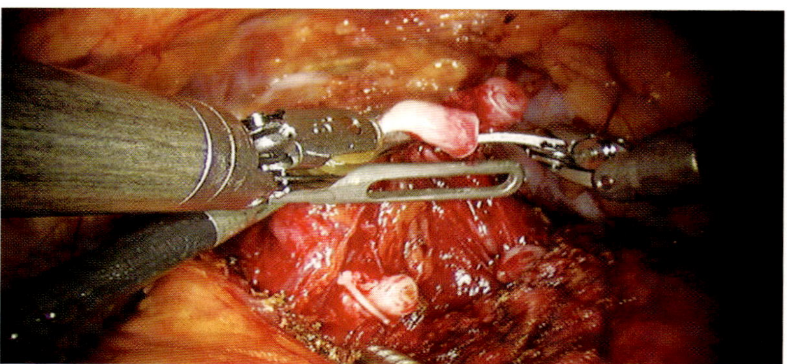

Fig. 13: The cut ends of the Vas Deferens is pulled anteriorly

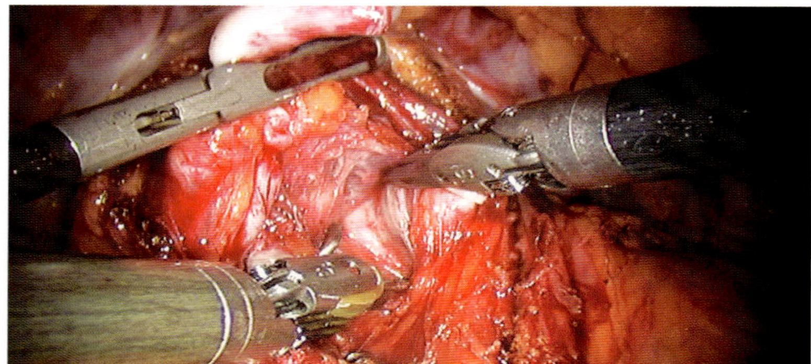

Fig. 14: Medial avascular plane is utilized for lateral dissection of the right seminal vesicle

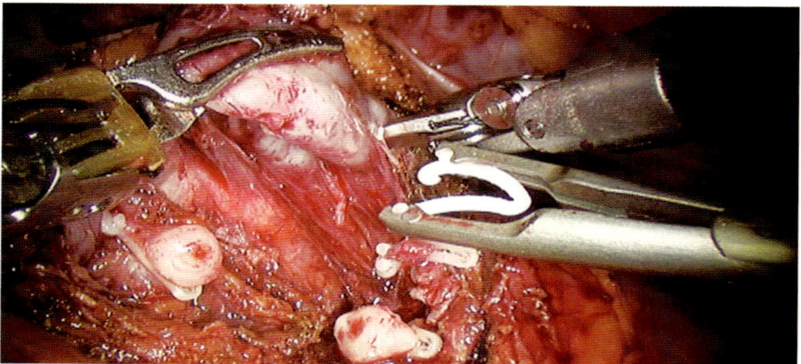

Fig. 15: Right seminal vesicle is mobilized athermally

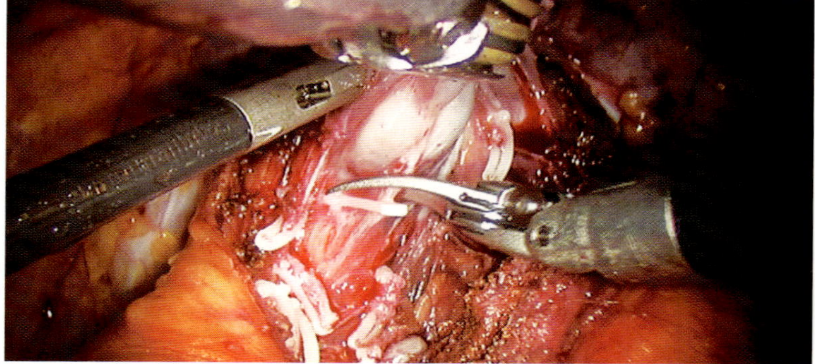

Fig. 16: Left seminal vesicle is mobilized athermally

Since most of the medial wall of a seminal vesicle lies adjacent to a nearly avascular space, this medial avascular plane serves as a safe starting point for lateral dissection of the seminal vesicles (Figs 14 to 16).

Posterior Dissection

Since cross-communicating nerve fibers have been demonstrated in the layers of the Denonvilliers' fascia, in appropriate cases with low-risk cancer, surgeon develops a plane just outside the prostatic capsule, leaving some layers of Denonvilliers' fascia in the patient. If there are concerns about oncologic safety, surgeon goes deeper and excise the fascia with the specimen. Keeping the undersurface of the prostate capsule under vision, the dissection proceeds laterally and a plane is developed that is either interfascial or intrafascial. At this point, tenting vessels entering the prostate base near the attachment of the SVs are controlled bilaterally with small clips. The transected distal ends of the VD are grasped by the left side assistant (or the fourth robotic arm) and pulled anteriorly, tenting the Denonvilliers' fascia occupying the retroprostatic space (Fig. 17). This fascia is incised in the midline and the opening is enlarged laterally toward the medial edge of the pedicles (Figs 18 and 19). A cave-like space is created behind the prostate and dissection is deliberately extended distally to release the apex and the urethra from deeper tissue (Fig. 20).

Lateral Pedicle Control

Upward traction is exerted on the VD and SVs by the left side assistant and the pedicles are easily differentiated from the predominant neurovascular bundle (Fig. 21). Selective clipping or ligation of the prostatic vessels is performed. The pedicles are controlled close to the base. Electrocautery and mass ligature are avoided, with small clips to control individual pedicles being preferred (Fig. 22).

Release of Neurovascular Bundles

Next, surgeon releases the neurovascular tissue using both our trizonal-neural-hammock-release technique and our athermal approach. Surgeons employ sharp athermal dissection of the prostatic pedicles, controlling arteries and veins with Hem-o-Lok® clips (Teleflex Medical Inc, Research Triangle Park, NC) as they enter the prostatic base (Fig. 23). The lack of use of cautery results in preservation of natural tissue texture and the predominant neurovascular bundle can often be identified and differentiated from

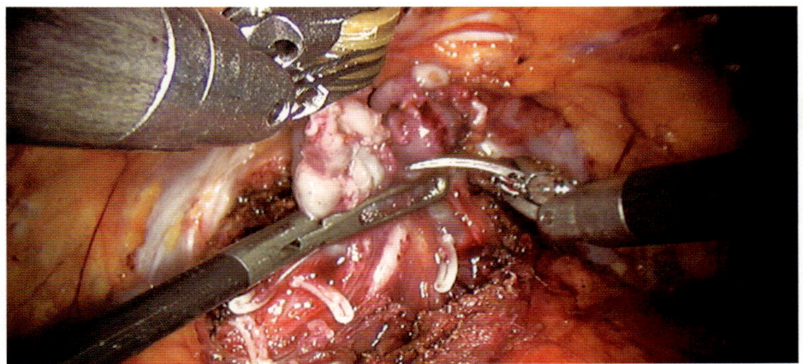

Fig. 17: The transected distal ends of the VD are grasped by the left side assistant (or the fourth robotic arm) and pulled anteriorly, tenting the Denonvilliers' fascia

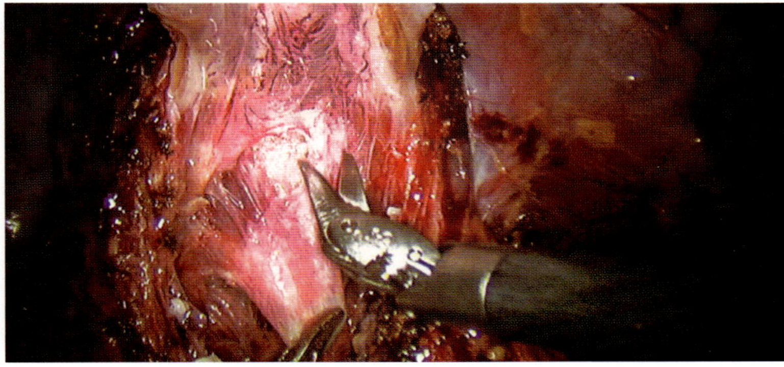

Fig. 18: Denonvilliers' fascia is incised in the midline

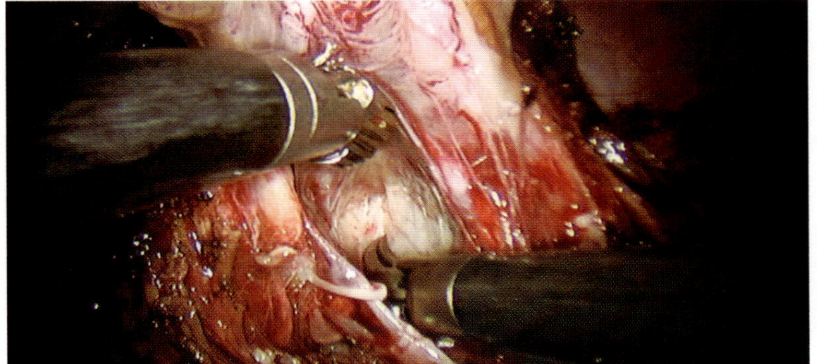

Fig. 19: The opening in Denonvilliers' fascia is enlarged laterally toward the medial edge of the pedicles

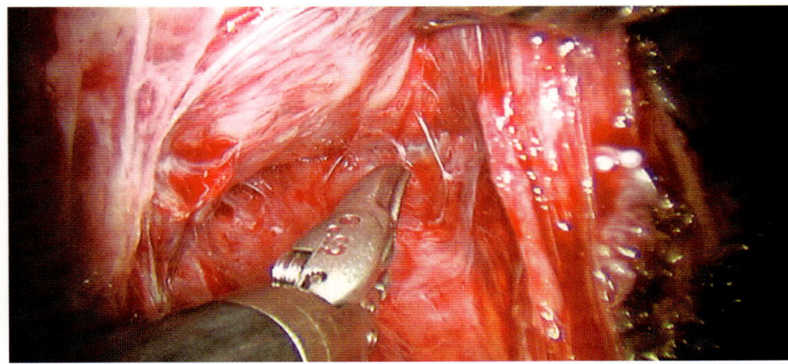

Fig. 20: A cave-like space is created behind the prostate and dissection is deliberately extended distally to release the apex and the urethra from deeper tissue

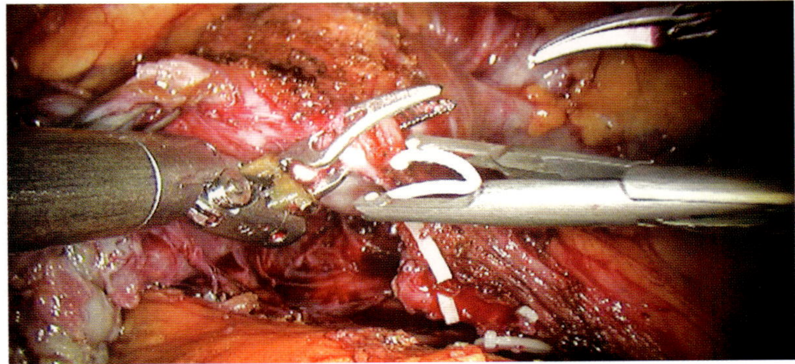

Fig. 21: Upward traction is exerted on the VD and SVs by the left side assistant and the pedicles are easily differentiated from the predominant neurovascular bundle. Selective clipping or ligation of the prostatic vessels is performed

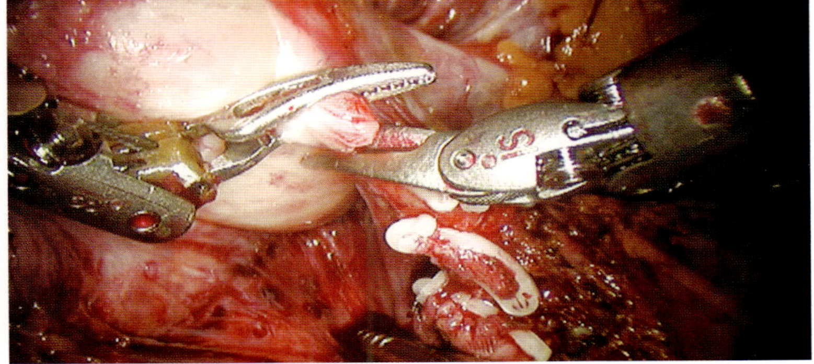

Fig. 22: The pedicles are controlled close to the base

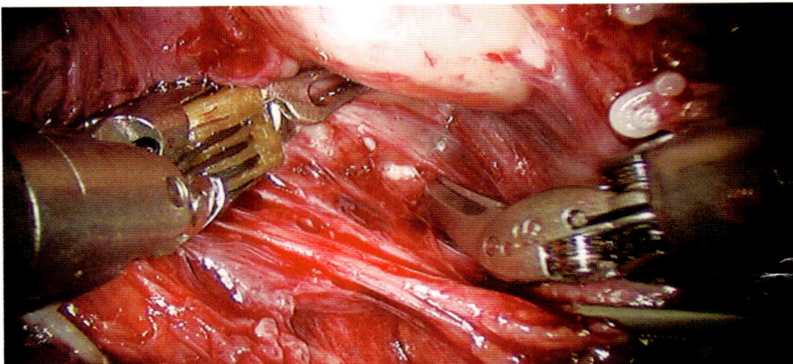

Fig. 23: Sharp athermal dissection of the prostatic pedicles is performed controlling arteries and veins with Hem-o-Lok® clips as they enter the prostatic base

the vascular pedicle. Depending on the preoperative decision about the extent of cancer, the authors' developed a plane very close (just on the prostatic capsule: more aggressive nerve sparing/intrafascial/Grade 1 Nerve Sparing) (Fig. 24) or close (outside the prostatic fascia—moderate nerve sparing: most commonly performed/interfascial/Grade 2 Nerve Sparing) or farther (leaving a few medial layers of lateral pelvic fascia on the specimen: partial/incremental nerve sparing/Grade 4 Nerve Sparing).

In appropriate cases, surgeons also preserve the retroapical nerve plexus by leaving a distal layer of superficial Denonvilliers' fascia. In authors' practice, the predominant neurovascular bundles are usually released in an antegrade fashion; that is, dissection continues from the bladder neck to the prostate apex (Figs 25 and 26).

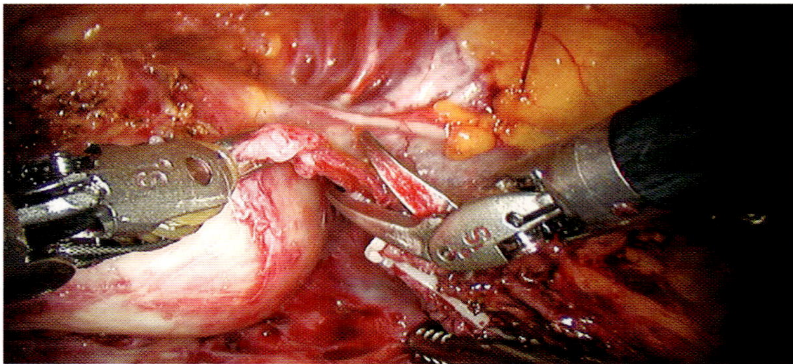

Fig. 24: Grade 1 nerve sparing (Intrafascial)

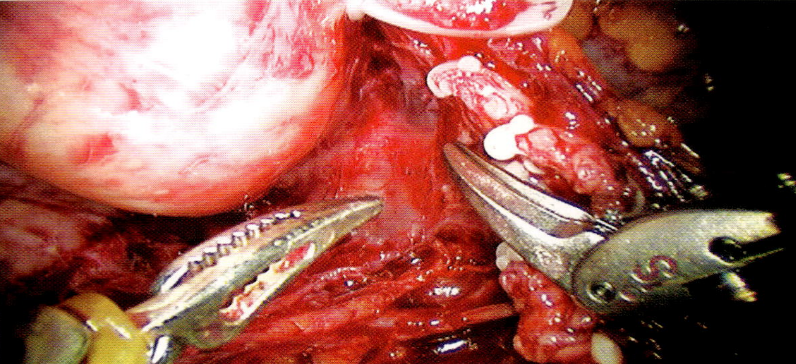

Fig. 25: Nerve sparing on the right side

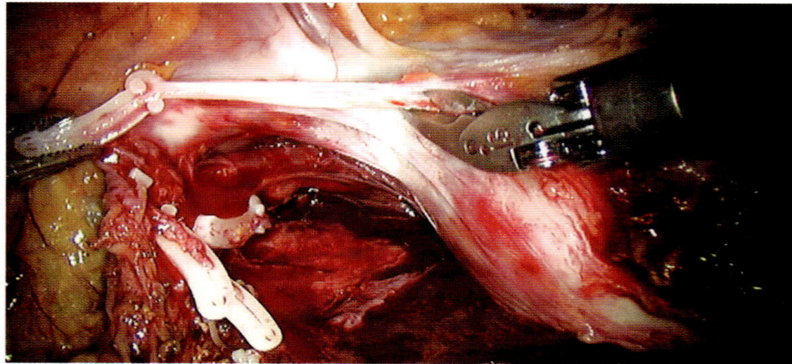

Fig. 26: Nerve sparing on the left side

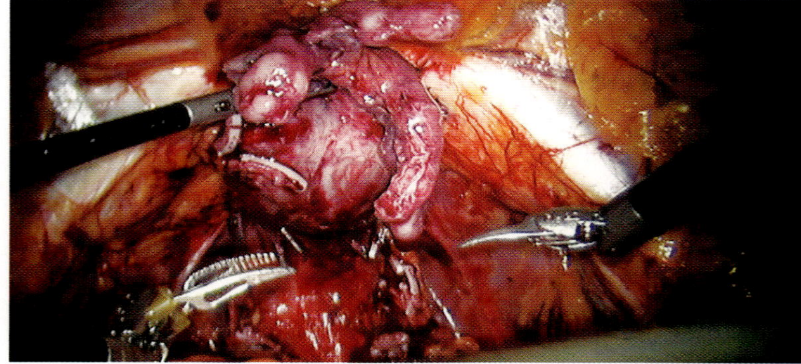

Fig. 27: The prostate is lifted anteriorly towards the anterior abdominal wall and pubic symphysis

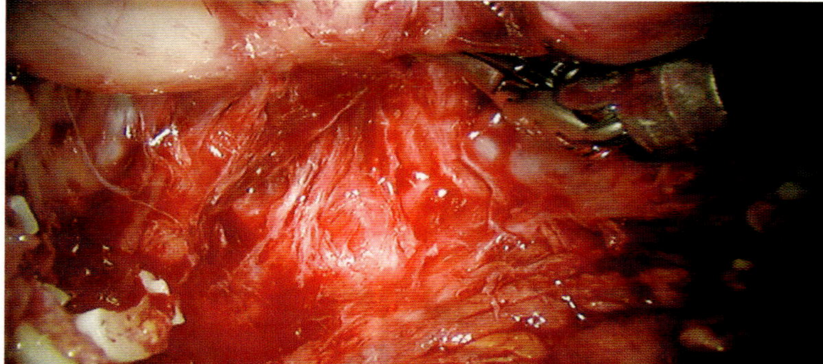

Fig. 28: Denonvilliers' fascia is covering the posterior surface of the prostate, and the membranous urethra is posteriorly supported by the rectourethralis muscle

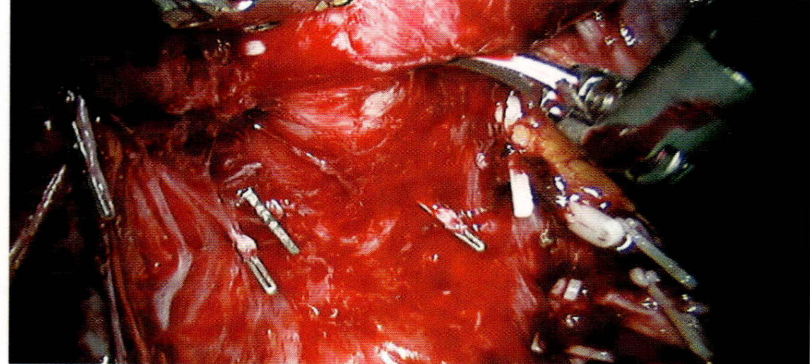

Fig. 29: Superficial layers of the Denonvilliers' fascia are dissected and the precise prostatourethral junction is exposed

Retroapical Dissection

This portion of the robotic prostatectomy poses several challenges to the surgeon, its execution having a significant impact on the primary outcomes of margin positivity, continence and sexual function. These challenges include significant variations in the size and shape of the prostate gland and its relationship to the functional rhabdosphincter complex, nerves and urethra. In surgeons experience, the prostatic apex either tapers like a spin top, or forms a ledge over the membranous urethra. To overcome this difficulty we have developed an anatomic retroapical technique. Using this approach our positive apical margin rates have dropped fourfold.

The prostate is completely freed postero-laterally on either side. At this point it is quite mobile and is lifted anteriorly towards the anterior abdominal wall and pubic symphysis. This action opens up the space behind the urethra and apex and torques and angles the DVC, thus temporarily occluding it (Fig. 27). The camera lens is changed to 30° upward-facing for a retro-apical approach to the apical-urethral junction. Once positioned at the perfect vantage point the glistening white surface of apex can be differentiated from the membranous urethra. The transition from prostatic apex into urethra is further appreciated by manipulating the 20Fr Foley catheter in and out of the apical-urethral junction.

The prostate has a few layers of Denonvilliers' fascia covering its posterior surface and the membranous urethra is posteriorly supported by the rectourethralis muscle (Fig. 28). Using sharp, curved scissors we dissect the superficial layers of the Denonvilliers' fascia and expose the precise prostatourethral junction (Fig. 29).

Next, the posterior hemicircumference of the urethra is sharply incised 1 mm distal to the apex (Fig. 30). The Foley catheter is exposed and positioned with its tip at the distal urethral opening (Fig. 31).

This permits appreciation of the anterior urethral hemicircumference, with urethral mucosa and muscular wall being seen clearly. Using blunt and sharp dissections, the urethra is divided circumferentially (Fig. 32). At this point all the muscle fibers are transected and the DVC is left attached to the anterior surface of the prostate.

DVC Control and Transection

Management of the DVC now depends upon the width and thickness of the anterior tissue. If the remaining tissue is thin, we increase the pneumoperitoneum to 20 cm water column pressure and inflate the Foley catheter balloon to 30 cc behind the prostate. The Foley balloon is placed on caudal traction, resulting in partial occlusion of the DVC and developing the space behind the prostate.

The lens is now changed to 0° and the prostatic apical dissection is continued anteriorly. The prostate is retracted cephalad by the left assistant grasping the SVs and distal ends of the transected VD.

Employing robotic Maryland dissectors on the left arm, the anterior tissue is grasped between its two jaws to ensure that only venous tissue and some parts of the ligaments are grabbed. We sharply cut distally to the grip and can see the sharp scissors cutting through the venous sinuses (Fig. 33).

Bleeding is minimal due to the inflated Foley balloon placed under traction or suture used. The prostate is freed with a 1 mm hood of ligaments and venous tissue still on the prostatic apex. Care is taken in preserving the puboprostatic ligaments and arcus tendineus for later reconstruction (Fig. 34).

If the remaining tissue is broad and thick, surgeons ligate the DVC using a CT-1 needle and an O-Polyglactin suture using a slipknot (Figs 35 and 36).

Once the prostate is freed, surgeon performs lymph node dissection, limited/standard or extended depending on the D'Amico risk grouping of the patient and place the specimen in a laparoscopic entrapment bag (Figs 37 and 38).

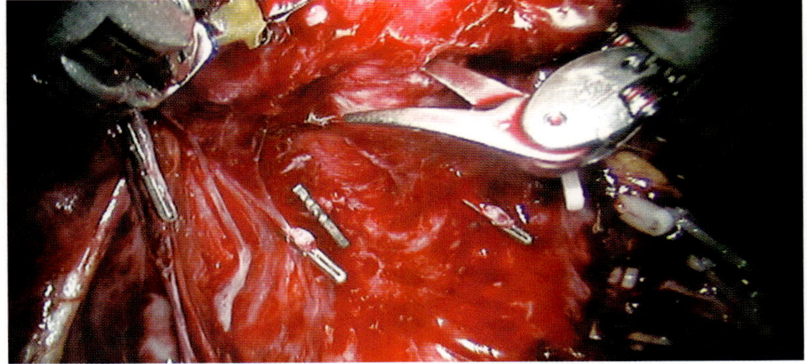

Fig. 30: The posterior hemicircumference of the urethra is sharply incised 1 millimeter distal to the apex

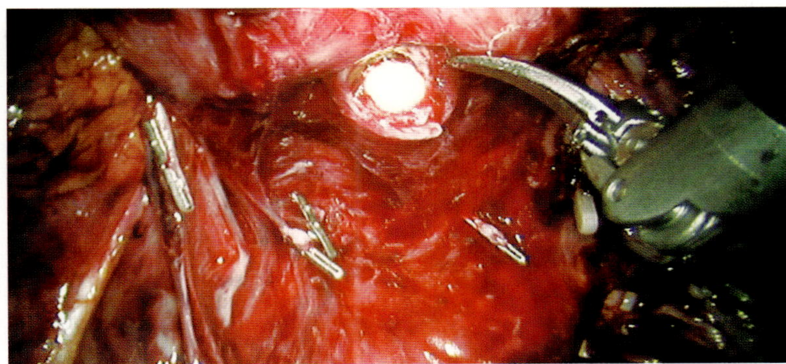

Fig. 31: The Foley catheter is exposed and positioned with its tip at the distal urethral opening

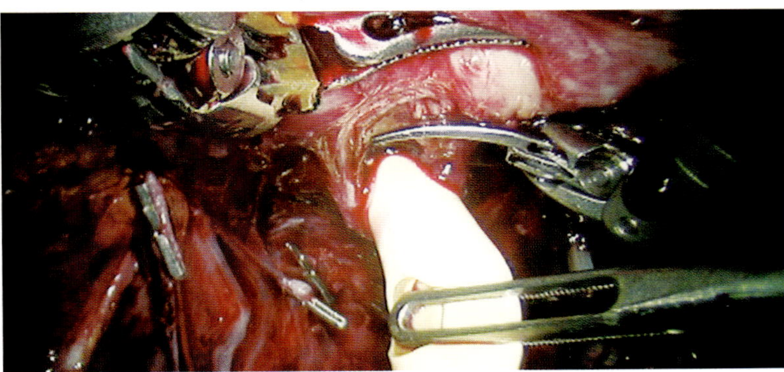

Fig. 32: Using blunt and sharp dissections, the urethra is divided circumferentially

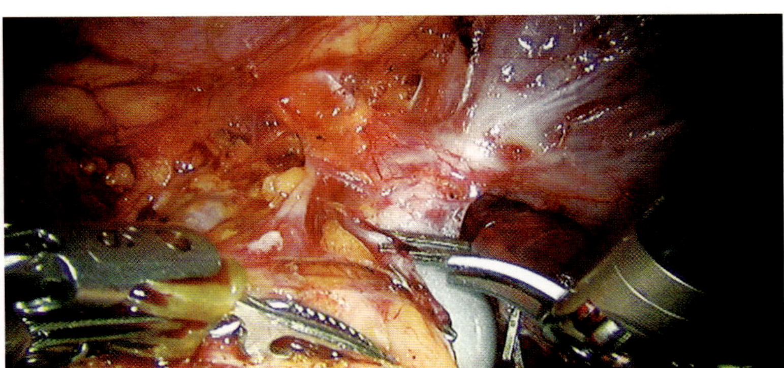

Fig. 33: The Foley balloon is placed on caudal traction and the anterior tissue is sharply cut distally to the grip

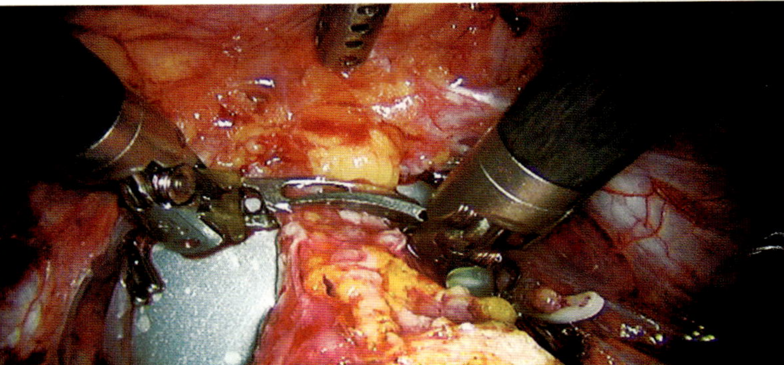

Fig. 34: The prostate is freed with a 1mm hood of ligaments and venous tissue still on the prostatic apex

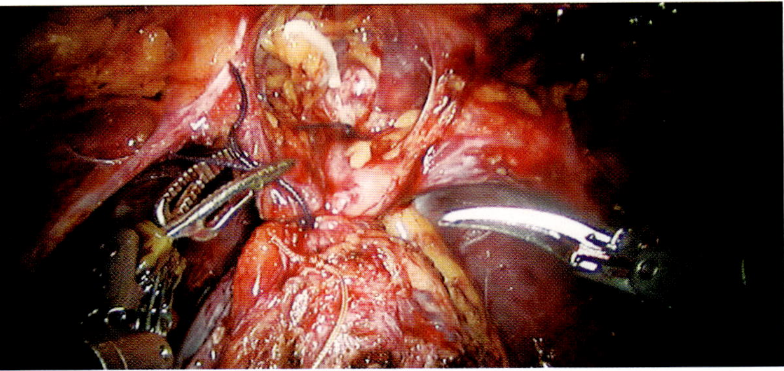

Fig. 35: If the remaining tissue is broad and thick, the DVC is ligated using a CT-1 needle and an O-Polyglactin suture using a slipknot

Total Anatomic Reconstruction

The authors' routinely reconstruct the posterior bladder neck as well as the Denonvilliers' musculofasical plate before performing the vesicourethral anastomosis. This technical modification serves to relieve tension on the anastomosis and provide suspensory support for the posteriorly deficient Ω-shaped rhabdosphincter to contract effectively against (Figs 39 to 50).

Surgeons complete the bladder neck reconstruction anteriorly by taking partial thickness sutures of the anterior bladder neck to the preserved arcus tendineus and puboprostatic ligaments for all round suspensory support (Figs 51 and 52).

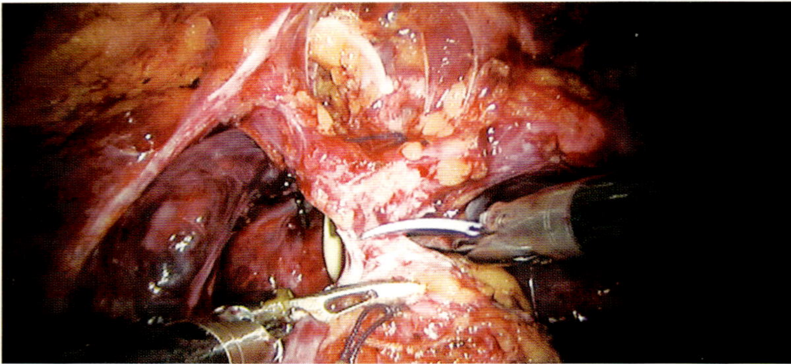

Fig. 36: DVC is transected distal to the slipknot using sharp scissors

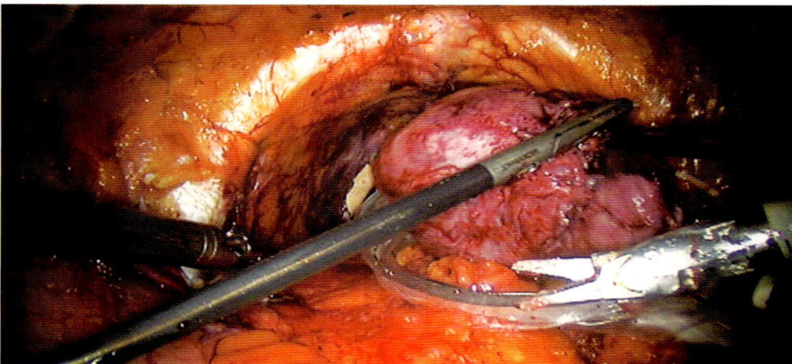

Fig. 37: Dissected lymph nodes and prostate are placed in laparoscopic entrapment bag

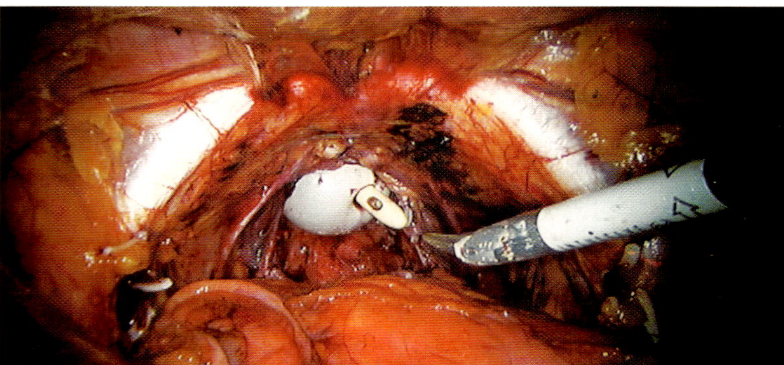

Fig. 38: Field of view after prostate is removed; balloon tamponade prevents excessive bleeding through the DVC

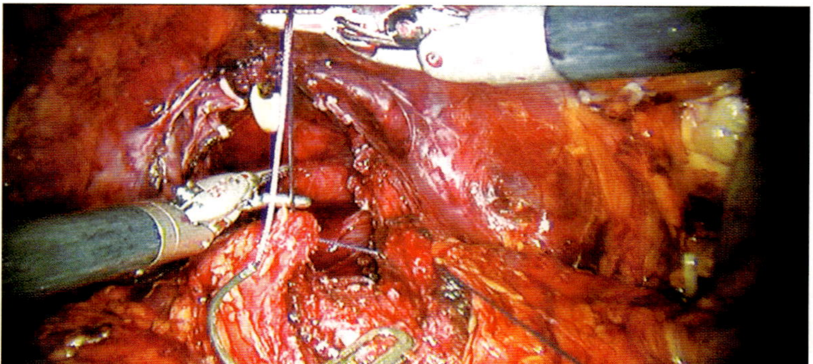

Fig. 39: Imbrication of the right and left posterior edges of the bladder around the retracted retrotrigonal flap with a running 3-0 polyglactin suture

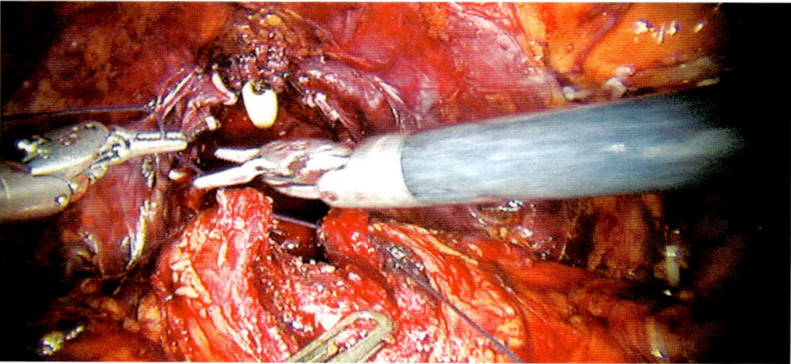

Fig. 40: Imbrication of the posterior bladder edges is completed. This will be followed by imbrication of the right and left edges of the retrotrigonal flap (RTL) to form a retrotrigonal stump

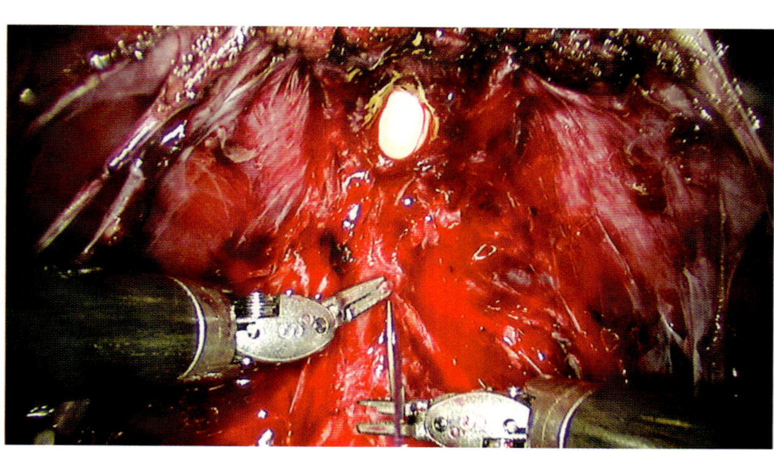

Fig. 41: Posterior reconstruction using the V-Loc 180 barbed suture

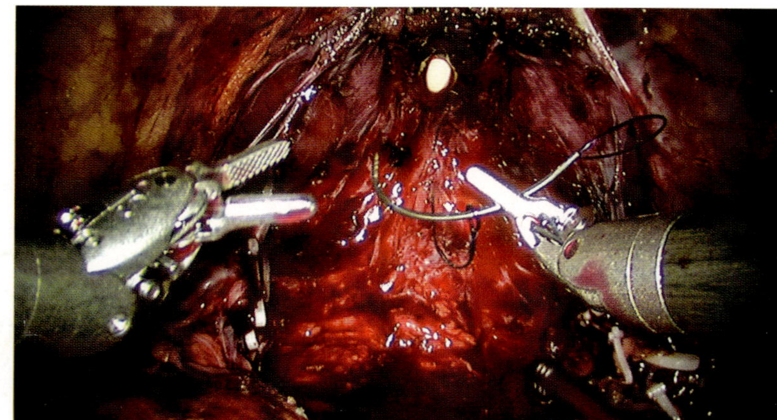

Fig. 42: Bites are taken from the rectourethralis muscle, posterior musculofascial plate and the retrotrigonal layer

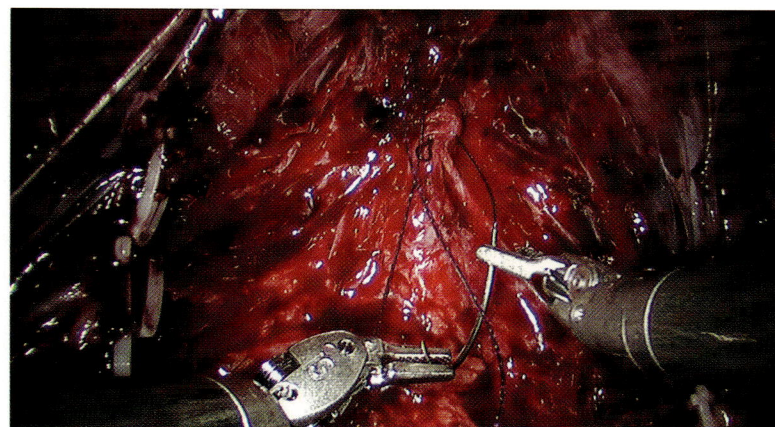

Fig. 43: Reconstruction of the posterior musculofascial plate is completed

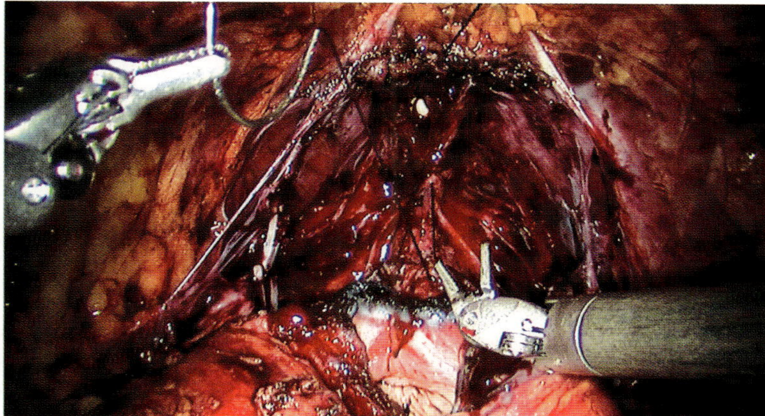

Fig. 44: The V-Loc 180 suture is lifted anteriorly, with the right needle driver holding the suture close to the tissue

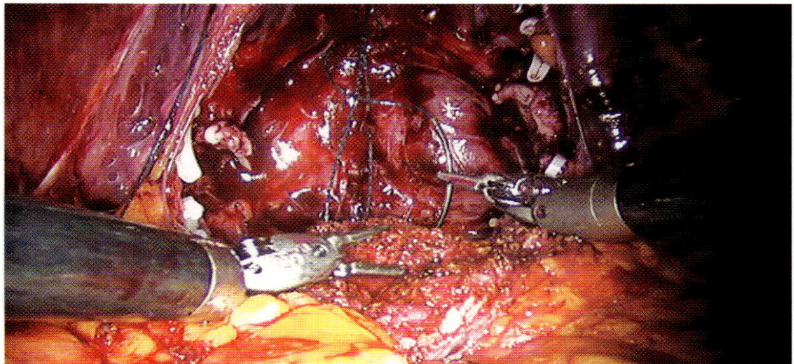

Fig. 45: Additional bite is taken from retrotrigonal layer before bringing the bladder close to the urethra

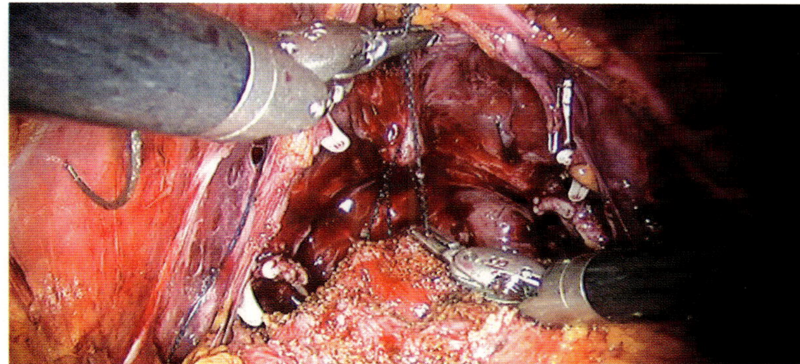

Fig. 46: The left needle driver pulls the suture while the right one pushes the tissue distally toward the urethra

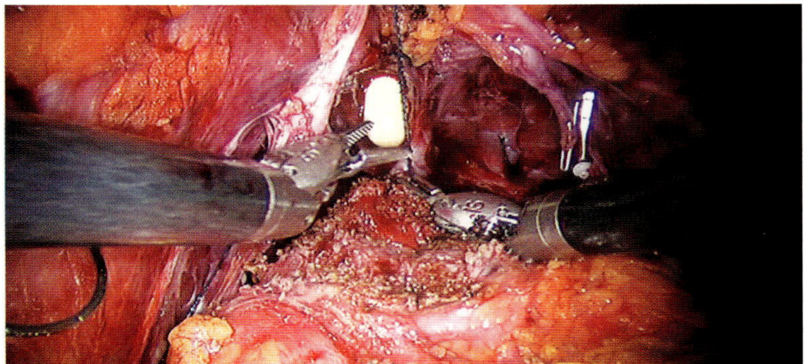

Fig. 47: Synchronized pull and push technique cinches the retrotrigonal layer close to the rectourethralis muscle. This process is repeated until the tissue is cinched down, and there is no gap between the rectourethralis and retrotrigonal layer

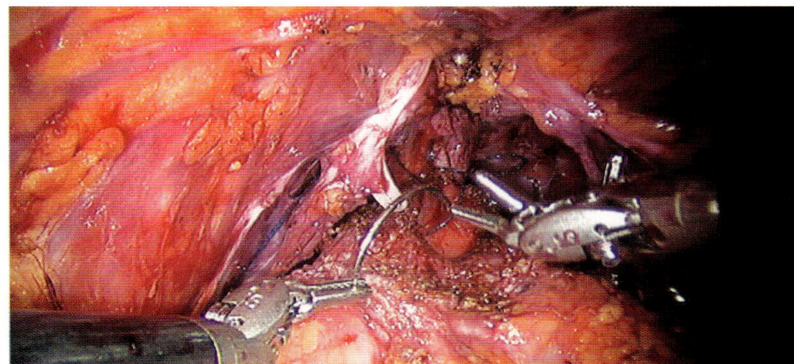

Fig. 48: An inside-out bite is then taken through the urethra on the right side and care is taken to include mucosa

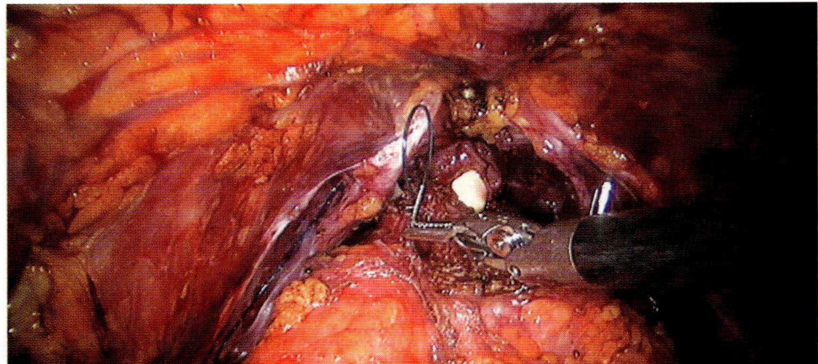

Fig. 49: The suture is brought to the anterior side after finishing the entire left wall of the anastomosis

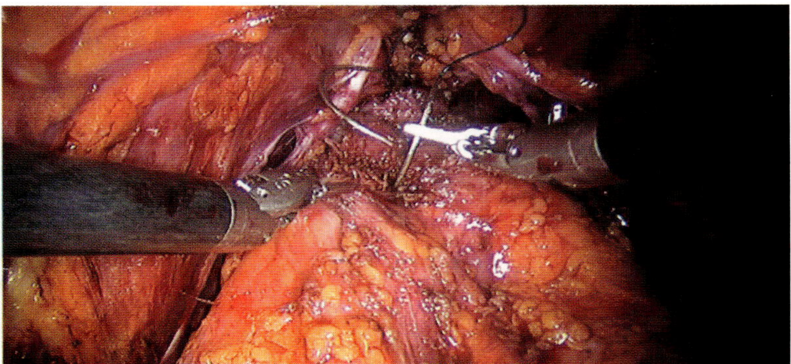

Fig. 50: A second V-Loc 180 suture is used for the right side of the bladder and the anastomosis is completed. The two V-Loc 180 sutures are then tied to each other

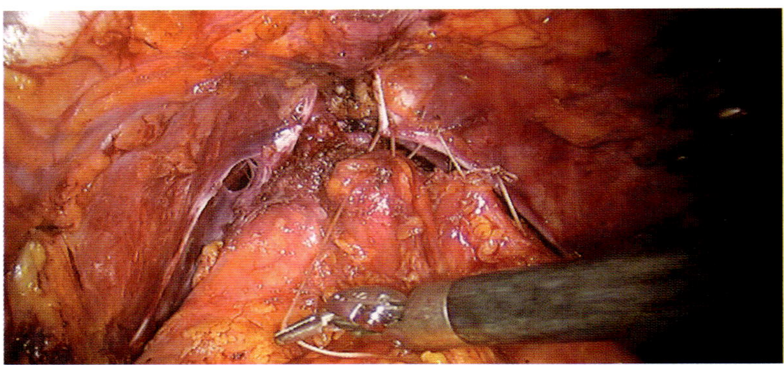

Fig. 51: The anterior bladder neck reconstruction begins by taking partial thickness sutures of the anterior bladder neck to the preserved arcus tendineus and puboprostatic ligaments for all round suspensory support

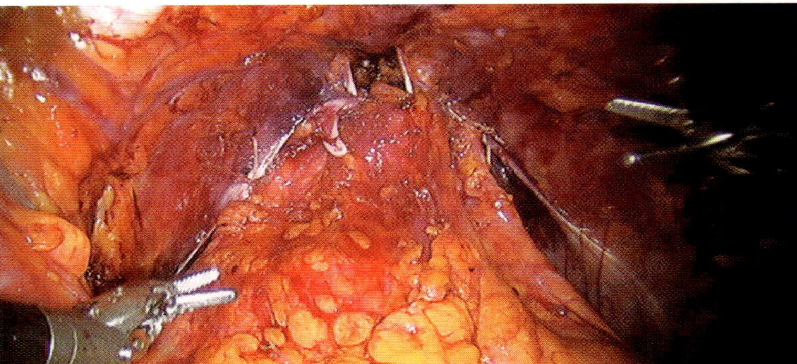

Fig. 52: Anterior reconstruction is completed

13 Chapter Extraperitoneal Robot-Assisted Radical Prostatectomy

Ahmed Ghazi, Jean Joseph

INTRODUCTION

Extraperitoneal laparoscopic prostatectomy was initially described by Raboy in 1997, the same year Schuessler reported on the transperitoneal approach in the United States.[1,2] In 2001 and 2002, Bollens and Stolzenburg respectively reported on their initial series with the extraperitoneal approach.[3,4] Robot assistance was first utilized during an extraperitoneal laparoscopic prostatectomy in 2003, with 4 cases performed in Creteil, France.[5]

In 2003, after prior experience with laparoscopic extraperitoneal prostatectomy, we converted from a pure laparoscopic to a robot-assisted approach. Our group later reported on 325 patients, who underwent extraperitoneal robot-assisted radical prostatectomy.[6] The procedure was initially performed using a three-arm robot with two assistants. With the four-arm robot it is performed with a single bedside assistant, with no difficulty maneuvering instruments in the extraperitoneal space. Both extraperitoneal and transperitoneal approaches are now routinely performed as standard first line approaches for the surgical management of prostate cancer at several institutions.

ADVANTAGES OF THE EXTRAPERITONEAL APPROACH

Once the extraperitoneal space is created, the steps involved in the radical prostatectomy are similar to those performed during a transperitoneal approach, with some technical modifications described in this chapter. The extraperitoneal approach is similar to the open retropubic radical prostatectomy, as it avoids entering the peritoneal cavity. With the bowel cavity isolated from the operative field, the extraperitoneal approach is often associated with a lower risk of ileus, which is often described as a major advantage of this approach.[7] Urine and blood from the operative field remain contained in the extraperitoneal space. The peritoneum also serves as a natural barrier preventing bowel from entering into the surgical field. This is particularly advantageous in obese patients with a redundant sigmoid colon, which can easily enter the operative field, at risk for injury.

The extraperitoneal approach is most suitable for patients where avoidance of the abdominal cavity is desirable. Patients with prior upper abdominal surgeries and internal scarring are excellent candidates for this approach. There is no need for lysis of adhesions with the associated risks of bowel or intra-abdominal injuries. Furthermore, when the operation is performed in the extraperitoneal space, the risk of subsequent intra-abdominal adhesions, which can complicate subsequent laparoscopic procedures, is eliminated. Similarly, in patients requiring subsequent radiotherapy, the bowel remains away from the radiation field, limiting the risk of radiation related complications. It is also an excellent approach in patients with conditions that preclude a steep Trendelenburg positioning. The peritoneum serves as a natural retractor, keeping the bowels out of the operative field, negating the need for any significant Trendelenburg positioning.

CONTRAINDICATIONS

The surgical indications and contraindications are similar to the transperitoneal approach for robot-assisted radical prostatectomy except in one setting. A history of prior bilateral extraperitoneal inguinal hernia mesh repair is often considered a contraindication, as it makes development of the space of Retzius a troublesome task. Prior creation of the space, in addition to the inflammatory reaction from the mesh, leads to scarring which obliterates the potential extraperitoneal space. When the space creation is attempted, peritoneotomy often ensues causing pneumoperitoneum which itself further limits visualization. Should this occur conversion to the transperitoneal approach is generally necessary

INSTRUMENTATION

Nondisposable

- da Vinci surgical system (Intuitive Surgical Inc.): four arms
- 0 and 30° binocular telescope
- EndoWrist PK dissecting forceps or Maryland bipolar graspers
- EndoWrist Prograsp forceps
- EndoWrist monopolar scissors
- Two EndoWrist needle drivers (1 suture cut device)
- Three 8 mm robotic trocars
- Hem-o-lok™ clip applier

Disposable

- Two 12 mm, long (150 mm), smooth Laparoscopic trocars
- One standard 5 mm Laparoscopic trocar
- Balloon dilator trocar (OMS-XB2 ExtraView™ or SpaceMaker™)
- Suction/irrigation device
- Laparoscopic grasper
- Hem-o-lok™ clips

PROCEDURAL STEPS

The steps of the procedure are depicted sequentially in Figures 1-56.

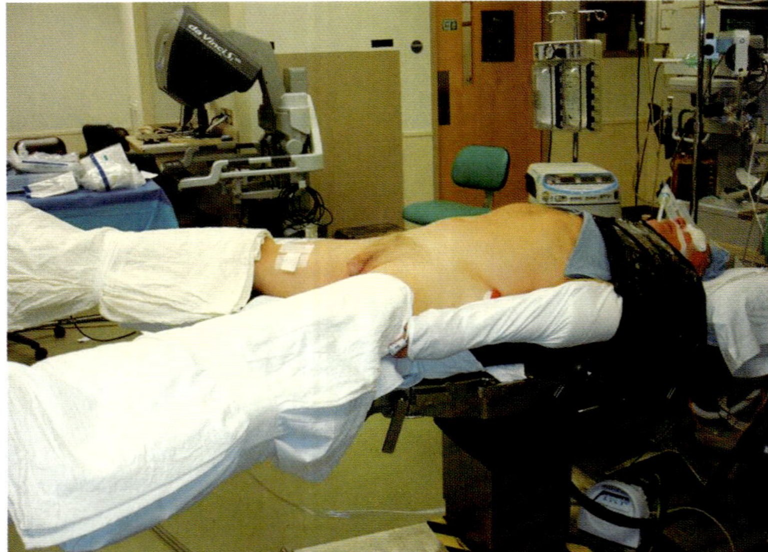

Fig. 1: Patient positioning. Padded chest straps are used to secure the patient to the operating table. The legs are abducted, with care taken to avoid overextending the hips. Only a mild Trendelenburg position (less than 10°) is required

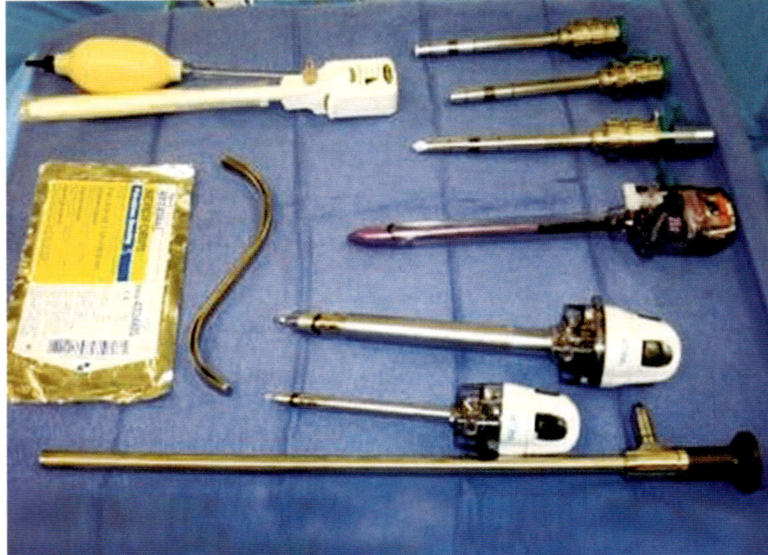

Fig. 2: Instruments required for extraperitoneal pelvic access. From upper left clockwise: Balloon dilatation trocar (OMS-XB2 ExtraView™ balloon dilator, or a SpaceMaker™); Three 8 mm robotic trocars; One 150 mm, smooth trocar (10/12 mm 512 XD, Ethicon Endo-Surgery, Cincinnati, Ohio); A 10/12 mm assistant trocars; A 5 mm assistant trocar; A zero degree 10 mm endoscope; S-shaped retractors; Petroleum gauze

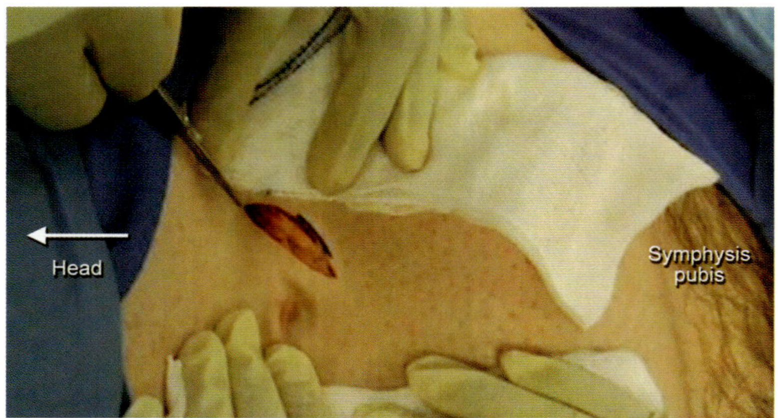

Fig. 3: A 3-5 cm left periumbilical incision for initial access

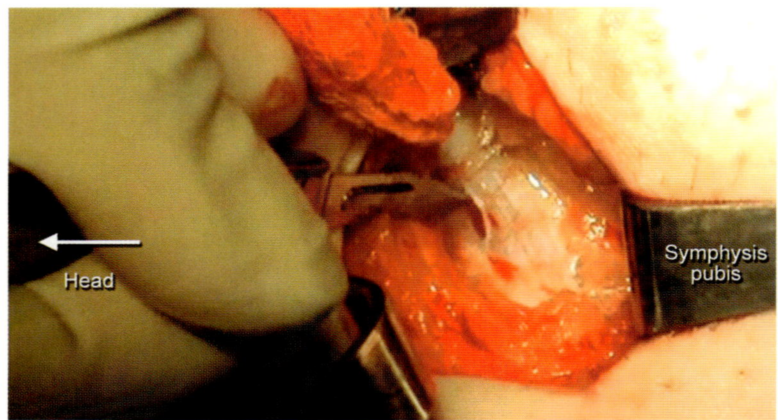

Fig. 4: A 1 cm incision made in the anterior rectus sheath

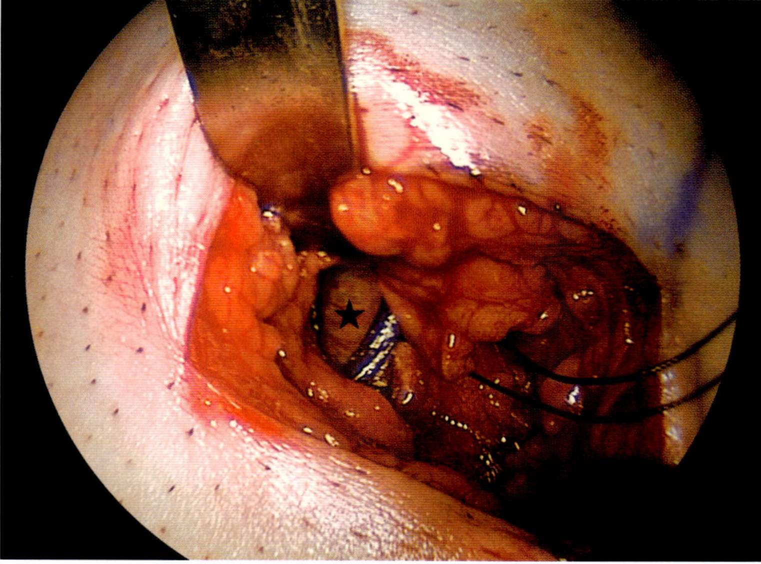

Fig. 5: Exposure of posterior sheath (★) following retraction of the rectus muscle laterally. A purse string suture is used to tighten the fascia around the trocar

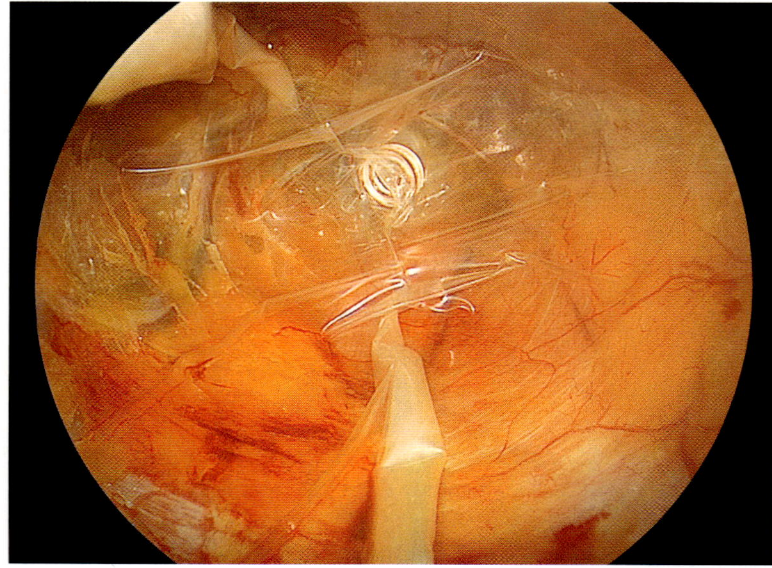

Fig: 6: Zero degree scope placed through balloon dilator, at start of inflation

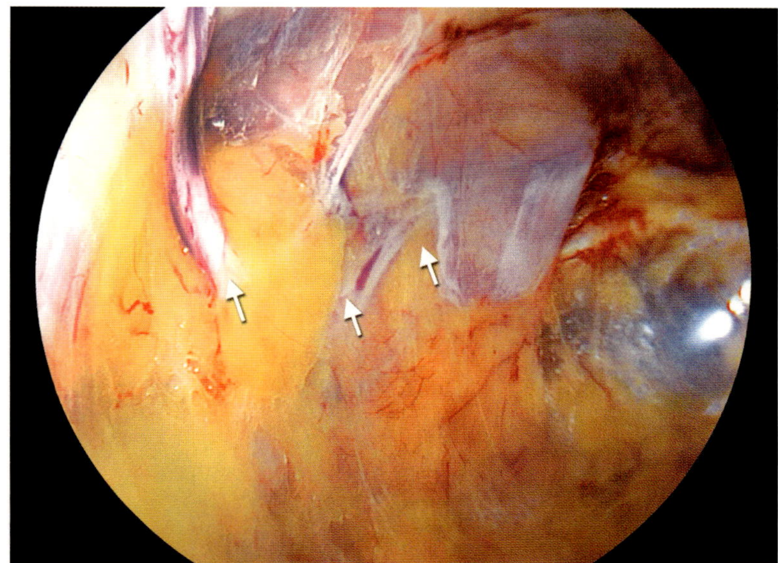

Fig. 7: View of left epigastric vessels through balloon dilator

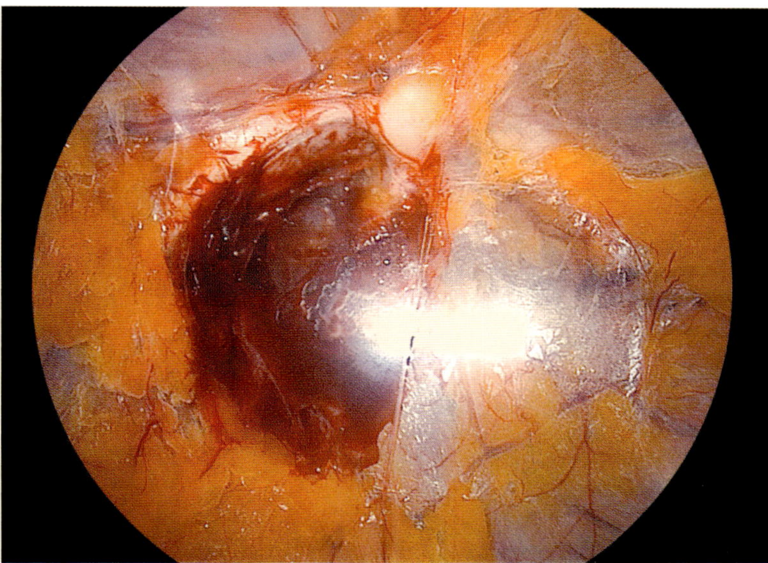

Fig. 8: Pubic symphysis visualized through balloon dilator

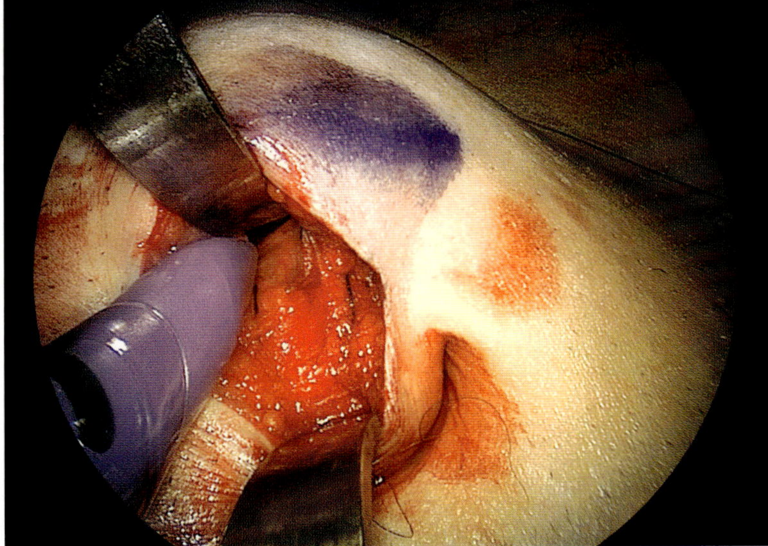

Fig. 9: Following deflation and removal of the balloon dilator, a 'S' retractor is used to retract rectus muscle upward for placement of dissecting smooth trocar (between rectus and posterior sheath) used to create the extraperitoneal space further cephalad and lateral

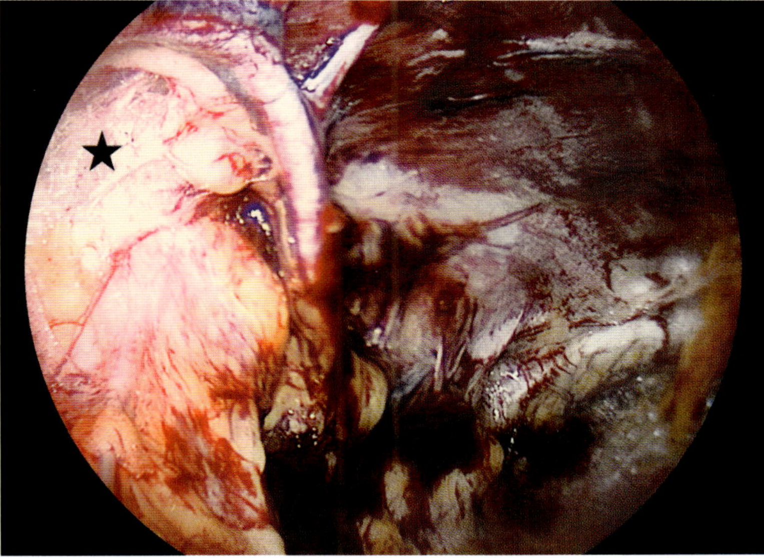

Fig. 10: Space lateral to left epigastric vessels for lateral dissection to accommodate lateral trocars (★)

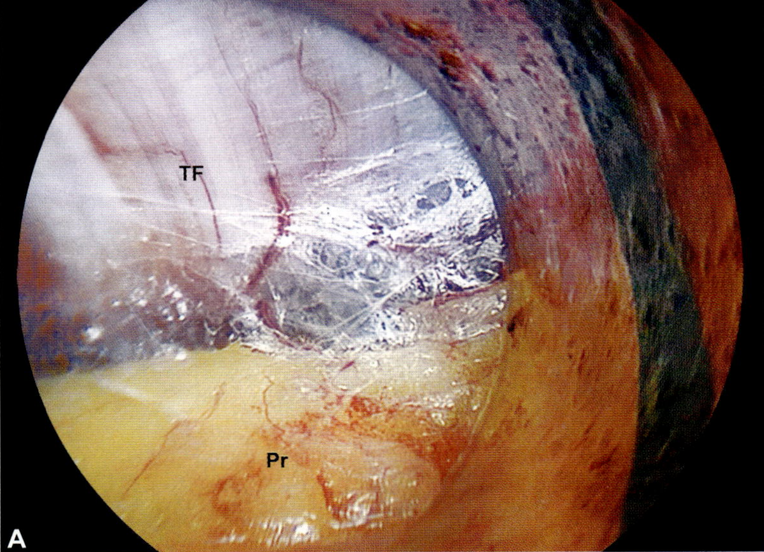

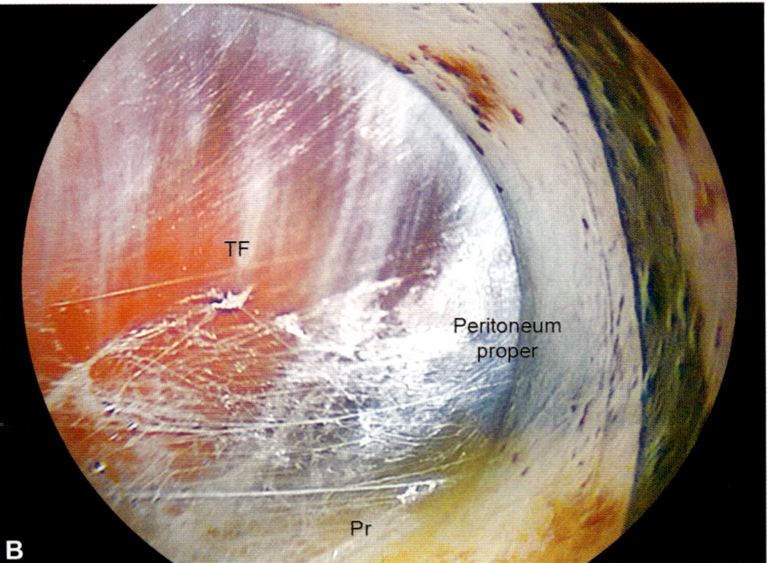

Figs 11A and B: Development of the extraperitoneal space lateral and cephalad between the transversalis fascia (TF) above and preperitoneal (Pr) layer below. The beveled edge of the dissecting trocar used to bluntly develop the space is seen to the right of the picture

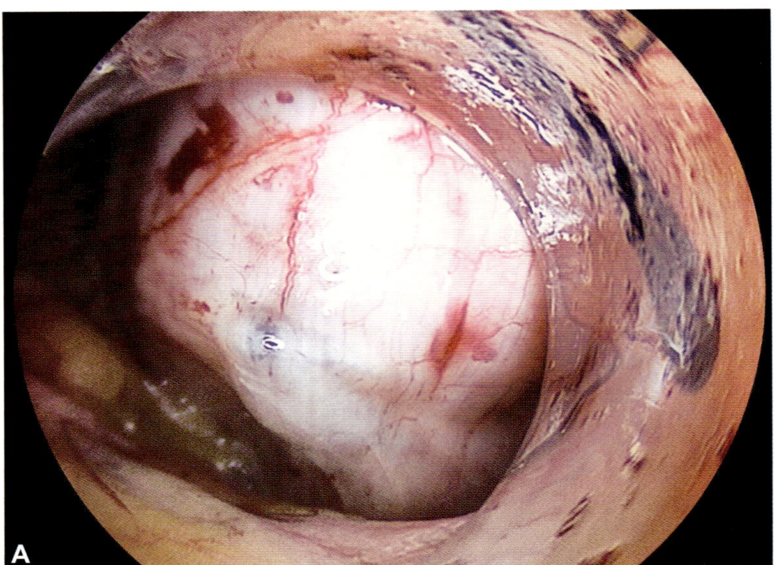

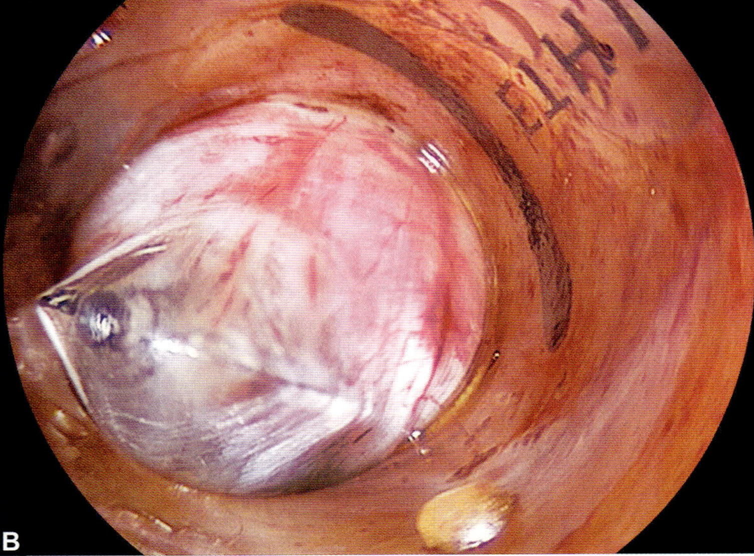

Figs 12A and B: Insertion of the right 12 mm lateral assistant trocar using the smooth dissecting trocar as a guide to prevent peritoneal injury

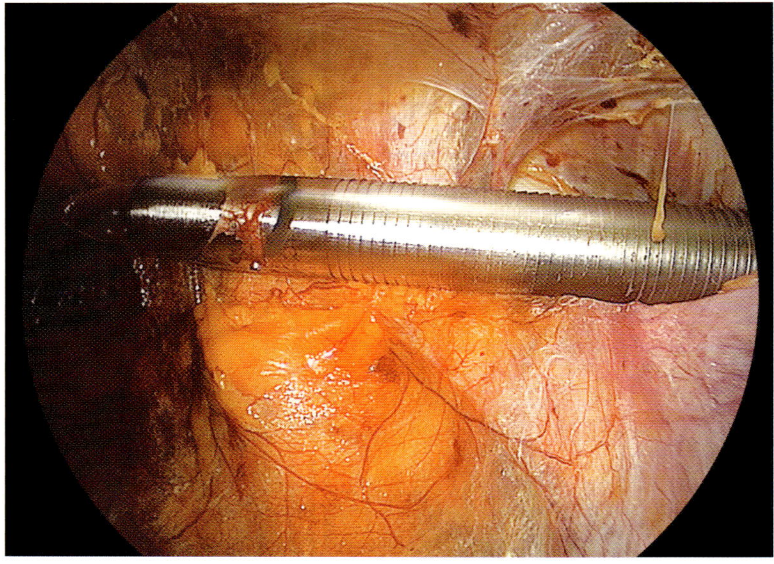

Fig. 13: View of right side. Long trocar passed over peritoneum toward the space of Retzius

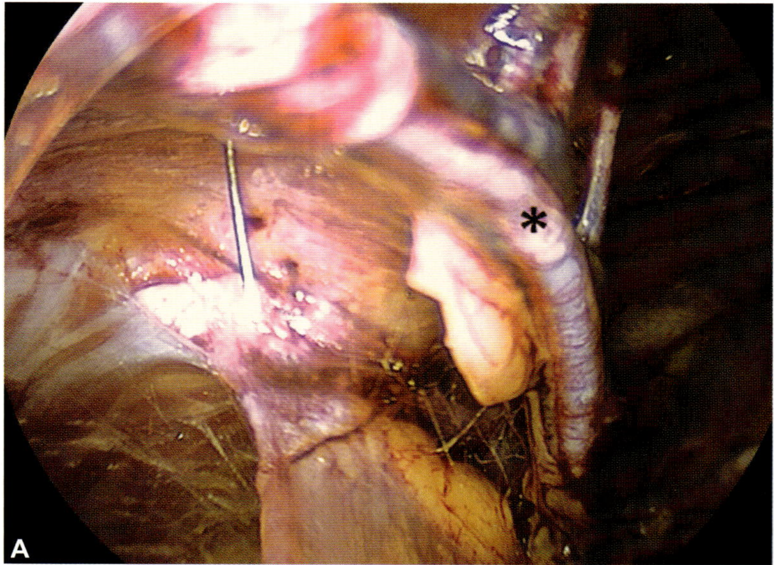

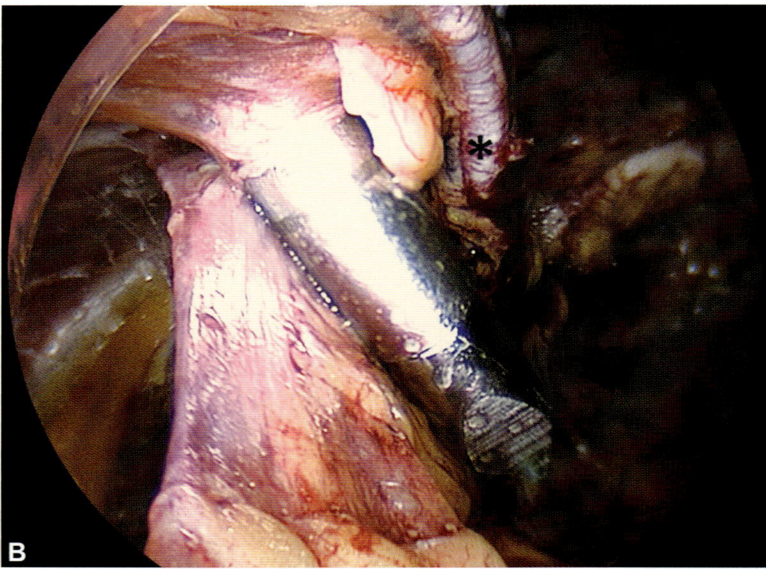

Figs 14A and B: Use of spinal needle to localize the site for the left robotic arm trocar preventing injury to the epigastric vessels (*) during introduction of the trocar for left robotic arm

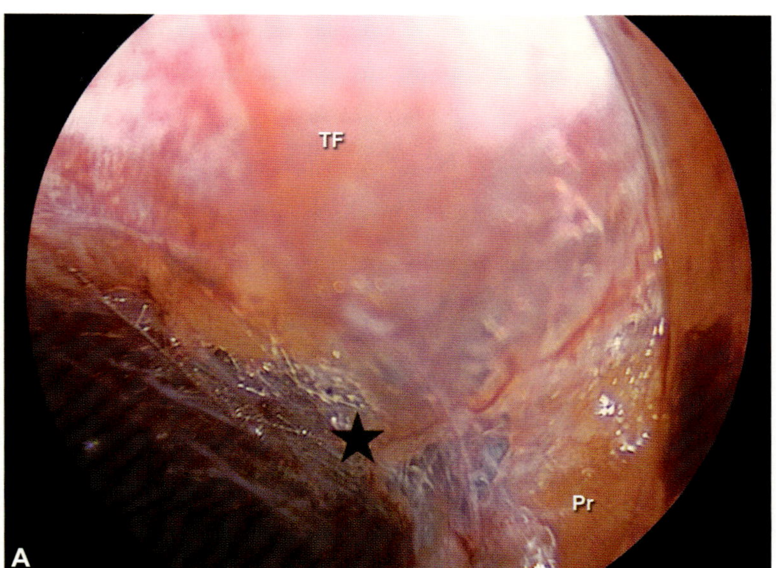

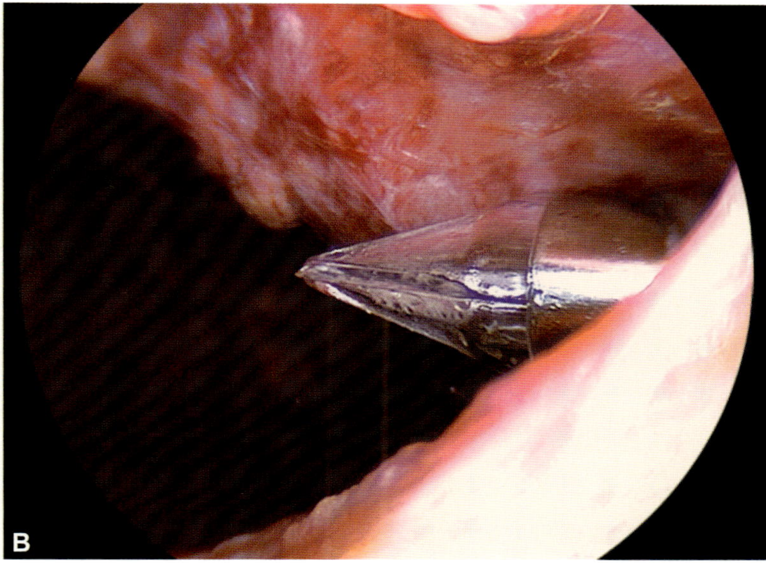

Figs 15A and B: Creation of space (★) for insertion of 5 mm assistant trocar between the transversalis fascia (TF) above and peritoneal (Pr) layer below

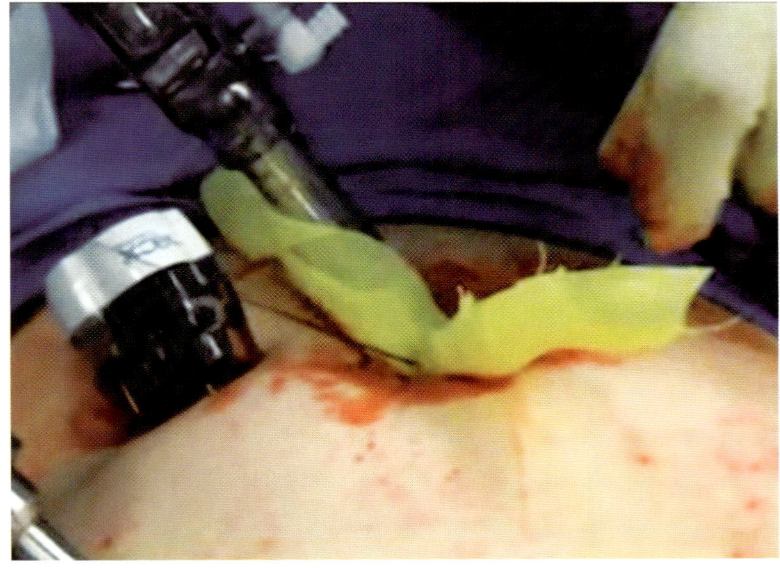

Fig. 16: Petroleum gauze secured around camera trocar (at periumbilical incision) to reduce gas leakage

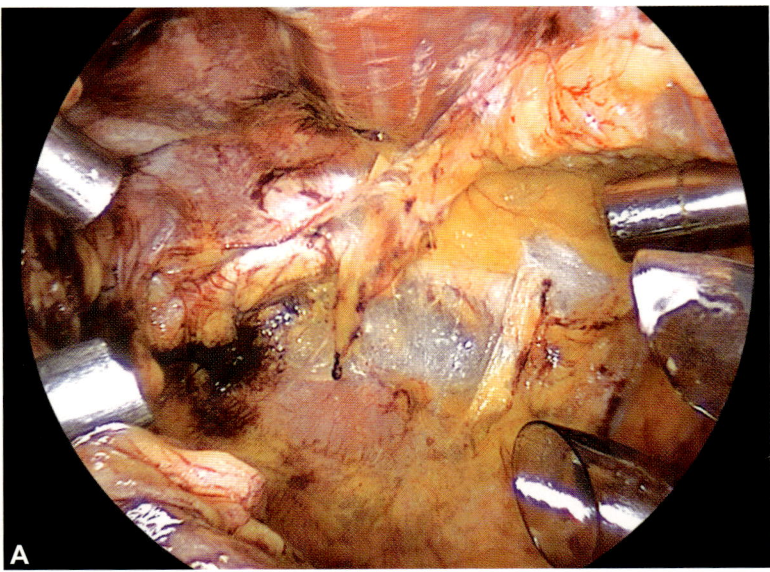

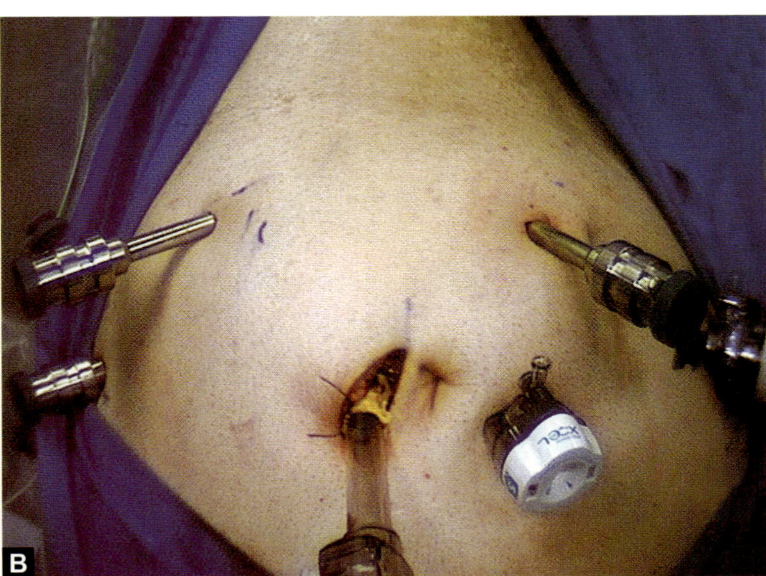

Figs 17A and B: Final 6-port trocar arrangement for 4-arm robot-assisted extraperitoneal radical prostatectomy. (A) insert endoscopic view, and (B) insert external view

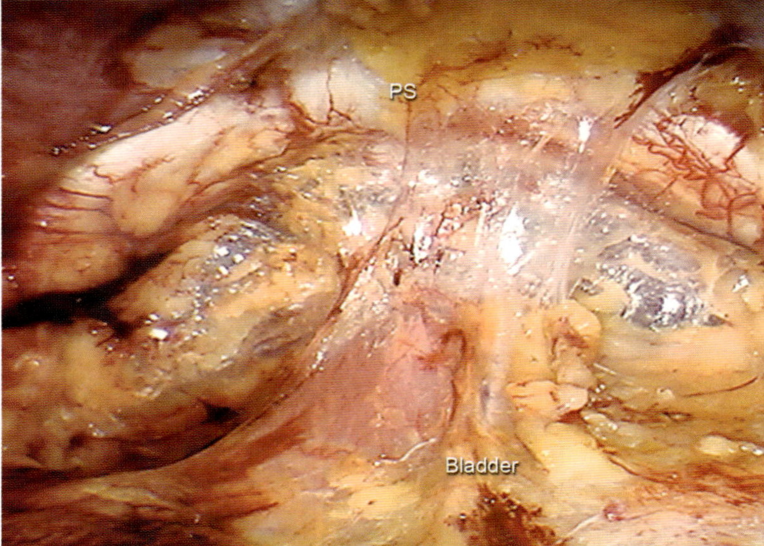

Fig. 18: View of Retzius space following access (PS: pubic symphysis). The first step following access is to clear the endopelvic fascia from overlying loose fatty tissues, all vessels are cauterized to ensure hemostasis

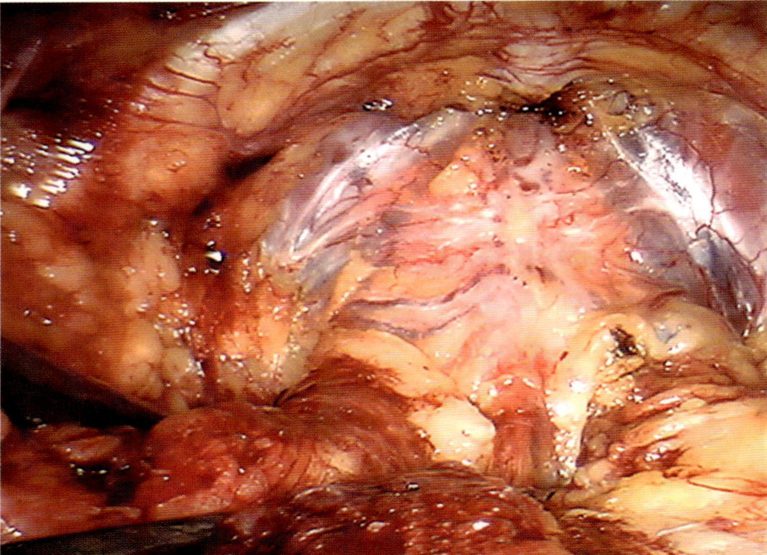

Fig. 19: Exposure of endopelvic fascia

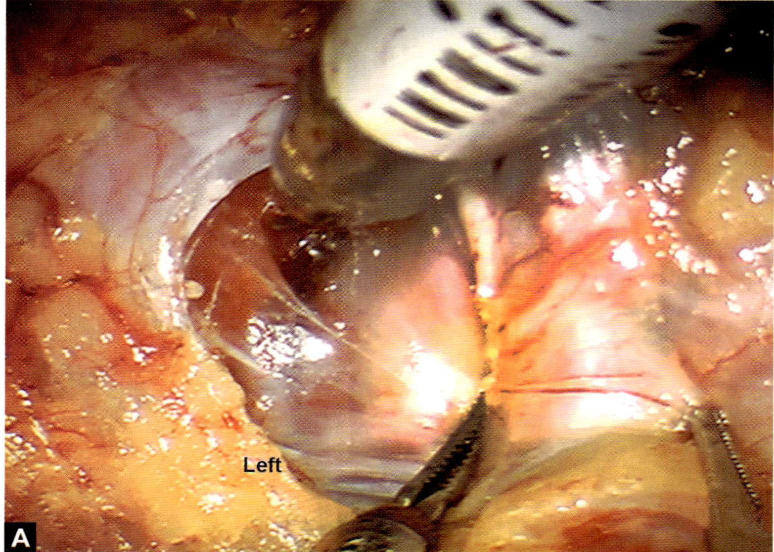

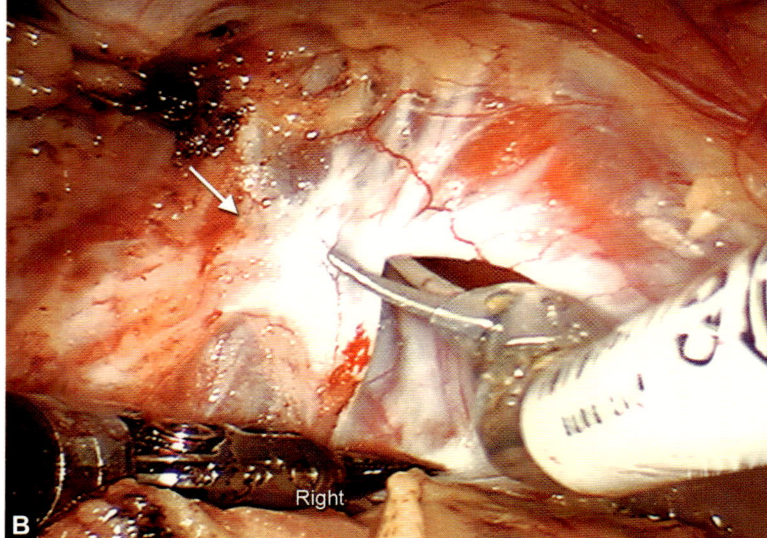

Fig. 20: Incision of endopelvic fascia. Opening the fascia along the midportion of the prostate provides an avascular plane and can be done without cautery. The incision extends from the base of the prostate to the puboprostatic ligaments (arrow head)

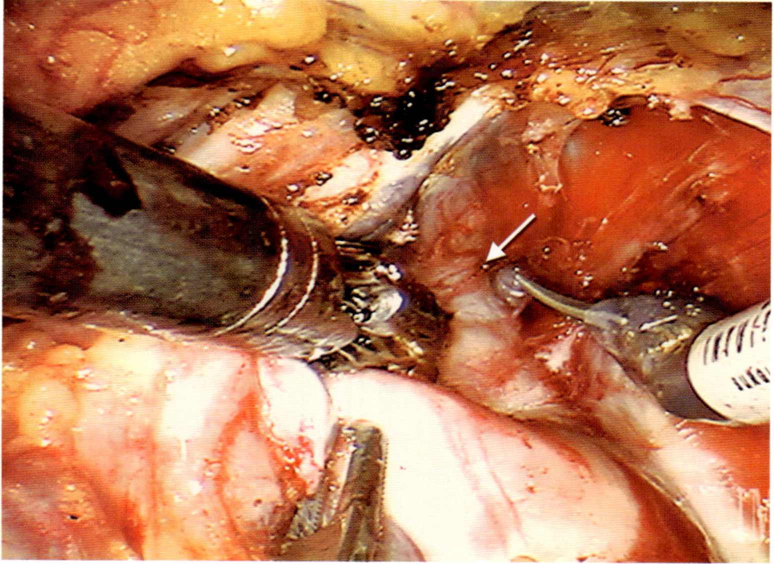

Fig. 21: Exposure of notch between dorsal venous complex (DVC) and urethra for needle placement during DVC suture

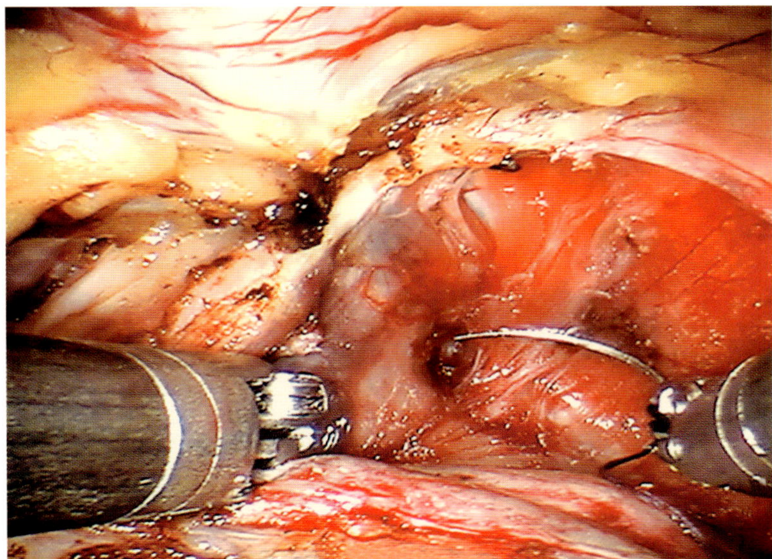

Fig. 22: Placement of dorsal venous complex (DVC) stitch. A 2-0 Polygalactin suture on an SH needle is used for ligation. The needle is placed from left to right parallel to the urethra. Positioning the needle driver at the proximal 1/3 of the needle at a perpendicular angle optimizes suture placement

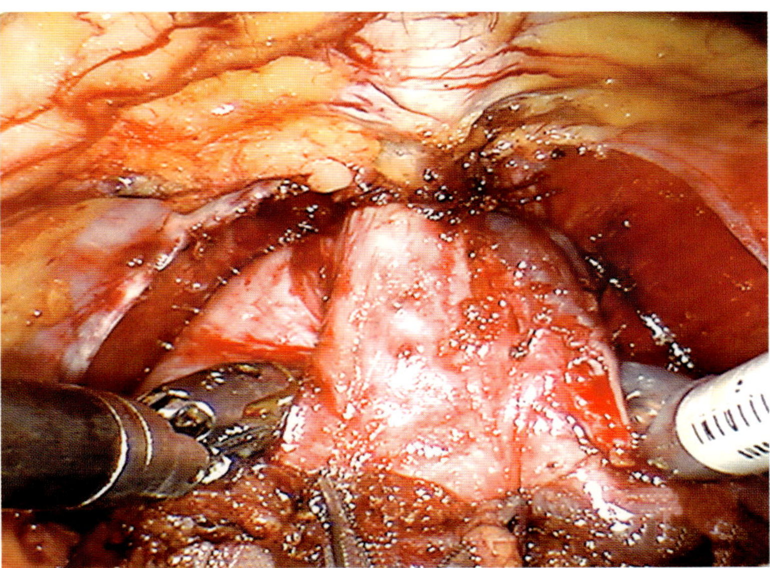

Fig. 23: Final dorsal venous complex (DVC) stitch. Inadvertent suturing of the catheter may occur if the knot does not hold

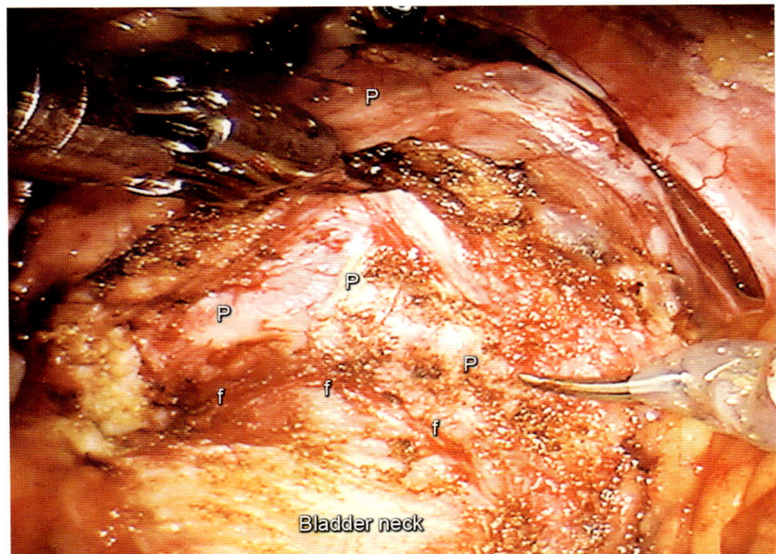

Fig. 24: Developing the plane between the anterior bladder neck fibers (f) and prostate (P)

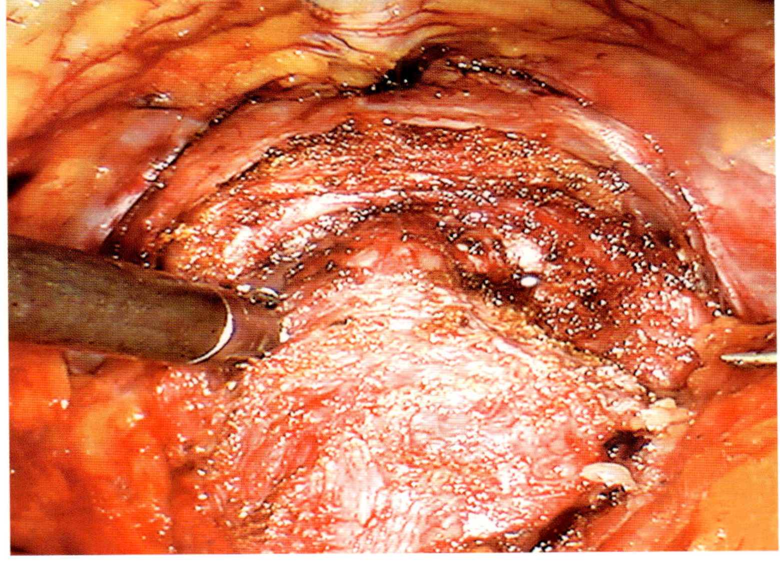

Fig. 25: View of bladder neck funnel prior to transection

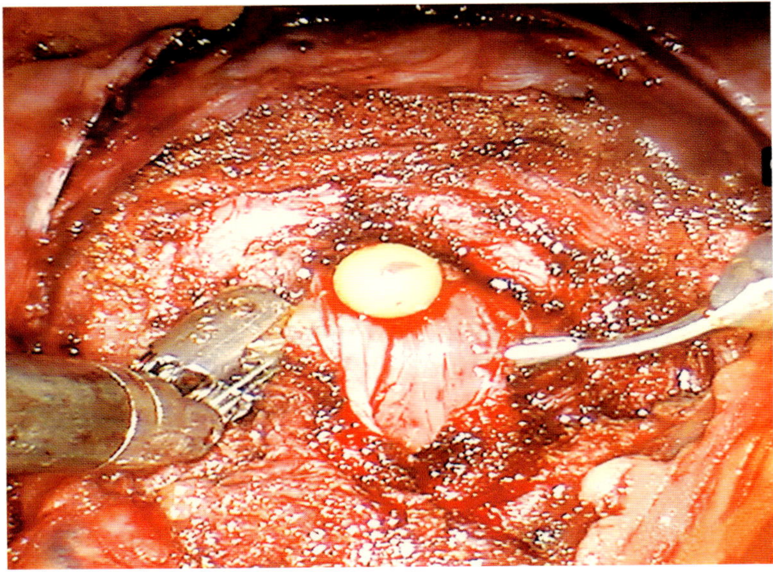

Fig. 26: Transection of anterior bladder neck, retraction of the catheter and identification of posterior bladder neck

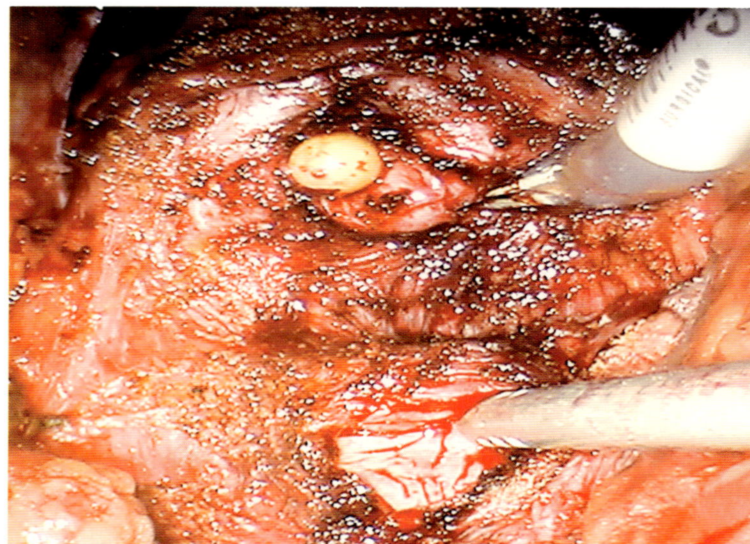

Fig. 27: View after transection of bladder neck. The plane between the bladder neck and prostate can be followed posteriorly, with the posterior bladder neck dissection

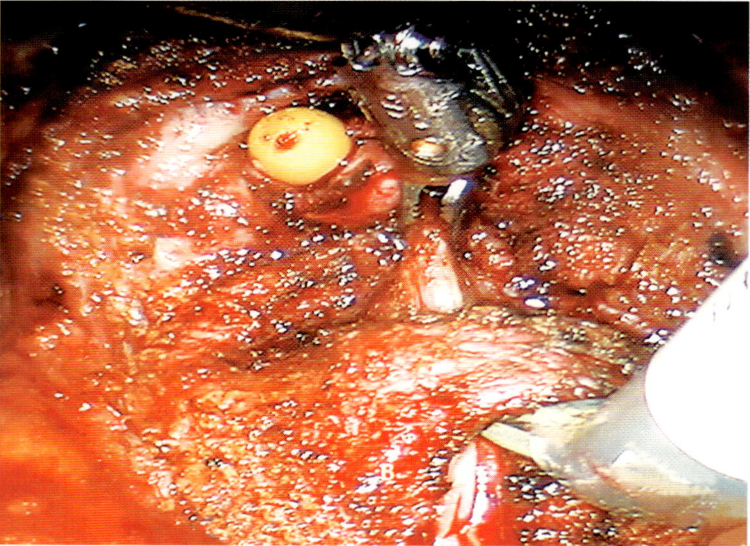

Fig. 28: Identification of the posterior plane between the posterior bladder wall and prostate. An instrument placed inside the transected bladder neck to aid in delineation of the extent of the posterior bladder wall. Care should be taken not to inadvertently place a hole in the posterior bladder, risking injury to the ureteral orifices. The 4th arm can be used to either retract the bladder cephalad, or to retract the Foley catheter anteriorly

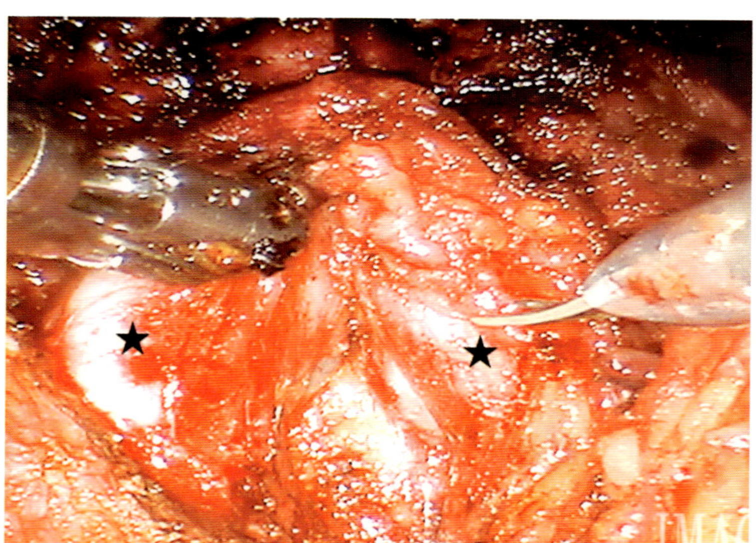

Fig. 29: Exposure of both ampullae of the vas deferens (★) following opening of the longitudinal muscle fibers crossing posterior to the bladder

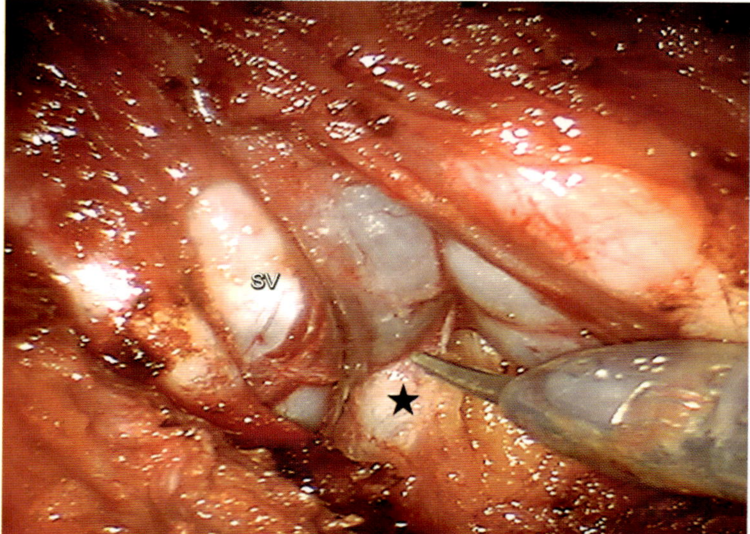

Fig. 30: Prior to transection of the vas deferens we prefer to expose the underlying seminal vesicles (SV). Denonvilliers' fascia (★) is pushed posteriorly, leading to complete visualization of the SVs in a relatively avascular plane

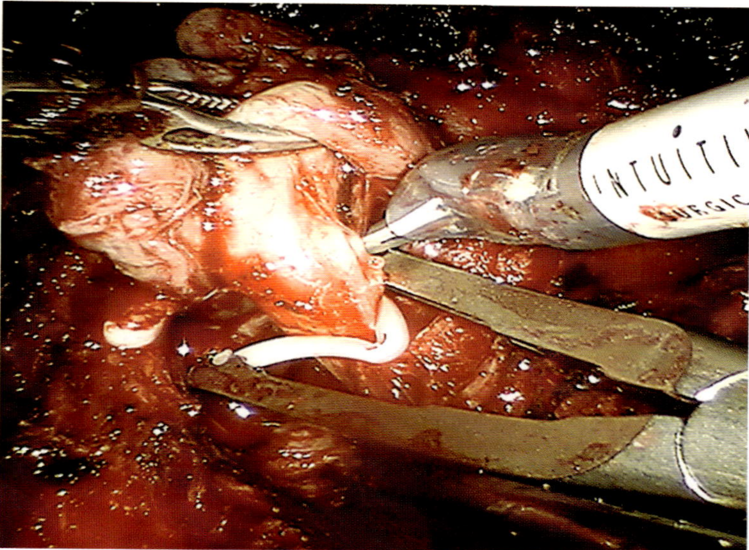

Fig. 31: Clipping of right ampulla with artery to the vas en bloc. The visible vas is grasped and dissected cephalad, until it courses laterally. At this point, it is clipped en bloc with the adjacent artery to the vas

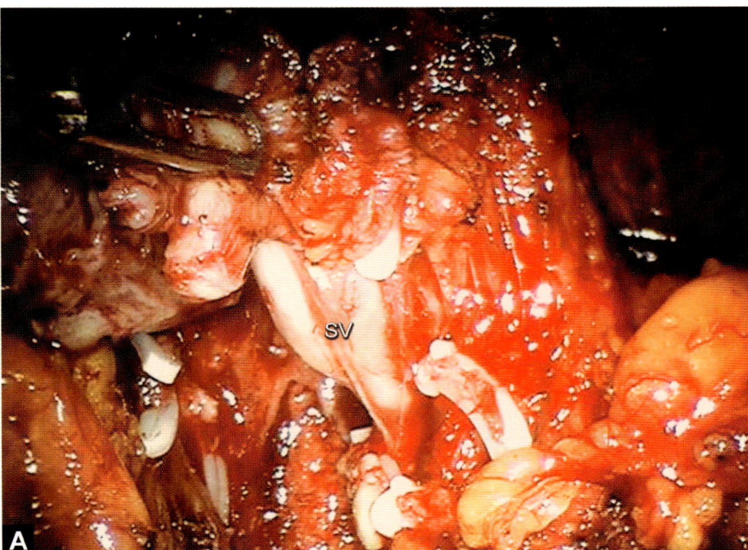

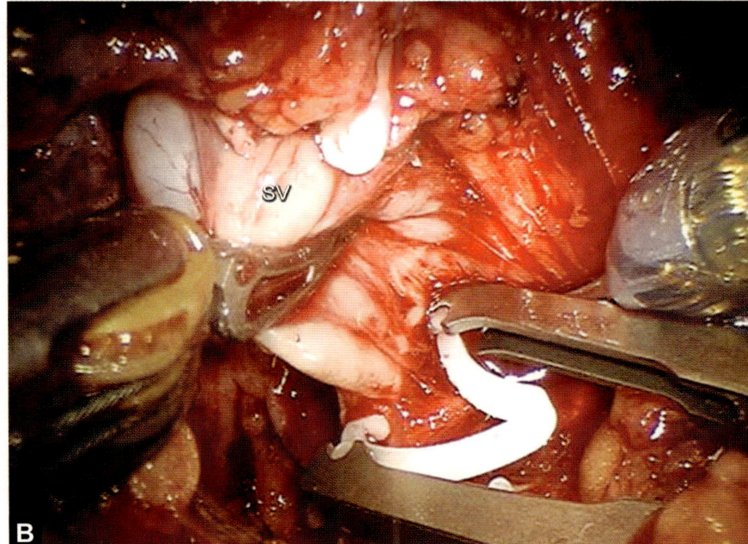

Figs 32A and B: Clipping of the posterolateral remaining seminal vesicles (SV) attachment. (A) Retraction of the SV medial and cephalad using 4th arm for ideal exposure; (B) Energy avoidance is recommended near the tip of the seminal vesicles, in nerve sparing cases, to avoid damage to the adjacent neurovascular bundles

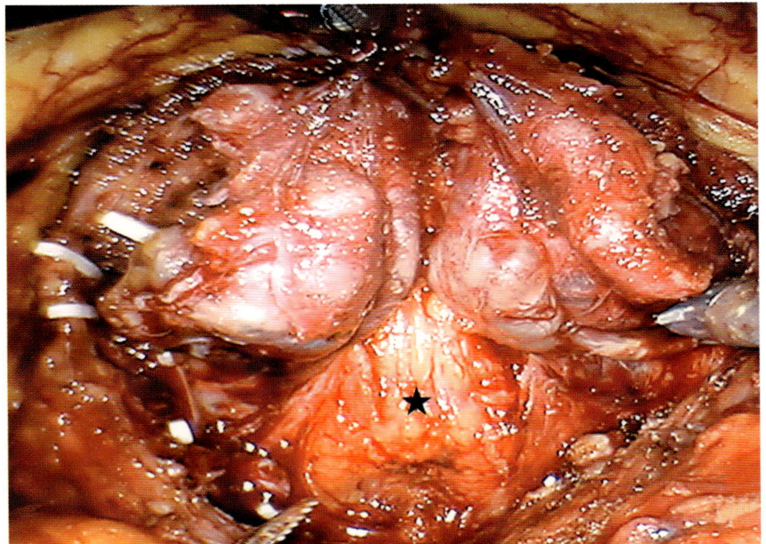

Fig. 33: Retraction of dissected seminal vesicles and prostate using 4th arm to expose Denonvilliers' fascia (★)

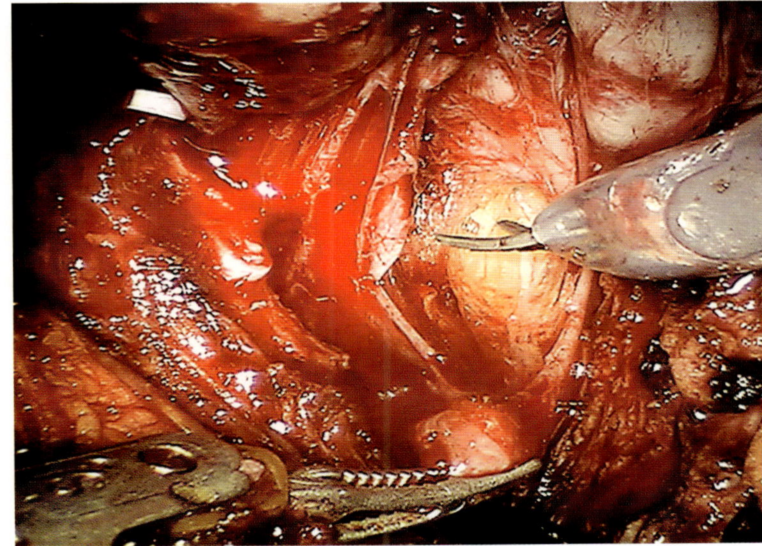

Fig. 34: Opening of Denonvilliers' fascia, exposing perirectal fat

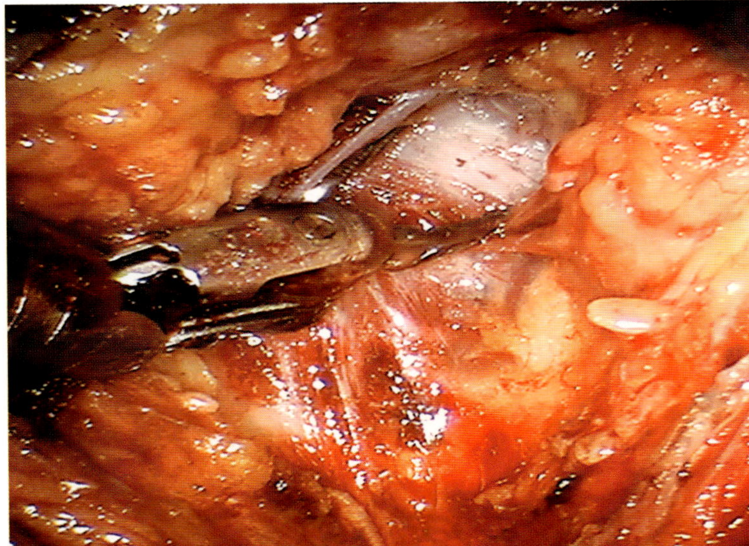

Fig. 35: The plane between Denonvilliers' fascia and the prostatic fascia is developed bluntly using the bipolar forceps, spread open and pushing posteriorly away from the prostate

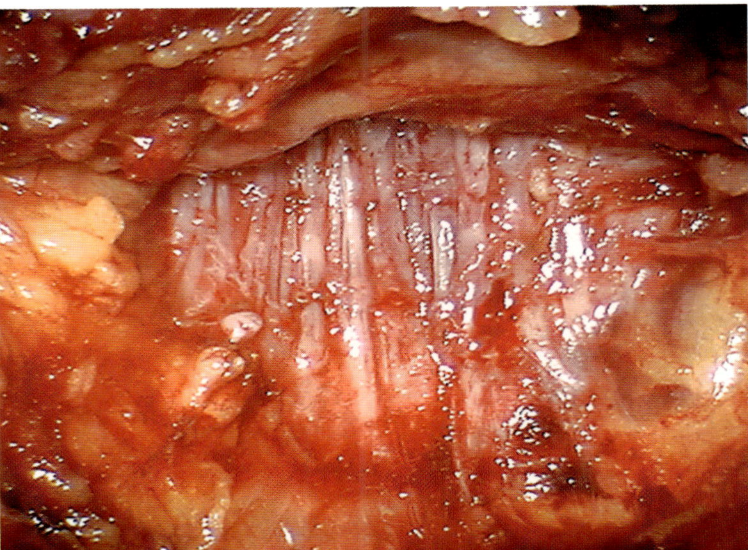

Fig. 36: View following posterior dissection between prostate and perirectal fat

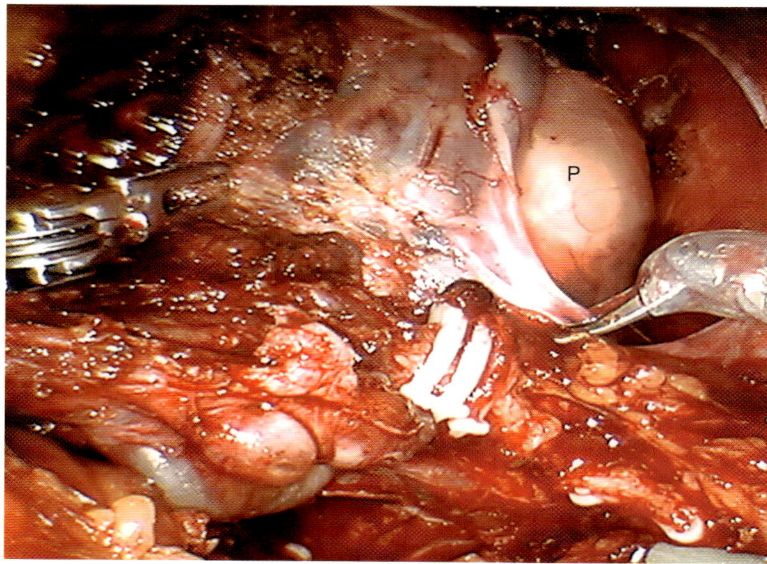

Fig. 37: Retraction of the prostate (P) cephalad and to the contralateral side (4th arm) to expose the plane for neurovascular bundle (NVB) dissection (right side)

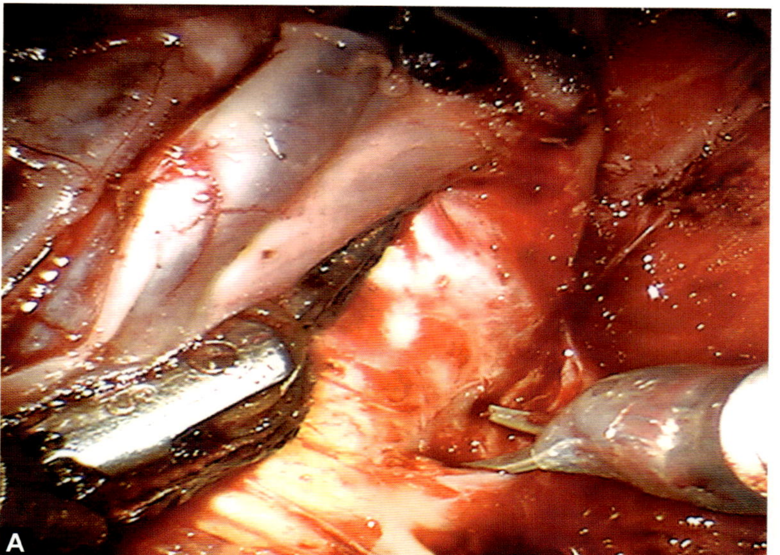

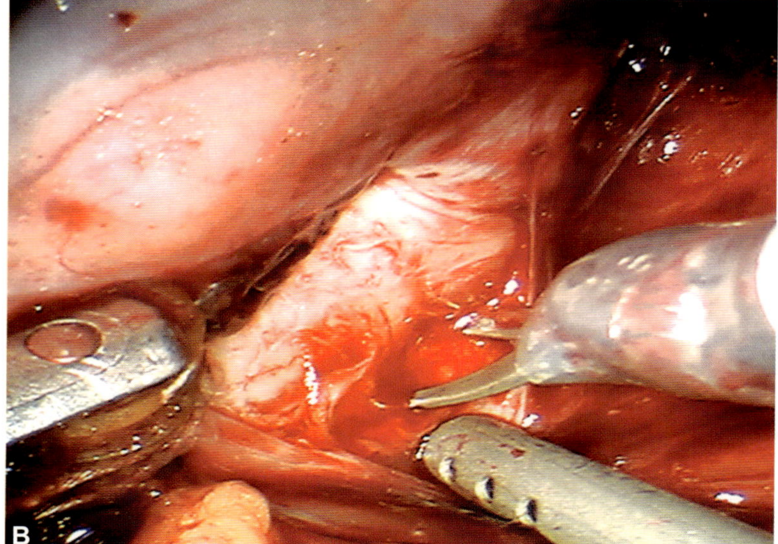

Figs 38A and B: Development of the interfascial plane laterally for retrograde right neurovascular bundle (NVB) dissection. The left instrument rolls the prostate medially to aid in exposure of the plane

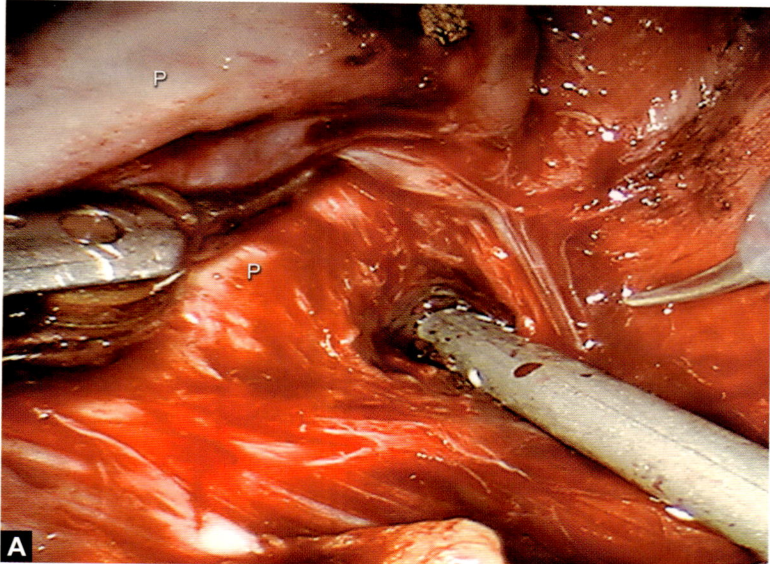

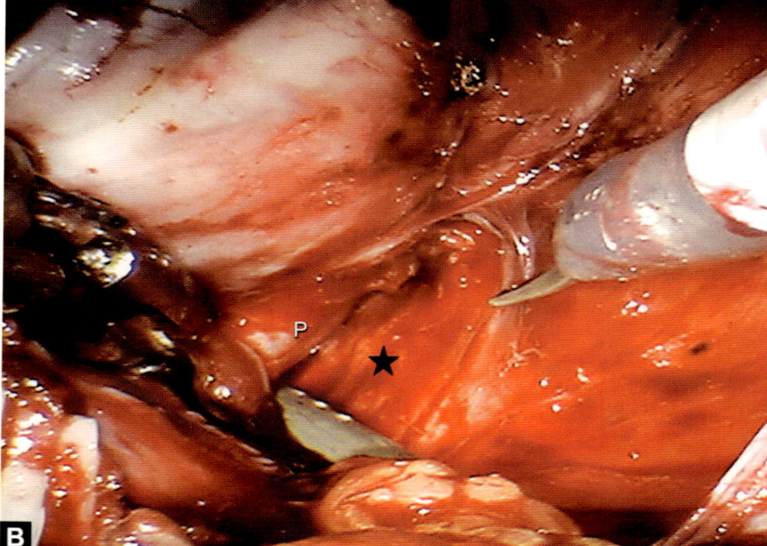

Figs 39A and B: Right neurovascular bundle (NVB) (★) lateral release (retrograde dissection)

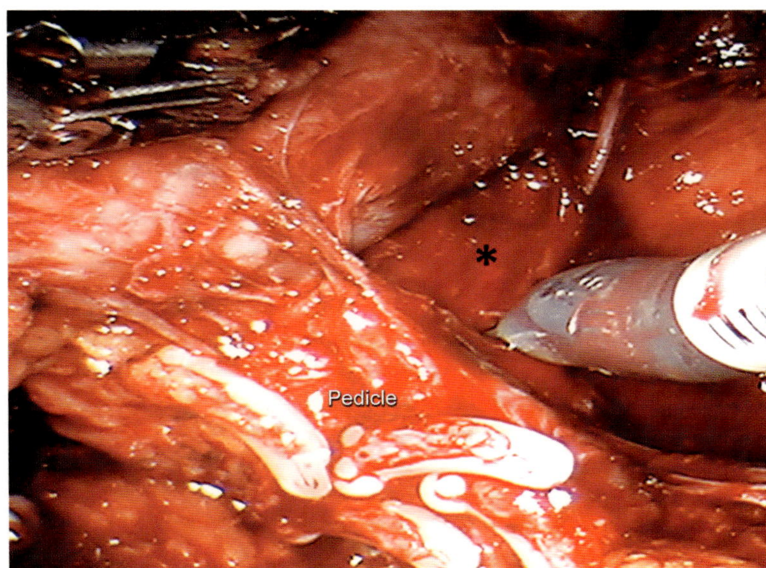

Fig. 40: Right prostate posterior neurovascular bundle (*) release. The vessels are pushed posterolaterally, until entry into the previously dissected plane posterior to the prostate, over the rectum

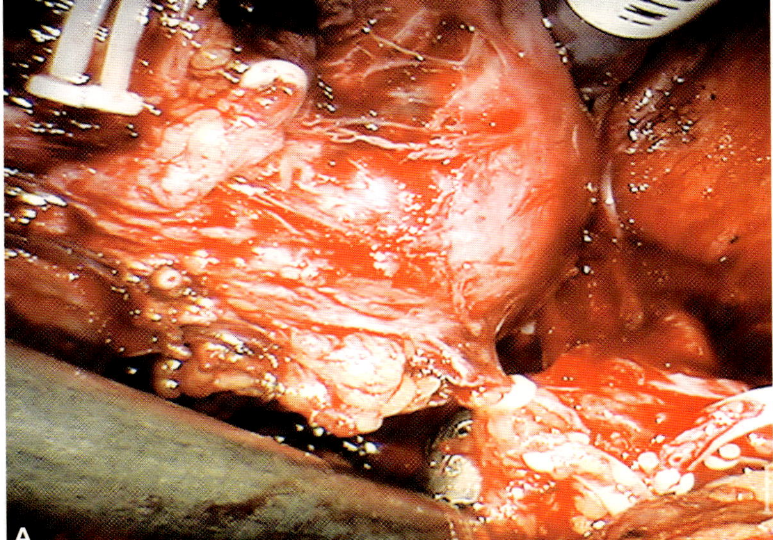

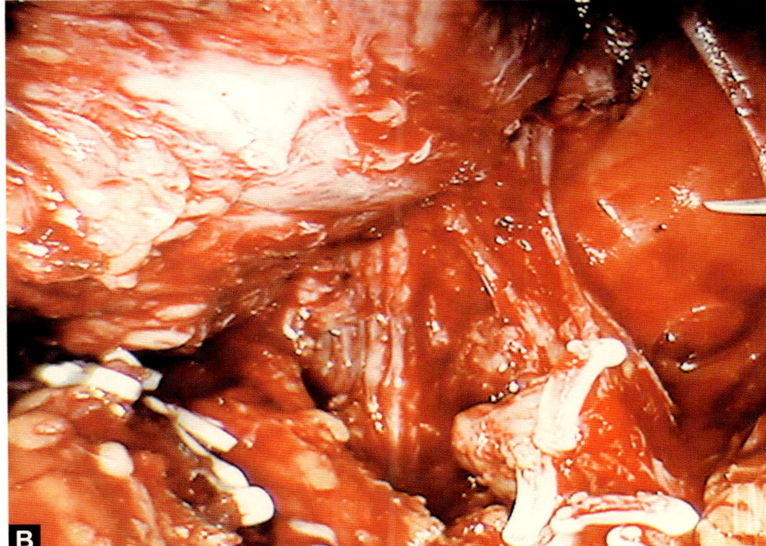

Figs 41A and B: Antegrade neurovascular bundle (NVB) release. Antegrade clipping of prostate pedicle connecting previously created lateral and posterior planes while preserving the structures coursing posteriorly, to later form the cavernous vessels and nerves (antegrade dissection)

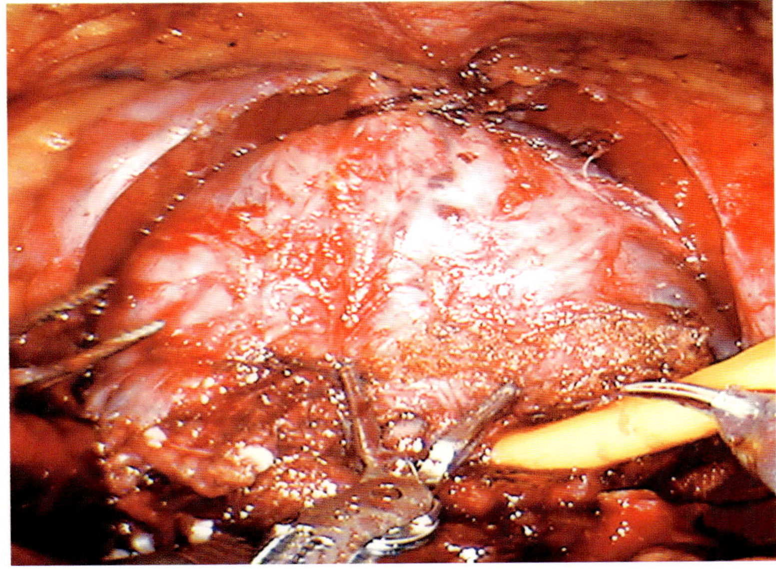

Fig. 42: Insertion of Foley catheter and retraction of prostate cephalad prior to dorsal venous complex (DVC) division

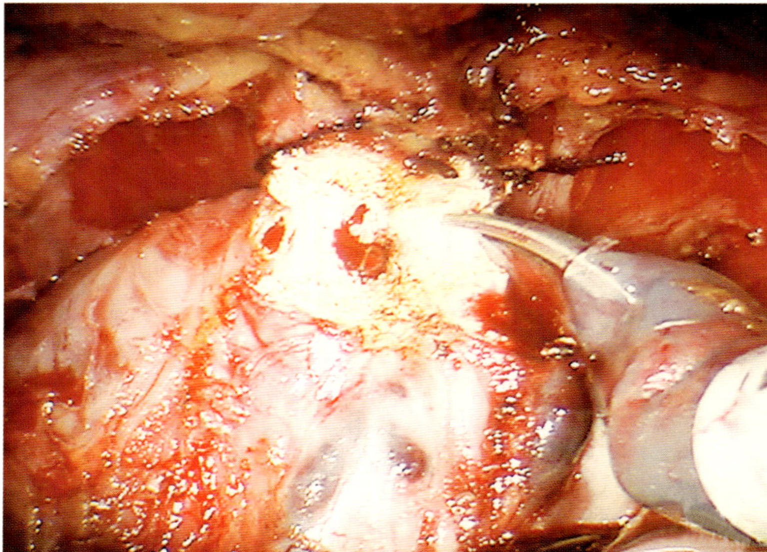

Fig. 43: The ligated dorsal vein is transected down to the level on the longitudinal urethral fibers. Occasionally, the dorsal vein suture falls due to the posterior traction. The dorsal vein can be oversewn without difficulty. To facilitate this and limit bleeding, the intra-abdominal pressure can be elevated temporarily to 20 mm Hg

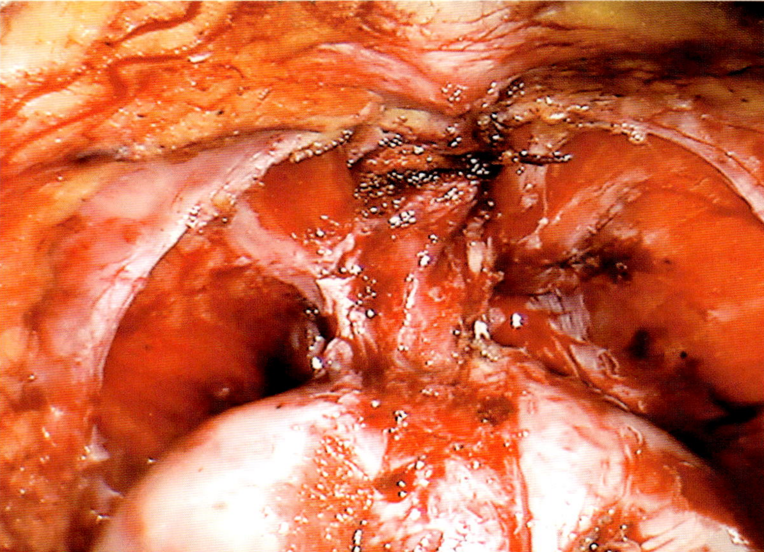

Fig. 44: Exposed urethra

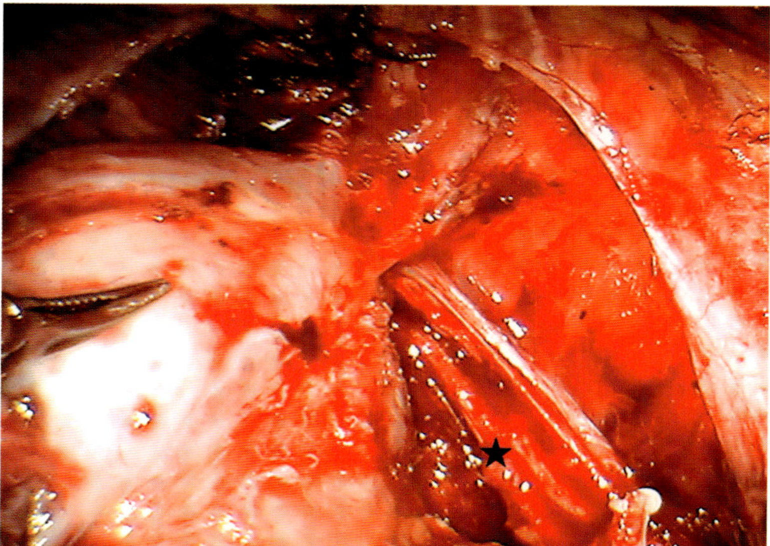

Fig. 45: Prior to transection of the urethra, the prostate is rotated medially and neurovascular bundles (NVBs) (★) inspected, or further dissected from the prostate apex to avoid injury

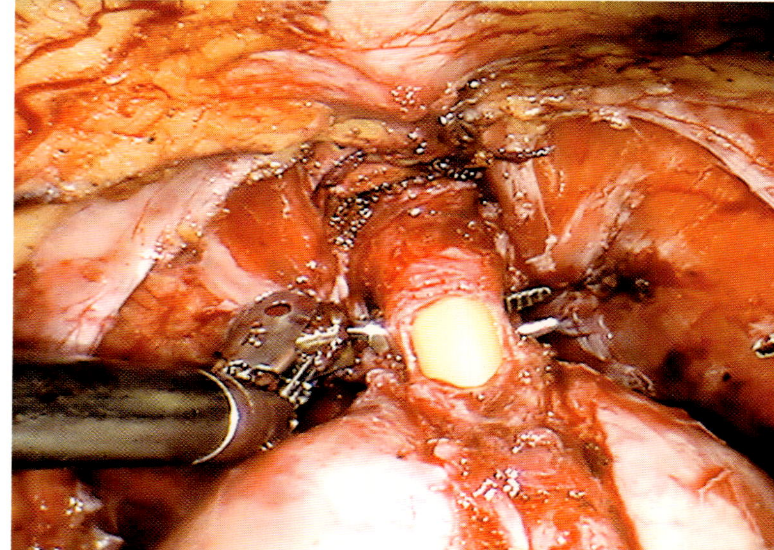

Fig. 46: Exposure of Foley catheter following sharp transection of anterior urethra

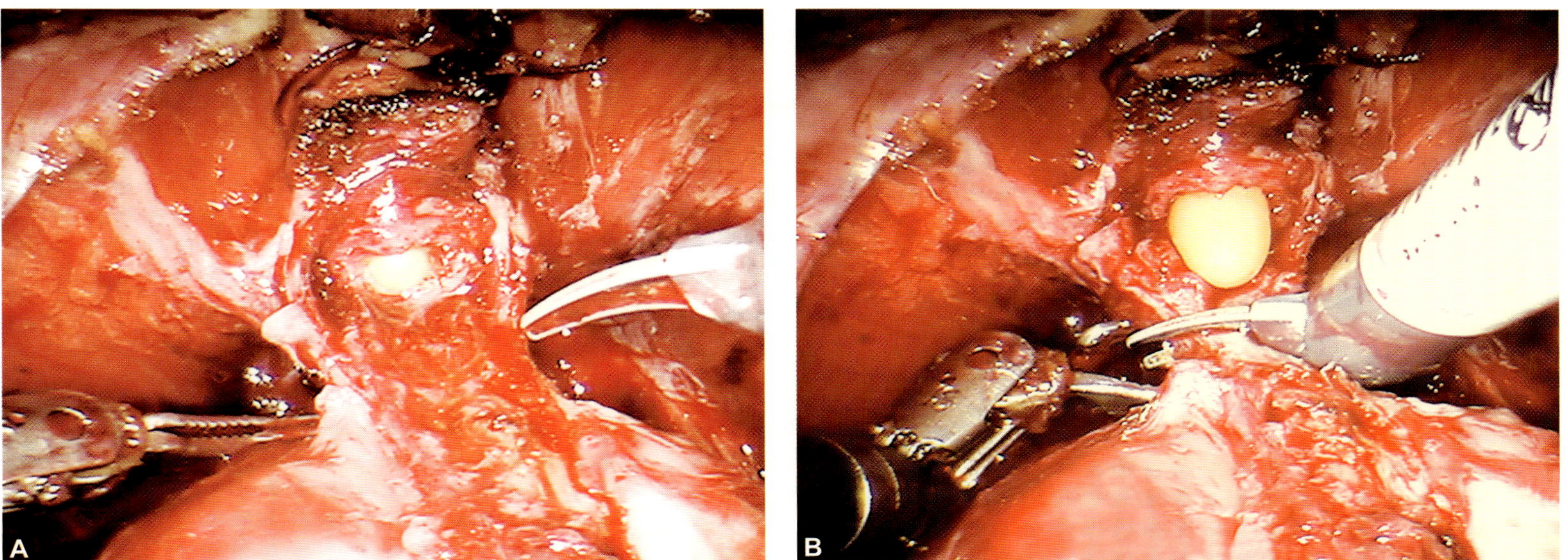

Figs 47A and B: The posterior prostate often extends more caudally than the anterior aspect. The transection should therefore follow the contour of the prostate

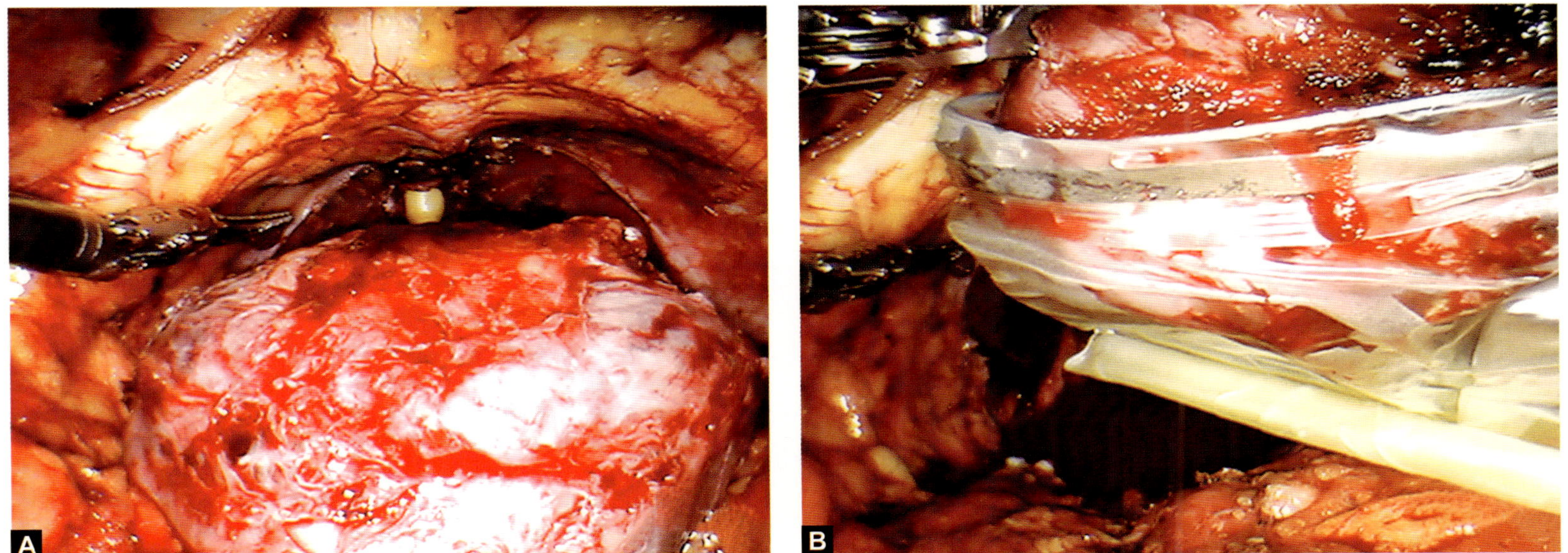

Figs 48A and B: (A) The specimen is inspected and (B) Placed in an entrapment bag

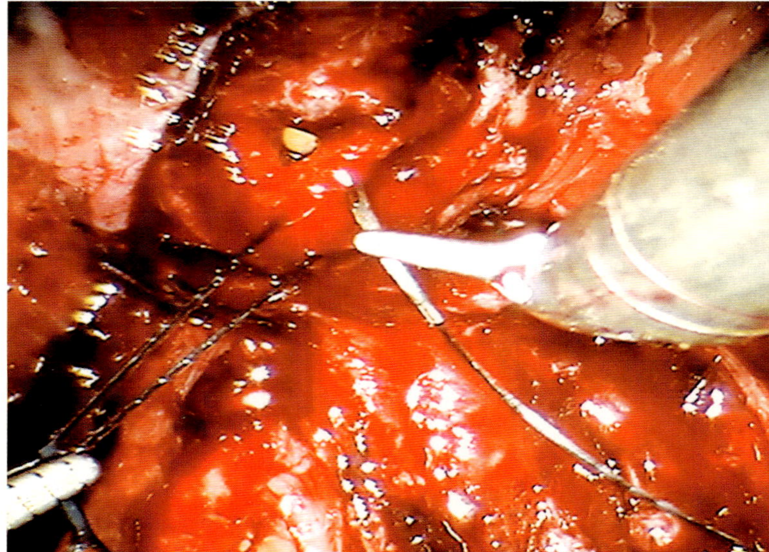

Fig. 49: Posterior reconstruction. A 2-0 barbed suture (V-LOC, Glycolic acid-trimethylene carbonate, Covidien, Norwalk, CT, USA) is used for this step

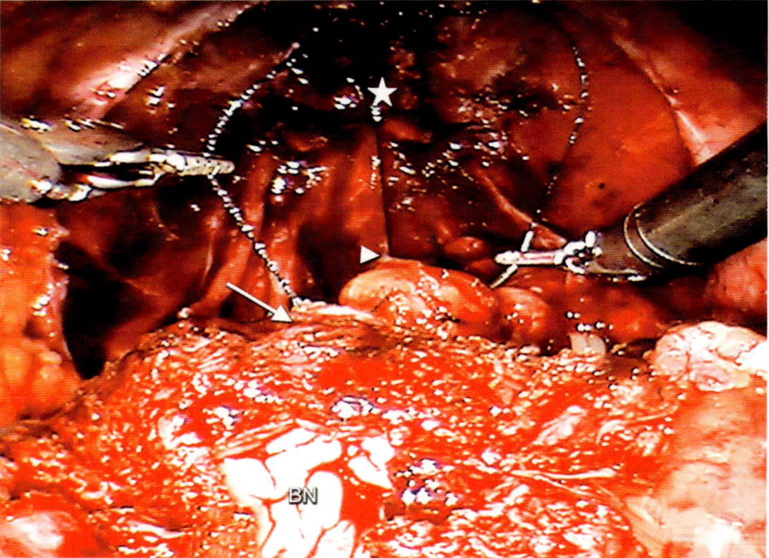

Fig. 50: Posterior reconstruction. Approximation of the posterior rhabdosphincter (★) with Denonvilliers' fascia (arrow), posterior to the bladder neck (BN). We prefer to also include the longitudinal fibers posterior to the bladder which were previously covering the seminal vesicles (arrow head)

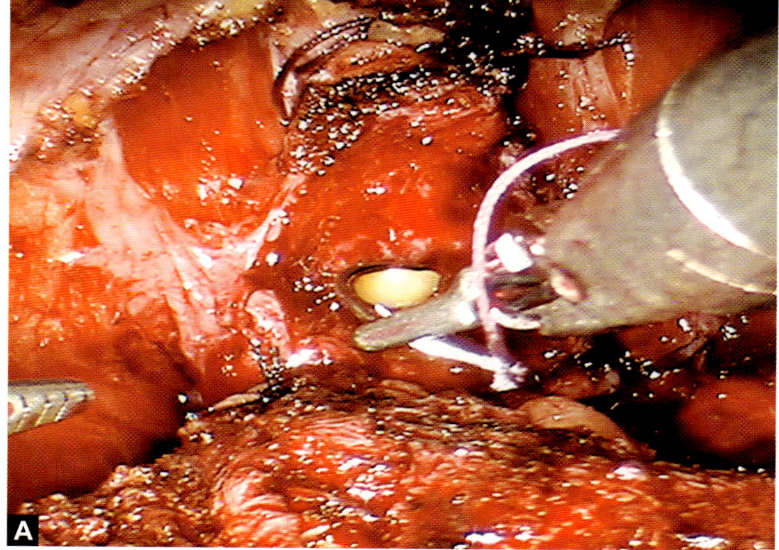

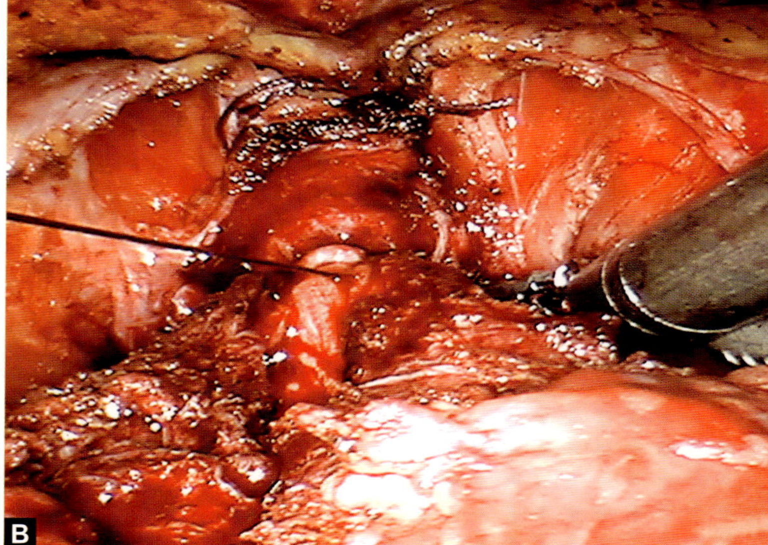

Figs 51A and B: Urethrovesical anastomosis. Two 2-0 Polygalactin sutures on an RB-1 needle (Ethicon) are used to complete the anastomosis. The posterior layer starts at the 5 o'clock position

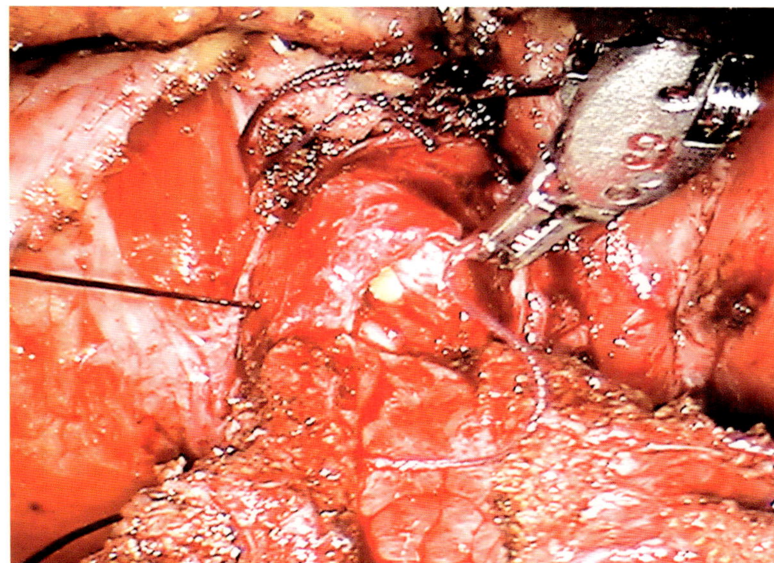

Fig. 52: The posterior layer is carried out in a clockwise direction from the 5 o'clock to the 11 o'clock position

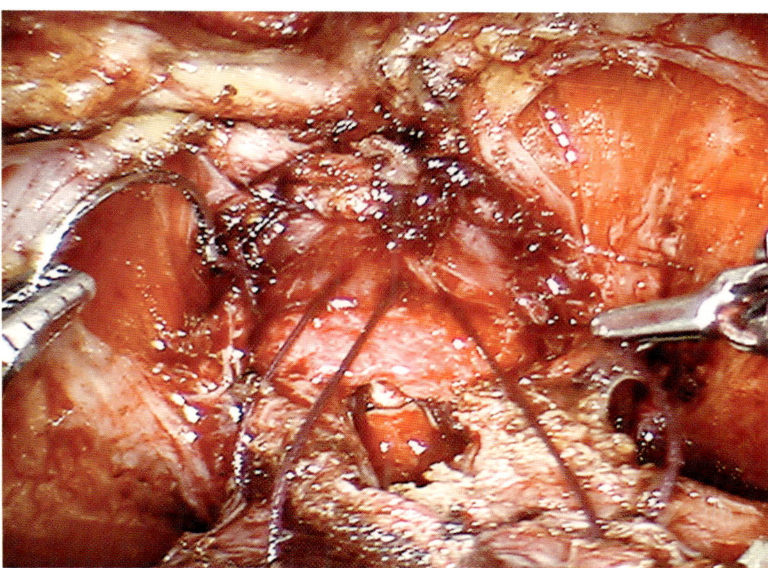

Fig. 53: The anterior layer is completed in the opposite direction

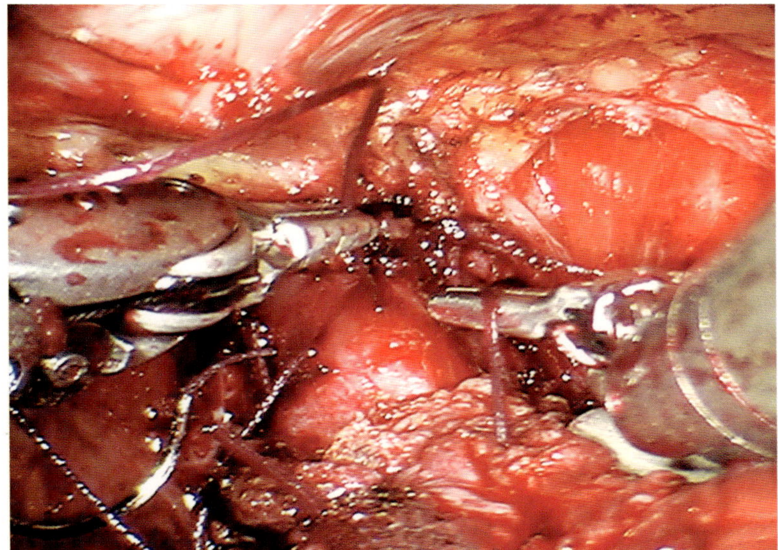

Fig. 54: The anterior layer sutures are cinched down perpendicular to the urethra and not toward the bladder to avoid tearing of the urethra, following introduction of the Foley catheter under vision

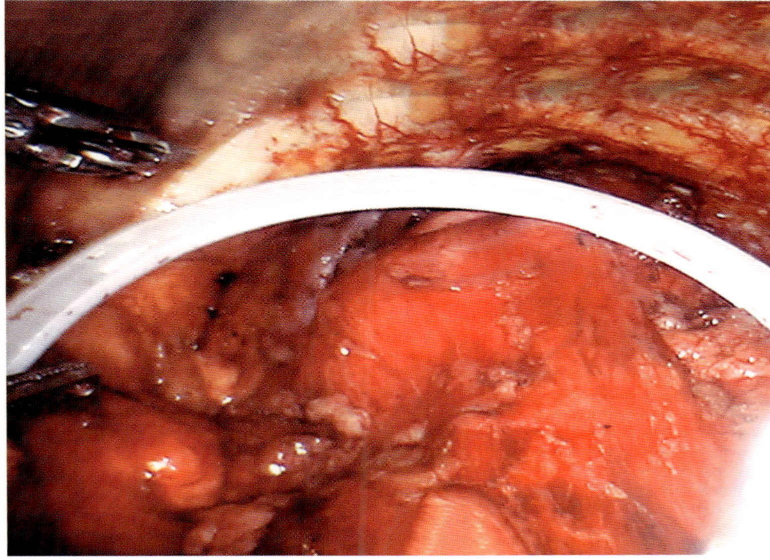

Fig. 55: Drain in place

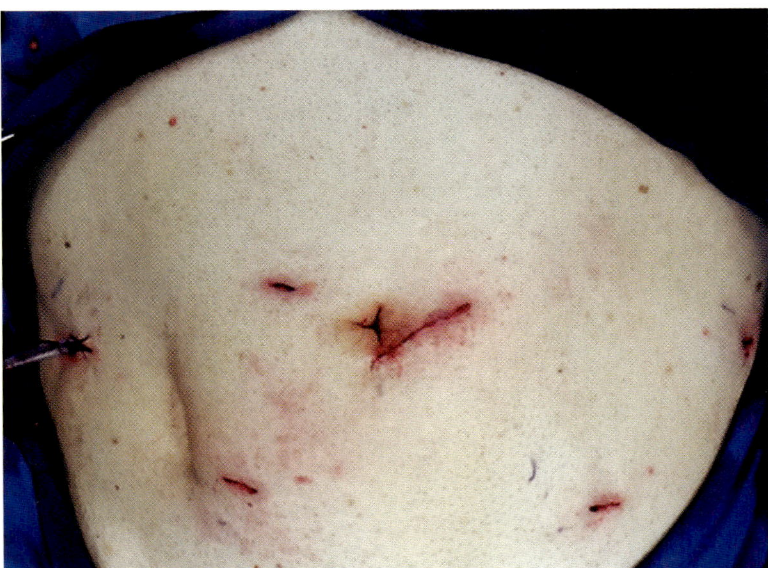

Fig. 56: The drain exits from the right lateral assistant trocar. Only the midline umbilical trocar opening is closed using 0 Polygalactin interrupted sutures to reconstruct the fascial anatomy. The anterior rectus sheath opening is enlarged to allow removal of the specimen. The skin incisions are closed using 4-0 monocryl subcuticular sutures

REFERENCES

1. Raboy A, Ferzli G, Albert P. Initial experience with extraperitoneal endoscopic radical retropubic prostatectomy. Urology. 1997; 50:849-53.
2. Schuessler WW, Schulam PG, Clayman RV, et al. Laparoscopic radical prostatectomy: initial short-term experience. Urology. 1997;50:854-7.
3. Bollens R, Vanden Bossche M, Roumeguere T, et al. Extraperitoneal laparoscopic radical prostatectomy. Results after 50 cases. Eur Urol. 2001;40:65-9.
4. Stolzenburg JU, Do M, Pfeiffer H, et al. The endoscopic extraperitoneal radical prostatectomy (EERPE): technique and initial experience. World J Urol. 2002;20:48-55.
5. GettmanMT, Hoznek A, Salomon L, et al. Laparoscopic radical prostatectomy: description of the extraperitoneal approach using the da Vinci robotic system. J Urol. 2003;170:416-9.
6. Joseph JV, Rosenbaum R, Madeb R, et al. Robotic Extraperitoneal Radical Prostatectomy: an Alternative Approach. J Urol. 2006;175:945-51.
7. Stolzenburg JU, McNeill A, Liatsikos EN. Nerve-sparing endoscopic extraperitoneal radical prostatectomy. BJU International. 2008;101: 909-28.

14 Chapter Laparoscopic Radical Prostatectomy

Boris Gershman, Douglas M Dahl

PATIENT SELECTION AND PREOPERATIVE PREPARATION

Laparoscopic radical prostatectomy is indicated in patients who are appropriate candidates for surgical therapy of prostate cancer—that is, patients with clinically organ-confined disease who are not expected to succumb to competing causes of death. Contraindications to laparoscopic surgery are relative with current experience, and may include inability to tolerate pneumoperitoneum, severe cardiac or pulmonary disease, uncorrected bleeding diathesis and morbid obesity. The authors generally employ an extraperitoneal approach, although patients who have had prior laparoscopic inguinal hernia repair may require a transperitoneal approach to facilitate dissection. Preoperative preparation includes a clear liquid diet the day prior to surgery as well as a mechanical bowel preparation that evening. Patients should have an active blood bank sample.

OPERATING ROOM SETUP AND PATIENT POSITIONING

The operating room is positioned as shown in Figure 1 with the surgeon standing to the patient's left and the assistant to the patient's right. Video monitors are placed at the foot of the bed in direct line of sight with the surgeon and laparoscopic instruments. Compression stockings and intermittent pneumatic compression devices are applied in the preoperative area for thromboembolism prophylaxis and intravenous antibiotics are given. General endotracheal anesthesia is induced and the patient is positioned supine with the arms tucked at the sides (Fig. 1). The patient is secured to the table with the shoulders padded to prevent movement in Trendelenburg position. The abdomen is shaved, prepped and draped in the usual fashion. An 18 Fr Foley catheter is inserted on the field.

OBTAINING ACCESS—EXTRAPERITONEAL APPROACH

The authors perform the majority of laparoscopic radical prostatectomies via an extraperitoneal approach. A 12 mm incision is made in the midline below the umbilicus and carried down to the rectus fascia. A small incision is made in the anterior rectus sheath, 1 cm lateral to the midline, to accommodate the distention balloon (PDB-S2 distention balloon, Auto Suture-Covidien). A heavy Kelly clamp is passed to the pubic symphysis and then withdrawn open to bluntly develop the extraperitoneal space. The balloon is then used to develop the retropubic space and the space is insufflated with CO_2 to 15 mm Hg (Fig. 2). One 11 mm port is placed lateral to the right rectus border and two 5 mm ports are placed in the lower abdomen

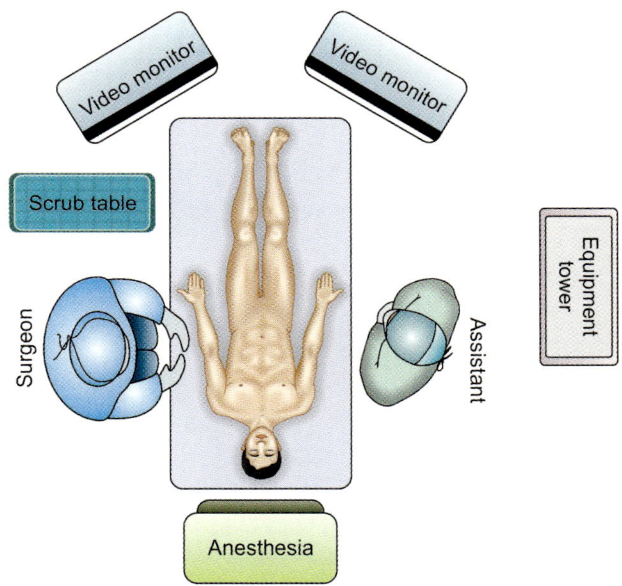

Fig. 1: Operating room and patient positioning

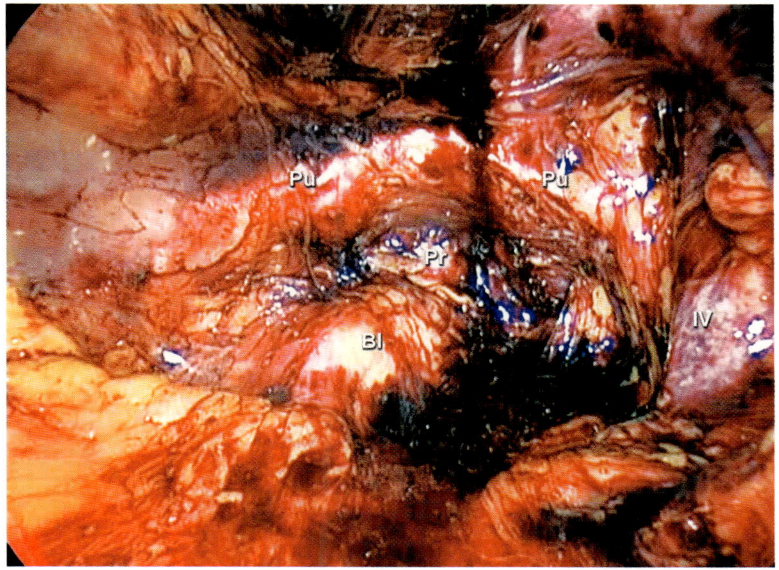

Fig. 2: Overview of pelvis following development of retropubic space (Pu: pubic ramus; Pr: prostate; Bl: bladder; IV: iliac vein)

bilaterally (Fig. 3) under direct vision using the VersaStep™ (Auto Suture-Covidien) system.

OBTAINING ACCESS—TRANSPERITONEAL APPROACH

The transperitoneal approach is employed in patients with prior extraperitoneal pelvic surgery or prior laparoscopic inguinal hernia repair, from which the potential retroperitoneal space is rarely feasible to develop. A 12 mm incision is made in the midline below the umbilicus and carried down to the rectus fascia. The rectus fascia is grasped with an Allis clamp and a Veress needle is used to enter the peritoneum. Saline drop test and aspiration of air confirm proper location. After CO_2 insufflation to 15 mm Hg, a 12 mm port is placed for the camera. One 11 mm port is placed lateral to the right rectus border and two 5 mm ports are placed in the lower abdomen bilaterally (Fig. 3) under direct vision using the VersaStep™ system.

PELVIC LYMPH NODE DISSECTION

Bilateral pelvic lymph node dissection is performed for patients with intermediate- or high-risk disease (Gleason > 6, prostate specific antigen (PSA) > 10 or clinical stage ≥ T2). Attention is drawn to the pelvic sidewall and the external iliac vein is identified. All fibro-fatty and lymphatic tissue bordered by the external iliac vein, obturator nerve and pelvic sidewall is grasped with grasping forceps (Clickline, Karl Storz) (Fig. 4). Surgical clips (Hem-o-Lok, Weck) are placed at the proximal and distal ends of the tissue before transection with laparoscopic scissors (Fig. 5).

Dissection of Endopelvic Fascia and Dorsal Venous Complex Ligation

The endopelvic fascia is cleaned of all adipose tissue overlying it using the Harmonic scalpel (Fig. 6). The endopelvic fascia is then opened sharply bilaterally and careful blunt dissection is used to sweep the

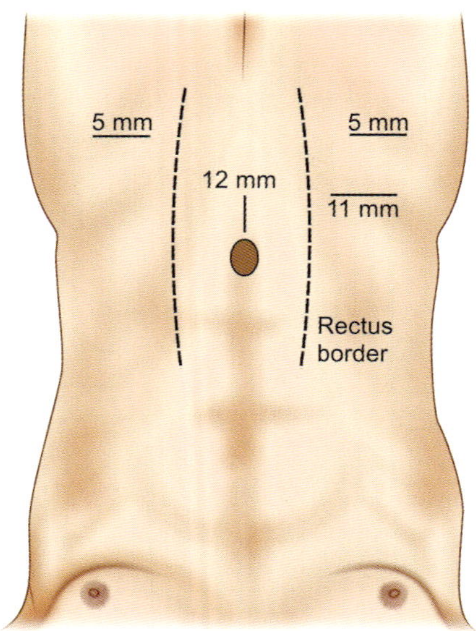

Fig. 3: Port placement

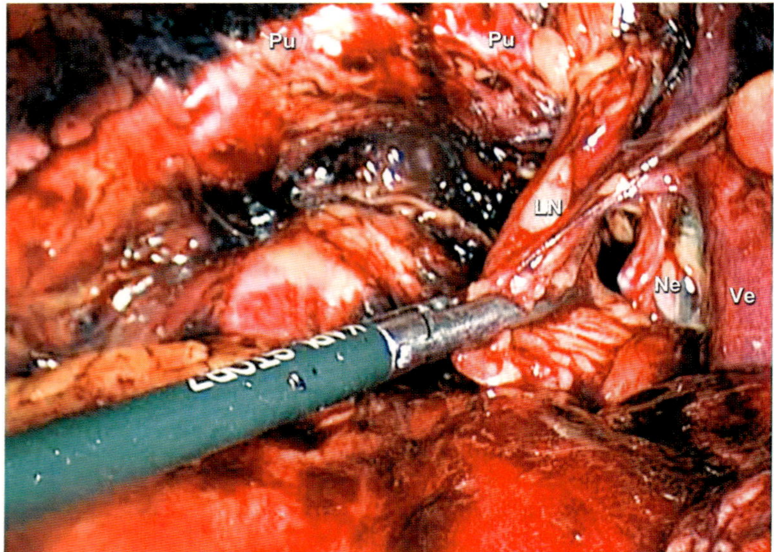

Fig. 4: The lymphatic tissue bordered by the external iliac vein, obturator nerve and pelvic sidewall is dissected (Pu: pubic bone; LN: lymph nodes; Ne: obturator nerve; Ve: external iliac vein)

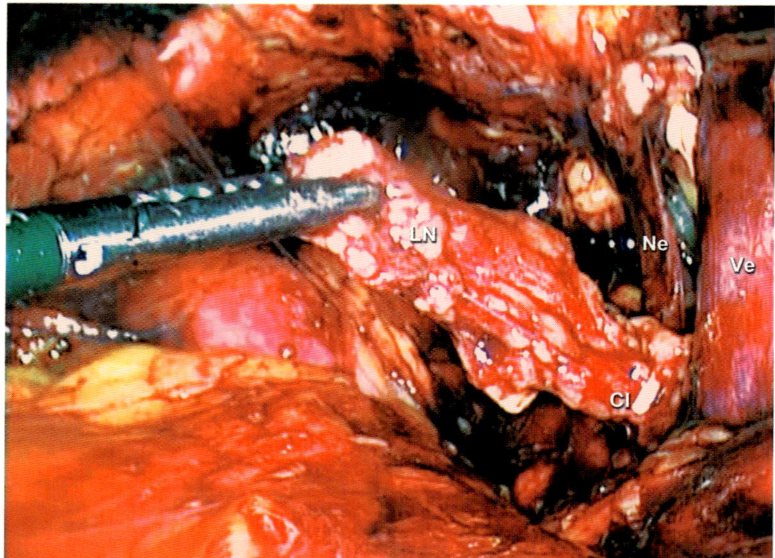

Fig. 5: Surgical clips are placed at the proximal and distal ends of lymphatic tissue before transection with laparoscopic scissors (LN: lymph nodes; Ne: obturator nerve; Ve: external iliac vein; Cl: Hem-o-Lok clip)

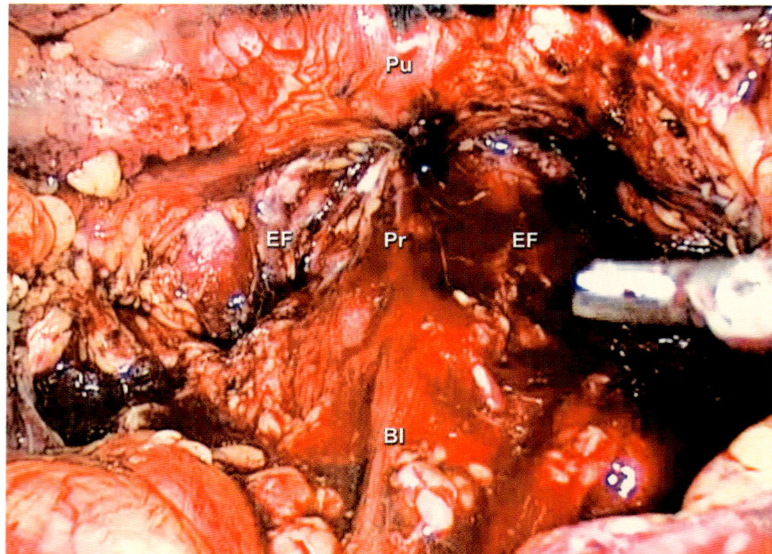

Fig. 6: The endopelvic fascia is cleaned of all adipose tissue overlying it using the Harmonic scalpel (EF: endopelvic fascia; Pr: prostate; Bl: bladder; Pu: pubic bone)

neurovascular bundles laterally (Figs 7A and B). A 0-Vicryl suture ligature is then placed to ligate the dorsal vein complex (Fig. 8).

Bladder Neck and Posterior Dissection

Attention is next turned to the anterior bladder neck. The location of the bladder neck is identified by several maneuvers, including gentle traction on the Foley catheter to visualize the bladder neck-prostate junction, identification of the detrusor apron overlying the bladder neck, and medial approximation of two instruments to identify the prostate base (Fig. 9). The vascular and connective tissue in the area between the prostate and the bladder neck is taken down with the Harmonic scalpel (Fig. 10). The catheter is removed and a urethral sound is placed to retract the prostate superiorly and expose the bladder neck (Fig. 11). The bladder neck is then carefully dissected from the base of the prostate anteriorly, laterally, and posteriorly using the Harmonic scalpel (Fig. 12). This exposes the seminal vesicles and vas deferens. Each vas deferens is lifted and carefully dissected from surrounding structures prior to division with the Harmonic scalpel (Fig. 13). The seminal vesicles are then dissected free from surrounding attachments, again taking care to divide vascular attachments with the Harmonic scalpel (Fig. 14). Once the vas deferens and seminal vesicles are entirely freed, they are lifted superiorly with grasping forceps to expose the posterior plane of the prostate (Fig. 15). Judicious use of the laparoscopic suction irrigator can provide helpful countertraction during this dissection.

Lateral and Apical Dissection

Denonvillier's fascia is incised and sharp dissection is used to develop the lateral pedicles (Fig. 16). A tumescent solution consisting of buffered Ringer's lactate with lidocaine and epinephrine is infiltrated just underneath the lateral prostatic fascia to hydrodissect the lateral prostatic fascia from the lateral aspect of the prostate and lateral pedicles (Figs 17A and B). The Harmonic scalpel is used to ligate and divide the major pedicles at the prostate base with judicious

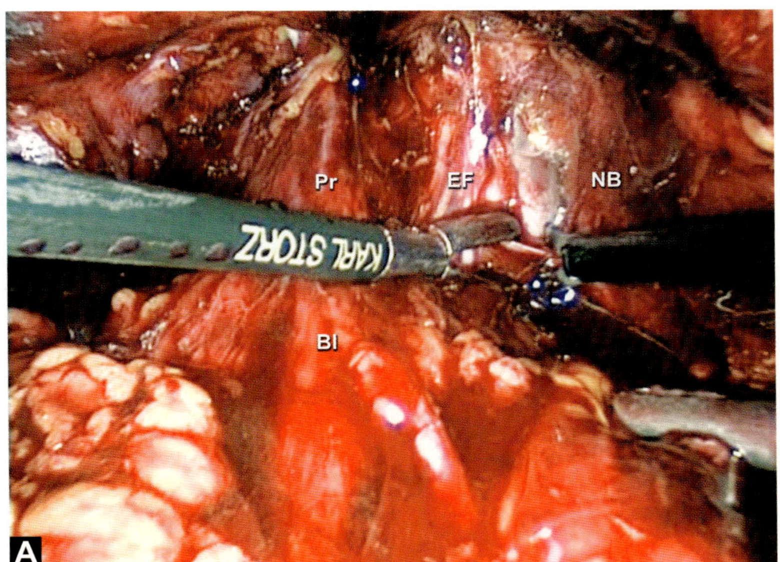

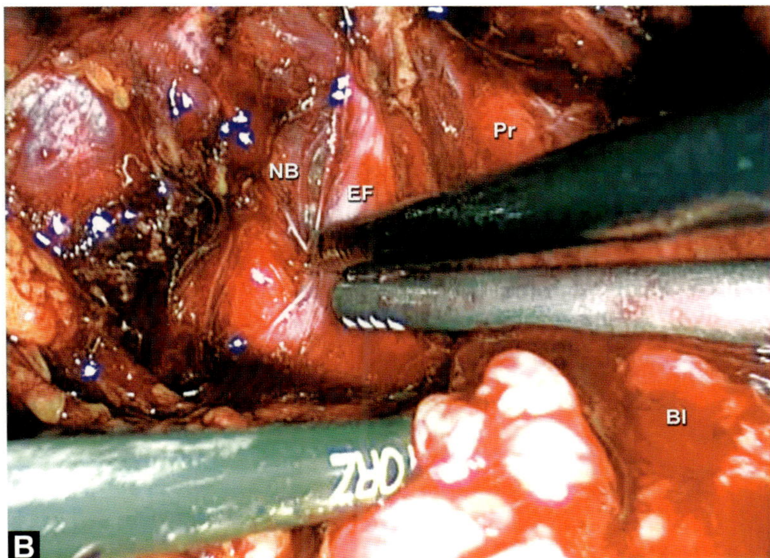

Figs 7A and B: The endopelvic fascia is then opened sharply bilaterally and careful blunt dissection is used to sweep the neurovascular bundles laterally (Pr: prostate; EF: endopelvic fascia; NB: neurovascular bundle; Bl: bladder)

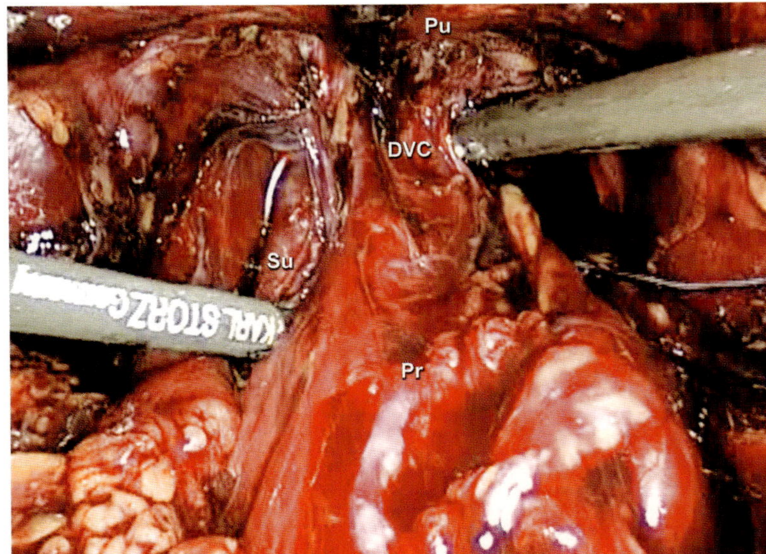

Fig. 8: A 0-Vicryl suture ligature is then used to ligate the dorsal vein complex (Pr: prostate; DVC: dorsal vein complex; Su: suture ligature; Pu: pubic bone)

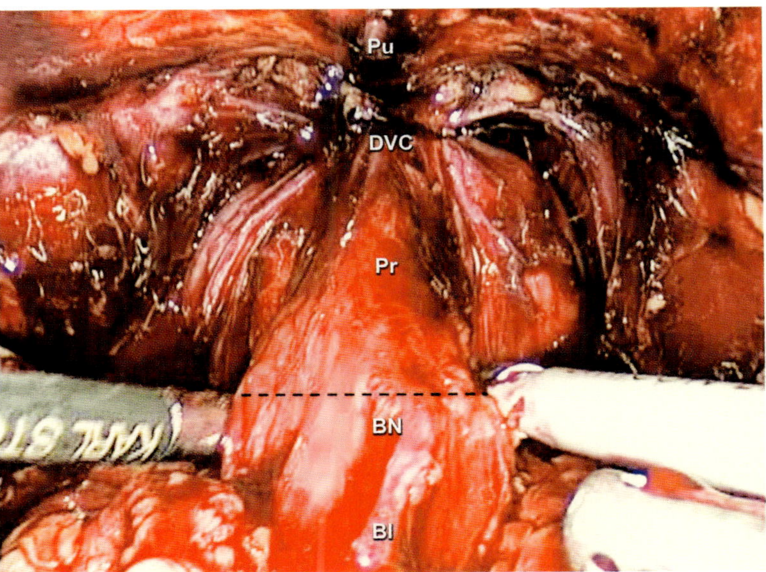

Fig. 9: The location of the bladder neck is identified by medial approximation of two instruments to identify the prostate base (Pr: prostate; DVC: dorsal vein complex; Pu: pubic bone; Bl: bladder; BN: bladder neck; dotted line: junction of prostate and bladder neck)

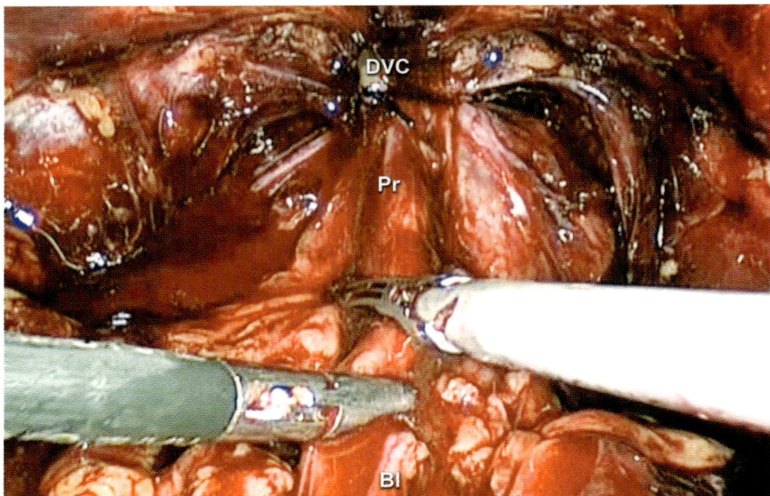

Fig. 10: The vascular and connective tissue in the area between the prostate and the bladder neck is taken down with the Harmonic scalpel (Pr: prostate; Bl: bladder; DVC: dorsal vein complex)

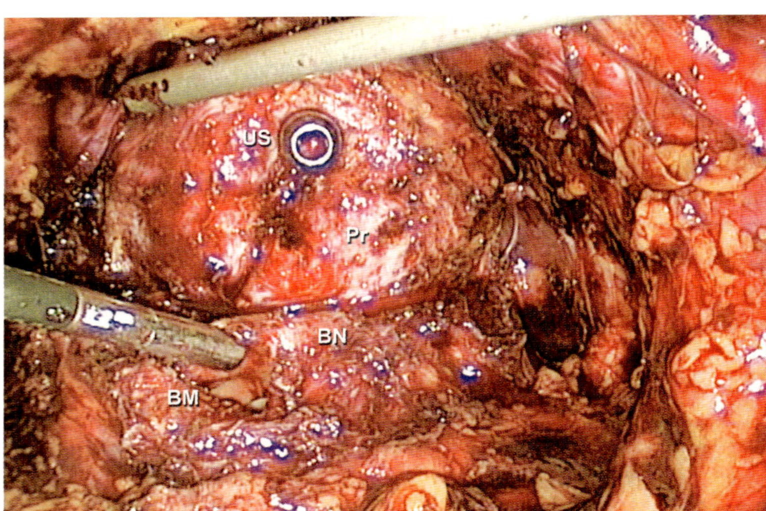

Fig. 11: The catheter is removed and a urethral sound is placed to retract the prostate superiorly and expose the bladder neck [Pr: prostate; US: urethral sound; BN: bladder neck; BM: bladder mucosa (visible below grasping forceps)]

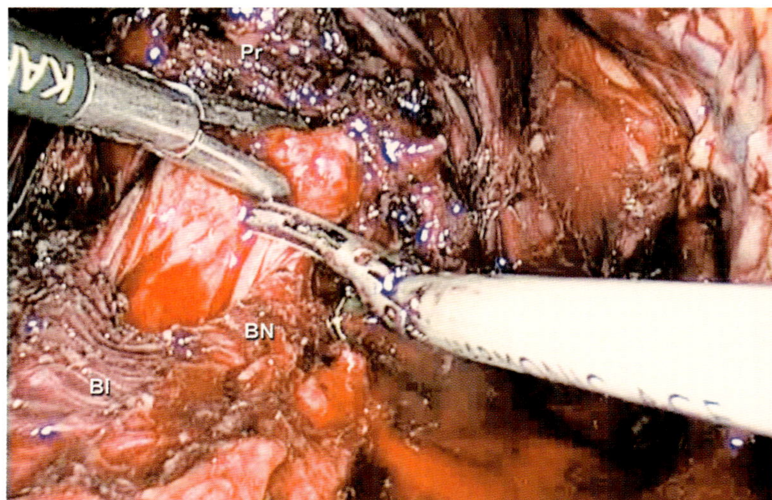

Fig. 12: The bladder neck is then carefully dissected from the base of the prostate anteriorly, laterally, and posteriorly using the Harmonic scalpel (Pr: prostate; Bl: bladder; BN: bladder neck)

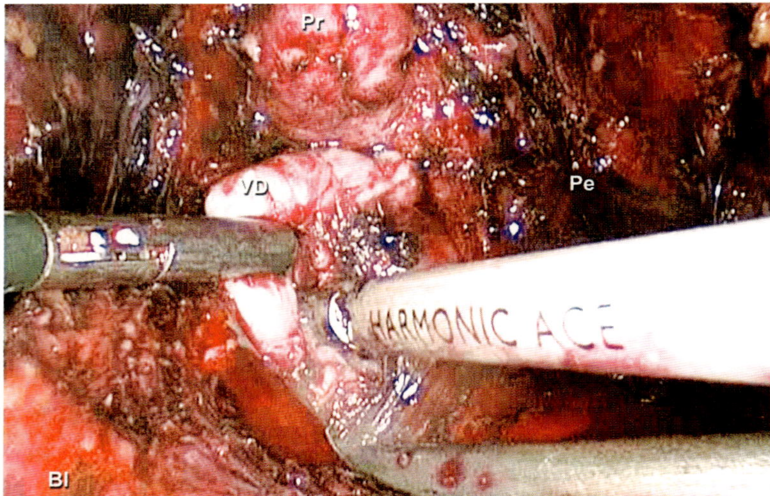

Fig. 13: Each vas deferens is lifted and carefully dissected from surrounding structures prior to division with the Harmonic scalpel (Pr: prostate; Bl: bladder; VS: vas deferens, Pe: lateral pedicle)

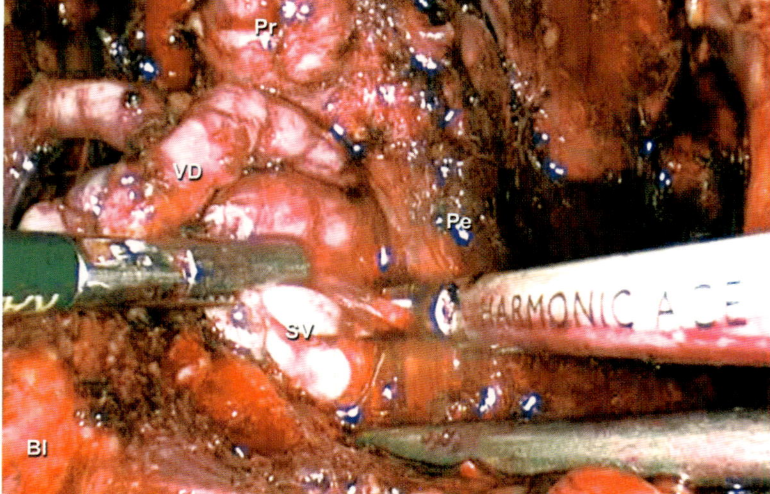

Fig. 14: The seminal vesicles are then dissected free from surrounding attachments, again taking care to divide vascular attachments with the Harmonic scalpel (Pr: prostate; Bl: bladder; VD: vas deferens; SV: seminal vesicle; Pe: lateral pedicle)

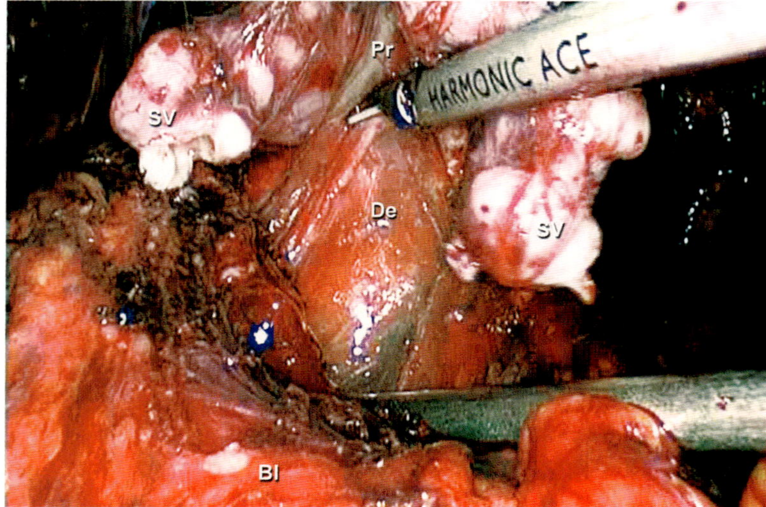

Fig. 15: The vas deferens and seminal vesicles are lifted superiorly with grasping forceps to expose the posterior plane of the prostate (Pr: prostate; Bl: bladder; SV: seminal vesicle; De: Denonvillier's fascia)

application of surgical clips as necessary (Figs 18A to C). Thermal dissection is limited to avoid injury to the neurovascular bundle, and after reaching approximately two-thirds the distance to the urethra, careful sharp dissection with laparoscopic scissors is used to free the neurovascular bundle bilaterally to the apex until the urethra is visualized (Figs 19A to C). The previously ligated dorsal venous complex is now divided using the Harmonic scalpel, and the urethra is transected sharply with scissors (Fig. 20). Once the specimen is freed it is entrapped in a laparoscopic specimen bag.

Vesicourethral Anastomosis

The vesicourethral anastomosis is then performed using interrupted 2-0 Vicryl sutures with the aid of a urethral sound (Figs 21A to D). Anastomotic sutures are placed posteriorly to anteriorly. Typically five to seven sutures are required depending on size of the anastomosis. The bladder neck is narrowed when necessary using figure-of-eight sutures. A 20 Fr Foley catheter is inserted after placement of the last two anastomotic sutures prior to tie-down (Fig. 22). The Foley catheter is irrigated to ensure a watertight anastomosis. Insufflation pressure is then lowered to 4 mm Hg and the surgical field is inspected for hemostasis. A 19 Fr Blake drain is introduced into the retropubic space through the 5 mm right lower quadrant trocar. The trocars are then removed under direct vision, the specimen is removed through the subumbilical incision, and the wounds are closed.

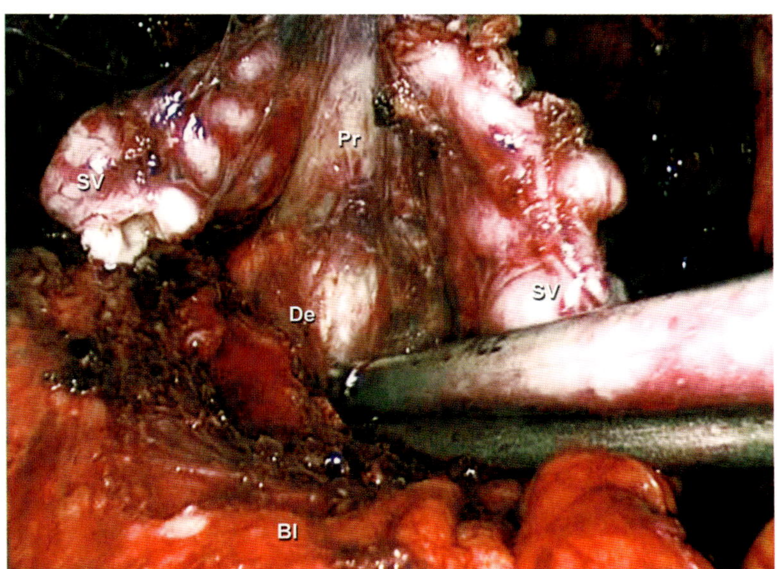

Fig. 16: Denonvillier's fascia is incised and sharp dissection is used to develop the lateral pedicles (Pr: prostate; Bl: bladder; SV: seminal vesicle; De: Denonvillier's fascia)

POSTOPERATIVE CARE

Patients are admitted to the inpatient floor following surgery. On postoperative day 1, patients are advanced to a clear liquid diet, transitioned to oral pain medications, and encouraged to ambulate. If the Blake drain has low output, it is removed and the patient is discharged later that afternoon.

COMPLICATIONS

Intraoperative and immediate postoperative complications include hemorrhage, bowel injury, vascular injury, urinary leak, ileus, thromboembolism and myocardial infarction. Delayed complications include persistent urinary leak, rectourethral fistula and lymphocele. Urinary control and erectile function can improve for up to 12 months following surgery.

SURGICAL ADJUNCTS

Laparoscopic radical prostatectomy can be technically facilitated with special equipment and instrumentation. We employ a voice-activated robotic arm (AESOP, Intuitive Surgical, Inc., and ViKY, EndoControl) to maneuver the laparoscopic camera (Figs 23 and 24). In addition, we use a laparoscopic instrument holder (Civco Medical Corporation) to immobilize urethral sounds used in dissection and vesicourethral reconstruction (Fig. 25).

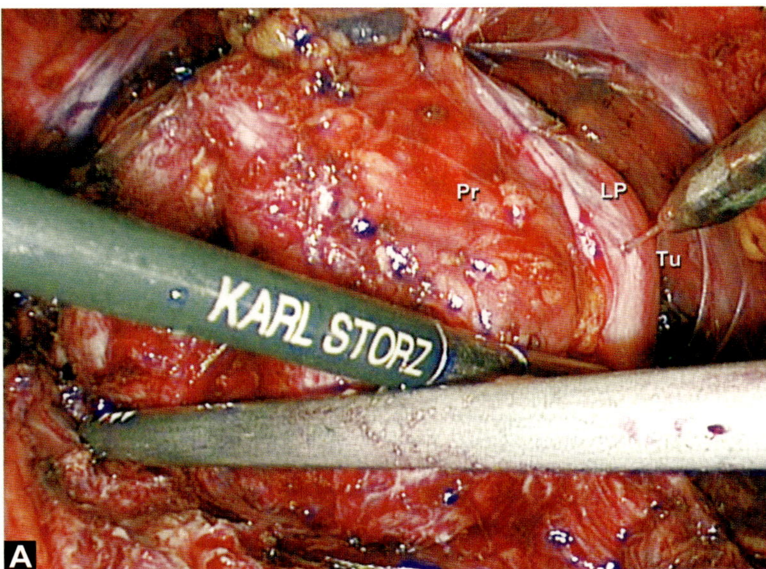

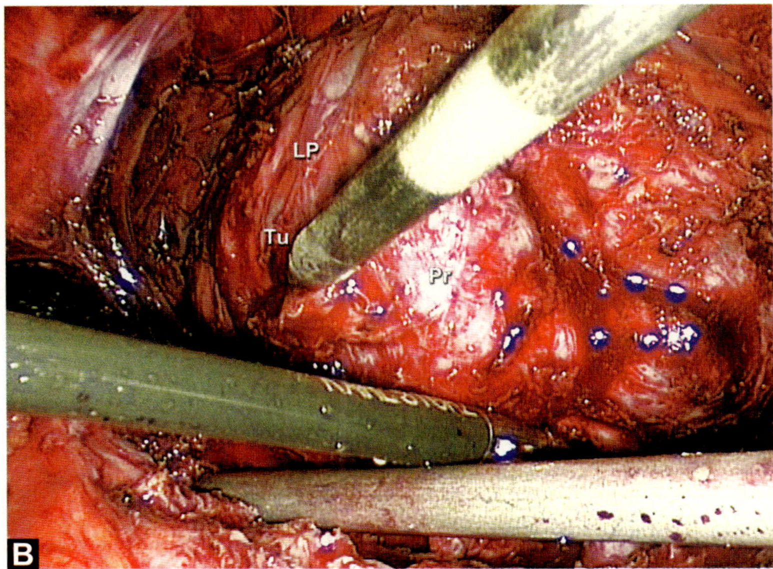

Figs 17A and B: A tumescent solution consisting of buffered Ringer's lactate with lidocaine and epinephrine is infiltrated just underneath the lateral prostatic fascia to hydrodissect the lateral prostatic fascia from the lateral aspect of the prostate and lateral pedicles (Pr: prostate; LP: lateral prostatic fascia; Tu: tumescent solution via laparoscopic needle)

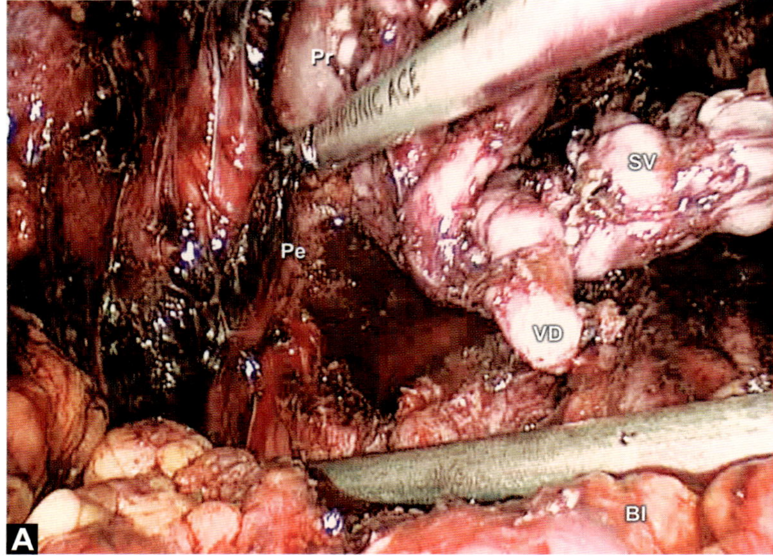

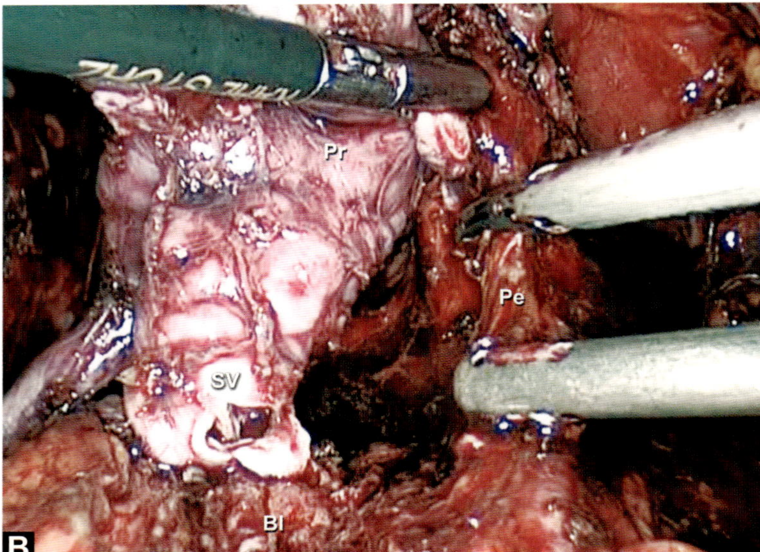

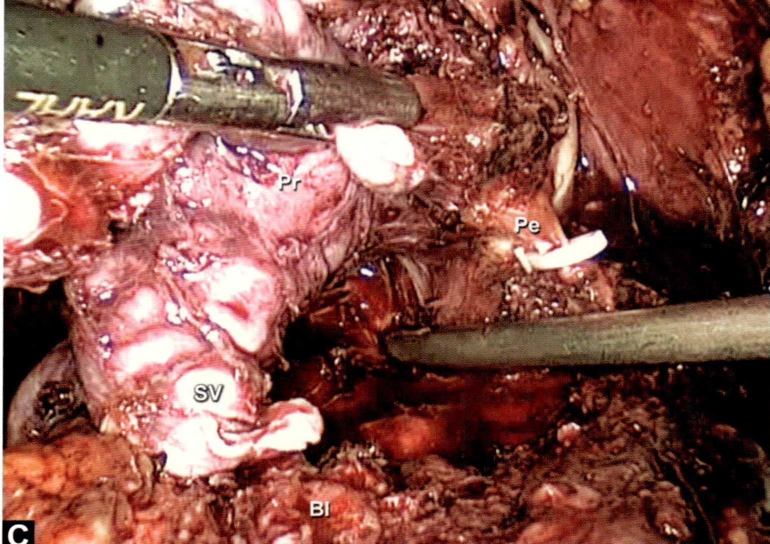

Figs 18A to C: The Harmonic scalpel is used to ligate and divide the major pedicles at the prostate base with judicious application of surgical clips as necessary (Pr: prostate; Bl: bladder; SV: seminal vesicle, VD: vas deferens; Pe: prostatic pedicle)

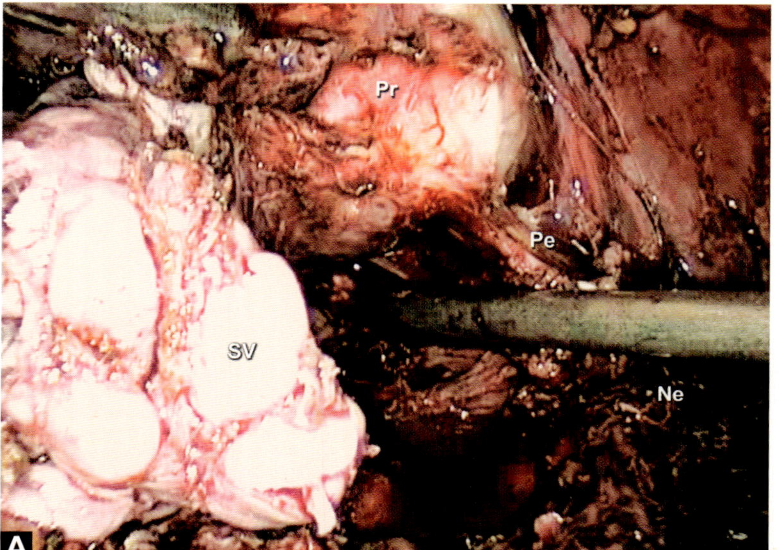

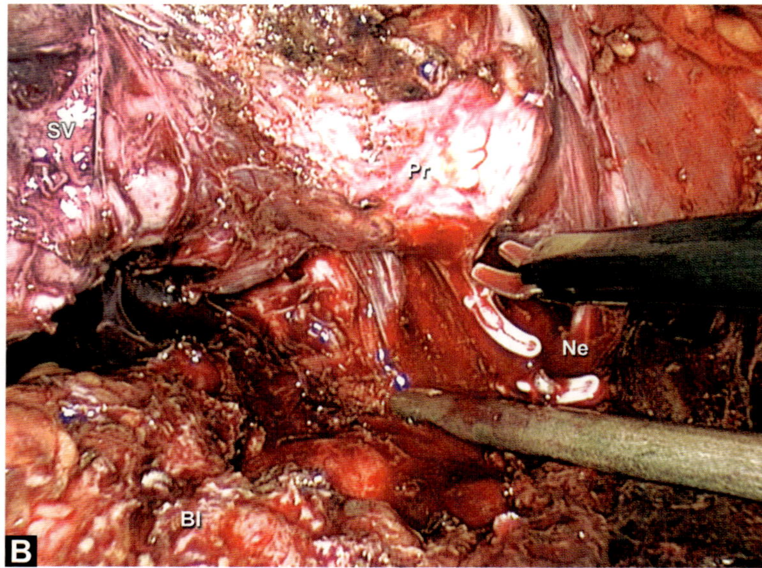

Figs 19A and B

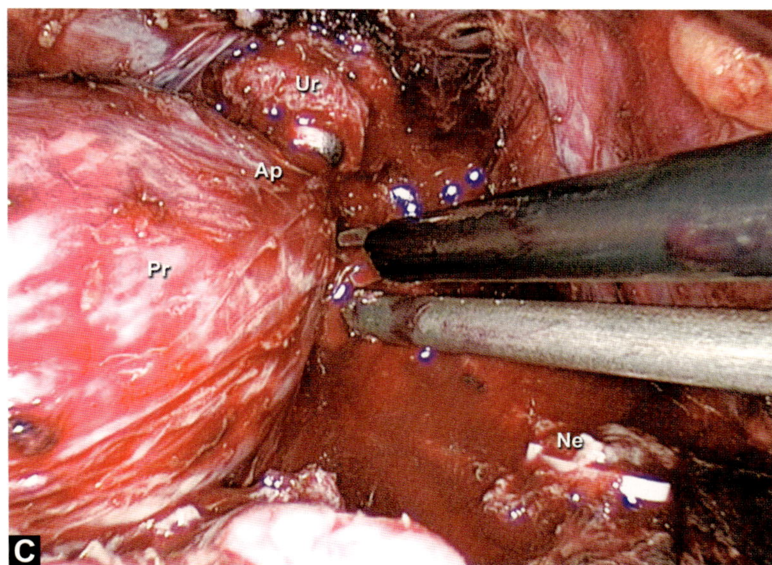

Figs 19A to C: Approximately two-thirds the distance to the apex, careful sharp dissection with laparoscopic scissors is used to free the neurovascular bundle bilaterally to the apex until the urethra is visualized (Pr: prostate; Bl: bladder; Ne: neurovascular bundle; Pe: lateral prostatic pedicle; Ap: apex; Ur: urethra, SV: seminal vesicle)

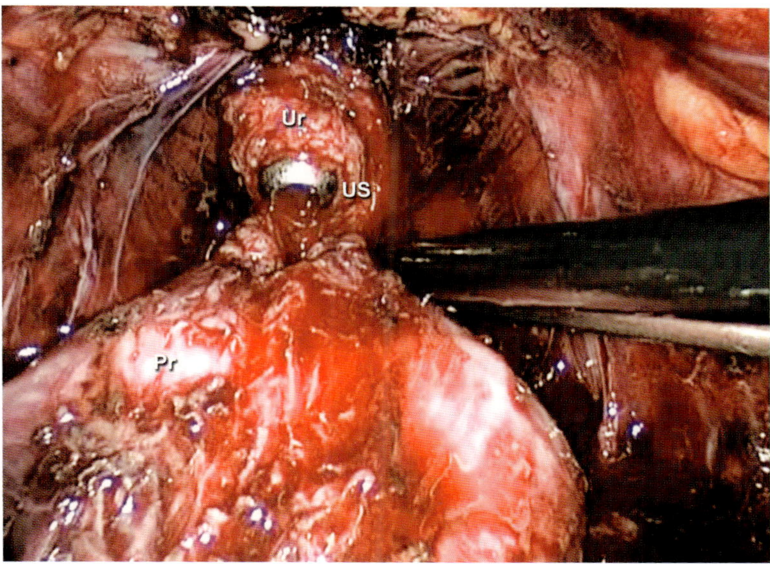

Fig. 20: The urethra is transected sharply with scissors (Pr: prostate; Ur: urethra; US: urethral sound)

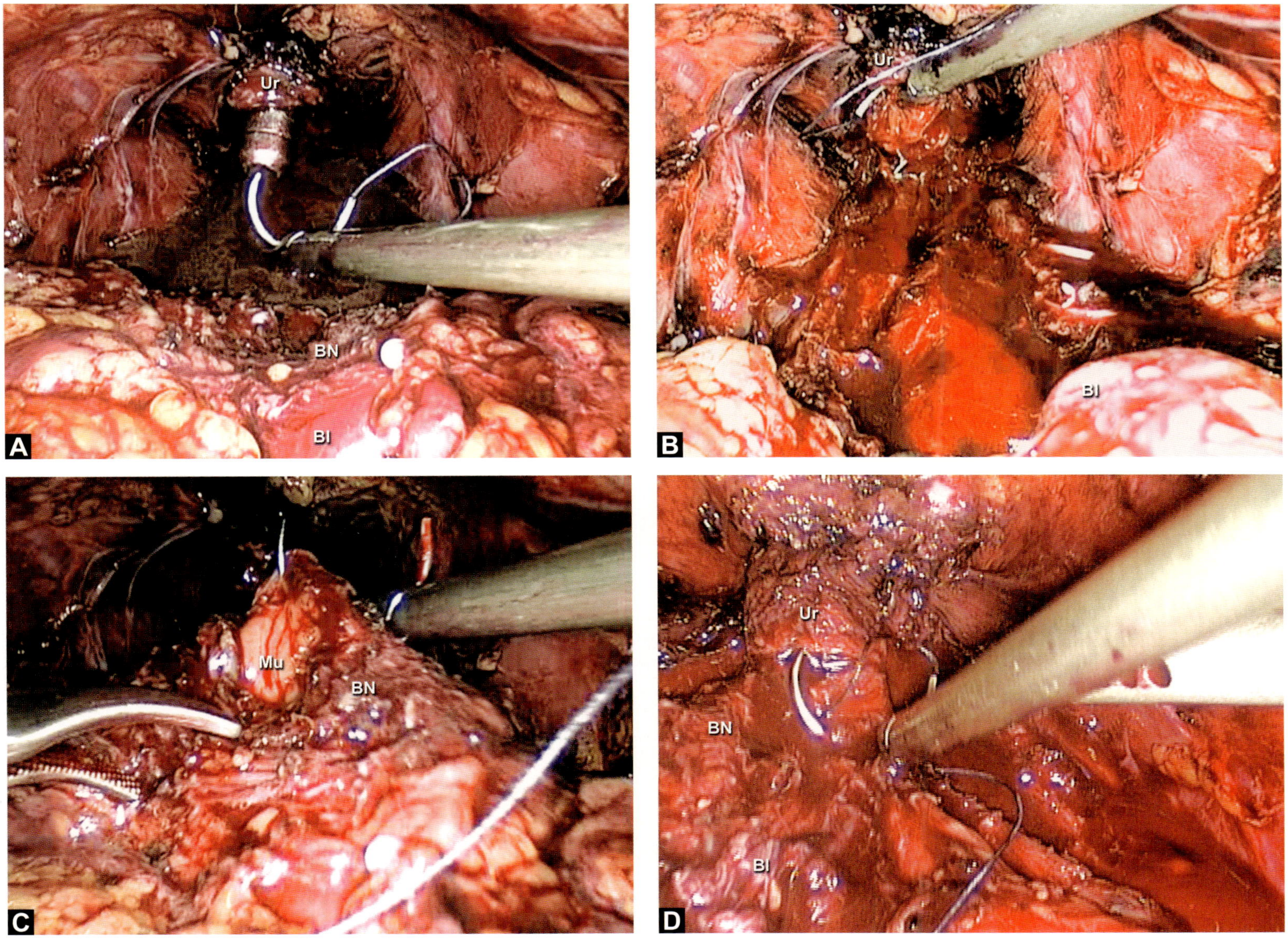

Figs 21A to D: The vesicourethral anastomosis is then performed using interrupted 2-0 Vicryl sutures with the aid of a urethral sound [Pr: prostate; Bl: bladder; Ur: urethra; BN: bladder neck; Mu: bladder mucosa (everted)]

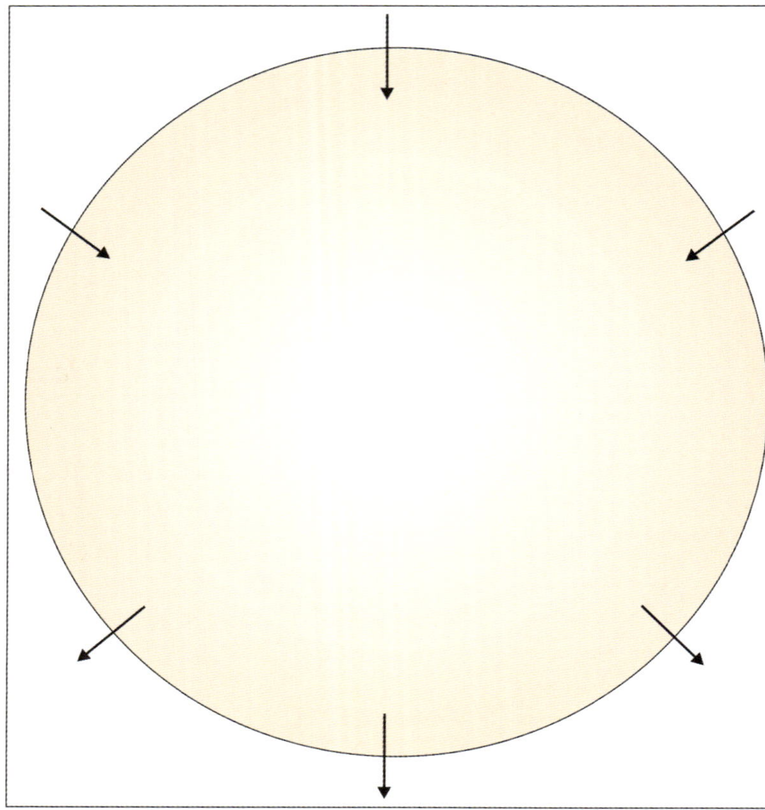

Fig. 22: Location of anastomotic sutures along urethral stump (arrowhead indicates direction of suture)

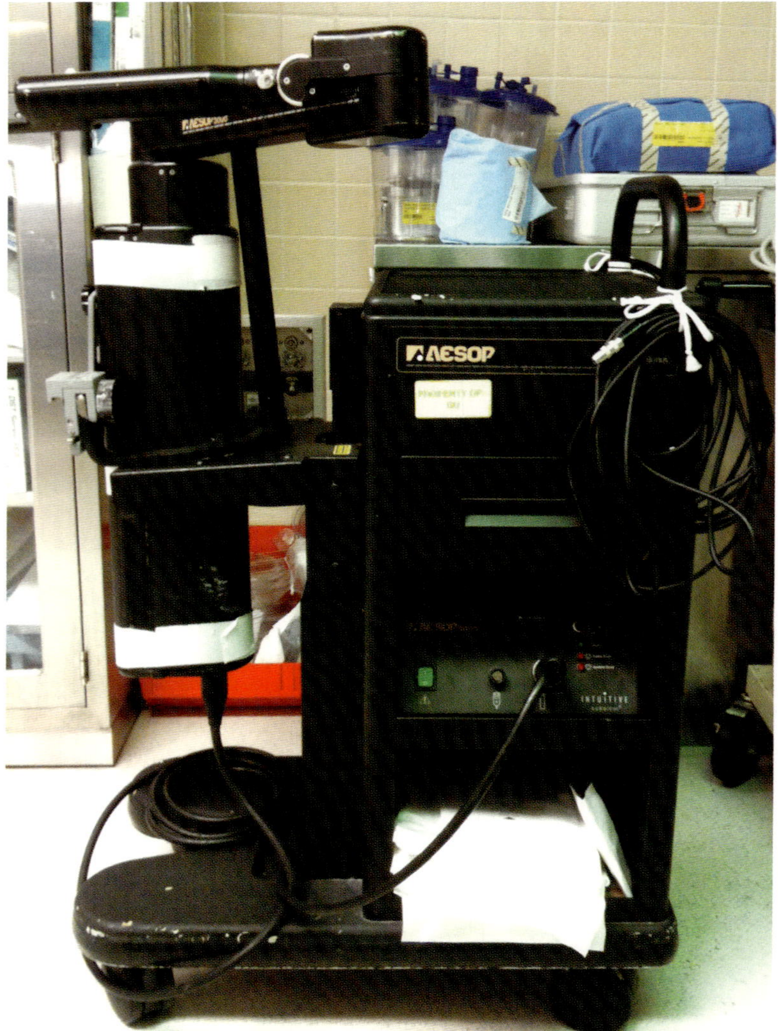

Fig. 23: The AESOP voice-activated robotic arm is used to maneuver the laparoscopic camera

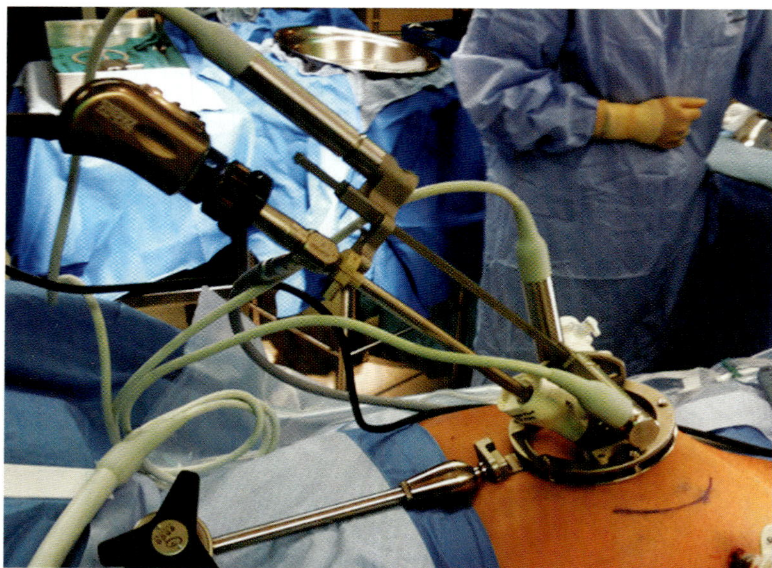

Fig. 24: Alternatively, the ViKY voice-activated robotic arm may be used to maneuver the laparoscopic camera

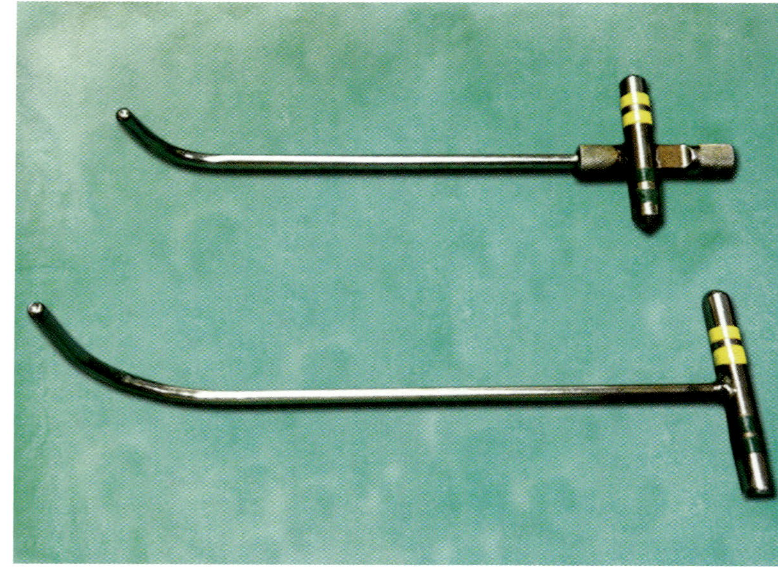

Fig. 25: Urethral sounds used for dissection and vesicourethral reconstruction

Chapter 15

Laparoscopic Radical Cystectomy and Urinary Diversion

Iqbal Singh, Reza Ghavamian, Ashok K Hemal

INTRODUCTION

Laparoscopic radical cystectomy (LRC) was first performed by Para et al. in 1992[1] for pyocystis in a case of retained neurogenic bladder. Later in 1993, Sanchez de Badajoz et al.[2] reported on LRC for bladder cancer and later Gill et al. described the operative technique of LRC with the urinary diversion [orthotopic neobladder (ONB)] performed completely intracorporeally demonstrating the initial feasibility of the laparoscopic technique.[3,4] Subsequently Turk et al. reported the technique of LRC with continent urinary diversion (rectal sigmoid pouch) performed completely intracorporeally in their initial five cases for muscle invasive localized bladder cancer.[5] From Asia, Hemal et al. in 2003[6] reported their preliminary experience of LRC concluding that the procedure was feasible and was associated with lower blood loss and analgesic requirement. Subsequently LRC was also successfully reported from select centers by other workers.[7-9] In most series, urinary diversion (ileal conduit, ileal or sigmoid ONB) was performed extracorporeally through a mini-incision while some highly skilled laparoscopic surgeons have also performed it completely intracorporeally.[4,5] The main constraints for LRC and urinary diversion were longer operating time, long learning curve morbidity and complications.

INDICATIONS

Radical cystoprostatectomy in the male and anterior pelvic exenteration in the female are operative procedures of choice for muscle invasive bladder cancer in order to provide the best chance for long-term cancer control and eradication of the disease. Laparoscopic radical cystectomy is contraindicated in patients with coexisting extensive comorbidity and prior abdominal surgery/bowel adhesions/peritonitis sepsis and/or prior radiotherapy.

Table of Equipment and Instruments

The laparoscopic instruments are depicted in Figure 1 and Table 1.

PREPARATION

Detailed informed consent and counseling is a mandatory step before patients are taken up for laparoscopic radical cystectomy. Preoperative preparation generally includes bowel preparation with antibiotic cover. A suitable polyethylene glycol-based osmotic purgative is given to drink orally the night before along with oral neomycin and metrogyl. Perioperative antibiotic prophylactic cover with parenteral cephazolin, amikacin, ciprofloxacin and metrogyl are also desirable as per hospital policy. Urethral Foley catheterization and general anesthesia with a naso- or orogastric tube are essential to the procedure. A liberal lithotomy position with a 30° Trendelenburg position is desirable. At the time of pelvic lymphadenectomy an ipsilateral tilt may be performed during the procedure on the respective side.

LAPAROSCOPIC TECHNIQUE (SURGICAL METHODS)

Trocar Placement

Generally a six or five port intraperitoneal technique is employed. The authors generally prefer an extracorporeal ileal conduit reconstruction via the site of specimen retrieval (mini laparotomy) as previously described elsewhere by Hemal & others.[10] The port placement is depicted in Figures 2 to 4. Pneumoperitoneum is established by inserting a Veress needle by using a closed technique in the supraumbilical region. Initially a zero degree laparoscope is inserted through a disposable 12 mm primary port to perform a detailed inspection of the entire peritoneal cavity in order to rule out any visceral injury and also to reconfirm operability and rule out any metastatic disease. The second 12 mm port is inserted via the proposed site of the future ileal conduit, generally via the right rectus muscle bulk a few centimeters below the level of the primary camera port. A third 12 mm camera port is also inserted at the same level of the second port through the contralateral rectus muscle. Two additional 10 mm ports are each placed bilaterally about 2.5 cm superomedial to the respective anterior superior iliac spines. An optional sixth port

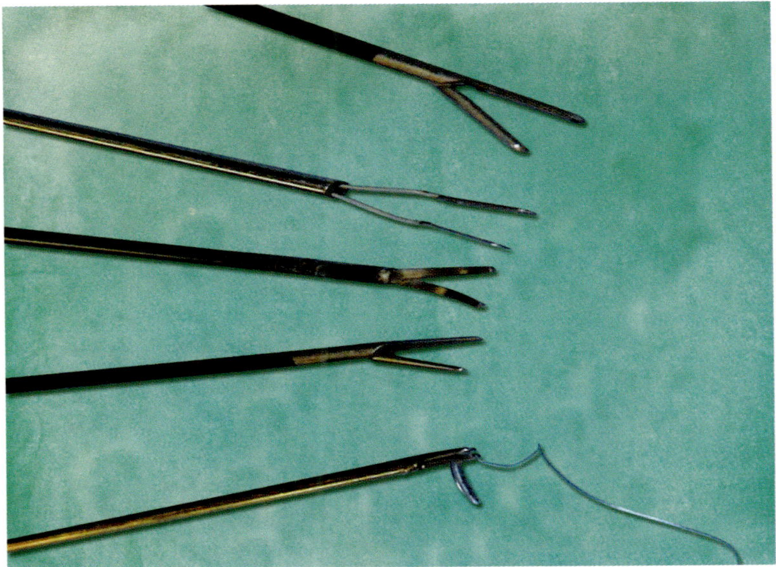

Fig. 1: Picture depicting the hand held laparoscopic needle holder, dissector, scissors, atraumatic grasper and grasping forceps depicted from left to right

Table 1: Table of instruments needed for laparoscopic radical cystectomy
Laparoscopic Instruments
Veress needle (Disposable or reusable)
Hasson's blunt tip cannula (For transperitoneal open access for ensuring air tight seal at entry site)
Laparoscopic trocars (Blunt blade disposable) 10 mm -2, 12 mm -3, 5 mm -1 (optional) (Ethicon Endo-Surgery™, Cincinnati, OH, USA)
Laparoscopic metzenbaum scissors-1
Laparoscopic atraumatic grasping forceps-2
Laparoscopic bipolar forceps-1
Laparoscopic needle driver -10 or 12 mm -1
Laparoscopic suction irrigation cannula (disposable or re-usable)-1
Laparoscopic Endo GIA™ stapler 10 mm -1
Laparoscopic Endosac/Endocatch bag or bag-1 (for 10 mm or 12 mm port)-1
Harmonic scalpel and or Ligasure for 10 mm forceps-1 (Tyco Healthcare™)
Laparoscopic multiload clip applicator -10 mm -1
Hem-o-lok™ (Teleflex, Research Triangle Park, NC) clip OR lapraTy™ (Ethicon, Cincinnati, OH,USA) -Desirable
Surgicel™ (Ethicon Inc., Somerville, NJ) bolster (Optional)
Basic Laparoscopic Equipment
3-CCD Camera or HDTV Camera System-1
Cold Light (Xenon) 300 W-1
12 mm and or 10 mm Endoscope 0° and 30° (1 each desirable)
High flow CO_2 insufflator system-1

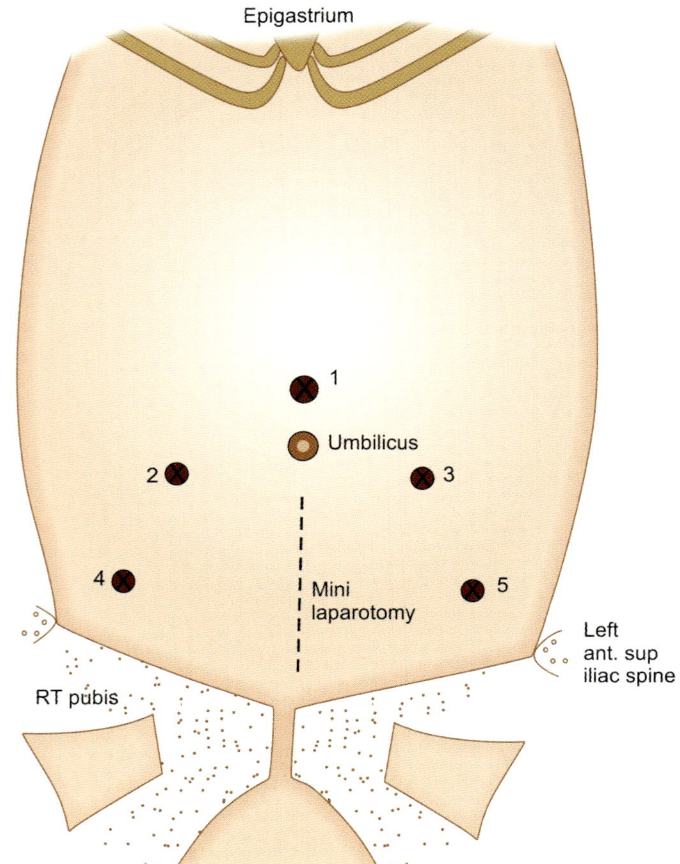

Fig. 2: Diagrammatic sketch depicting the placement of the ports for laparoscopic radical cystectomy; 1-Primary 12 mm camera port, 2/3–10 mm, Secondary working ports, and 4/5–10 mm additional ports

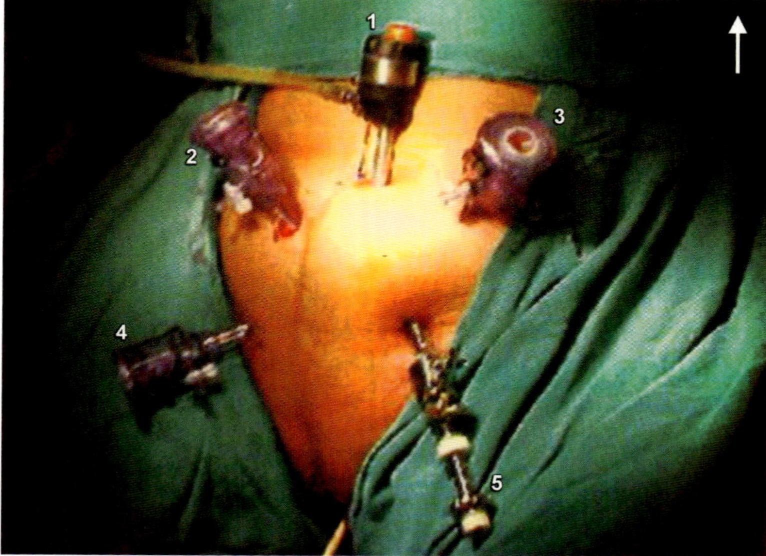

Fig. 3: An external view depicting the laparoscopic port placement in one such female patient undergoing laparoscopic radical cystectomy. Top arrow depicts the cranial left side of the patient in supine position with pointers 1–5 depicting the serial number of the respective ports inserted for laparoscopic assisted radical cystectomy

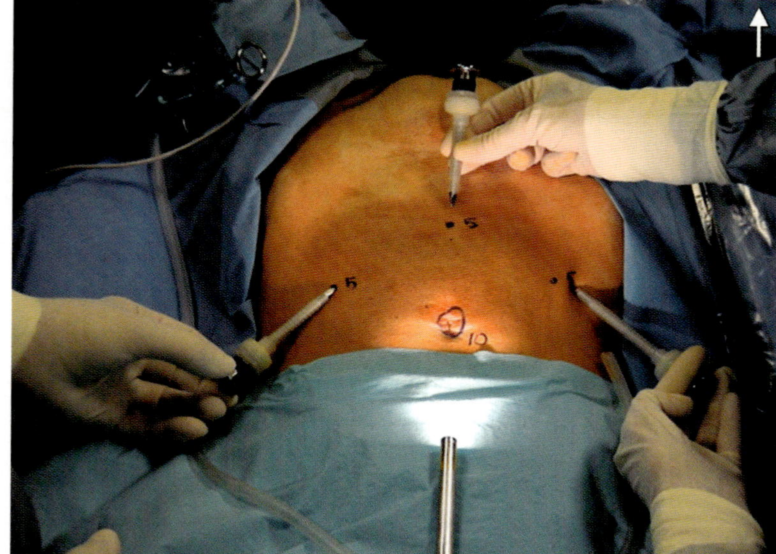

Fig. 4: External view of another patient showing the planning for placement of the laparoscopic ports for laparoscopic assisted radical cystectomy with the arrow depicting the caudal right side of the patient in supine position

may be inserted suprapubically in the midline if one plans to do an intracorporeal ileal conduit reconstruction.

Lateral Dissection and Pelvic Lymphadenectomy

Ideally pelvic lymphadenectomy (PLND) should be able to clear the entire lymph node (LN) drainage basin of the bladder. It must respect the anatomical boundaries of dissection, that demands a high degree of meticulousness of the surgeon and it should be capable of providing a specimen yield of a high LN density.

Four types of PLND have been described in the literature; (a) Limited PLND: which includes removal of LNs of primarily the obturator region; (b) Standard PLND: It includes removal of all LNs from the bifurcation of common iliac vessels proximally, from the genitofemoral nerves laterally, with the tissue around deep circumflex iliac vein, node of Cloquet and femoral canal up to the hypogastric vessels distally and obturator fossa posteriorly; (c) Extended PLND which in addition includes a standard PLND with a cephalad extension to the level of aortic bifurcation including the presacral nodes; (d) Superextended PLND: This is a more extensive PLND that extends more proximally up to the level of inferior mesenteric artery (Singh et al. 2010).[11]

Laparoscopic bilateral pelvic lymphadenectomy is performed by baring the pelvic vessels proximally up to the level of pelvic bifurcation superiorly, lateral rectal fascia medially and the obturator nerve laterally. A split and roll technique with liberal use of Hem-o-lok™ (Teleflex, Research Triangle Park, NC) clip(s) or titanium clips or bipolar energy is recommended in order to minimize the risk of any oozing and lymphocele formation in the postoperative period. The left and right pelvic nodes are labeled and sent separately for histopathological/frozen section analysis to the pathologist.

Pelvic Dissection

This involves incising the parietal pelvic peritoneum and dividing it in the plane between the bladder and the rectum (Figs 5A and B). This enables identification of the bilateral vas deferens on either side of the bladder. The vas are individually clipped and divided in between on either side. The ejaculatory organs are left en-bloc with the specimen and held anteriorly to separate the rectum from the specimen (Fig. 5C). Laparoscopic fan retractor(s) are inserted via the 2nd/3rd ports and this is used to sweep away the sigmoid colon out of the way, as well as to simultaneously retract the urinary bladder anteriorly. This enables an unobstructed clear view of the bladder and the pelvic cavity in order to identify, dissect and expose both ureters. The ureter is identified in the retroperitoneum as it crosses over the common iliac artery and the posterior peritoneum is divided (Figs 6A and B). The ureter is retracted with a vessel loop and dissected towards the muscular hiatus of the bladder (Fig. 7). After mobilization of the ureters inferiorly to the level of the ureterovesical junction, they are carefully clipped and divided individually on either side (Fig. 8). The resected ends of both the ureters are also labeled separately and sent for histopathological evaluation by frozen section in order to ensure the cut ends are free of any residual tumor. Next the superior vesical pedicles are identified on each side by tracing the median umbilical ligament, which continues as superior vesical artery and terminate to internal iliac vessels, these are then mobilized, clipped with Hem-o-lok clips [alternatively a multifire Endo GIA™ 30 Stapler with 2.5/3.5 mm staple size or Endo GIA™ Universal 12 mm staple, (Covidien Surgical) may be used if the superior pedicles are wide and thick] and divided sequentially on either side (Fig. 9). The dissection now proceeds more distally deep into the pelvis by entering the plane between the bladder base and the prostate. Subsequent dissection is performed freeing the seminal vesicles and their attachment

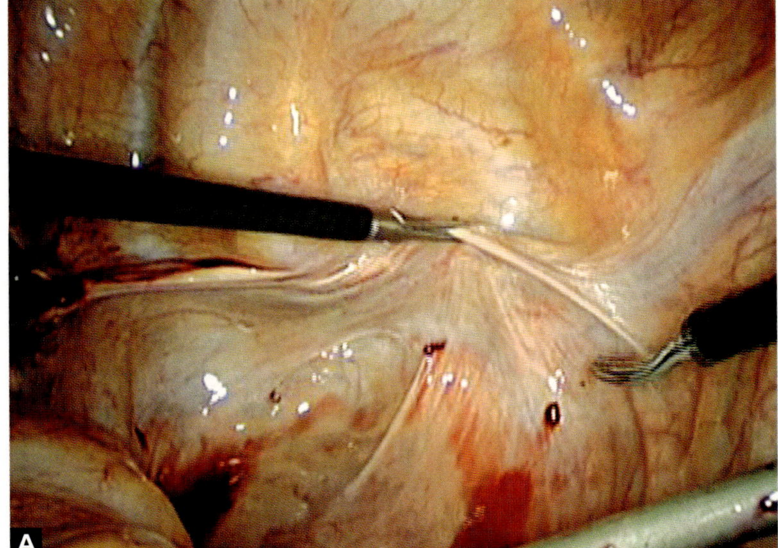

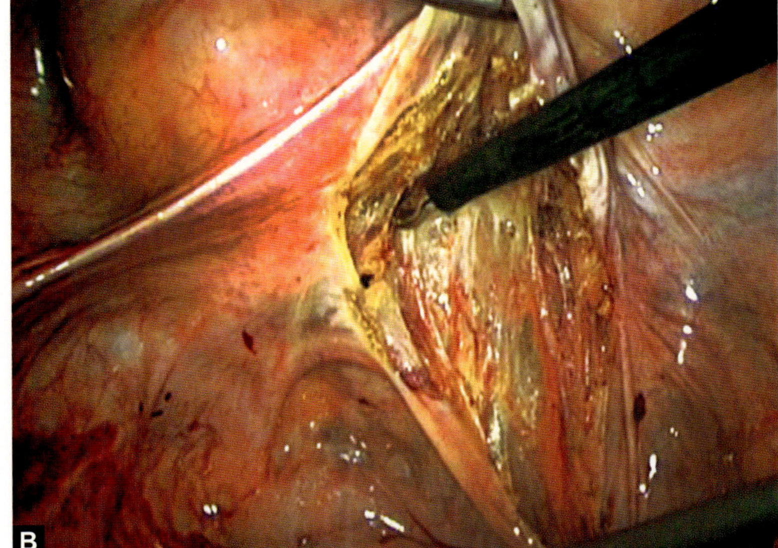

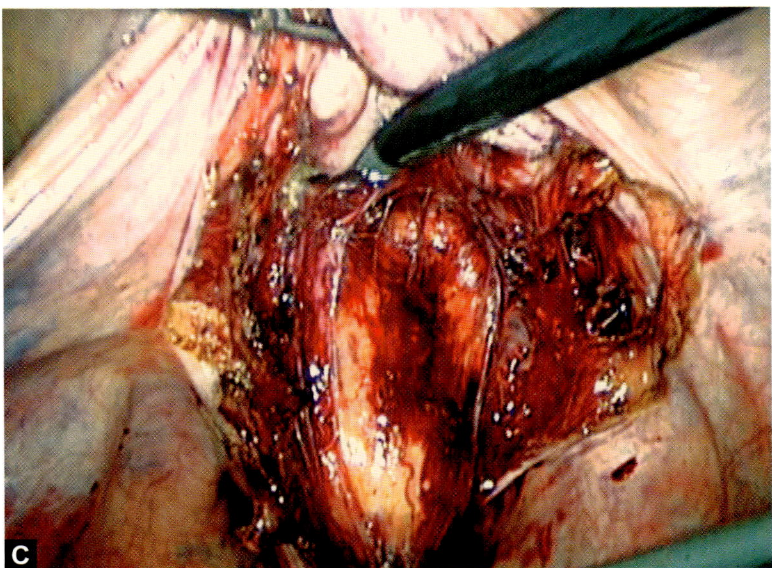

Figs 5A to C: Laparoscopic endoview of the patient depicting incision, exposure of retrovesical peritoneum and Dennonvillier's fascia
Courtesy: Reza Ghavamian

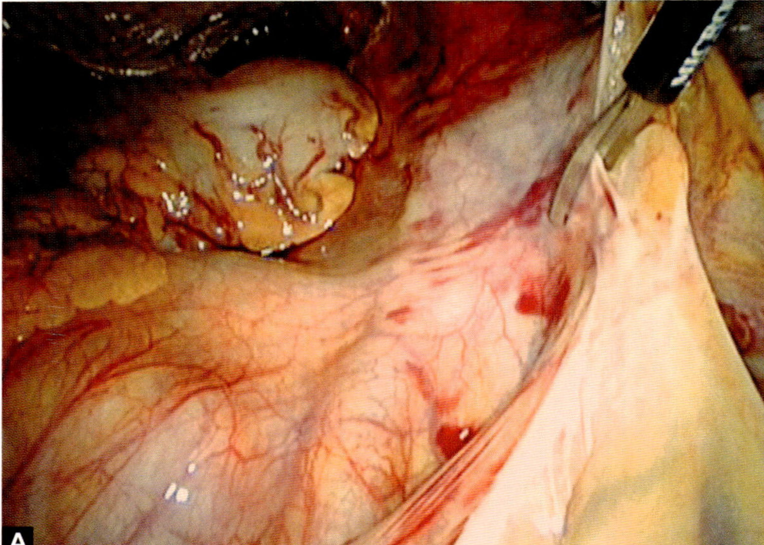

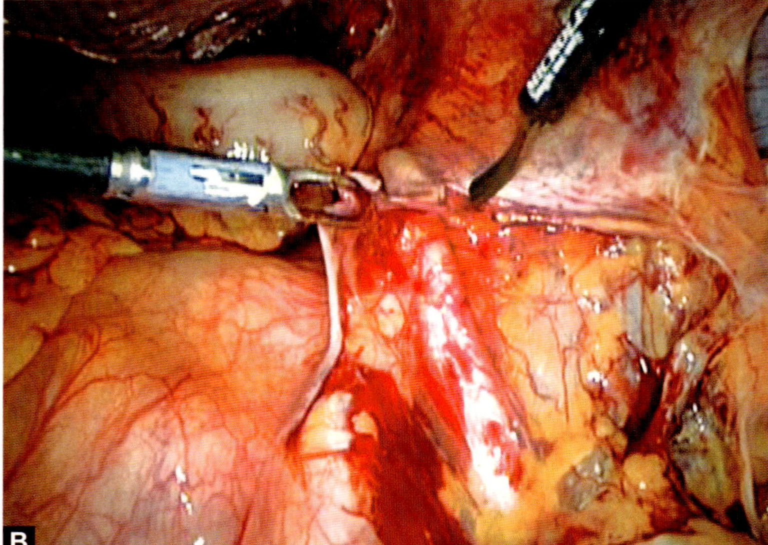

Figs 6A and B: Laparoscopic endocamera view of the patient with the panel images depicting (A) dissection, (B) division of the right ureter in progress
Courtesy: Reza Ghavamian

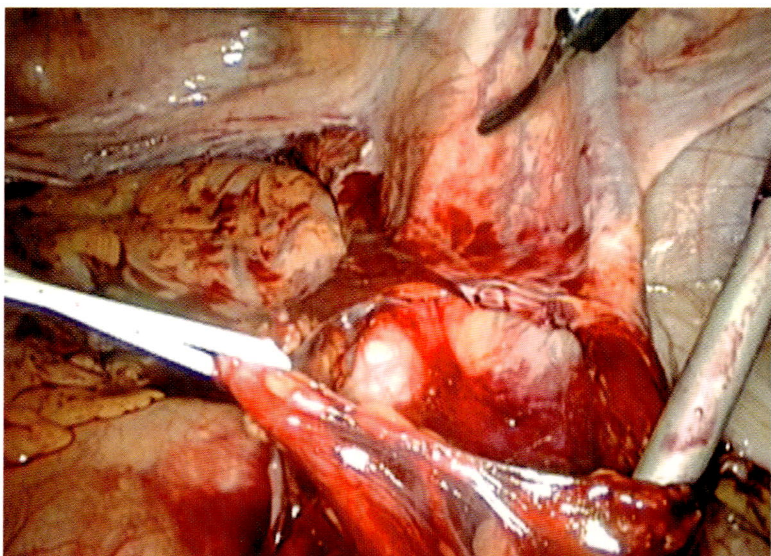

Fig. 7: Laparoscopic view showing dissection of right ureter towards its insertion in the bladder (*Courtesy:* Reza Ghavamian)

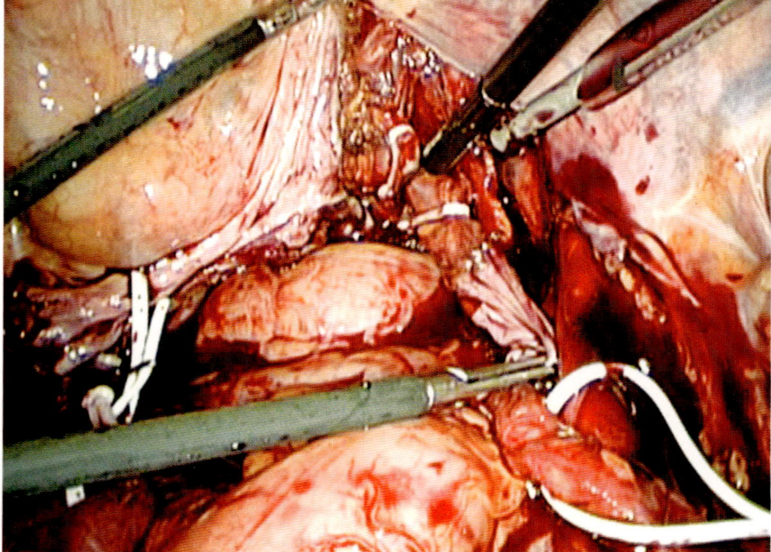

Fig. 8: The ureter is doubly clipped with Hem-o-Lok® clips and divided
Courtesy: Reza Ghavamian

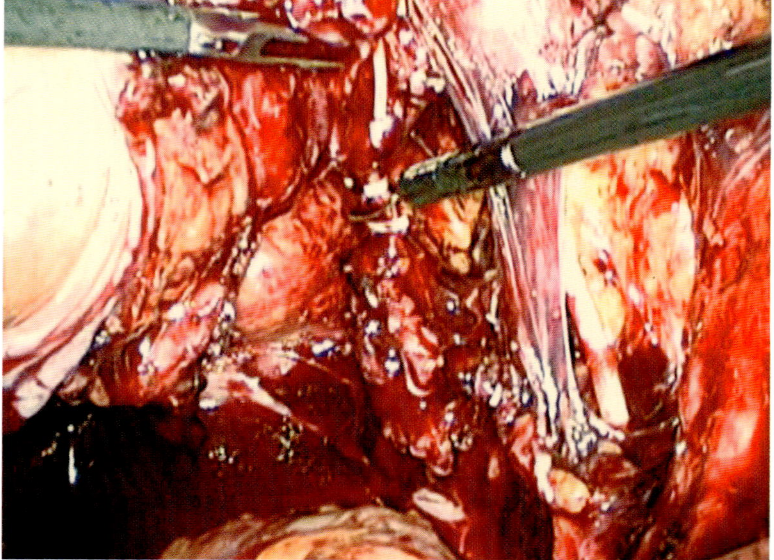

Fig. 9: Division of the superior vesical pedicles
Courtesy: Reza Ghavamian

with the Denonvillier's fascia and adjacent tissues (Fig. 10). It is essential to incise and or divide the plane of Denonvilliers in order to ensure dissection in this avascular plane. Precise entry into this plane is essential in order to ensure visualization of the posterior and inferior vesical pedicles. These pedicles are mobilized, dissected and divided using the Endo GIA™ stapler. Auxillary titanium and or Hem-o-lok™ clips (Teleflex, Research Triangle Park, NC) or intracorporeal suturing may be used to control additional bleeding vessels if any. Bipolar energy, LigaSure™, plasmakinetic energy and ultracision are other alternatives.

Dissection of the Retrovesical Space

The bladder is now distended by instilling about 200 ml of distilled water so as to facilitate dissection and freeing up of the attachment of the urachus (Fig. 11) and the vesical peritoneum. This step helps during initial learning curve. The retropubic space is exposed by depressing the bladder so as to expose the glistening white endopelvic fascia on either side of the prostate as this allows complete mobilization of the bladder (Fig. 12). It is important to clean the space of Retzius and

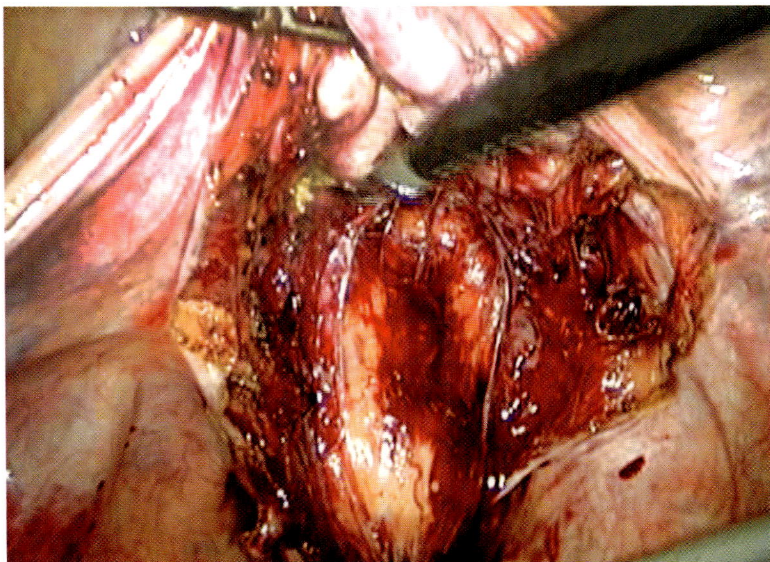

Fig. 10: The ejaculatory organs are held anteriorly and the plane between the bladder and the rectum is developed
Courtesy: Reza Ghavamian

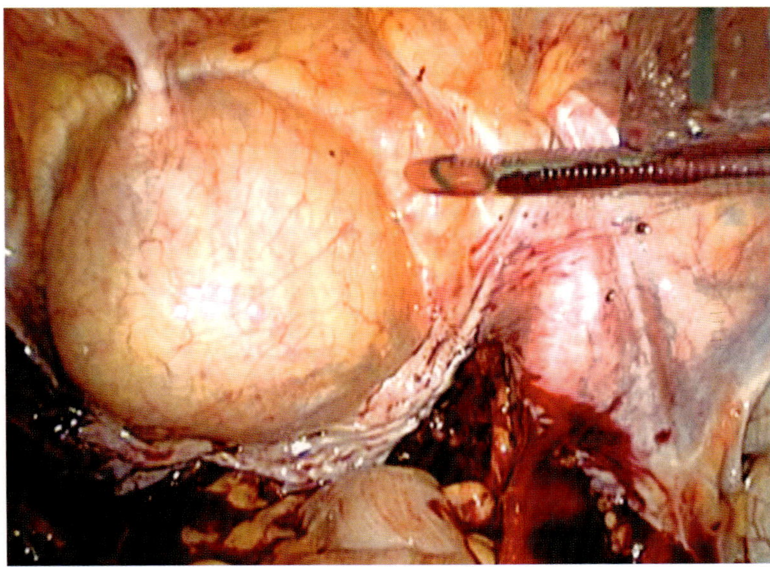

Fig. 11: The bladder is distended to allow for easy, anterior dissection
Courtesy: Reza Ghavamian

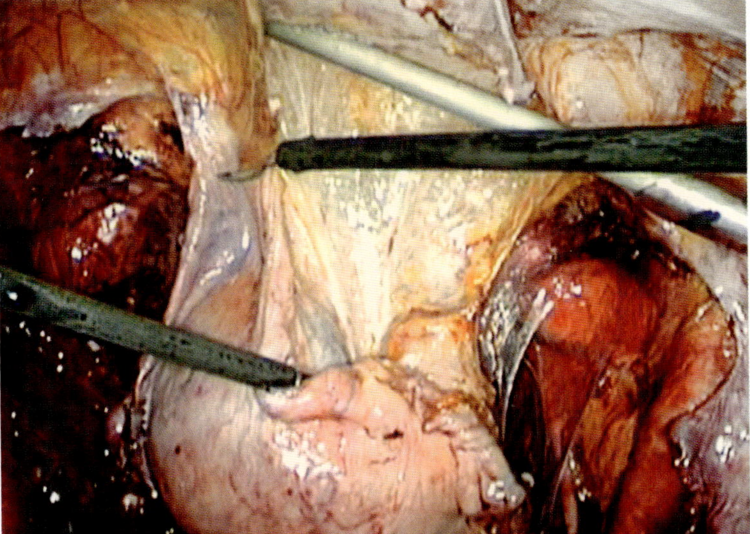

Fig. 12: The space of Retzius is developed
Courtesy: Reza Ghavamian

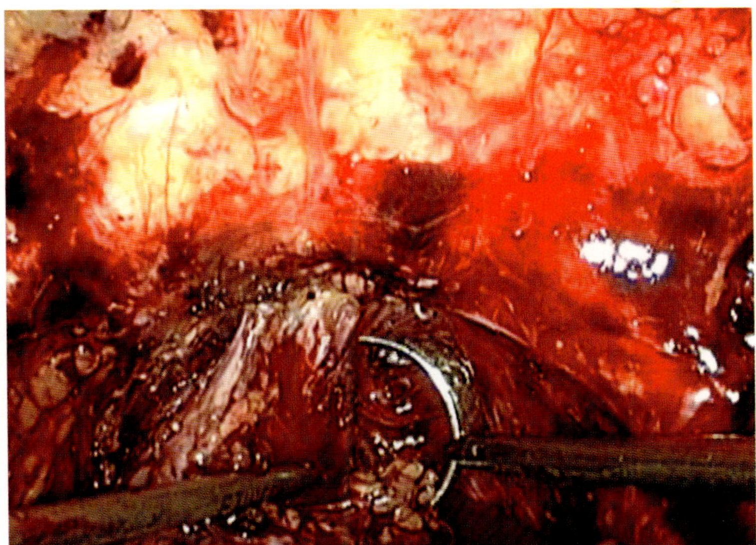

Fig. 13: Ligation of the dorsal venous complex (DVC)
Courtesy: Reza Ghavamian

superficial dorsal vein to expose the anterior surface of the prostate. The exposed endopelvic fascia is now incised bilaterally to expose the puboprostatic ligaments on either side. The dorsal venous complex is gently dissected with a laparoscopic right angled forceps and can be divided with a vascular Endo GIA™ (Covidien Surgical) stapler or suture ligated (Fig. 13). Alternatively, the dorsal vein complex may be sutured and ligated intracorporeally. The urethra is now dissected at a point just distal to the apex of the prostate. The progress of cysto-prostatectomy is depicted in Figure 14.

Nerve Sparing Technique of LRC

For this technique the lateral aspect of prostate is dissected and exposed placing counter traction on the prostatovesical junction so as to expose it accurately. The important nerve branches from hypogastric plexus are located below the vesicoprostatic pedicles. The visceral pelvic fascia is exposed on the lateral aspect of the prostate and the neurovascular prostate bundle is dissected and periprostatic fascia is dissected off the prostate up to the apex of the prostate on either side using a bipolar plasma kinetic (PK™) forceps or a harmonic scalpel.

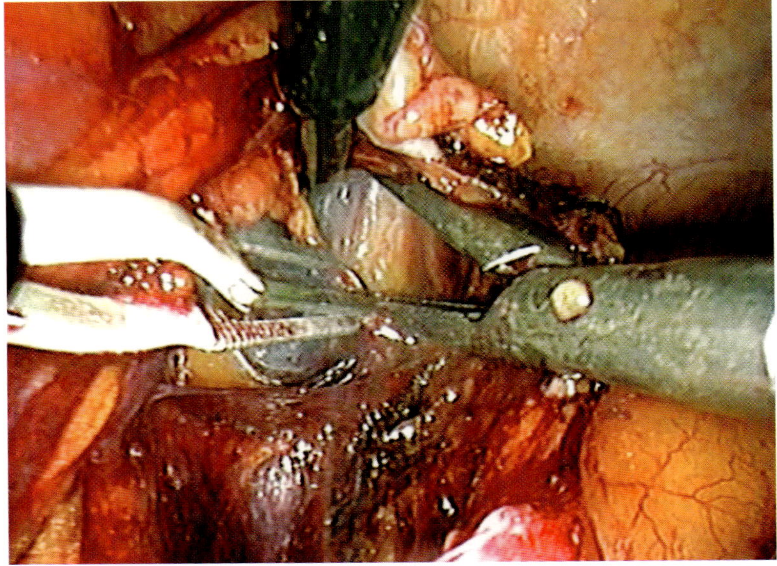

Fig. 14: The cystectomy is completed

Specimen Retrieval

In the female patients, posterior vesicovaginal plane is dissected to expose the anterior vaginal wall, the umbilical ligaments, urachus and the pubourethral ligaments are divided to expose the anterior bladder wall, anterior vaginal wall and the bladder neck. Swab on sponge stick in the vagina or uterine manipulator may help in better delineation. The endopelvic fascia is opened to complete the lateral urethral dissection and finally the urethra is transected in between the clips as low as possible. The rectovaginal space is exposed by both blunt and sharp dissection. Here the dissection extends to both the ischiorectal fossae. In women the entire specimen comprising the urinary bladder, urethra and the anterior vaginal wall is delivered en-bloc via an incision in the anterior vaginal wall or through a lower midline incision which will be utilized for the urinary diversion. In male patients, the radical cystoprostatectomy specimen is delivered via a small 5–6 cms midline infraumbilical laparotomy incision or transverse incision including ileostomy site, which is used for subsequent urinary diversion (extracorporeal ileal conduit with stented ureteroileal anastomoses). The specimen is bagged in to an EndoCatch™ bag for retrieval (Fig. 15A). The ports are removed under vision and the pneumoperitoneum is terminated. After delivering the specimen (Fig. 15B) a number 20 two-way Foley catheter inflated to 50 cc is placed perurethrally in the pelvis that is kept on mild traction for 24 hours, if there is bleeding from the prostatic bed. It also serves as a pelvic drain. The ileostomy is created in the previously marked stoma site along the middle of the right spino-umbilical line (Fig. 16A). The pelvis is drained via a Jackson Pratt ™ drain or any other suitable tube drain (Fig. 16B) that may be removed 72 hours later. The port sites are closed with a 1-0 vicryl™ interrupted suture and the abdominal wound is closed with a running suture of No-1 vicryl™.

URINARY DIVERSION

The authors' patients are given the choice of an ONB or ileal conduit based on their disease status. The authors have performed urinary diversion both intracorporeally (Figs 17 to 20), as well as extracorporeally. Pure laparoscopic intracorporeal urinary diversion may lead to some complications during initial learning curve.[12]

On the contrary, with robot assistance, this may involve less operative time and may be more ergonomic for the surgeon. In authors' opinion, pure laparoscopic intracorporeal urinary diversion should be performed in patients with better performance status and minimal comorbidities, and by experienced surgeons at high volume centers. In search for minimally invasive urinary diversion, doctors should not jeopardize the option of offering a neobladder in suitable select patients.[13]

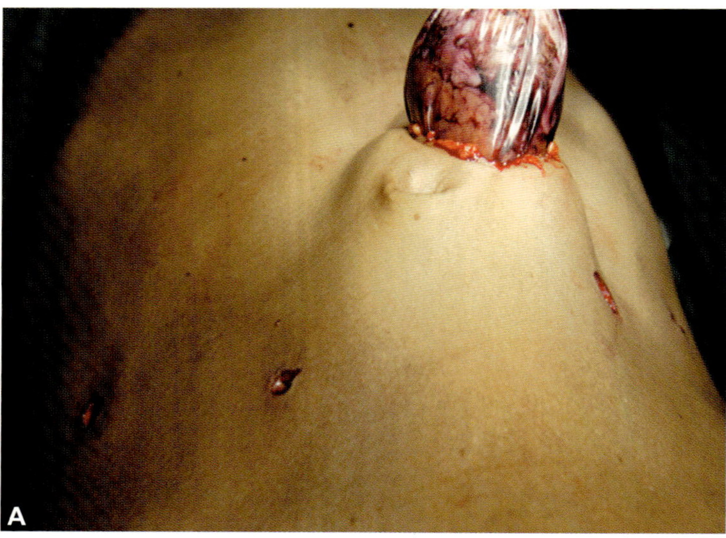

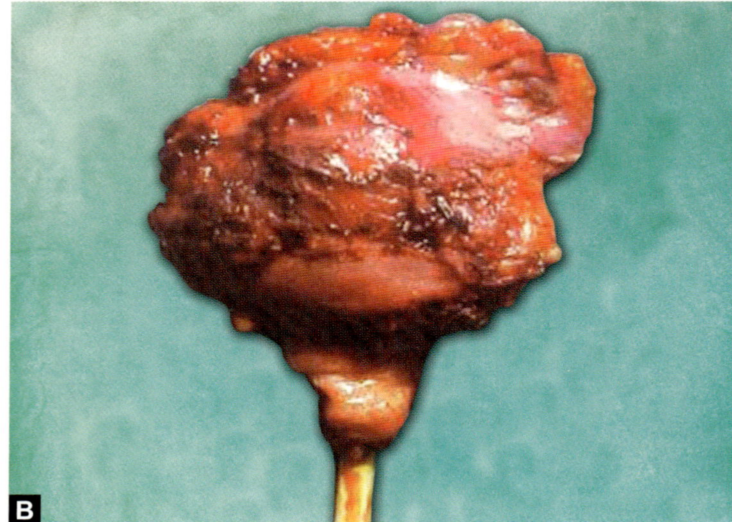

Figs 15A and B: (A) Depicting the specimen retrieval in progress; (B) and the complete excised cystoprostatectomy specimen

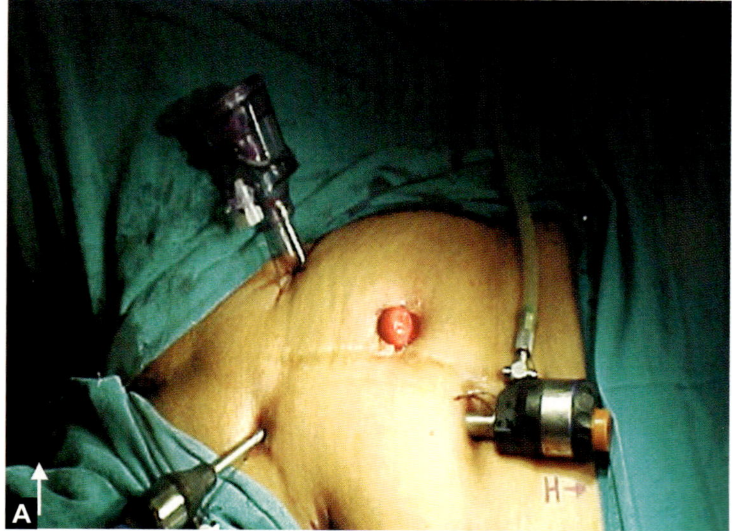

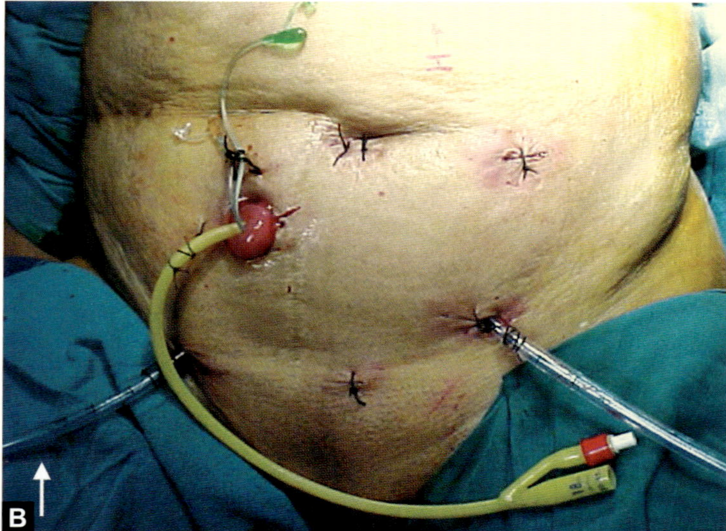

Figs 16A and B: Showing the final completed view: (A) The ileal conduit with the ports in position for an intracorporeal ileal conduit reconstruction and with the ports closed; (B) Drains placed

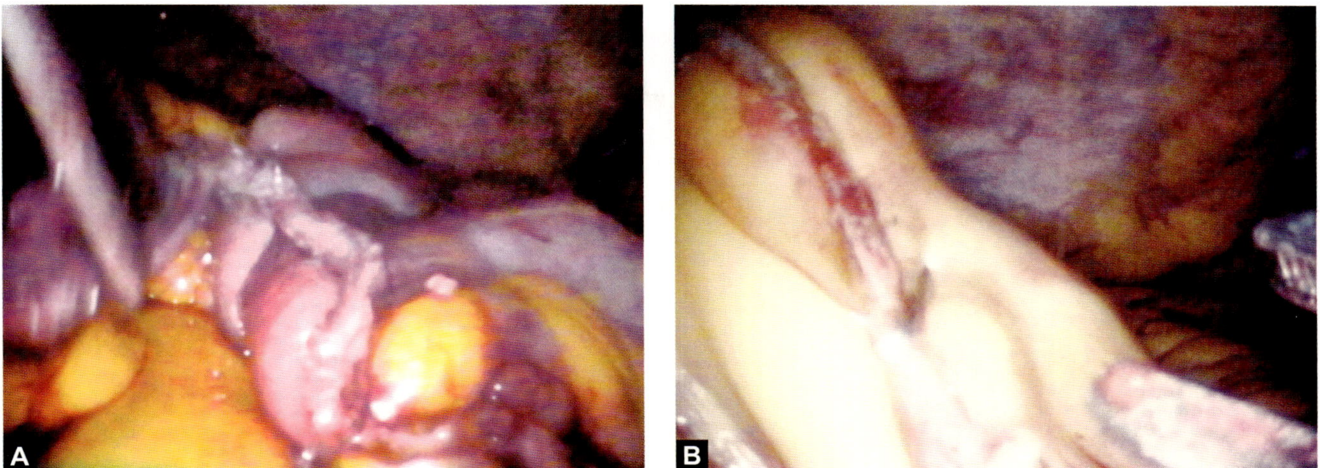

Figs 17A and B: Laparoscopic endocamera view showing: (A) The preparation of the bowel; (B) The division in the mesentery for constructing an ileal conduit in progress

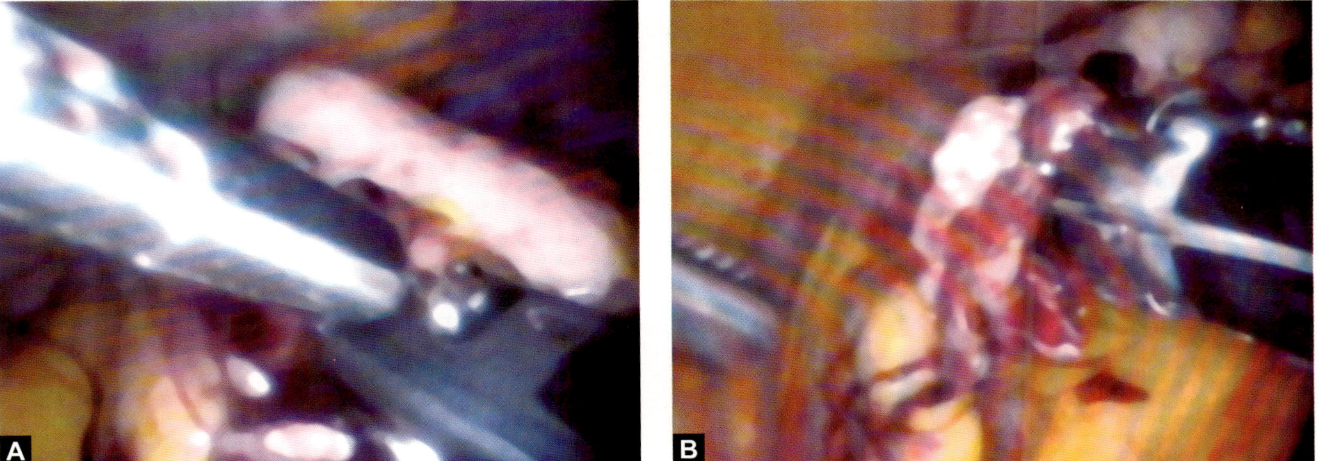

Figs 18A and B: Laparoscopic endocamera view showing: (A) The sequential application of the Endo GIA™ stapler; (B) The ileo-ileal anastomosis in progress

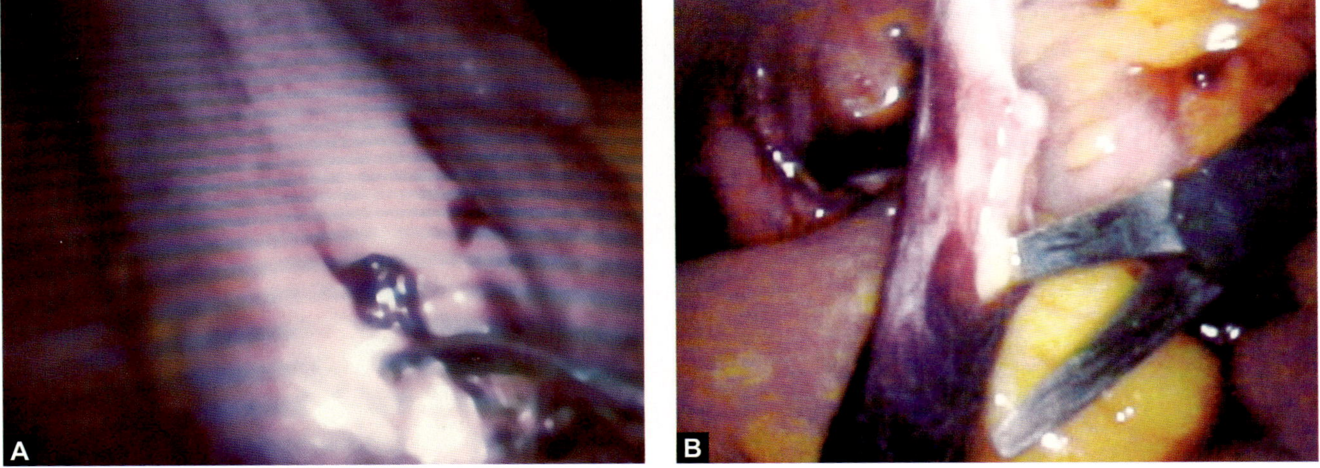

Figs 19A and B: Laparoscopic endocamera view showing: (A) The ileostomy; (B) Ureterotomy in progress for the uretroileal anastomosis for an ileal conduit

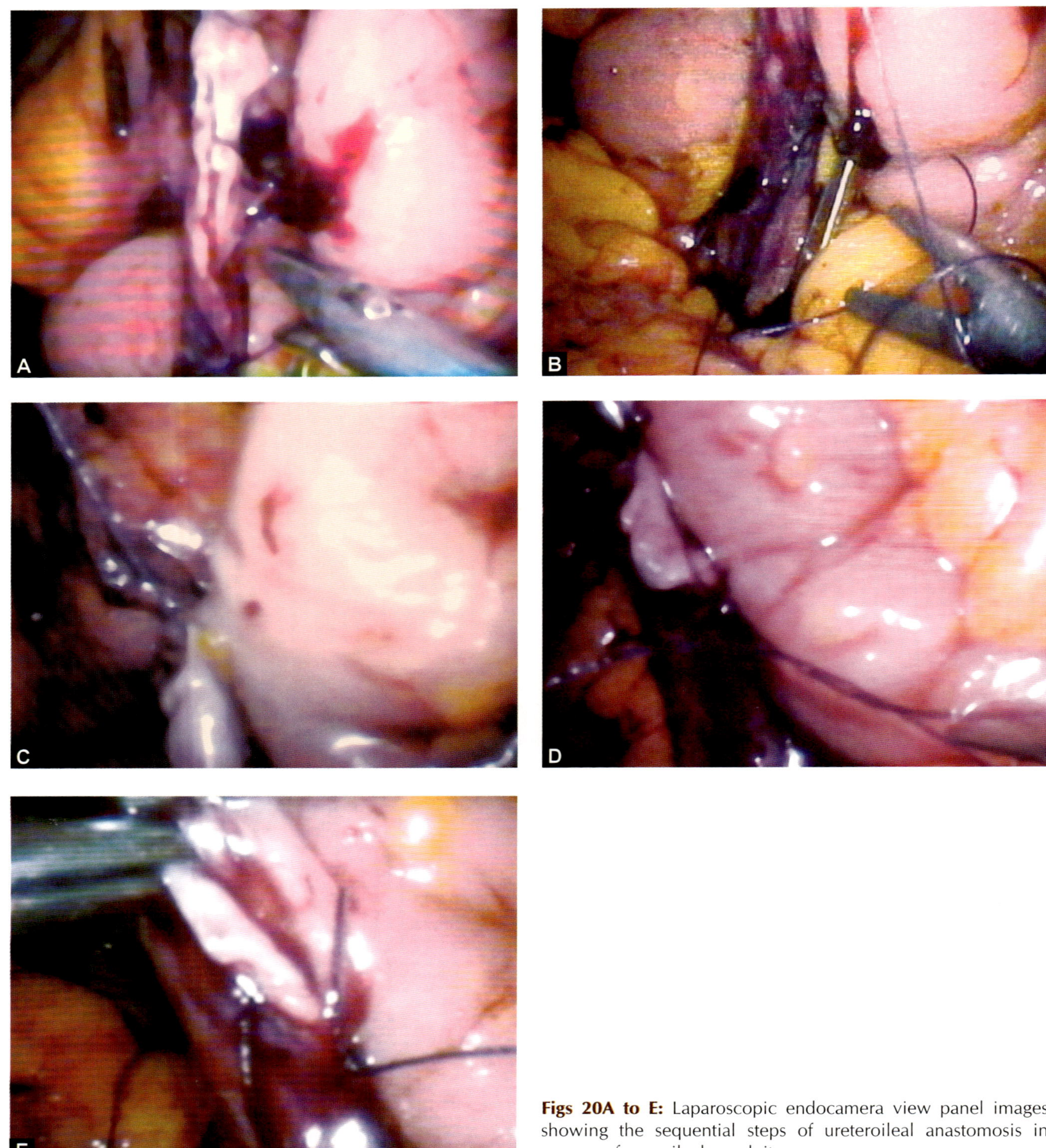

Figs 20A to E: Laparoscopic endocamera view panel images showing the sequential steps of ureteroileal anastomosis in progress for an ileal conduit

REFERENCES

1. Para RO, Andrus CH, Jones JP, et al. Laparoscopic cystectomy: initial report on a new treatment for the retained bladder. J Urol. 1992;148:1140-4.
2. Sanchez de Badajoz E, Galleo Perales JL, Reche Rosado A, et al. Radical cystectomy and laparoscopic ileal conduit. (Spa). Arch Esp Urol. 1993;46:621-4.
3. Gill IS, Kaouk JH, Meraney AM, et al. Laparoscopic radical cystectomy and continent orthotopic ileal neobladder performed completely intracorporeally: the initial experience. J Urol. 2002;168(1):13-8.
4. Gill IS, Fergany A, Klein EA. Laparoscopic radical cystectomy with ileal conduit performed completely intracorporeally:the initial 2 cases. Urol. 2000;56:26-30.
5. Turk I, Deger S, Winkelmann B, et al. Laparoscopic radical cystectomy with continent urinary diversion (rectal sigmoid pouch) performed completely intracorporeally. The initial 5 cases. J. Urol. 2001;165:1863-6.
6. Hemal AK, Singh I, Kumar R. Laparoscopic Radical Cystectomy and Ileal Conduit Reconstruction: Preliminary Experience. J. Endourol. 2003;17(10):911-6.
7. Rassweiler J, Frede T, Teber D, et al. Laparoscopic radical cystectomy with and without orthotopic bladder replacement. Minim Invasive Ther Allied Technol. 2005;14(2):78-95.
8. Hemal AK, Singh I. Hand assisted laparoscopic radical cystectomy for cancer bladder. Int Urol Nephrol. 2004;36(2):191-5.
9. AK Hemal, Singh I. In: Contemporary trends in Laparoscopic Urologic Surgery, Hemal. AK (Ed.). Laparoscopic bladder surgery Procedures, Ch.-19, New Delhi; BI Churchill Livingstone. 2002. pp. 161-77.
10. Menon M, Hemal AK, Tewari A, et al. Nerve-sparing robot-assisted radical cystoprostatectomy and urinary diversion. BJU Int. 2003; 92:232-6.
11. Singh I. Robot assisted pelvic lymphadenectomy for bladder cancer—Where have we reached by 2009. Urology. 2010;75(6):1269-74.
12. Gupta NP, Gill IS, Fergany A, Nabi G. Laparoscopic radical cystectomy with intracorporeal ileal conduit diversion: five cases with a 2-year follow-up. BJU Int. 2002;90(4):391-6.
13. Hemal AK. Editorial comment. Urology. 2010;76(4):866-71.

Chapter 16 Robot-Assisted Radical Cystectomy and Intracorporeal Ileal Conduit

Faris S Azzouni, Khurshid A Guru

BOWEL PREPARATION

The patient is started on clear liquid diet the day prior to surgery. Mechanical bowel preparation is started the day before surgery as well. Some surgeons utilize enemas only, whereas others use oral solutions, e.g. polyethylene glycol electrolyte solution (GoLYTELY®). Recent studies have found no significant difference in the rate of postoperative wound infections, clinical anastomotic leaks, or intra-abdominal abscesses between patients with and without antegrade bowel rinses. Such preparations can also increase the risk of fluid imbalances. In the elderly patient, this can produce cardiovascular instability due to intravascular volume depletion and can potentially place the patient in a catabolic state prior to surgery. The authors don't use any mechanical or oral antibiotic bowel preparation.

PREOPERATIVE PREPARATION

The patient is placed on the operating room table in a modified lithotomy position where the legs are gently abducted and placed in Stirrups, in a steep Trendelenburg position (Fig. 1). The arms are kept close to the body and padded. All pressure points are padded to prevent pressure sores. Broad-spectrum antibiotics covering Gram-positive, Gram-negative and anaerobic pathogens are administered intravenously. A nasogastric tube and a Foley catheter are placed. In females, the vagina is prepped and included in the surgical field.

TECHNIQUE OF ROBOT-ASSISTED RADICAL CYSTECTOMY IN THE MALE PATIENT (TECHNIQUE OF SPACES) (TABLE 1)

The authors' technique involves identifying the 4 spaces located anterior, lateral and posterior to the bladder, before division of the ureters and vascular pedicles. The authors believe that this technique (technique of spaces) helps reduce the risk of positive surgical margins and the risk of inadvertent bladder entry by facilitating exposure of important perivesical structures early in the course of the operation, specially since tactile feedback is not available. These spaces are the periureteral spaces, the lateral pelvic spaces, the anterior rectal space and the retropubic space.

The anterior rectal space is separated from the right and left lateral pelvic spaces by the two periureteral spaces.

Port Placement

After creation of pneumoperitoneum with a veress needle, a 12 mm port is placed at the supraumbilical area for the camera. On the right side, an 8 mm port is placed just lateral to the rectus muscle for the right robotic arm. A 12 mm right assistant port is placed about 5 cm above the right anterior superior iliac spine in the anterior axillary line (replaced by a 15 mm port at the end of the cystectomy part to facilitate insertion of the specimen retrieval bag and the Endo-GIA stapler). A 5 mm port is placed midway between the robotic arm port and the camera port approximately 2.5 cm above the camera port. This is used by the right sided assistant for suction. On the left side, an 8 mm port is placed just lateral to the rectus muscle for the left robotic arm. An 8 mm port is placed about 5 cm above the left anterior superior iliac spine for the 4th robotic arm port.

The robot is docked between the patient's legs. Inspection of the pelvic cavity reveals the bladder anteriorly in the pelvis, the sigmoid colon posteriorly and the paracolic gutters on both sides. The pulsating iliac arteries can be seen bilaterally. The gutters should be assessed for adhesions which should be lysed. A cobra grasper in the 4th robotic arm is used to hold/retract the sigmoid colon away from the site of the ureteral dissection.

Development of the Periureteral Space

Peristalsis of the ureter with the aid of 10x magnification and 3-dimensional vision helps define the site of posterior peritoneal incision (Figs 2 and 3). The authors prefer to incise the posterior peritoneum medial to the ureter since the origin of ureteral pelvic blood supply is mostly lateral. The periureteral dissection proceeds distally to the ureterovesical junction (UVJ) and proximally to the bifurcation of the common iliac vessels. Preservation of the periureteral tissue is critical to insure viability of the ureter. The periureteral space is developed by gently sweeping the areolar tissue away from the ureter and cauterizing the small vessels present. The internal iliac (hypogastric) artery can be identified pulsating underneath, lateral to the ureter. Typically used instruments in this part of the dissection are round tip cold scissors and bipolar forceps, with the occasional use of blunt monopolar hook cautery. The developed spaces reveal pearly white tissue planes. After dissecting the periureteral space, one should be able to identify the edge of posterior peritoneum medial to the ureter, the ureter, the hypogastric artery, the external iliac artery and vein, all lateral to the ureter.

Development of the Lateral Pelvic Space (Figs 4 to 6)

This space follows the medial curve of the pubic rami. It is bound laterally by the bony pelvis, covered by the Psoas major muscle (above), obturator internus and pelvic floor (below). Anteriorly, there is the anterior abdominal wall and the peritoneal reflections over the inferior epigastric vessels and obliterated umbilical arteries (lateral and medial umbilical ligaments respectively). Medially is the urinary bladder and posteriorly is the ureter. The contents of this space are the vas deferens crossing between the internal inguinal ring

Table 1: Male radical cystectomy: technique of spaces

Surgical step	Lens	Right robotic instrument	Left robotic instrument	Fourth robotic arm	Right assistant port
Port placement/Lysis of adhesions	30 angled up	—	—	—	Microfrance grasper/Non Ratcheted curved scissors
Periureteral space	0	Round tip scissors	Precise bipolar	Cobra retracts the sigmoid	Suction
Lateral pelvic space	0	Monopolar cautery hook	Precise bipolar	Cobra retracts the bladder	Suction
Anterior rectal space	0	Round tip scissors	Precise bipolar	Cobra lifts the bladder anteriorly	Suction
Control of vascular pedicle and division of ureters	0	Round tip scissors	Precise bipolar	—	Hem-o-lok® Weck Clip/Endovascular stapler
DVC Control	0	Needle driver	Needle driver	Cobra grasper, Retracts bladder specimen	Suction

Accessory Instruments
- Allen stirrups (yellow finsR)
- Egg crates and gel pads customized to cover pressure points
- Scope Warmer (Applied Medical)
- Endo-catch II (Tyce, Auto suture); 15 mm (bladder specimen)
- Endo-pouch retriever (Ethicon); 10 mm (lymph nodes)
- Rectal Tube (Kendall) Seamless 24 French
- Foley Catheter (Bardex) Hematuria 24 French 30 cc balloon
- Hem-o-lok® (Weck Clip); (ML, L, XL)
- Irrigation Suction System (ACMI Surgi-wave XP Pump)
- Suction Irrigation probe (Reusable 5 mm x 45 cm)

Laparoscopic Instruments and Trocars
- Pneumo-needle insufflation needle with luer lock (Ethicon PN 120)
- MicroFrance grasper (CEV 525); (Medtronic/XOMED)
- Needle holder (Karl Storz 26178 MC or 26178 ML)
- Non-Ratcheted curved scissors (Olympus)
- 10/12 mm Bladeless Trocar (Ethicon-512 NT) (1)(Camera port)
- 5 mm Trocar (XCEL) (1) (Suction port)
- 15 mm Trocar (XCEL) (1) (Right assistant port)
- Seal Reducer cap for 10/12 mm Ethicon port (Ethicon)(1)

Robotic Instruments
- Endo-wrist precise bipolar (400110) (1)
- Round Tip Scissors (400007) (1)
- Hook Permanent cautery (400183) (1)
- Needle driver large (400006) (2)
- Cobra Grasper (400190) (1)

Sutures
- Vicryl CT-2 (control of dorsal venous complex)

Stapler (vascular)
- Endo GIA™ Roticulator (Universal) 45 mm; (4–6 refills available in OR room)

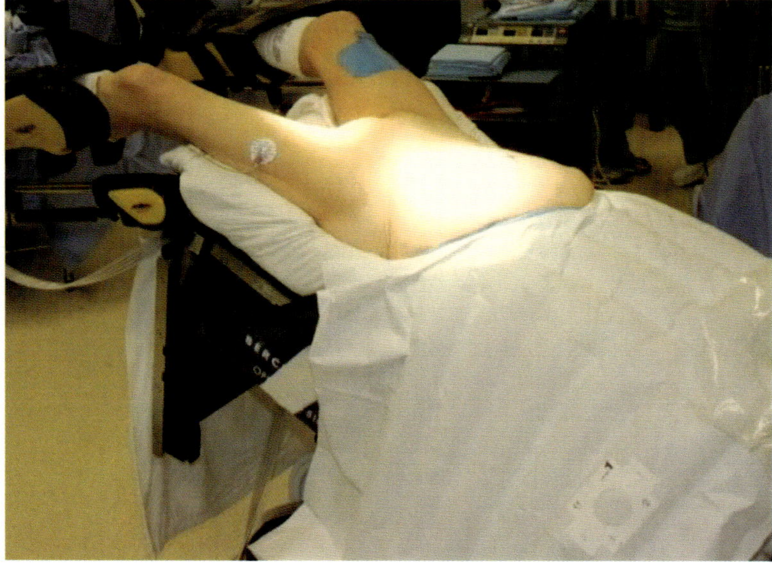

Fig. 1: Patient positioning in dorsal lithotomy and steep Trendelenburg

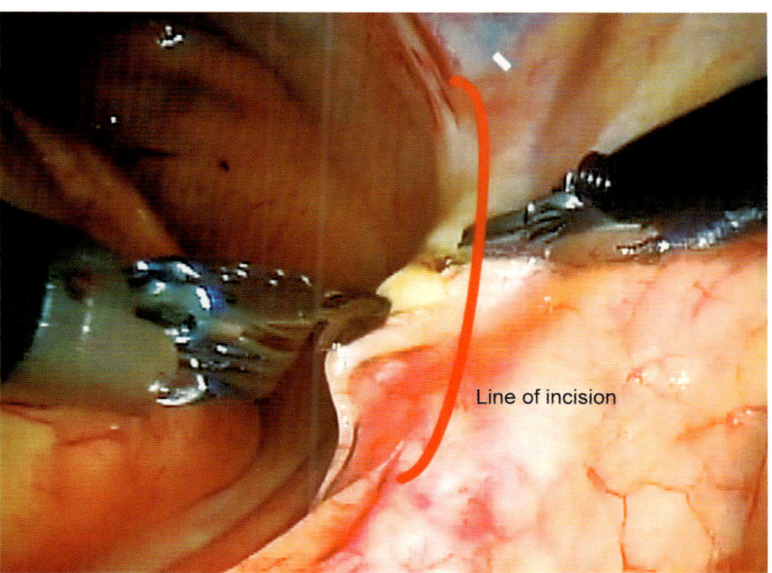

Fig. 2: Line of posterior peritoneal incision over the right ureter

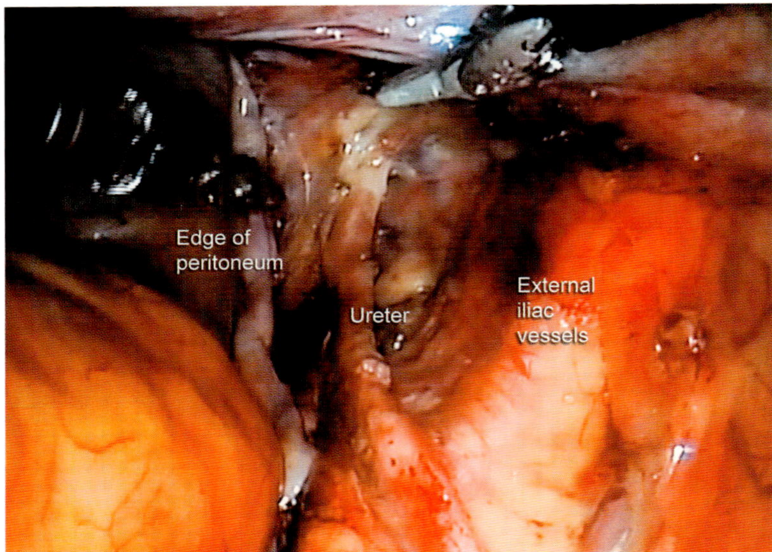

Fig. 3: Right periureteral space

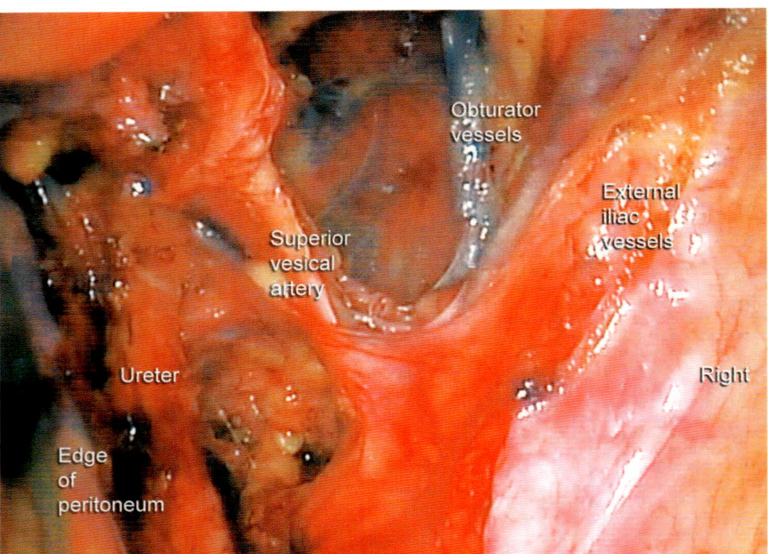

Fig. 4: Right lateral pelvic and periureteral spaces

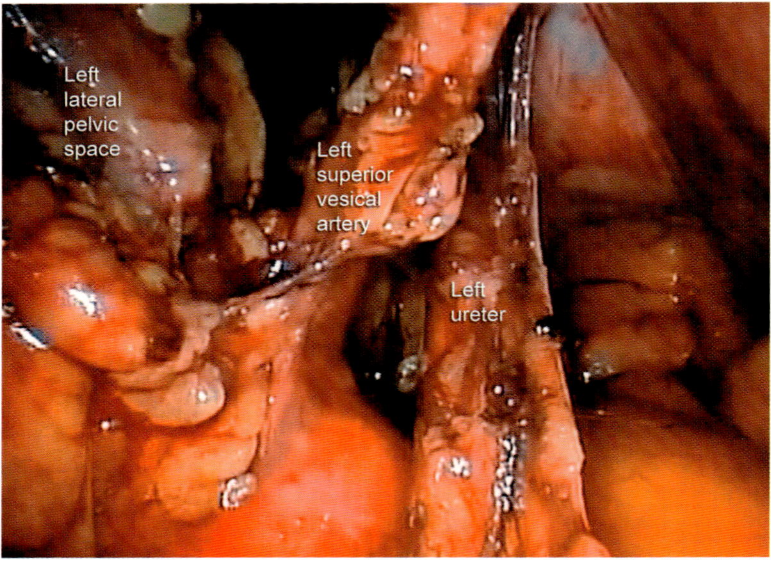

Fig. 5: Left ureter and superior vesical artery

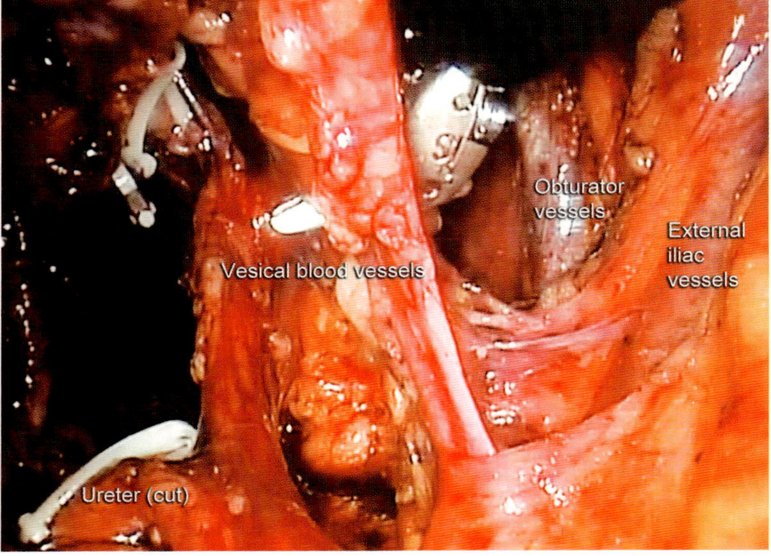

Fig. 6: Right lateral pelvic and periureteral spaces

(anterolaterally) toward the bladder base (posteromedially). Below the vas are the obturator nerve, obturator vessels and the internal iliac vessels. The inferior vesical artery arises from the anterior trunk of the internal iliac artery and with its surrounding pelvic fascia; it constitutes the lateral vesical ligament (pedicle). At the medial edge of the Psoas muscle, the external iliac vessels descend, with the artery being anterior to the vein.

The lateral pelvic space is developed by incising the posterior peritoneum lateral to the medial umbilical ligament toward the already-incised posterior peritoneum around the ipsilateral ureter. The vas is clipped and divided. The loose areolar tissue is gently swept away to identify the important landmarks in this space. The bladder is still attached to the anterior abdominal wall and this provides natural anterior retraction. Deep in this space, one should be able to identify the endopelvic fascia and the loose areolar tissue in the paravesical space along the lateral wall of the bladder. During blunt dissection in the lateral pelvic space, one should encounter only tiny vessels in the areolar tissue which should be point-cauterized to avoid bothersome bleeding. Once the lateral pelvic space is opened, one should be able to identify the lateral pelvic sidewall, the external iliac vessels, the obturator vessels and nerve.

Development of the periureteral and lateral pelvic spaces is similarly done on the opposite side.

Development of the Anterior Rectal Space

Once the periureteral and lateral pelvic spaces have been prepared bilaterally, attention is turned to the rectovesical pouch and development of the anterior rectal space is performed. The remaining segment of posterior peritoneum between the two ureters is incised in the midline. This way the incised posterior peritoneum around the two ureters will be connected. Blunt dissection is carried out to isolate the plane between the fascia of Denonvilliers' and the rectum. The seminal vesicles should not be dissected separately and should stay attached to the bladder. This dissection is performed utilizing a 0° lens and a combination of sharp and blunt dissection, all the way down to the posterior apex of the prostate. It is preferable not to use cautery in this dissection to avoid thermal injury to the rectum. The superior vesical artery, arising from the anterior trunk of the internal iliac artery passes toward the bladder in this space. It is located posteromedial to the ureter and constitutes the posterior vesical ligament (pedicle).

After the development of these spaces, the ureters are clipped with Hem-o-lok™ (Weck) clips and the distal ends of the proximal ureteral edges are sent for frozen section. Anterior and sideway traction on the bladder via its attachments to the anterior abdominal wall and the cobra grasper in the 4th robotic arm, respectively facilitate exposure of the vascular pedicles. Each vascular pedicle is clipped with Hem-o-lok™ clips and divided. The vessels are divided close to the base of the bladder when a nerve-sparing procedure is intended. Patients expected to have a more locally advanced (T3, T4) disease should undergo a wider, non-nerve sparing resection, in which the endo GIA™ vascular stapler can be used to control the vessels. After the vessels are divided, the endopelvic fascia can be identified and it is incised bilaterally in an anteromedial direction, along with the Puboprostatic ligaments to provide access to the anterior apex of prostate, common trunk of the dorsal vein complex and the external urethral sphincter.

Development of the Retropubic Space (Anterior Exposure)

Attention is then turned to the anterior attachments of the bladder to the abdominal wall. The urachus and medial umbilical ligaments are divided high, allowing the bladder to fall down in the pelvis and providing access to the retropubic space of Retzius. The retropubic fat is dissected and the central (superficial) branch of the dorsal vein complex is cauterized. The urethra/apex of prostate are dissected and suture ligation of the DVC is performed. A back bleeding stitch is placed around the dorsal vein complex proximally over the anterior surface of the prostate. The DVC is divided, providing better access to the prostatic apex (Fig. 7). The Foley catheter is subsequently removed. A large Hem-o-lok™ (Weck clip) is applied proximal to the point of division of the urethra to prevent any urine spillage (Fig. 8). The full circumference of the urethra is subsequently divided. The specimen is placed in a large retrieval bag inserted through the 15 mm right assistant port (replaces the original 12 mm port inserted at the beginning of the case) and removed via a Pfannenstiel or a lower midline incision later in the case. The pelvic cavity is inspected for any bleeding points which are cauterized with the bipolar forceps. Irrigation is then done with 1 liter of sterile water. A frozen section of urethral tip can then be sent.

TECHNIQUE OF ROBOT-ASSISTED RADICAL CYSTECTOMY (ANTERIOR PELVIC EXENTERATION) IN THE FEMALE PATIENT (TABLE 2)

The classic (standard) female radical cystectomy is essentially an anterior pelvic exenteration. The urinary bladder, whole urethra, uterus, most of the anterior vaginal wall, fallopian tubes and ovaries are removed.

Recently, there has been interest in orthotopic neobladder reconstruction, sexual function-sparing and reproductive function-sparing radical cystectomy in females in order to preserve quality of life and since the risk of urethral involvement with TCC is less than equal to 2%.

The principles of the dissection are the same as in men. A similar six-port transperitoneal access is achieved using the Veress needle. The pelvic anatomic landmarks are observed (Fig. 9). Adhesions (if any) are lysed. The cobra grasper in the 4th robotic arm is used to retract the sigmoid colon.

Development of the Periureteral and Paravesical Spaces

The ureters are seen peristalsing as they cross anterior to the common iliac arterial bifurcation at the pelvic brim. The posterior peritoneum overlying the ureters is incised medially and the periureteral tissue is gently dissected distally toward the ureterovesical junction and proximally toward the common iliac arterial bifurcation, using cold-tip scissors and bipolar forceps. Occasionally, a monopolar hook cautery is used. Care is taken not to skeletonize the ureter of its surrounding loose tissue since this is important for insuring ureteral blood supply and viability. The uterine artery is seen to cross above the ureter from lateral to medial on its way to uterine sidewall. At this point, both the ureter and uterine artery are preserved (Fig. 10), until all anatomic landmarks are identified. Deep in the paravesical space (below the ureter-uterine artery intersection) is the paravaginal space where several vaginal blood vessels can be identified as they arise from the internal iliac artery laterally and pass to the lateral vaginal wall medially.

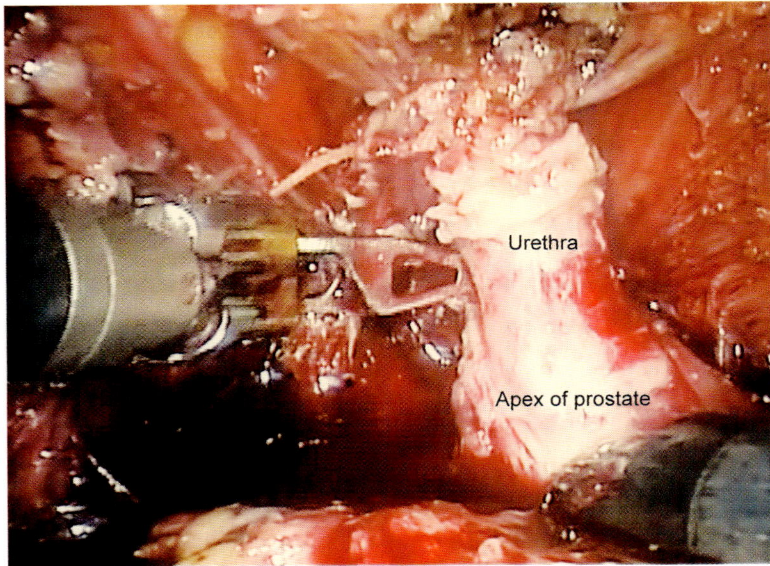

Fig. 7: Development of prostatic apex-urethral junction

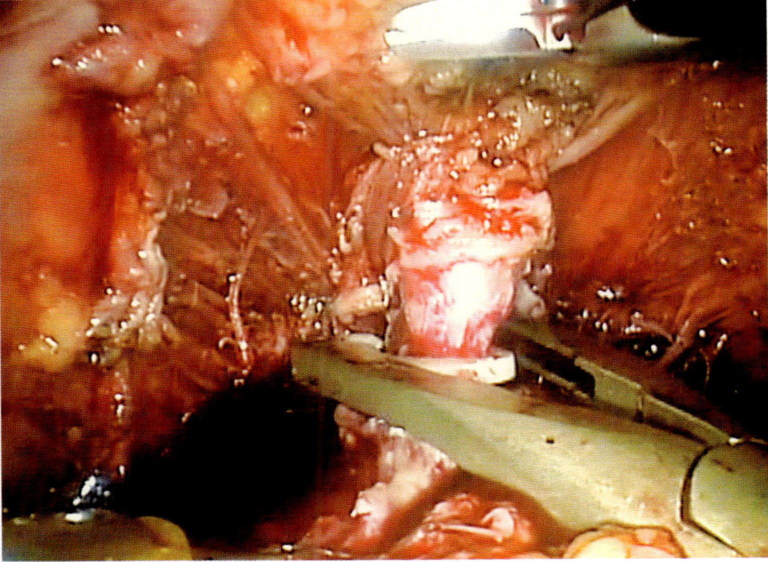

Fig. 8: Clip application at the prostatic apex, to prevent urine spillage

Table 2: Female radical cystectomy: technique of spaces

Surgical step	Lens	Right robotic instrument	Left robotic instrument	Fourth robotic arm	Right assistant port
Port placement/Lysis of adhesions	30 Angled up	—	—	—	Microfrance grasper/Non-Ratcheted curved scissors.
Periureteral space	0	Round tip scissors	Precise bipolar	Cobra retracts the sigmoid	Suction
Lateral pelvic space	0	Monopolar cautery hook	Precise bipolar	Cobra retracts the bladder	Suction
Anterior rectal space	0	Round tip scissors			
Precise bipolar	Cobra lifts the bladder anteriorly	Suction.			
Control of vascular pedicle and division of ureters	0	Round tip scissors	Precise bipolar		Hem-o-lok™ Weck Clip/ Endovascular stapler
DVC control	0	Needle Driver	Needle driver	Cobra Grasper retracts bladder specimen	Suction
Vaginal Reconstruction	0	Needle driver	Needle driver		
Extended pelvic lymph node dissection	0	Round tip scissors or monopolar cautery hook	Precise bipolar		Suction

Accessory Instruments
- Allen stirrups (yellow finsR)
- Egg crates and gel pads customized to cover pressure points
- Scope Warmer (Applied Medical)
- Endo-catch II (Tyce, Auto suture); 15 mm (bladder specimen)
- Endo-pouch retriever (Ethicon); 10 mm (lymph nodes)
- Rectal tube (Kendall) Seamless 24 French
- Foley catheter (Bardex) Hematuria 24 French 30 cc balloon
- Hem-o-lok™ (Weck Clip); (ML, L, XL)
- Irrigation suction System (ACMI Surgi-wave XP Pump)
- Suction irrigation probe (Reusable 5 mm x 45 cm)

Laparoscopic Instruments and Trocars
- Pneumo-needle insufflation needle with luer lock (Ethicon PN 120)
- MicroFrance grasper (CEV 525); (Medtronic/XOMED)
- Needle holder (Karl Storz 26178 MC or 26178 ML)
- Non-Ratcheted curved scissors (Olympus)
- 10/12 mm bladeless trocar (Ethicon-512 NT)(1)(Camera port)
- 5 mm trocar (XCEL)(1)(Suction port)
- 15 mm trocar (XCEL)(1)(Right assistant port)
- Seal reducer cap for 10/12 mm Ethicon port (Ethicon)(1)

Robotic Instruments
- Endo-wrist precise bipolar (400110)(1)
- Round tip Scissors (400007)(1)
- Hook permanent cautery (400183)(1)
- Needle driver large (400006)(2)
- Cobra grasper (400190)(1)

Sutures
- Vicryl CT-2 (control of dorsal venous complex)

Stapler (vascular)
- Endo GIA™ Roticulator (Universal) 45 mm; (4-6 refills available in or room)

Development of the Lateral Pelvic Space

The peritoneum lateral to the medial umbilical ligament (Fig. 11) is incised parallel to the medial curve of the pubic bone, toward the dissected posterior peritoneum overlying the ipsilateral ureter. The round ligament is seen to cross the lateral pelvic space from the internal inguinal ring toward the uterine sidewall. The round ligament is preserved. Blunt dissection is carried deep to the incised lateral peritoneum in this space from the pelvic sidewall toward the bladder wall. Once this space is dissected, the pelvic diaphragm, the obturator neurovascular bundle and the inferior vesical vessels can be identified.

A similar dissection to develop the periureteral, paravesical (Fig. 12) and lateral pelvic spaces is done on the opposite side.

Ligation of the Pedicles

The posterior peritoneum separating the infundibulopelvic ligament from the iliac blood vessels is incised. This ligament contains the ovarian blood vessels (Fig. 13) travelling anterior and lateral to the ipsilateral ureter. It is clipped with Hem-o-lok™ clips and divided. The medial umbilical ligament, ureter, uterine and vesical blood vessels are similarly clipped individually, with Hem-o-lok™ clips and divided. A piece of the distal part of the proximal ureteral stump is sent for frozen section analysis.

Development of the Rectouterine Pouch

The posterior peritoneum in the rectouterine pouch is incised. The loose areolar tissue between the posterior vaginal and anterior rectal

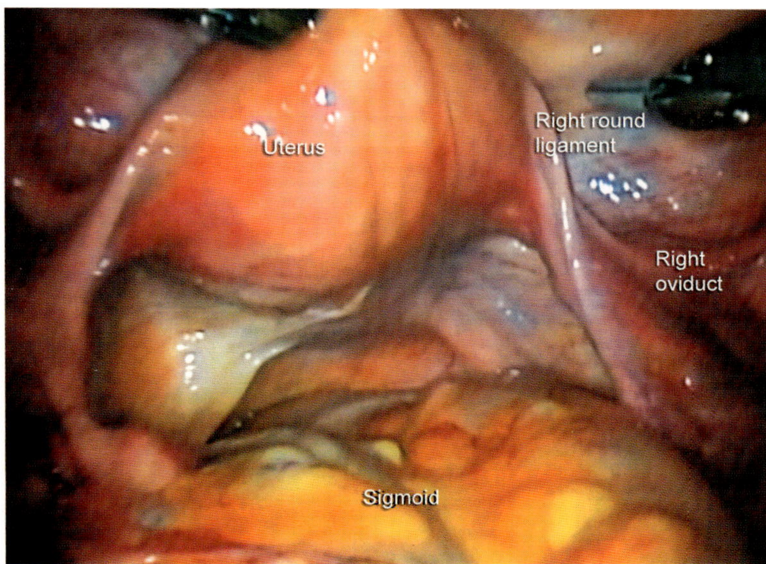

Fig. 9: Laparoscopic view of the female pelvis

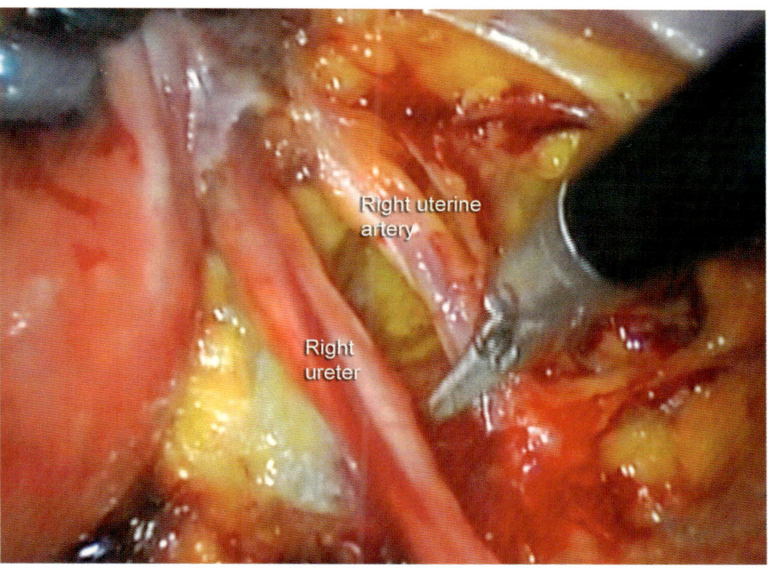

Fig. 10: Right uterine artery

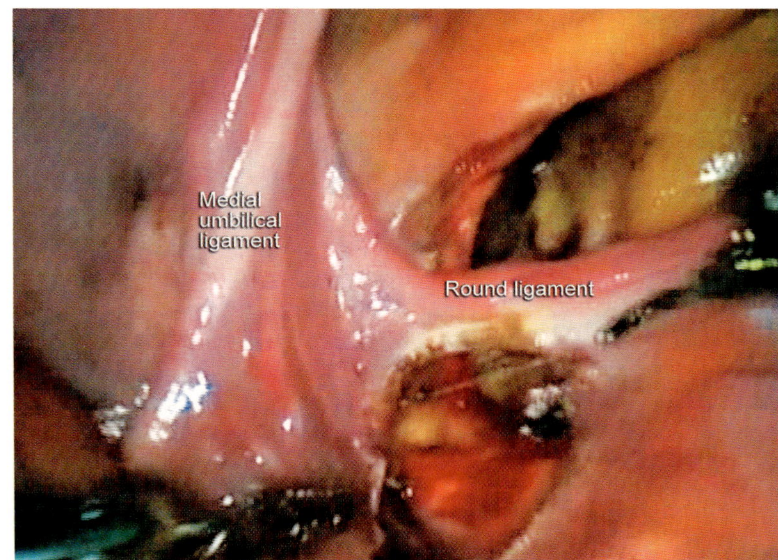

Fig. 11: Right medial umbilical and round ligaments

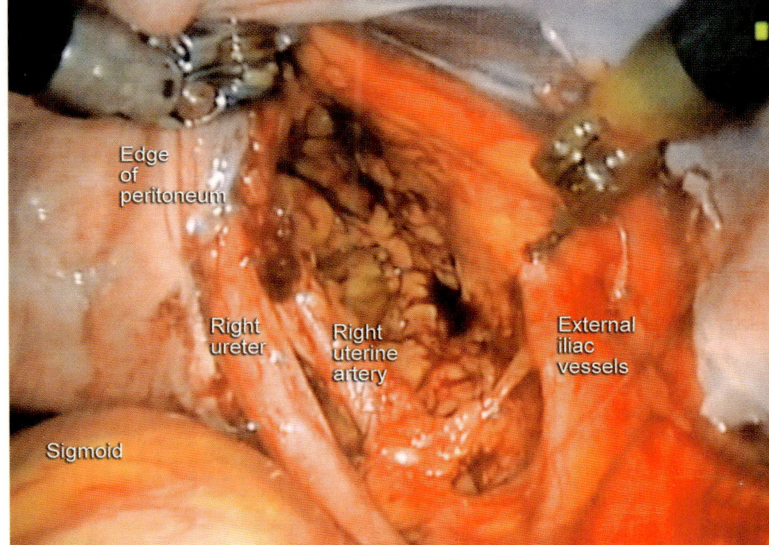

Fig. 12: Right paravesical space

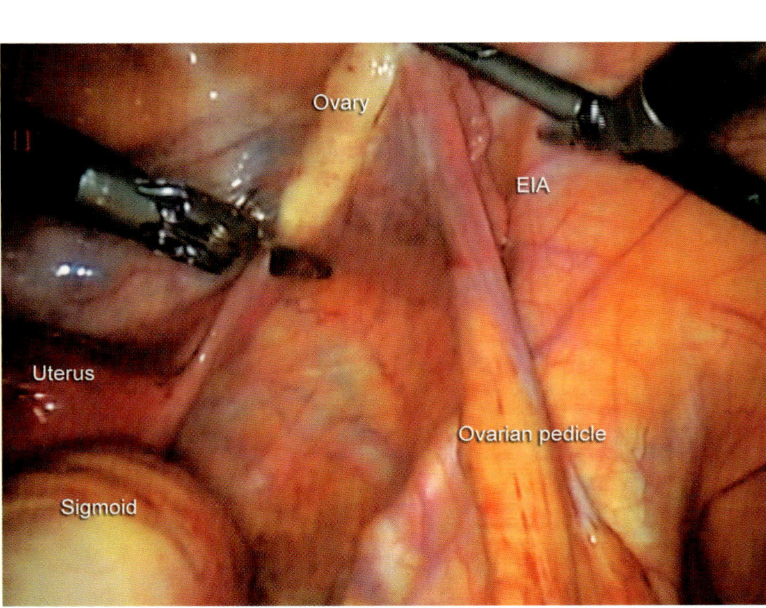

Fig. 13: Right ovarian pedicle

wall is dissected bluntly. A sponge stick placed in the vagina helps identify the posterior vaginal fundus. A hook monopolar cautery device is used to incise the posterior vaginal fornix transversely. This incision is continued anteriorly. Branches of the pelvic plexus supplying the vagina and urethra descend on the lateral vaginal walls therefore dissection is continued toward the anterior vaginal wall to preserve these nerves if an orthotopic neobladder is planned. The extent of resection of the anterior vaginal wall depends on whether the female patient is getting an anterior pelvic exenteration or an orthotopic neobladder since there is no intervening fascia between the anterior vaginal wall and the urinary bladder base (as is the case in the male patient who has Denonvilliers fascia) and since the anterior vaginal wall provides anatomic support important for urinary continence (Double hammock theory).

Development of the Retropubic Space

The urachus and medial umbilical ligaments are divided with a hook cautery so that the bladder drops inferiorly. The dorsal vein complex is cauterized or suture-ligated and divided. If the decision is to perform an anterior pelvic exenteration, the entire urethra and most of the anterior vaginal wall are resected. Otherwise, the urethra is divided 1 cm below the bladder neck along with the corresponding segment of anterior vaginal wall. The specimen is placed in an EndoCatch™ bag and removed either via the vagina or (if large) via an anterior abdominal wall (Pfannenstiel or lower midline) incision.

The vagina is closed with a running, interlocking Vicryl stitch in a transverse fashion (clam shell technique). Preservation of the pelvic autonomic nerves running on the lateral vaginal wall bilaterally is more important for female sexual function preservation than vaginal length since these nerves are important for vaginal lubrication and orgasmic function. Closure of the vagina in a side to side fashion is discouraged since it will create a dysfunctional narrow vagina.

ROBOT-ASSISTED INTRACORPOREAL ILEAL CONDUIT (MARIONETTE TECHNIQUE) (TABLE 3)

Isolation and Transfer of the Left Ureter to the Right Side

The left ureter is delivered to the right side under the sigmoid mesocolon using a Micro-France grasper (Figs 14 and 15).

Creation of the 'Marionette' Suture and Isolation of Bowel Segment

Once the bowel is examined, a 12 cm segment of small bowel is identified ≈ 15 cm proximal to the ileocecal valve. A 152-cm 1-silk suture using a Keith needle is brought through the anterior abdominal wall at a location inferior to the marked stoma site to allow more space for the mobility of the robotic arms (Figs 16 to 18). The silk suture is passed full-thickness through the marked distal end of the future ileal conduit and then brought back through the anterior abdominal wall. This suture is controlled with an instrument and not tied to allow for raising and lowering of the conduit like a 'marionette' during the procedure. A ≈ 12 cm segment of bowel is identified proximal to the 'marionette' suture (distal end of the conduit) and is held in place by the fourth-arm Cobra grasper. The hook cautery is used to incise the peritoneum of the bowel mesentery (Fig. 19), after which the small mesenteric vessels are controlled using bipolar cautery or a stapler. The two mesenteric windows are created to isolate the ileal conduit (Fig. 20).

Once adequate vascularity to the ileal conduit is ensured, a 45 mm Endo GIA™ stapler is introduced through the 15 mm right assistant-port to divide the bowel lumen on both sides of the conduit. The 'marionette' is maneuvered appropriately during this step.

The bowel continuity is not re-established at this point, but completed towards the end of the procedure. A single zero silk suture is used to bring the two ends of small intestine together at this stage, maintaining proper orientation and preventing malrotation (Fig. 21).

Bowel Washout and Set-Up for Anastomosis

An electrosurgical J-hook is used to create a small opening in the distal (stomal) portion of the conduit for irrigation of the bowel contents. The 'marionette' is lowered to easily place a Foley catheter

Table 3: Intracorporeal ileal conduit—Marionette technique

Surgical step	Lens	Right robotic instrument	Left robotic instrument	Fourth robotic arm	Right assistant port
Isolation of bowel segment	0	Hook cautery	Cardiere forceps	Cobra grasper	Suction
Bowel washout	0	Cardiere forceps	Cardiere forceps	Cobra grasper	Foley Catheter
Spatulation of ureters	0	Robotic scissors	Cardiere forceps	Cobra grasper	Suction
Uretero-enteric anastomosis	0	Needle driver	Needle driver	Cobra grasper	Suction
Re-establishment of bowel continuity	0	Cardiere forceps	Cardiere forceps	Cobra grasper	New assistant port and Endo GIA™ stapler
Closing of mesentery and reinforcement of bowel anastomosis	0	Needle driver	Cardiere forceps	Cobra grasper	Suction

Laparoscopic Instruments and Trocars
- 5 mm laparoscopic suction
- 5 mm laparoscopic locking grasper
- 5 mm laparoscopic scissors
- 5 mm laparoscopic needle driver
- 10 mm laparoscopic Hem-o-lok™ clip applier
- 15 mm laparoscopic EndoCatch™ bag
- Endo GIA™ stapling device–45 and 60 mm loads

Robotic Instruments
- Monopolar Curved Scissors
- Prograsp Forceps
- Cobra grasper
- Cardiere forceps
- Permanent Cautery Hook
- Large Needle Driver x2
- 0° or 30° down lens (for deep pelvis)

Suture
- #1 silk on Keith needle (full size) – Marionette stitch
- 4-0 vicryl (polyglactin 910) on SH (4 inches) and 4-0 vicryl on RB-1 (4 inches); tied together for ureteroileal anastomosis (can be done with two 4-0 monocryl sutures tied together)
- 4-0 vicryl (or 4-0 monocryl) for the interrupted ureteroileal anastomosis
- 3-0 chromic on SH needle to secure ureteral stents
- #0 Silk on CT1 needle to bring the 2 ileal ends together
- #0 Silk on CT1 needle to close the mesenteric window
- 2-0 Silk on SH needle to reinforce the stapled bowel anastomosis

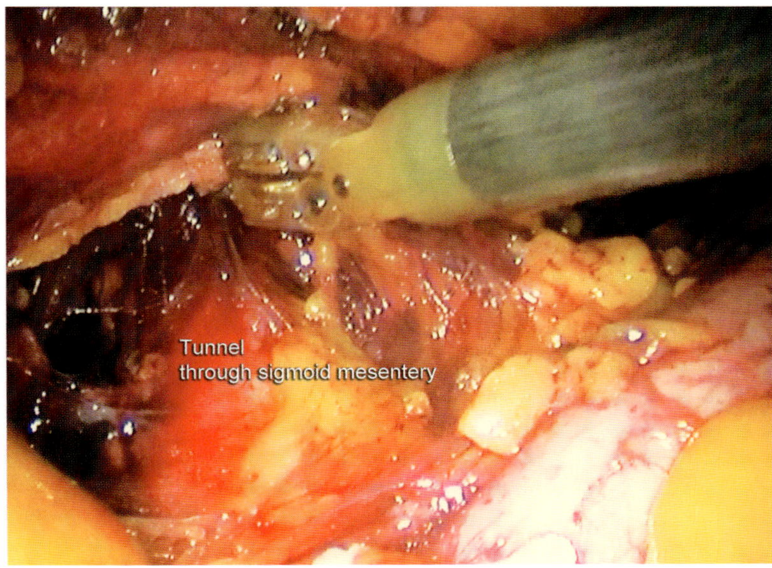

Fig. 14: Development of a tunnel for the left ureteral passage through the sigmoid mesentery

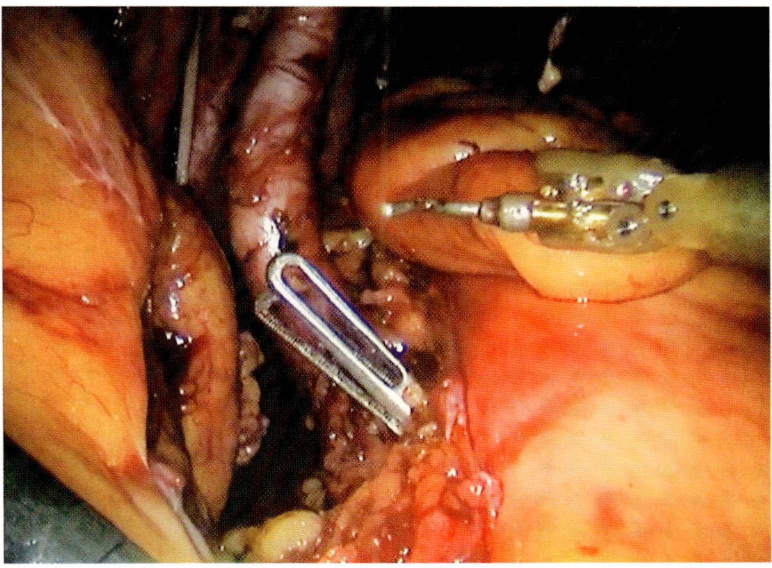

Fig. 15: Grasper catching the tip of the left ureter

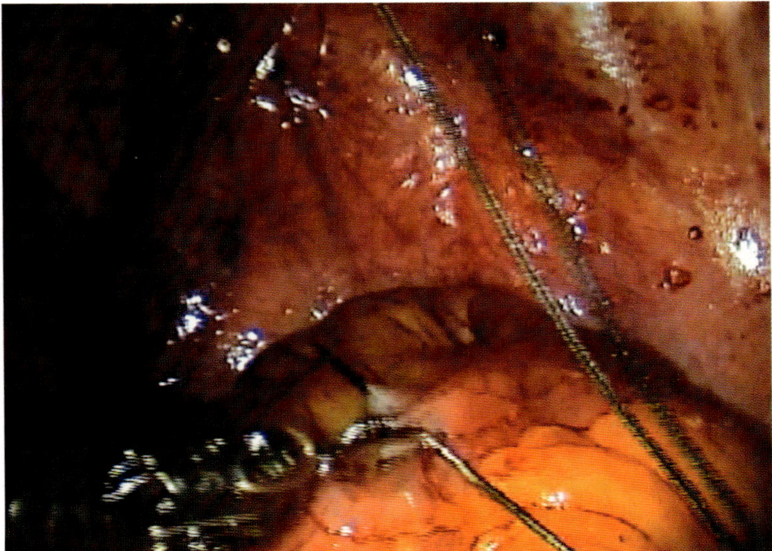

Fig. 16: Keith needle passed through the distal (stomal) end of future ileal conduit. This serves as the 'Marionette' handle

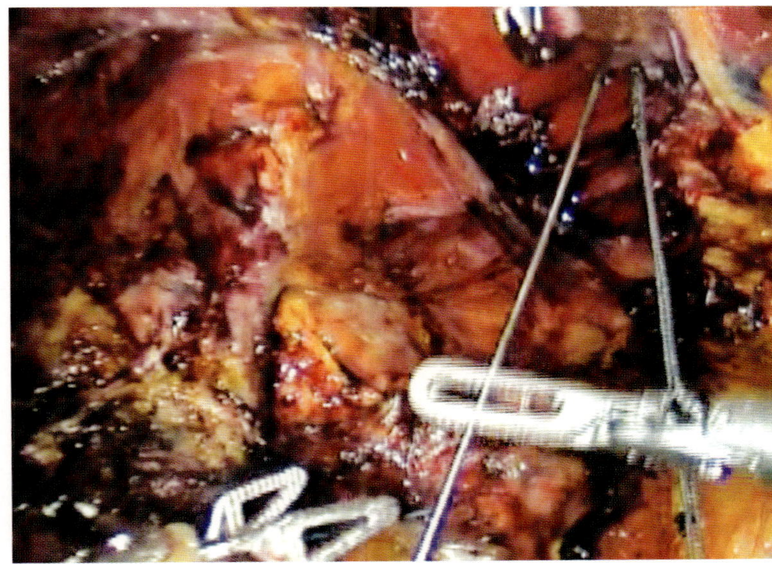

Fig. 17: Keith needle passed through the abdominal wall (to the outside)

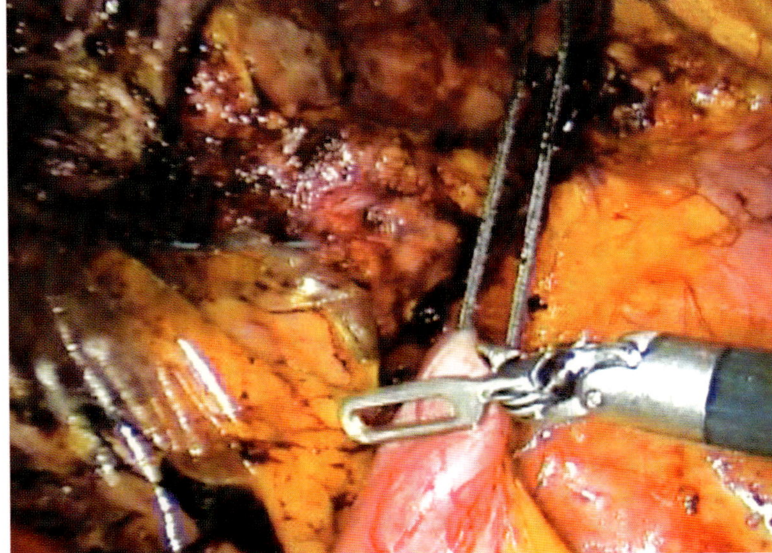

Fig. 18: Silk suture (Marionette) pulled toward the abdominal wall

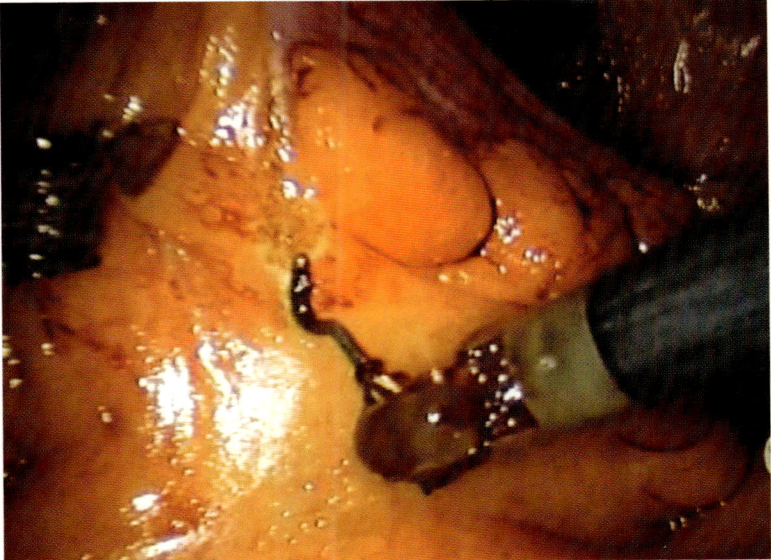

Fig. 19: Development of the mesentery of the future ileal conduit

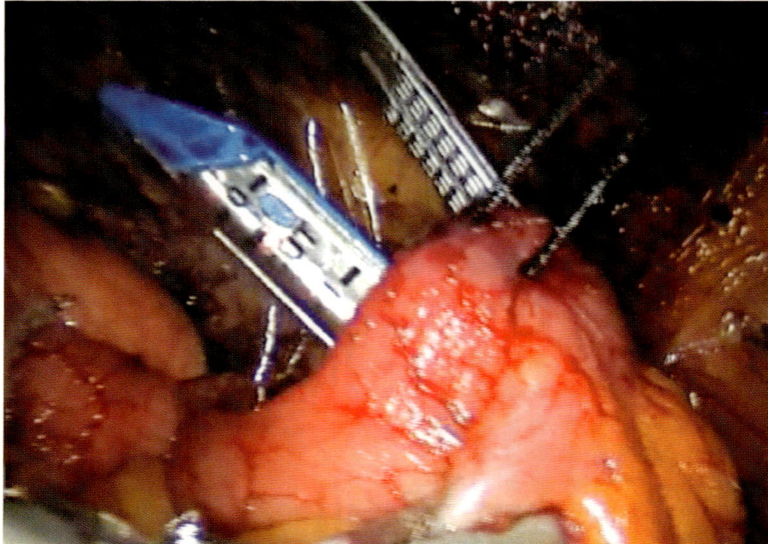

Fig. 20: 45 mm Endo GIA™ stapler used to isolate the ileal conduit

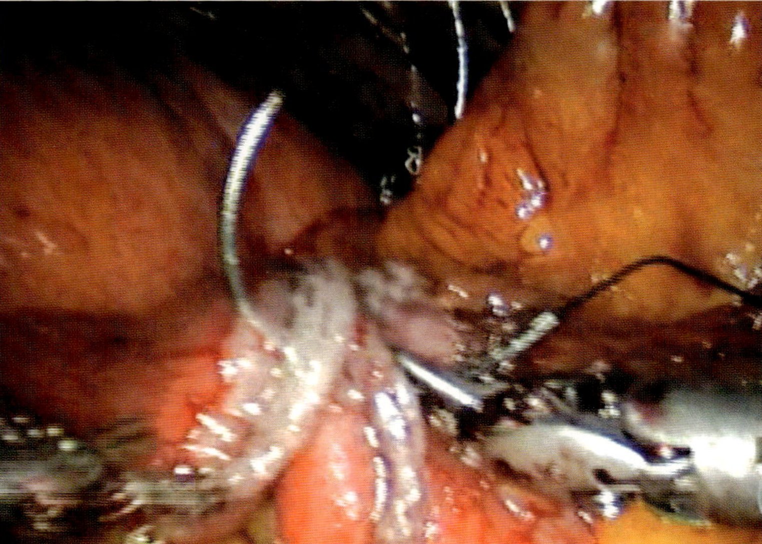

Fig. 21: The two ends of ileum are approximated with a single zero silk suture to maintain proper alignment and orientation. This facilitates future stapled bowel reanastomosis

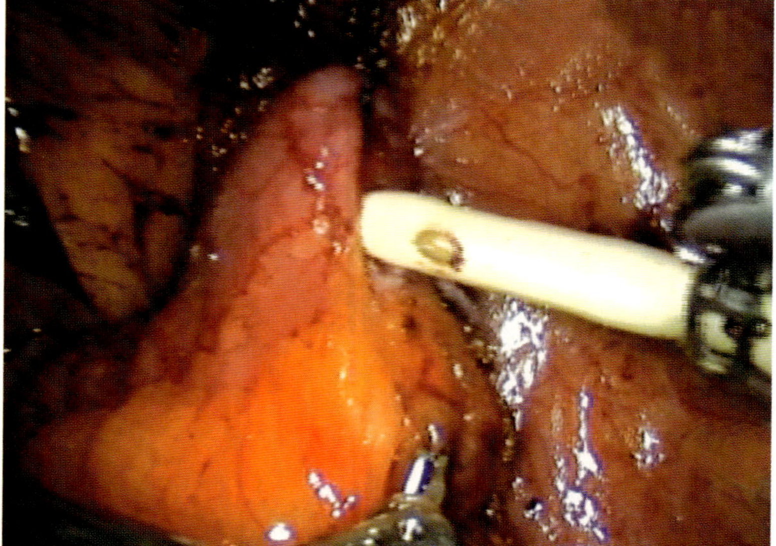

Fig. 22: Tip of Foley catheter being inserted into the ileal conduit

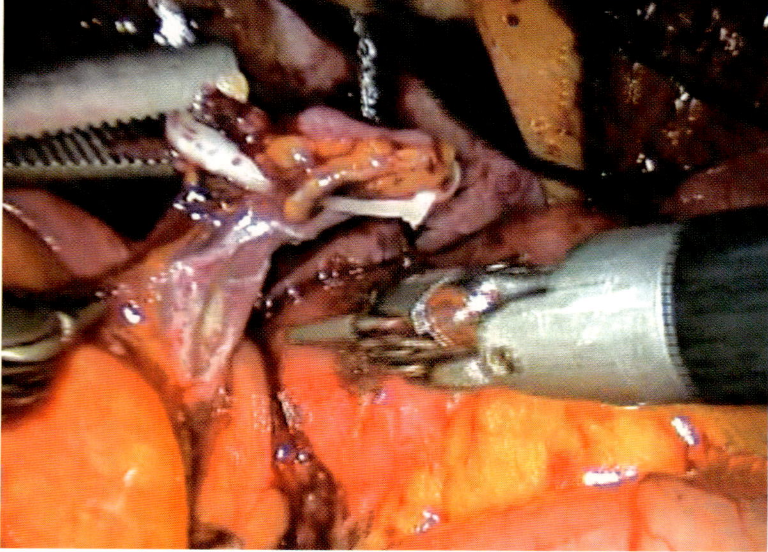

Fig. 23: Spatulation of ureter

into the conduit (Fig. 22). A 22 F catheter is introduced through the 15 mm right assistant-port and fed into the conduit through this enterotomy using a Cardier grasper in the right hand after lowering the 'marionette' suture. The catheter balloon is inflated with 5 ml of sterile water to prevent spillage while irrigating, the catheter is then used to irrigate the bowel segment. Once the irrigant is clear, the balloon is deflated and the catheter is removed.

Ureteroileal Anastomosis

Minimal proximal dissection and gentle handling of the ureter is crucial during ureteroileal anastomosis. The distal end of the ureter (Hem-o-lok™ clip) is held in position using the fourth robotic arm Cobra grasper. The robotic scissor is used to partially transect and spatulate the distal end of the ureter (Fig. 23). Scissors or an electrocautery hook is used to make two enterotomies in the proximal conduit segment on two opposite sides (Figs 24 and 25). The ureteroileal anastomosis can be performed in a running fashion (Van-Velthoven technique), using two 4-0 polyglactin 910 (or 4-0 monocryl) sutures tied together

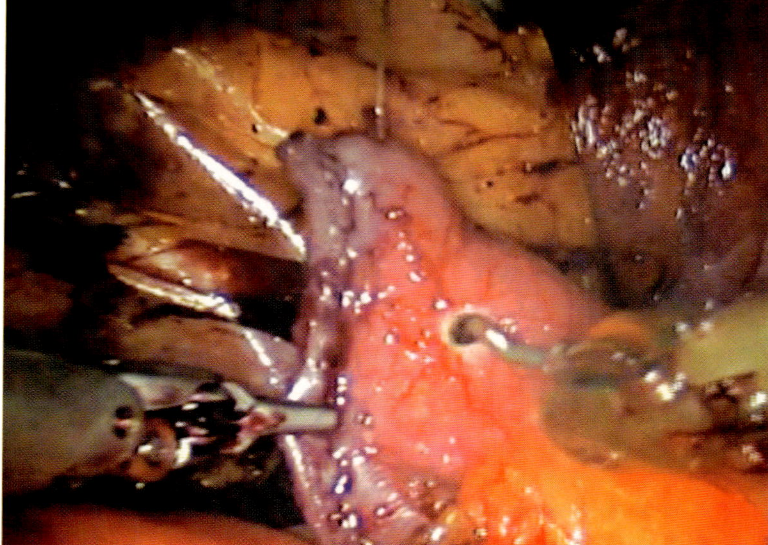

Fig. 24: Creation of enterotomy at proximal end of ileal conduit for ureteroileal anastomosis

(Fig. 26). The ureteroileal anastomosis can also be performed using simple interrupted stitches (4-0 vicryl or monocryl).

After half of the sutures have been placed, the ureteric stent is inserted. A metal laparoscopic suction tip is passed through the 15 mm assistant-side port and the 'marionette' is lowered to align for easy passage through the conduit. The tip of the suction is gently guided through the entire conduit, starting at the previously made opening at the distal conduit for irrigation. A 90 cm, 8.5 F single-J ureteric stent with a guidewire is passed through the suction tip and fed into the ureteric opening while holding the metal suction tip in place using the left robotic arm (Fig. 27). Once the single-J stent is positioned in the upper ureter, the suction tip is withdrawn while the robotic surgeon controls the stent with the guidewire. The guidewire is left in the stent to allow for easy identification of the stent inside the conduit.

A 3-0 chromic catgut suture is used to suture the stent to the conduit, preventing accidental dislodgement and the guidewire is removed.

The ureteroenteric anastomosis is then completed. A similar series of steps are undertaken for the other ureter. The distal ends of the two stents are left in the 15 mm side port, the ex vivo portions of these stents should not be clamped or attached to any instrument to prevent accidental dislodgement during maneuvering of the conduit. The 'marionette' can be raised and lowered as necessary, in combination with the manipulation using the fourth right robotic arm, to allow for optimal visibility and completion of the anastomosis.

Placement of a New 12 mm Suprapubic Port

This port is used to insert the 60 mm Endo GIA™ stapler for performing the side: side stapled ileo-ileal anastomosis and is extended to a Pfannenstiel incision, at the end of the case, for extraction of the specimen in the male patient (Fig. 28).

Re-establishment of Bowel Continuity

The fourth arm is used to hold the silk suture tagging the two stapled ends of the ileum and is raised up to the anterior abdominal wall.

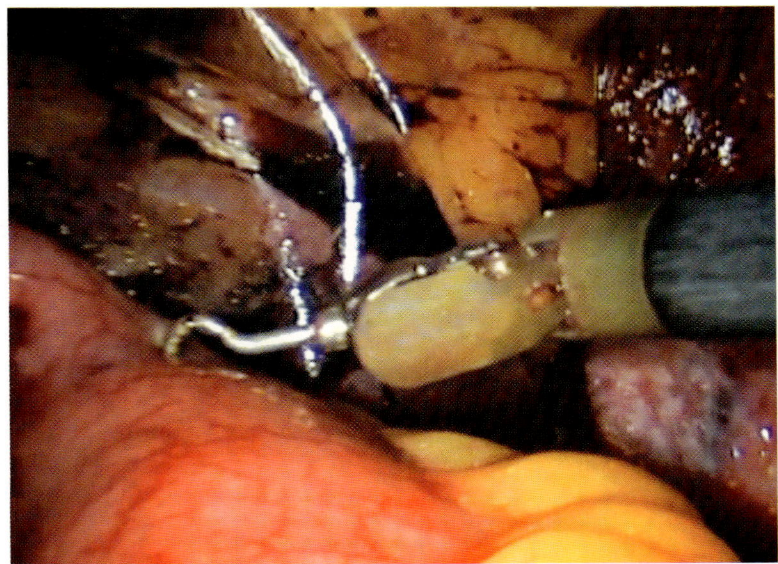

Fig. 25: Creation of a second enterotomy for the contralateral ureteroileal anastomosis

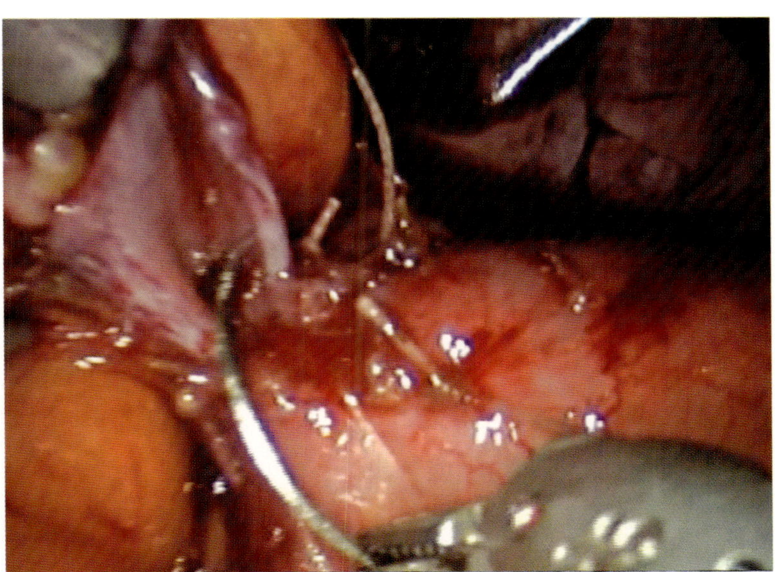

Fig. 26: Ureteroileal anastomosis

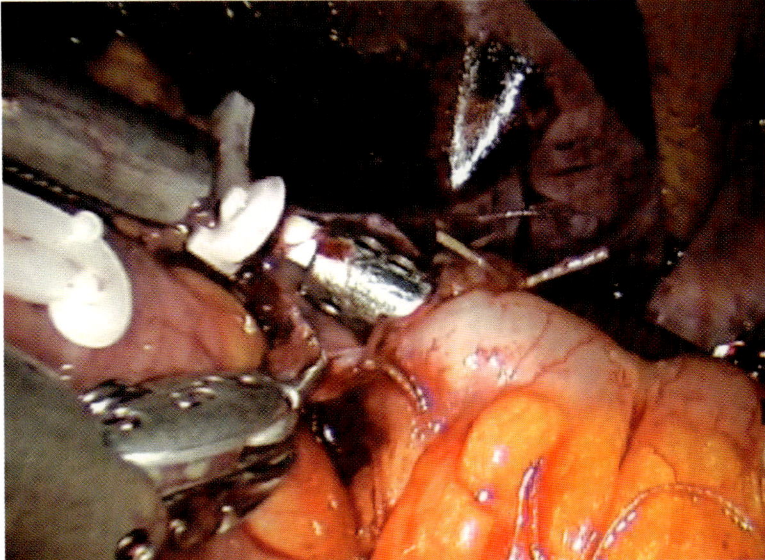

Fig. 27: Insertion of single J ureteral stent using the metal laparoscopic sucker

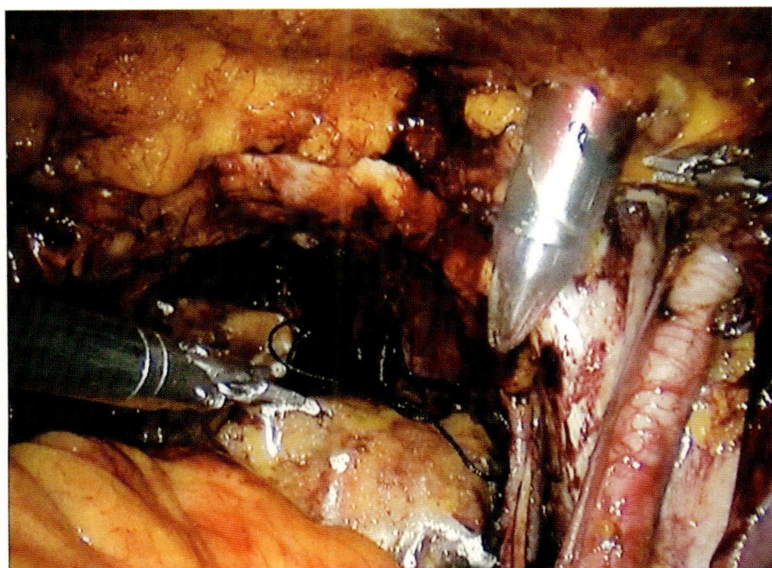

Fig. 28: New 12 mm port in the suprapubic area for the stapled bowel reanastomosis

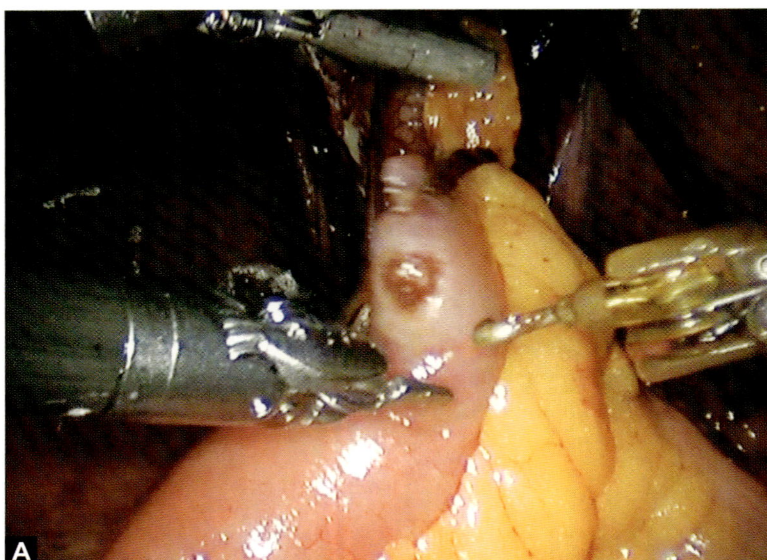

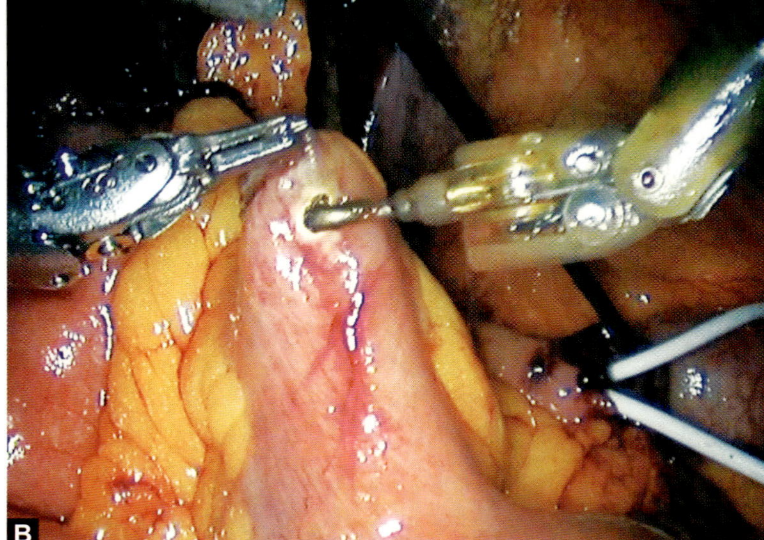

Figs 29A and B: Creation of 2 enterotomies in the 2 approximated ileal ends for the insertion of the stapler

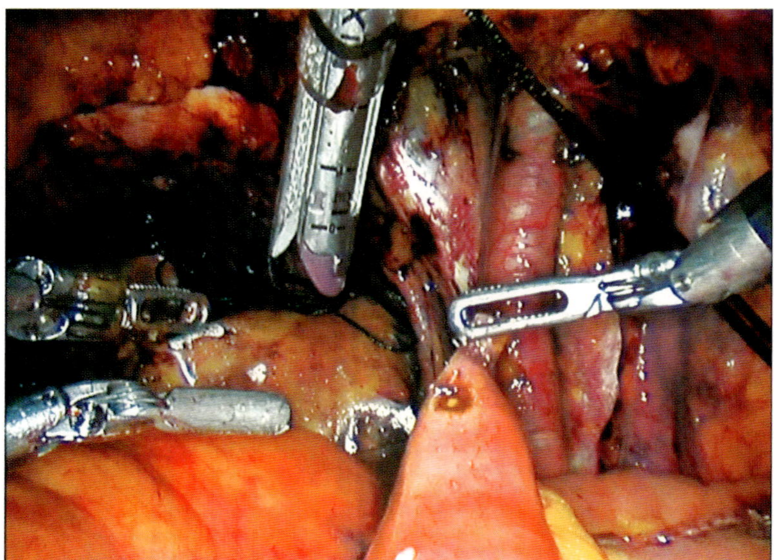

Fig. 30: Insertion of 60 mm Endo GIA™ stapler through the suprapubic port

This allows for proper orientation of the bowel and straightening the ileal segment, permitting the Endo GIA™ stapler to be passed without tension. A small enterotomy is created on the antimesenteric side of each segment of bowel, close to the previously placed staple lines (Figs 29A and B).

The silk suture tagging the two bowel ends is held by the fourth arm. A laparoscopic 60 mm Endo GIA™ stapler is passed through the 12 mm suprapubic port into the enterotomies (Fig. 30). After ensuring that the anti-mesenteric sides of the bowel are properly opposed, the stapler is fired and bowel continuity is re-established (Figs 31A and B).

The two open bowel ends are held with the robotic arms and a second firing of the Endo GIA™ stapler is performed transversely via

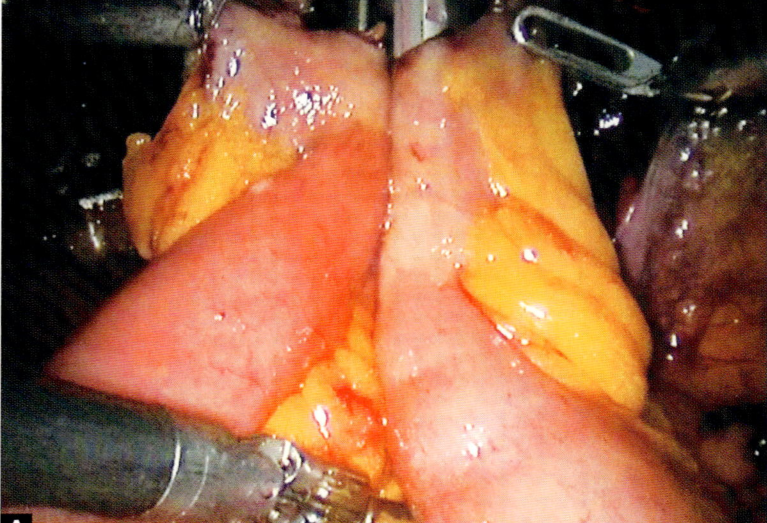

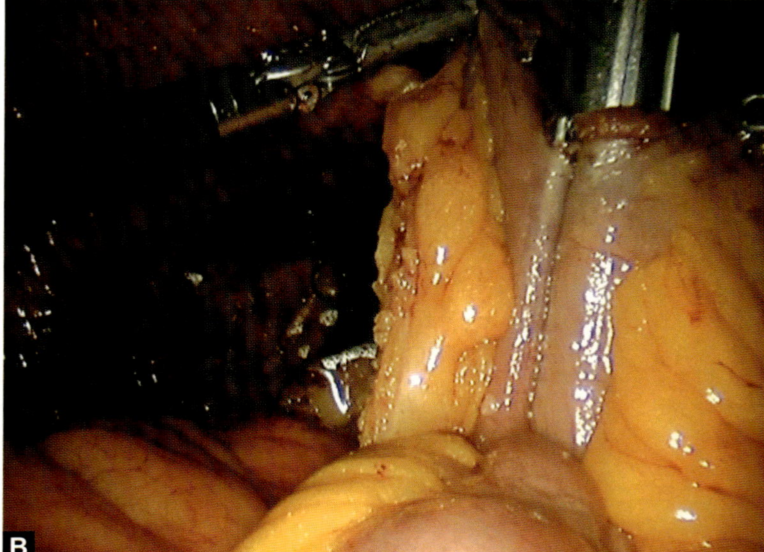

Figs 31A and B: Stapler introduced into the 2 opposed ileal ends and fired after correct alignment and orientation is ensured

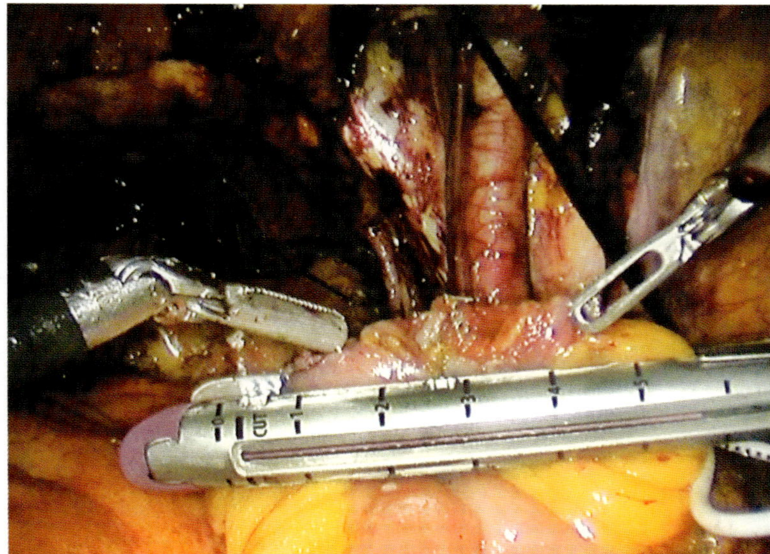

Fig. 32: The stapler is introduced the right assistant port and a second firing of the Endo GIA™ stapler is performed transversely across the 2 open ileal ends

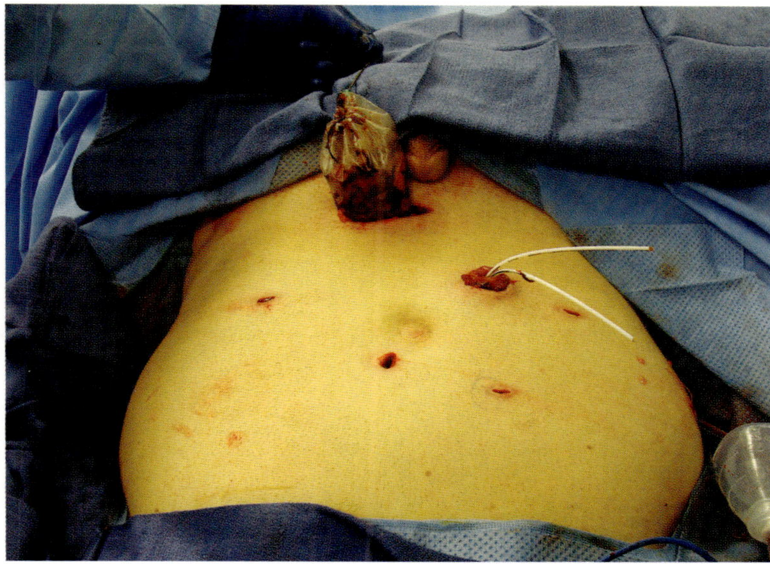

Fig. 33: Extraction of specimen in a male patient by extending the 12 mm suprapubic port transversely

the right assistant port (Fig. 32). The peritoneal window can then be closed using # 0 silk suture, and 1–2 simple interrupted reinforcement (2-0 silk) sutures can also be placed to reinforce the bowel anastomosis. The 12 mm suprapubic port is used to remove the specimen by extending it to a Pfannenstiel incision (Fig. 33). Specimen is removed via the vagina in female patients.

Creation of the Stoma

The marked stoma site is opened and a cylinder of fat is removed. A cruciate incision is made in the anterior rectus fascia, and a hemostat clamp is passed into the peritoneum. The distal end of the conduit and the stents are extracted using the 'marionette' suture and the stoma is fashioned according to the surgeon's preferences.

17

Chapter

Robotic Extended Pelvic Lymph Node Dissection for Bladder

Reza Ghavamian

INTRODUCTION

The rapid dissemination of robotic prostatectomy has led to a parallel increase in the incidence and interest in performing radical cystectomy for the treatment of bladder cancer. It has been suggested and shown that the adequacy of the nodal dissection in bladder cancer surgery is a surrogate for the oncologic efficacy of the procedure.[1,2] This adequacy is both reflected in the number of nodes resected and the comparable morbidity as well as complications of the robotic nodal dissection to open pelvic lymph node dissection.[3]

The boundaries of the nodal dissection, namely standard versus extended, have been the subject of study and it is now accepted that extended nodal dissection for urothelial carcinoma of the bladder is the procedure of choice. Whether robotic surgery with the da Vinci® surgical system can emulate the open procedure has also been the subject of recent debate.[4] Recent studies have now demonstrated adequate and equivalent nodal counts confirming the efficacy of the pelvic node dissection in robotic bladder cancer surgery. In fact, one study revealed that a robotic-assisted lymphadenectomy for bladder cancer followed by a second look open lymphadenectomy performed at the time of the diversion had a concordance of 93%.[5] The early concerns were mostly with the cephalad extent of the nodal dissection and whether the robot can access nodes at the aortic and vena caval bifurcation and whether, it can furthermore, reach the origin of the inferior mesenteric artery. While these were early concerns with the standard robot, the most recent model, the da Vinci® SI, allows for excellent access to these areas with the same trocar placement. The SI robot provides far more flexibility and hence improved cephalad range of motion of the robotic arms. The downward 30° lens further aids with the proximal portion of the operation and surgical field by allowing a downward panoramic view of the aortic bifurcation.

In this chapter, the technique of extended pelvic nodal dissection for bladder cancer is discussed. The cephalad boundary of the extended nodal dissection is the aortic bifurcation, and the distal extent is the node of Cloquet and the circumflex vessels coming off the external iliac artery. The lateral and medial borders are the genitofemoral nerve and the paravesical and pararectal nodes that are left after the cystectomy portion of the operation respectively. The posterior extent is the nodal tissue below the level of the obturator vessels and nerve. Also included in the template are the presacral nodes, the obturator nodes, the common iliac, external iliac and the internal iliac nodes. Finally, the nodal tissues in the triangle of Marcille are resected as part of the extended nodal template.

TECHNIQUE OF ROBOTIC EXTENDED PELVIC LYMPHADENECTOMY

The nodal dissection is usually performed after the cystectomy portion of the operation. The rationale for this is that in the era of advanced cross-sectional imaging, early diagnosis of bladder cancer and most importantly neoadjuvant chemotherapy, the patient who comes to cystectomy usually needs the cystectomy. Patients with bulky nodal disease and advanced bladder cancer undergo neoadjuvant chemotherapy. The occasion where the patient is surprisingly found to have bulky nodal involvement precluding cystectomy is now only rarely encountered.

A systematic dissection is preferred. The procedure is either begun distally and extended cephalad, or vice versa. This author begins the procedure by dividing the posterior peritoneal tissue from over the common iliac artery (CIA) with a split and roll technique. The descending colon is retracted medially with the fourth arm of the robot and the dissection is carried cephalad to identify the aortic bifurcation (Figs 1A and B).

Next, the nodes anterior to the bifurcation of the inferior vena cava (IVC) are dissected. The venal caval bifurcation is often more distal than the aortic bifurcation, and at times this nodal packet can be dissected en bloc with the presacral nodes (Figs 2A and B). In this area one has to be cautious of presacral venous branches that are flush with the sacrum and can be a source of significant bleeding if inadvertently injured.

The common iliac nodes are dissected next, removing the nodes anterior, and lateral and medial to the CIA (Figs 3A and B).

To perform the external iliac nodal dissection, the lateral border of the dissection template is identified. The genitofemoral nerve is identified lateral to the external iliac artery, by division of the posterior peritoneal tissue (Figs 4A to C).

The tissue is then lifted off the artery with a split and roll technique and the nodal tissue medial to the vessel is also dissected (Figs 5A and B).

Next attention is placed on dissection of the internal iliac nodal chain. As such, the bifurcation of the common iliac artery is targeted and the origin of the hypogastric artery is identified. Continued retraction is placed on the descending colon medially and the precise bipolar cautery is utilized in the left hand as the dissection is performed with the scissors in the right hand (Figs 6A and B).

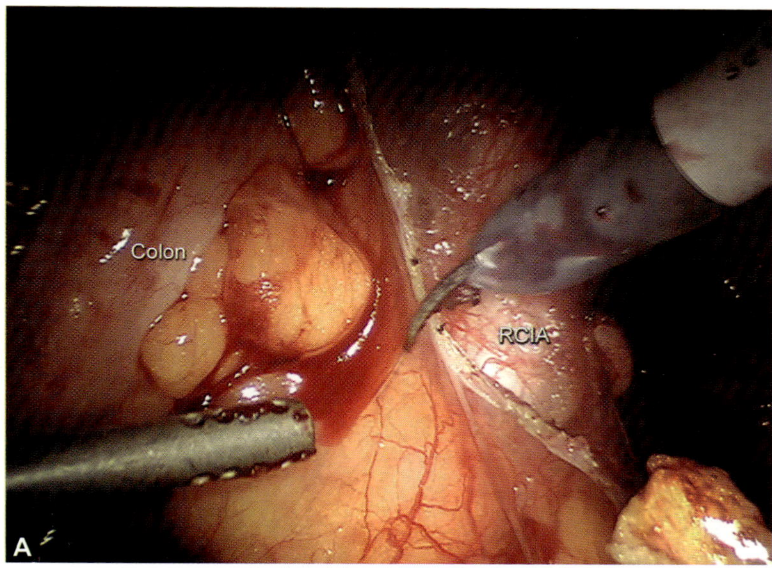

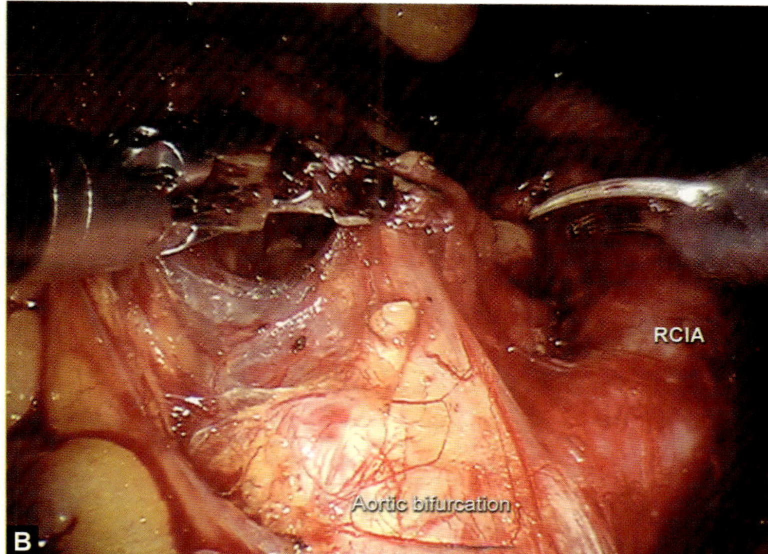

Figs 1A and B: (A) Split and roll over the right common iliac artery; (B) Identification of the aortic bifurcation and resection of lymph bearing tissue (RCIA: Right common iliac artery)

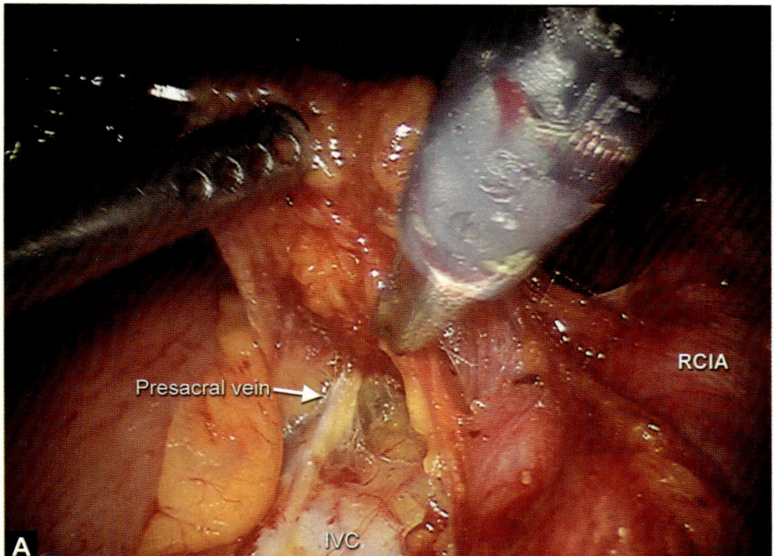

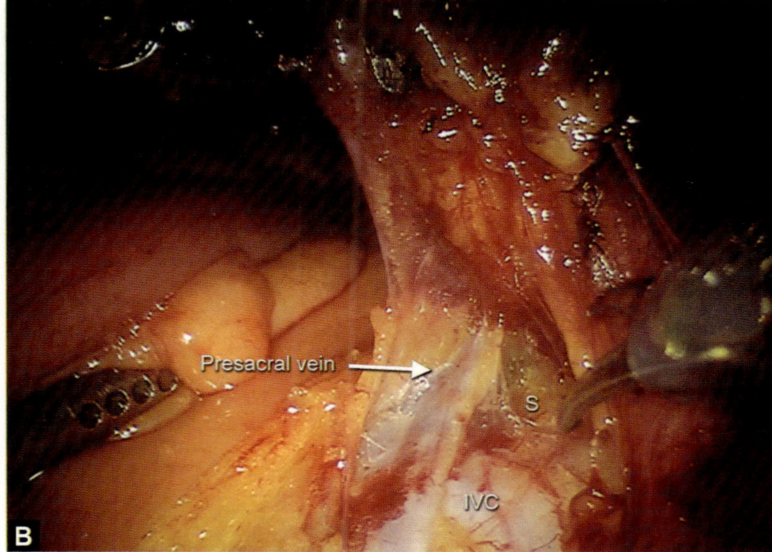

Figs 2A and B: Right-sided dissection of nodes anterior to the IVC and presacral nodes. Note a presacral vein that has to be preserved (IVC: Inferior vena cava; RCIA: Right common iliac artery, S: Sacrum)

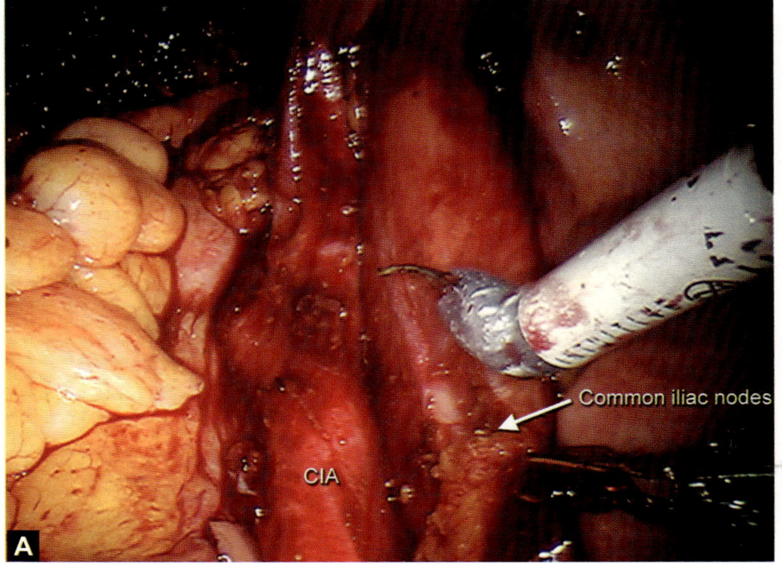

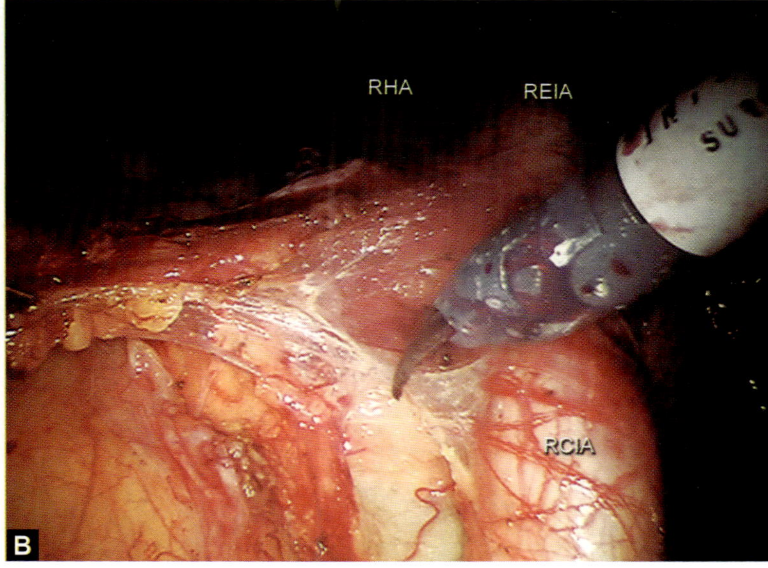

Figs 3A and B: Common iliac nodal dissection. Nodes lateral and medial to the common iliac artery are dissected. (CIA: Common iliac artery; RHA: Right hypogastric artery; REIA: Right external iliac artery; RCIA: Right common iliac artery)

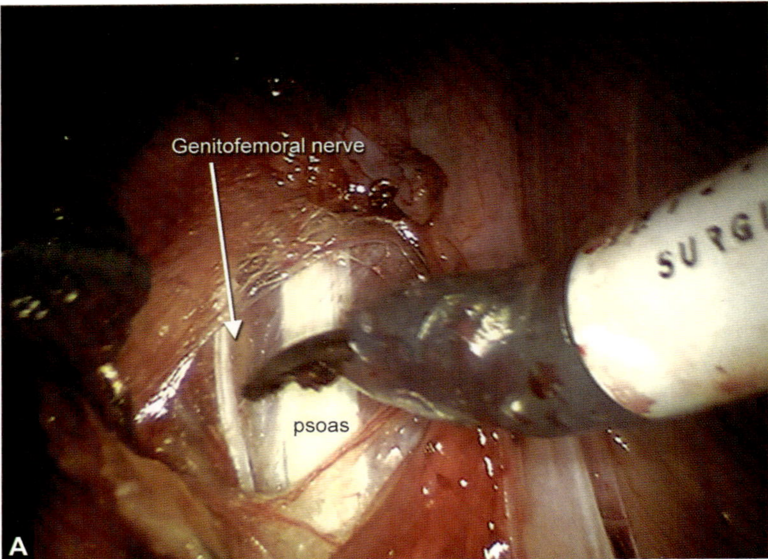

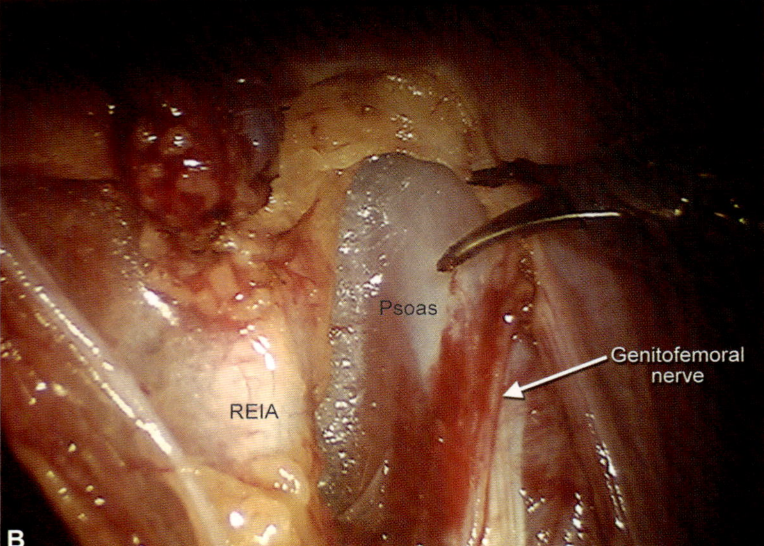

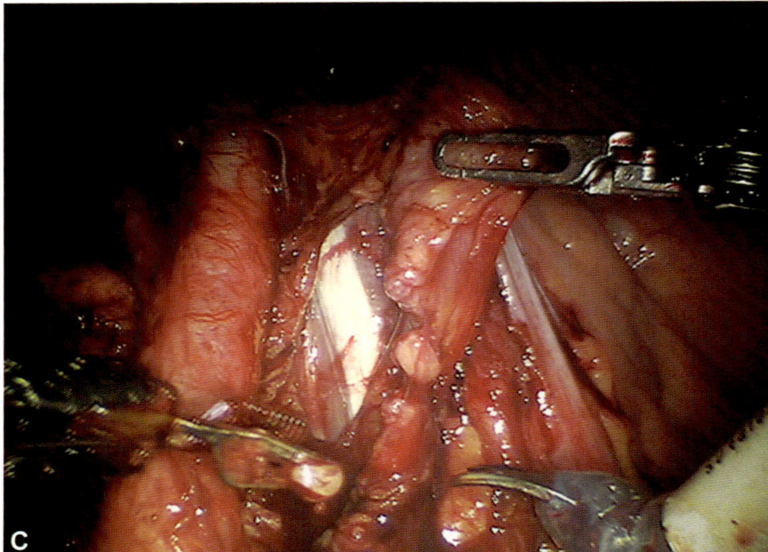

Figs 4A to C: External iliac nodal dissection. The genitofemoral nerve is identified lateral to the artery and medial to the psoas tendon and a split and roll maneuver is utilized (REIA: Right external iliac artery)

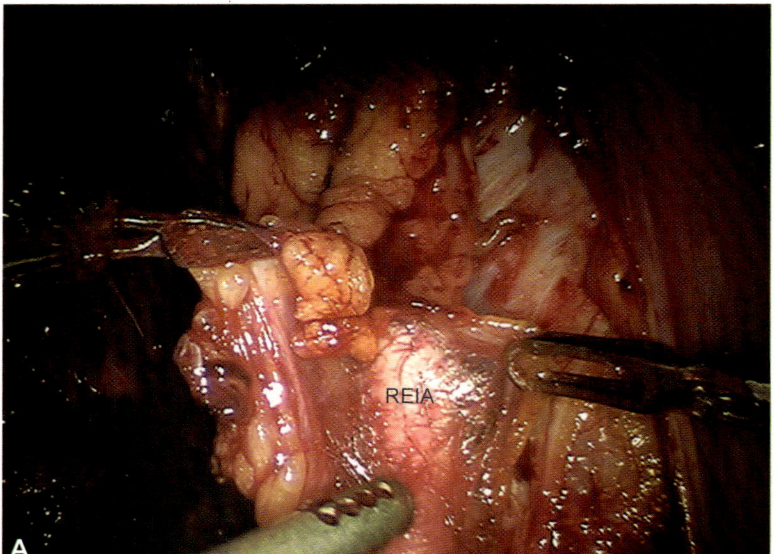

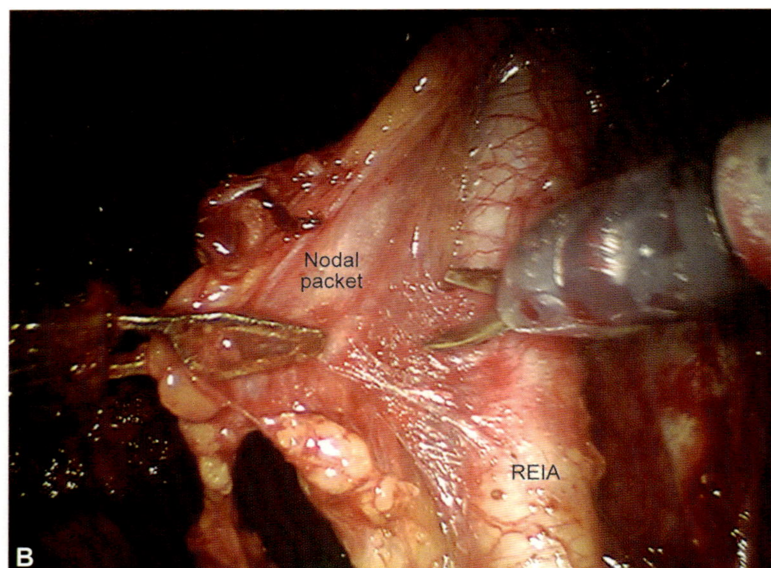

Figs 5A and B: External iliac nodal dissection. Nodes medial to the artery are dissected (REIA: Right external iliac artery)

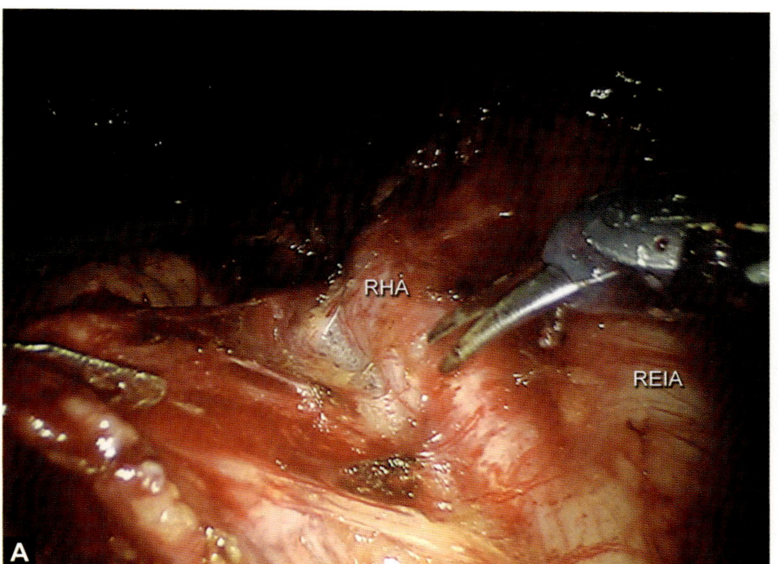

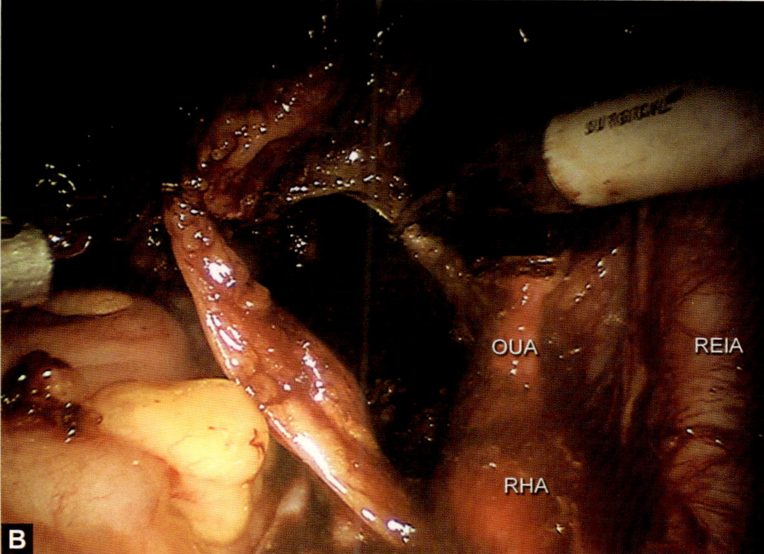

Figs 6A and B: Internal iliac nodal dissection. The surface of the internal iliac artery is cleared and the nodal tissue is removed. Note the origin of the obliterated umbilical artery in B (RHA: Right hypogastric artery; REIA: Right external iliac artery; OUA: Obliterated umbilical artery)

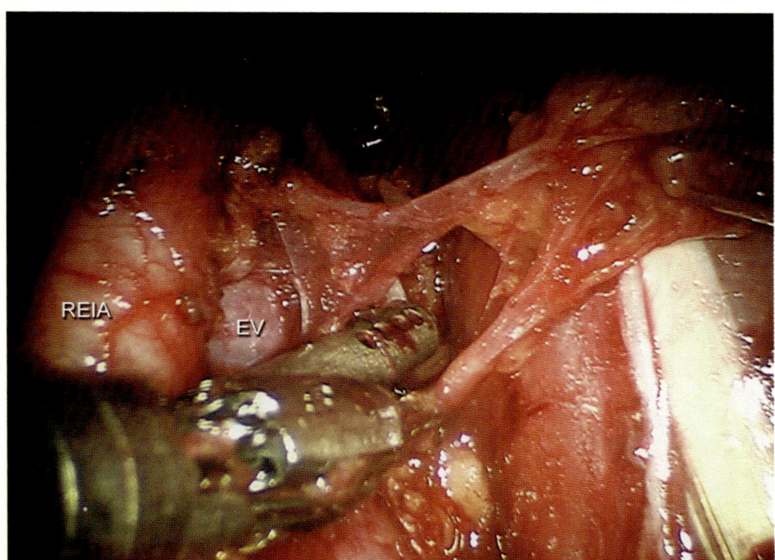

Fig. 7: Removal of the remainder of the nodes lateral to the external iliac artery (EV: External iliac vein; REIA: Right external iliac artery)

Then the dissection is carried out distally and the remainder of the node bearing tissue lateral to the external iliac vessels are removed (Fig. 7). Lymphatic vessels are identified, bipolar cauterized and divided. The dissection is carried distally over the pubic bone to the origin of the circumflex vessels.

At this point, the lateral aspect of the dissection at this level is complete and attention is then placed on performing the obturator nodal dissection. The most distal part of this dissection is the node of Cloquet. Careful attention must be placed on the circumflex vessels. These are easily injured with excessive traction or cautery. Bleeding at this location can be troublesome but easy to control with the excellent visualization afforded by the robot. The obturator nodes are grasped with the precise bipolar grasper, and all lymphatic channels are meticulously bipolar cauterized and divided with the robotic scissors. The assistant provides counter-traction when needed with the suction device. Large lymphatic channels can be ligated with the Hem-o-lok® clips placed by the assistant (Figs 8A to C).

Next, with the caudal aspect of the packet detached, the nodal packet is mobilized up to the origin of the bifurcation of the common iliac nodes (Figs 9A and B).

The completed obturator nodal dissection is presented in Figure 10. The nerve is skeletonized as well as the artery. At times, the obturator vein can be sacrificed to allow for a complete nodal dissection below the obturator nerve. Here, the obturator nodes merge with the paravesical nodes, which will be removed at a later step (Figs 11A and B).

Next, the nodes between the external iliac artery and vein are removed to allow for a full and complete dissection at this level skeletonizing the vessels (Fig. 12). In most patients, this area has scant amounts of lymph nodes.

Next attention is placed on the triangle of Marcille (Figs 13A to C). This is an area bound by the medial border of the psoas major, the lateral margin of the vertebral column and the iliolumbar ligament below. It is crossed by the obturator nerve. Access to this area is gained by careful medial retraction of the external iliac vessels. Extreme care is mandatory as the lack of tactile sensation with the da Vinci® robot can subject these vessels to excessive tension with retraction. In most patients undergoing cystectomy with peripheral vascular disease and calcification in the wall of the artery, the risk of vessel rupture and plaque embolization is present. Also undue stretch to the iliac vein can lead to intimal damage and place the patient at risk for subsequent deep vein thrombosis. Retraction is achieved with the fourth arm of the robot, and the precise bipolar and scissors are used for the dissection. Large lumbar veins are present in this area. Injury to these large vessels as noted in Figure 13B can be very troublesome and difficult to control robotically and open.

After the dissection of the triangle of Marcille, the remainder of lymph bearing tissue remaining below the level of the obturator vessels and nerve as they merge with the paravesical nodes in the lateral rectal sulci and deep pelvic sidewalls are removed (Figs 11A and B). The amount of nodal tissue in this area varies from patient to patient and depends on the lateral extent of the resection during the cystectomy portion of the operation.

Often, inspection of the contralateral presacral region (left side, if the dissection is started on the right and vice versa) reveals additional

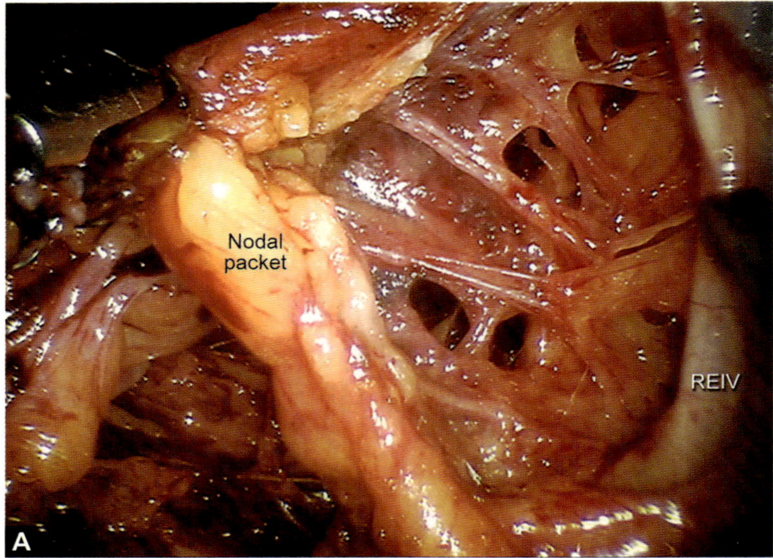

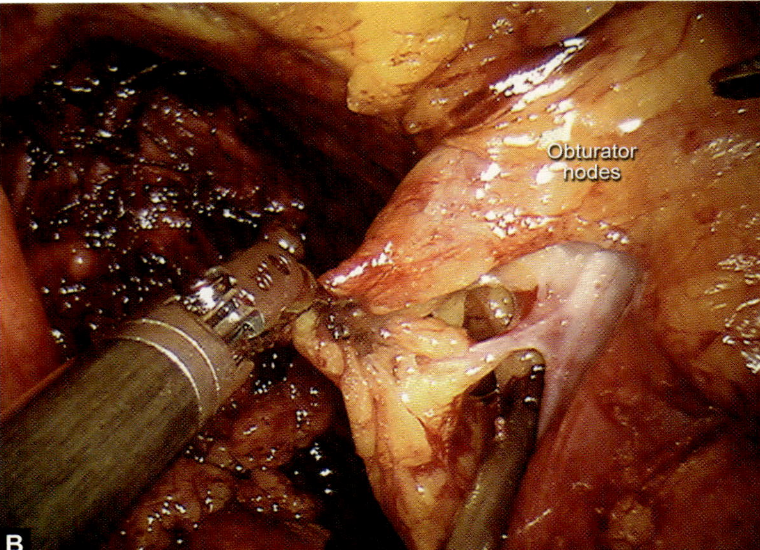

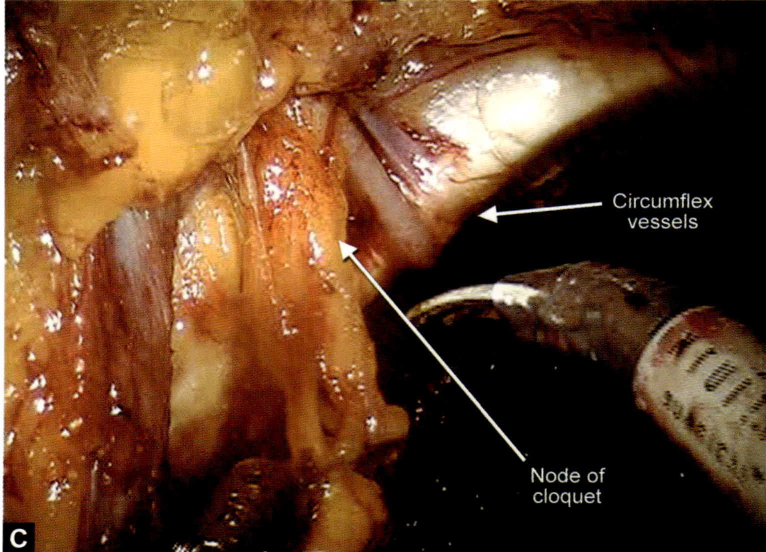

Figs 8A to C: Obturator nodal dissection. (A) The nodes are mobilized and the dissection carried out over the pubic brim. Excellent visualization of lymphatic vessels to be cauterized and/or ligated is provided; (B) Note the accessory obturator vein; (C) The node of Cloquet is dissected and delivered. It marks the most distal aspect of the nodal dissection. The distal extent is marked by the circumflex artery and vein (REIV: Right external iliac vein)

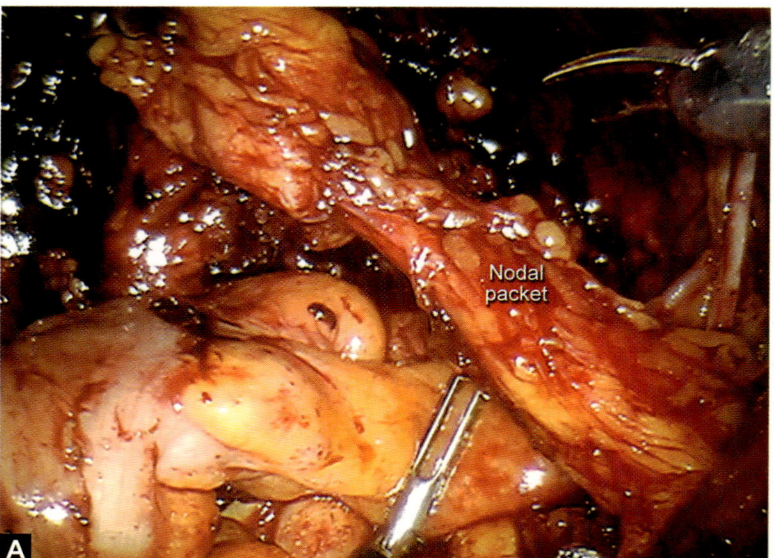

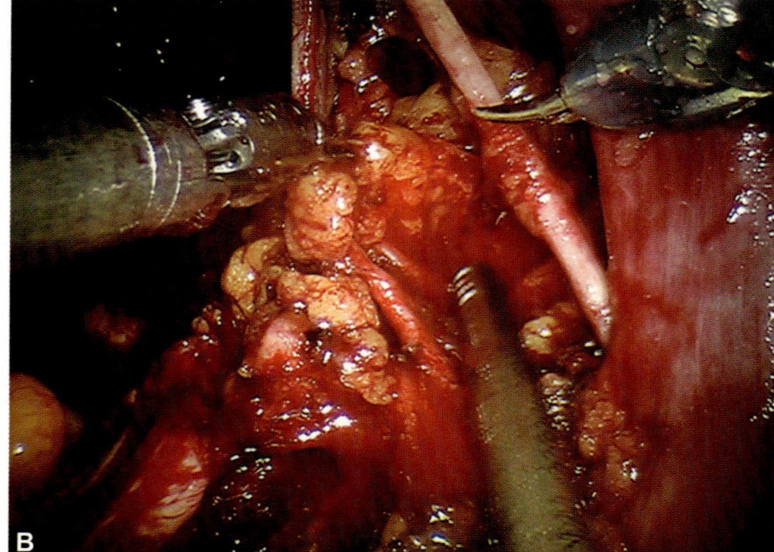

Figs 9A and B: (A) Completion of the obturator nodal dissection; (B) The origin of the obturator artery is visualized as well as the full length of the obturator nerve, the remainder of nodal tissue in between these structures are removed

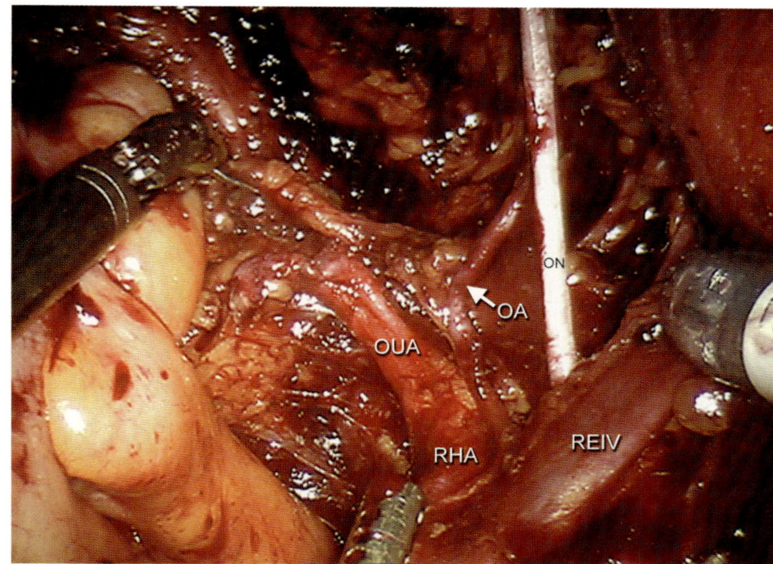

Fig. 10: Completed obturator node dissection (OUA: Obliterated umbilical artery; ON: Obturator nerve; REIV: Right external iliac vein; OA: Obturator artery, RHA: Right hypogastric artery)

nodal tissues that were hidden underneath the sigmoid mesentery which has to be rotated from side to side to allow full dissection in this area (Fig. 14).

An optional maneuver at this point is to apply Tiseel® fibrin glue to cover the external iliac vessels and the raw surface of the nodal dissection with a single layer of covering Surgicel® (Figs 15A and B) over the vessels and the deep obturator fossa. This author utilizes this maneuver in cases where large nodal packets and large lymphatic channels are encountered during the course of a major portion of the operation. This can potentially decrease the chance for lymphocele formation by sealing any potential small open lymphatic channel. The maneuver is also helpful in cases where small continuous oozing is encountered.

At this point, all areas defined by the template of extended pelvic node dissection for bladder cancer is removed and addressed. The completed dissection is depicted for two separate cases in Figures 16A and B. The bifurcations of the great vessels are clearly demonstrated, and all lymph bearing tissues are removed skeletonizing the vessels and clearing the sacrum. Note that in Figure 15A, only the tip of the

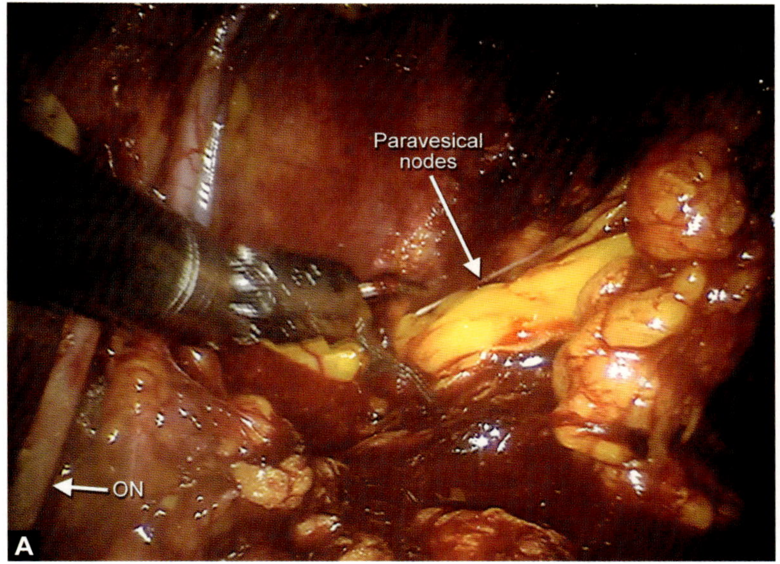

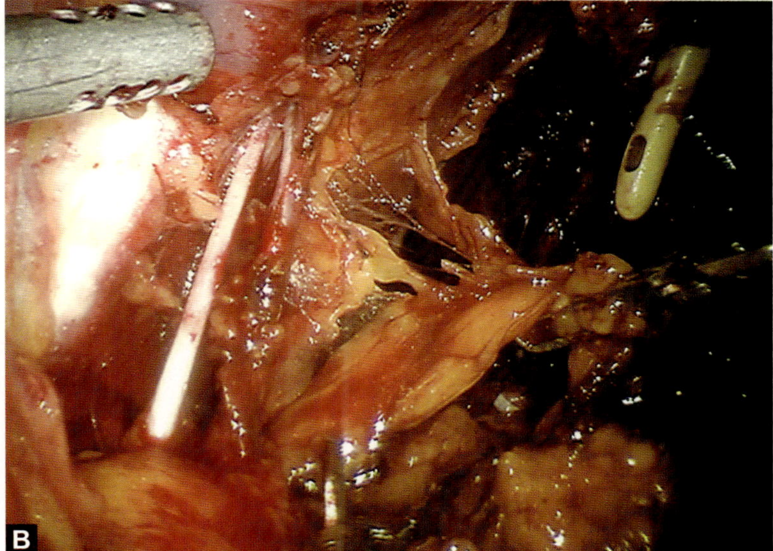

Figs 11A and B: (A) Removal of the paravesical nodes; (B) Nodes below the obturator vessels and nerve (ON: Obturator nerve)

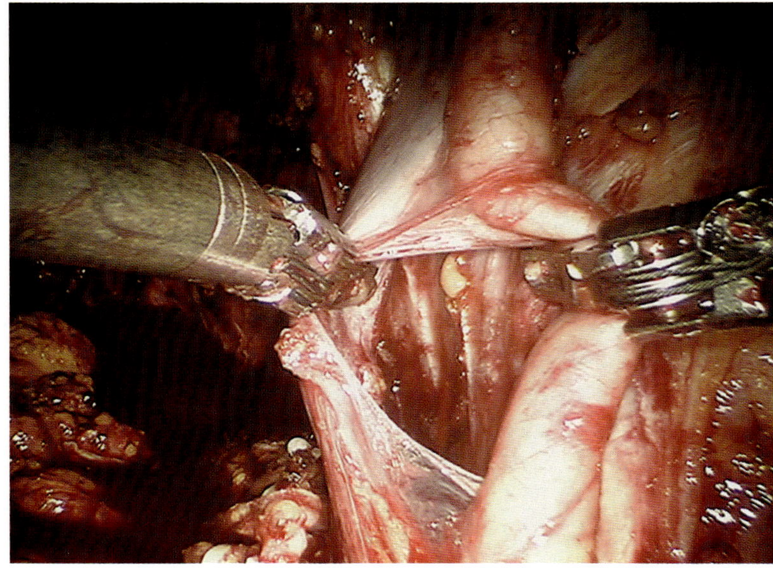

Fig. 12: Removal of nodes between the external iliac artery and vein

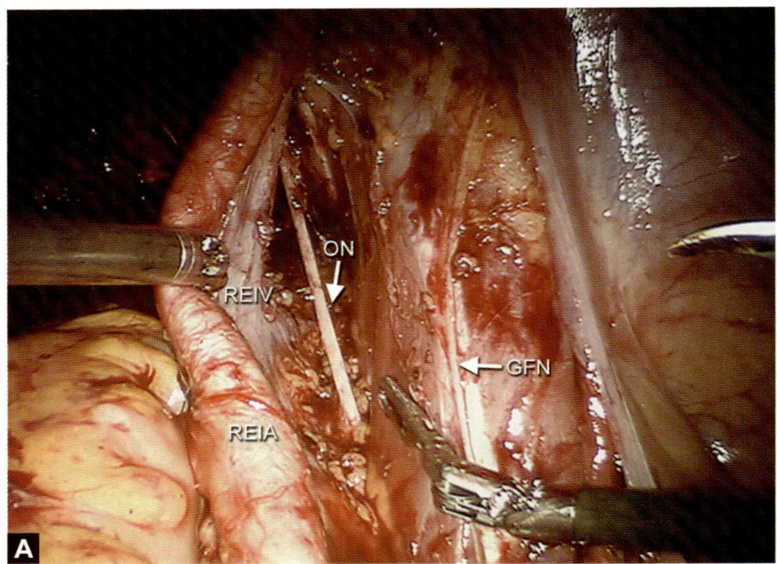

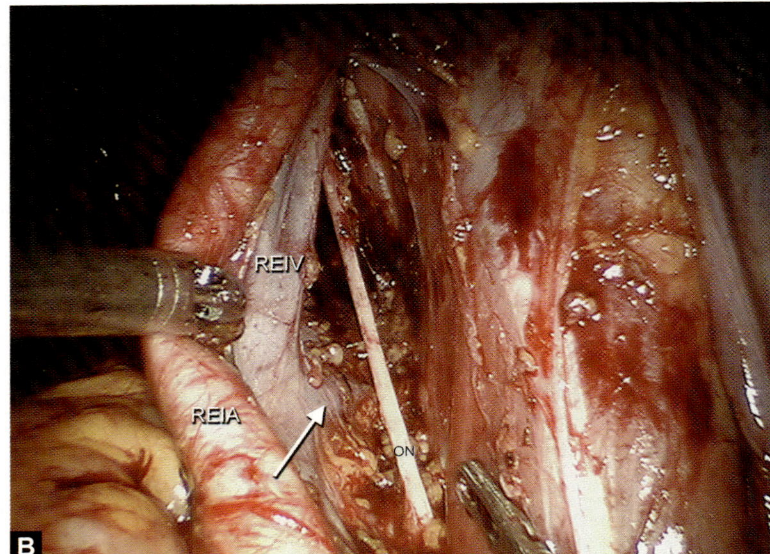

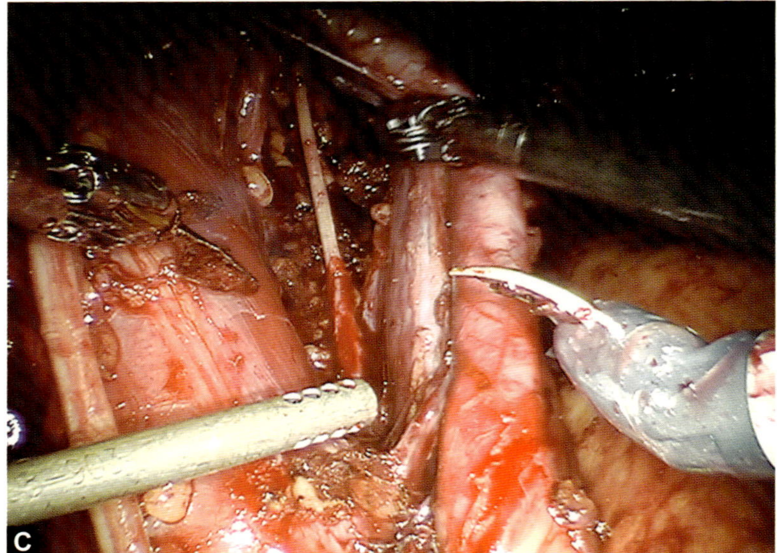

Figs 13A to C: (A and B) Dissection of the right triangle of Marcille. Note the obturator vein completely skeletonized along its course. All lymph nodes at the origin of the obturator nodes are removed in this area as it emerges from the belly of the psoas; (B) The large lumbar vein marked by an arrow; (C) Left-sided completed dissection (REIA: Right external iliac artery; REIV: Right external iliac vein; GFN: Genitofemoral nerve; ON: Obturator nerve)

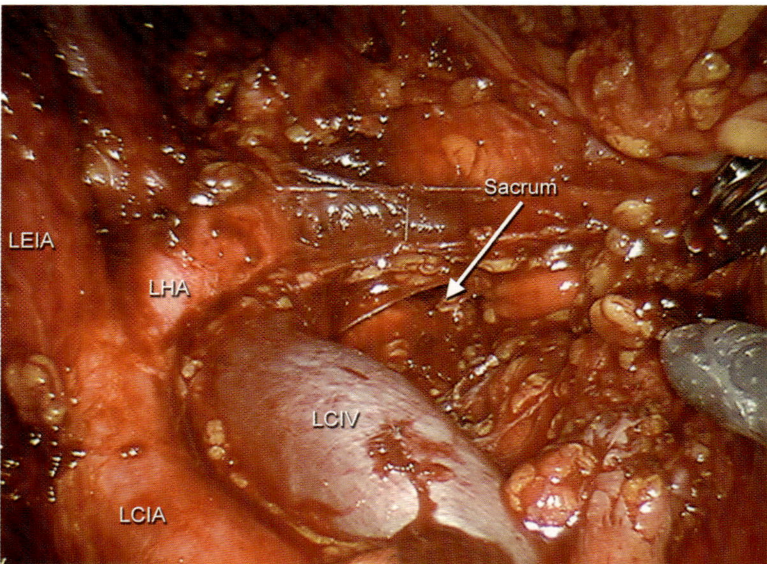

Fig. 14: Completion of left-sided presacral dissection (LCIV: Left common iliac vein; LHA: Left hypogastric artery; LEIA: Left external iliac artery; LCIA: Left common iliac artery)

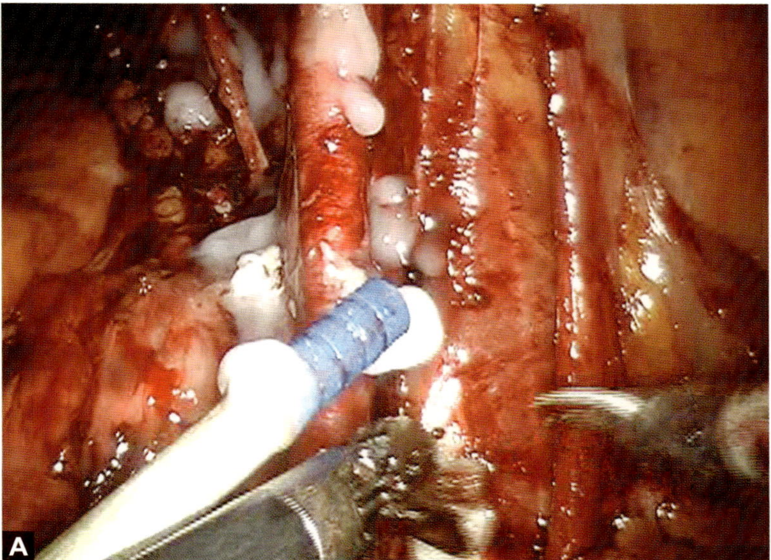
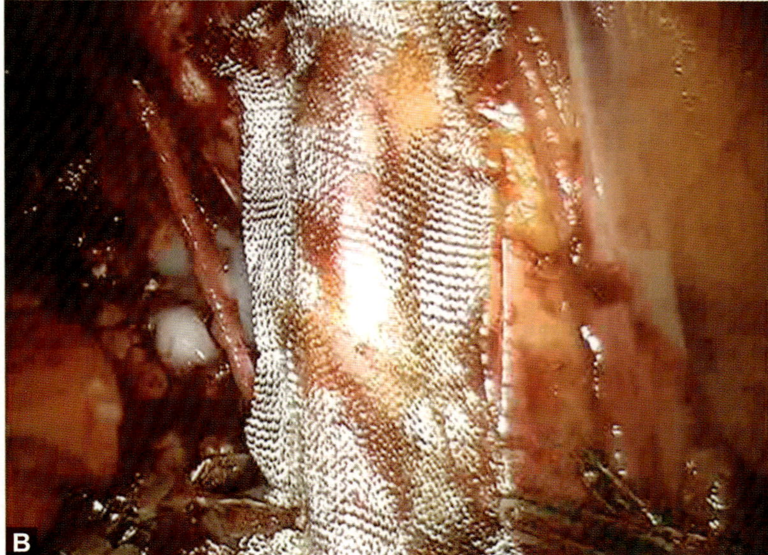

Figs 15A and B: Fibrin glue is applied and a layer of Surgicel® is applied over the vessels and in the deep obturator fossa

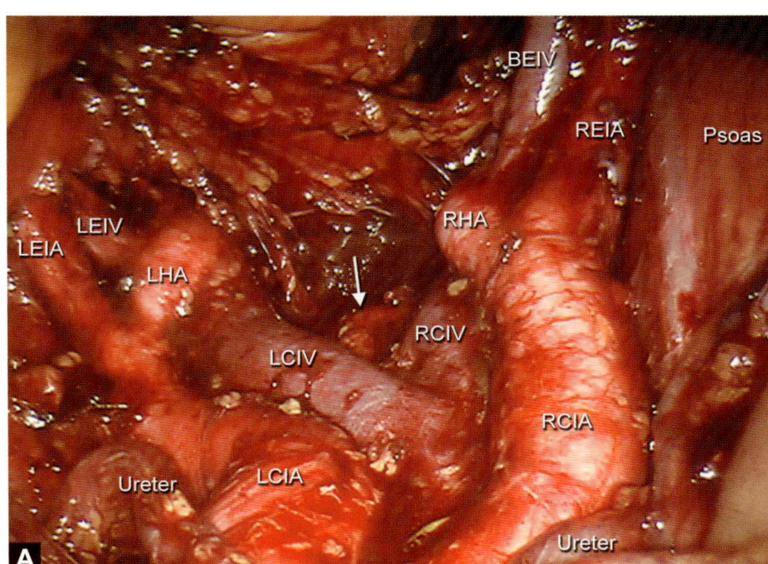

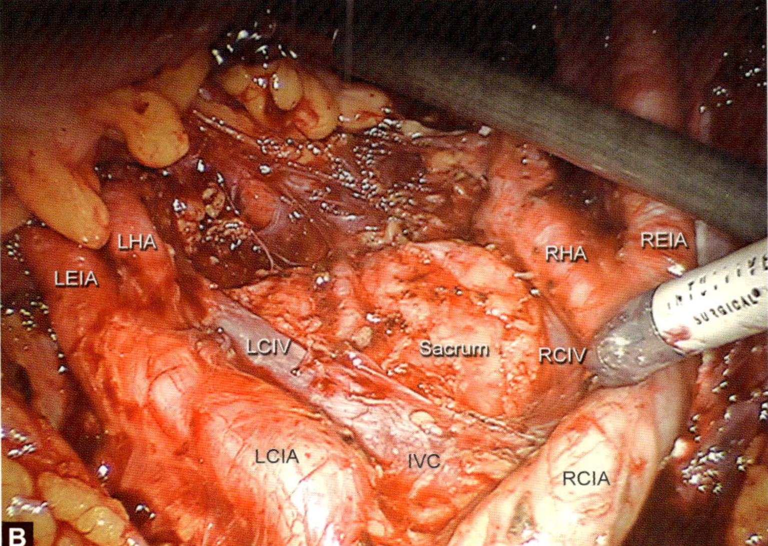

Figs 16A and B: Completed extended pelvic lymph node dissection (LEIA: Left external iliac artey; LEIV: Left external iliac vein; LHA: Left hypogastric artery; LCIV: Left common iliac vein; LCIA: Left common iliac artery; RCIV: Right common iliac vein; RHA: Right hypogastric artery; REIV: Right external iliac vein; REIA: Right external iliac artery; RCIA: Right common iliac artery; Arrow: Sacrum; IVC: Inferior vena cava)

sacrum is visualized below the bifurcation of the vena cava whereas in Figure 15B, the bifurcation of the great vessels are more superior and splayed allowing for visualization of a greater surface are of the bony protuberance.

CONCLUSION

Pelvic lymph node dissection for urothelial carcinoma of the bladder is feasible utilizing the robotic approach. Every step of the operation can be performed with robotic assistance and the open procedure can be emulated step by step. In fact, an argument can be made that due to the superior visualization afforded, the delicate small lymphatic vessels are easily identified, ligated or fulgurated with bipolar cautery. Close up visualization allows for careful dissection and identification of all potential lymph bearing tissue. Hard to access area in the deep pararectal sulci and pelvic sidewall, the triangle of Marcille and the nodes below the level of the obturator nerve are easily accessed with the robot.

REFERENCES

1. Sharir S, Fleshner NE. Lymph node assessment and lymphadenectomy in bladder cancer. J Surg Oncol. 2009;99(4):225-31.
2. Leissner J, Ghoneim MA, Abol-Enein H, et al. Extended radical lymphadenectomy in patients with urothelial bladder cancer: results of a prospective multicenter study. J Urol. 2004;171(1):139-44
3. Renard J, Billia M, Porpiglia F, et al. Open versus laparoscopy-assisted radical cystectomy: results of a prospective study. J Endourol. 2007;21:325-9.
4. Cha EK, Wiklund NP, Scherr DS. Recent advances in robot-assisted radical cystectomy. Curr Opin Urol. 2011;21(1):65-70.
5. Davis JW, Gaston K, Anderson R, et al. Robot assisted extended pelvic lymphadenectomy at radical cystectomy: lymph node yield compared with second look open dissection. J Urol. 2011;185(1):79-83.

18

Chapter

Robotic and Laparoscopic Partial Cystectomy

Rishi Nayyar, Ashok K Hemal

INTRODUCTION

Partial cystectomy for malignant lesions has always intrigued surgeons as an operation balancing principles of oncologic outcomes of treating bladder cancer with the prospects of functional loss and urinary diversion resulting from removal of entire urinary bladder. The operation per se may not be very demanding but it is extremely important to provide good oncological outcomes, especially in malignant tumors of urinary bladder. For carefully selected cases, it can provide similar oncological outcomes to radical cystectomy.[1] Partial cystectomy has never become very popular or widely acceptable due to high chances of locoregional recurrence given the multifocality (field change) of transitional cell carcinoma which is the most common tumor of urinary bladder.[2,3] The absence of any large randomized controlled trials to prove or disprove this makes the selection of cases of transitional cell carcinoma for partial cystectomy a more contentious issue. Other malignant tumors of bladder are uncommon and generally more aggressive, where a more radical approach is usually preferred at most centers. Urachal adenocarcinoma is another entity where partial cystectomy is often employed (Figs 1A and B) given its usual location at the dome, making it amenable to partial bladder resection.[4] A recent report has suggested that the use of partial cystectomy is more at nonacademic institutions, and very limited number of cases have a concomitant pelvic lymphadenectomy performed (23%).[2] A simultaneous ureteric reimplantation was used in 13% cases. In contrast to malignant tumors, partial cystectomy definitely provides a good option for benign tumors or conditions, amenable to complete resection by partial cystectomy, thereby simultaneously preserving as much bladder function as possible.[3,5]

Issues of concern with partial cystectomy are:

- *Good resection margins:* Classical anatomical extent of resection for en bloc partial cystectomy in cases of urachal adenocarcinoma includes the tumor with macroscopically (1.5 cm) and frozen section defined normal margins of the bladder and perivesical fat. The covering peritoneum extending lateral to the bilateral medial umbilical ligaments and preperitoneal fat over the posterior rectus sheath extending to the arcuate line are resected. The muscle fibers of the rectus muscle below the arcuate line, the urachus and the umbilicus have to be resected (Fig. 2).[6] Positive surgical margin is a poor prognostic marker for subsequent survival.[4]
- *What is the adequate bladder size that should be left behind?*: A very large bladder tumor may not leave adequate capacity (> 150 cc) after resection for the bladder to function without causing troublesome frequency. Augmentation should not be considered in the same sitting especially for malignant cases,

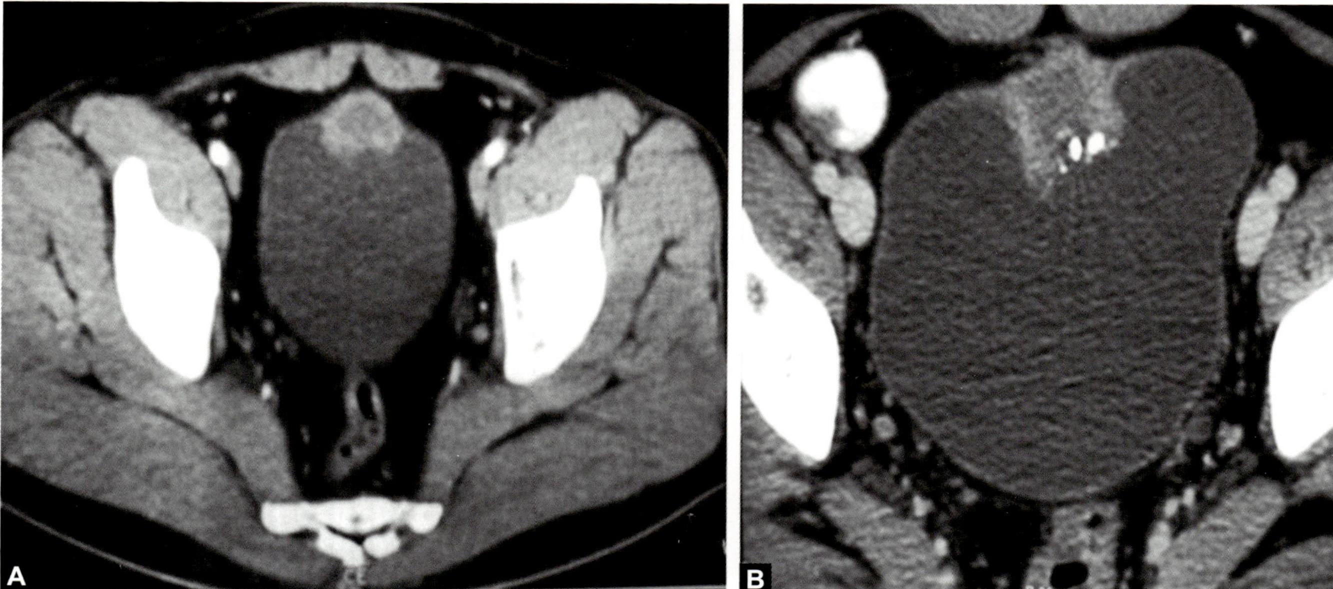

Figs 1A and B: CECT images showing urachal tumor at the dome of urinary bladder. Urachal pathologies are amenable to partial cystectomy, given their suitable location away from bladder neck and bilateral ureteric orifices

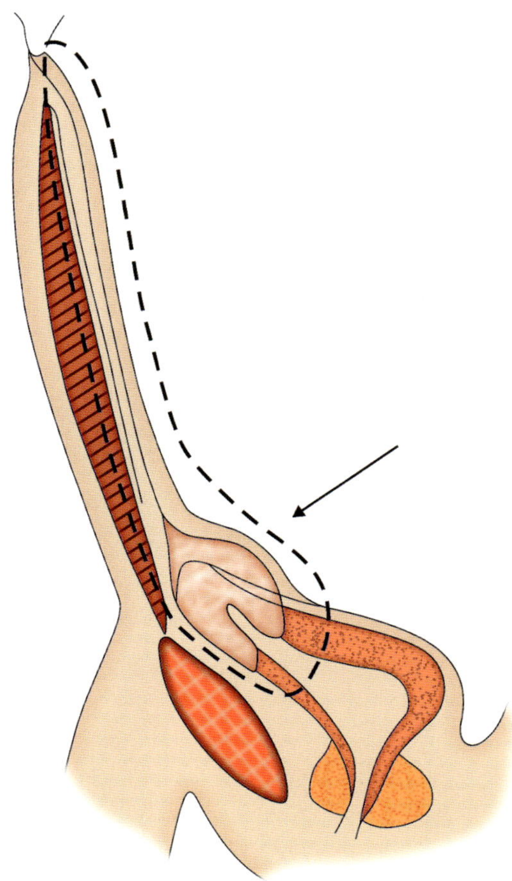

Fig. 2: Diagrammatic representation (sagittal section) depicting urachal tumor (black arrow) and limits of resection (interrupted line). Note, inclusion of posterior rectus sheath to arcuate line; below it, rectus muscle fibers (oblique line-shaded area) included in proposed resected specimen

particularly where there are reasonably strong doubts about locoregional recurrence of disease because subsequent need for redo surgery or radiation may jeopardize the augmented segment.

- *Proximity of tumor to bladder neck and prostate?*: Tumor involving bladder neck or prostate should not be considered a candidate for partial cystectomy. A safe margin of greater than 1 cm is advisable.
- *Should ureteric reimplantation be considered to achieve partial cystectomy?*: Ureteric reimplantation has been used in conjunction with partial cystectomy in cases where the patient is otherwise a good candidate except the tumor either encroaching or involving one ureteric orifice.[2] This is acceptable especially for clinically benign tumors.[7]
- *Extent of lymphadenectomy*: A bilateral pelvic lymph node dissection should be performed as a standard part of the procedure in all cases undergoing surgery for malignancy. The authors' standard template is bounded by bladder, genitofemoral nerve, femoral canal, lateral pelvic wall, obturator nerve and internal iliac vessels extending to the common iliac division.[6]

Partial cystectomy has been demonstrated both pure laparoscopically and using the robotic interface.[3,6,8-11] The use of surgical robot provides better ergonomics and perhaps more precise and controlled suturing during closure of the bladder or associated reimplantation of ureter.[7] The proposed advantages over conventional open technique are reduced blood loss and early recovery. There have been few reports of single port surgery through the umbilicus both pure laparoscopically and robotically, but the definitive advantage using this technique remains to be proven and extreme caution is required to be observed so as to prevent spillage.[12,13]

INDICATIONS

The indications for partial cystectomy as such are relatively few. Usually it is reserved for small unifocal tumors located near the dome or anterior wall with ureteric orifices or bladder neck sufficiently away from the resection margin and no concomitant carcinoma *in situ* elsewhere in the bladder. Solitary noninvasive bladder tumors in a diverticulum may also be amenable to partial cystectomy. Role of proper preoperative imaging and cystoscopy examination cannot be overemphasized in this regard. A variety of benign pathologies may be amenable to cure with partial cystectomy like benign tumors of bladder, urachal benign diseases, endometriosis, pelvic hydatid disease, etc.[14-16]

A preoperative cystoscopy is mandatory in most cases to ensure site, size, configuration and multiplicity of tumors. Cystoscopy also provides an opportunity to biopsy the tumor by transurethral resection. Multiple biopsies should also be taken from all macroscopically uninvolved walls of the bladder to rule out the presence of carcinoma *in situ*, in cases with urothelial carcinoma. It is also of utmost importance to properly assess proximity of the tumor from the bilateral ureteric orifices and the bladder neck. A ureteric catheter or stent may be placed at this time for definitive identification of the ureteric orifice if it lies close to resection margin.

STEPS OF SURGERY

The basic steps of the surgery are same as published earlier for laparoscopic partial cystectomy but strictly following oncologic principles.[6] The concepts of the surgery mimic those followed during open partial cystectomy. The following steps describe standard technique of laparoscopic or robot-assisted partial cystectomy.

Patient Preparation and Positioning

A steep Trendelenburg equivalent to that required for laparoscopic or robotic cystectomy or prostatectomy is not required for doing partial cystectomy, since access to confines of true pelvis are not needed. A 15–30 degree Trendelenburg is usually sufficient to keep the bowel away from surgical field. Bowel preparation is usually unnecessary. A urethral catheter is inserted and kept inside the surgical field for inflation of bladder during surgery. A lithotomy position is used for robot being brought in between the legs or supine position for being docked from the side. It also allows for a simultaneous cystoscopy to guide the proper surgical tumor margin, if needed.

Port Placement

Port placement is dependent upon the exact site of tumor and needs of surgery. Usually 4 or 5 ports are sufficient, including the camera port (Fig. 3). All ports are generally inserted slightly higher than the standard configuration used for laparoscopic or robotic radical prostatectomy. The camera port is placed 2–3 cm above the umbilicus, particularly for cases where the urachus is to be excised en bloc with the tumor. A transperitoneal approach is commonly followed. It is a good habit to quickly inspect the entire abdomen immediately after placing the camera port for adhesions, any injuries related to port placement, locoregional tumor spread and possible sites of intra-abdominal metastasis.

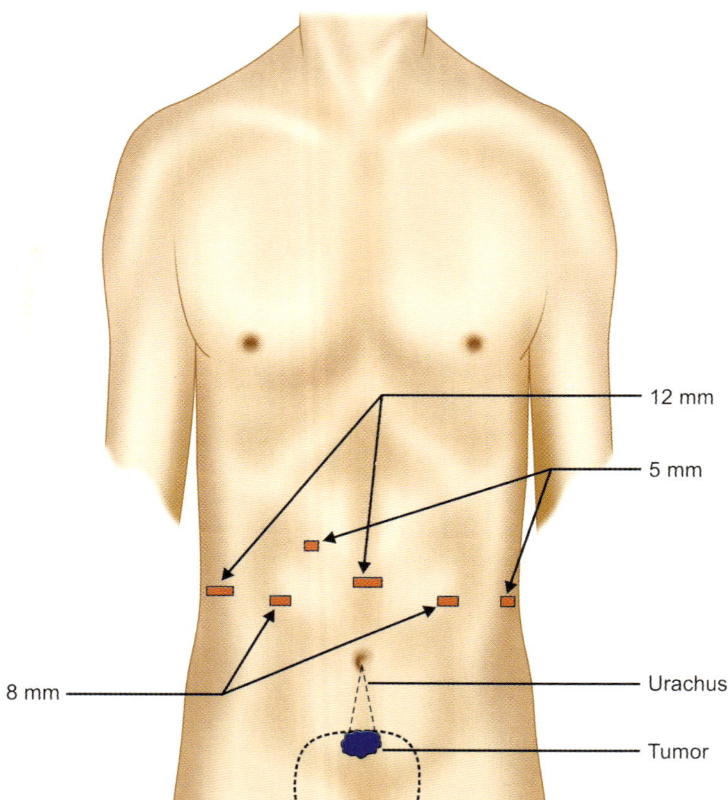

Fig. 3: Port site configuration for robotic partial cystectomy. A supraumbilical 12 mm midline port serves as the camera port. Two 8 mm robotic ports are placed one on each side about 8 cm from the camera port at a level about 2–3 cm below. Another 12 mm port placed far lateral in the anterior axillary line serves as the primary assistant port. Other 5 mm ports are optional. The lateral 5 mm port may be replaced by another 8 mm robotic port if using the 3rd working arm of the surgical robot. Port configuration remains essentially similar for laparoscopic partial cystectomy

Mobilizing the Urachus and Space of Retzius

Incision is made into the peritoneum along the lateral aspect of the medial umbilical ligaments bilaterally and deepened to lift off all the preperitoneal fat from the posterior rectus sheath or the muscle layer (Fig. 4). The incision lines from each side are made to join superiorly at the umbilicus so as to excise the entire urachus and its surrounding fat. Constant traction and countertraction provides easier and more precise appreciation of the proper avascular plane of dissection. A "twist and roll" action by the assistant using an atraumatic grasper is helpful in this regard while performing the laparoscopic procedure and the same can be performed with the 4th arm in the robotic procedure.[6] Dissection is continued in this plane deeper into the pelvis to develop the space of Retzius (Figs 5A to C). This space is continued around the lateral aspects of bladder. For larger tumors (> 5 cm), a posterior first approach has been described, where the anterior dissection as described above is done after completing a posterior cystostomy.[6]

Identifying and Marking Resection Margins

After initial dissection, the bladder is kept constantly empty in order to avoid spillage during cystostomy. To identify the correct site of incision into the bladder the following suggestions may be utilized:

- Prior cystoscopic scoring with Colling's knife (Cook Medical, Bloomington, IN).
- A simultaneous cystoscopic guidance may be the best during the initial cystostomy, especially in cases of malignancies where cutting through the tumor is unacceptable and achieving a proper and negative resection margin is oncologically important to ensure a good oncologic outcome. A simple transillumination through the bladder may guide the surgeon to the proper site of incision over the bladder.[17] Combination of both extravesical (robotically or laparoscopically) and intravesical (cystoscopically) approach has been used with the proposed advantage of better delineation of tumor margins (Figs 6A and B).[18-20] Authors always prefer multiple frozen sections from the remnant margin of the bladder in order to ascertain negative surgical margins for tumor.

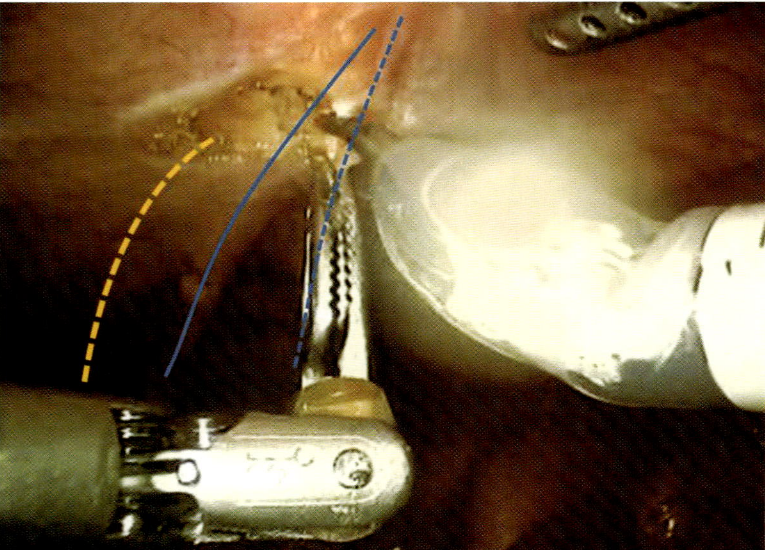

Fig. 4: Initial step for partial cystectomy after placing the ports.The yellow-dashed line depicts the incision line on the peritoneum along lateral aspect of medial umbilical ligament (blue line). The two incision lines are joined in the midline at the umbilicus. The urachus (blue-dashed line) and its surrounding fat is excised en masse with the surgical specimen

Excision of Tumor

The tumor is then completely excised all around taking care to minimize spillage into the general peritoneal cavity (Figs 7A and B). Some reports suggest the use of a stapling device to enable simultaneous suturing with excision.[21] Authors do not recommend such use due to the possibility of stone formation over the staples and blind excision with this technique. During this step, authors make sure that bladder is constantly empty. Once the specimen is free, it is immediately entrapped into a retrieval bag prior to embarking on the next step and kept aside until the completion of the procedure.

Closure of Bladder with or without Ureteric Reimplantation

Bladder closure has been perfomed using different approaches over an 18 Fr urethral catheter in place:

- A full thickness continuous closure with an absorbable suture using 3-0 polyglactin or poliglecaprone suture can be used. Authors have been recently using 2-0 unibarbed suture [V-Loc™, absorbable wound closure device (Covidien, Mansfield, MA, USA)].
- Two layers closure while performing robotic repair. For the first layer, a 5-0 poliglecaprone suture is used to close the mucosa. The second layer can be closed with 3-0 unibarb suture or polyglactin or poliglecaprone suture.

For large tumors, further mobilization of lateral bladder walls may be essential for closure without tension on the suture line

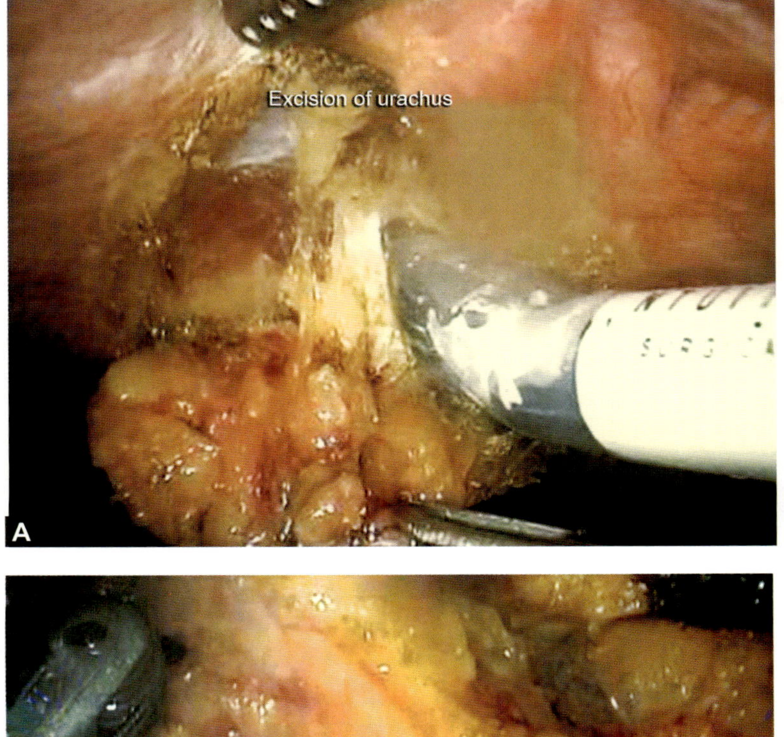

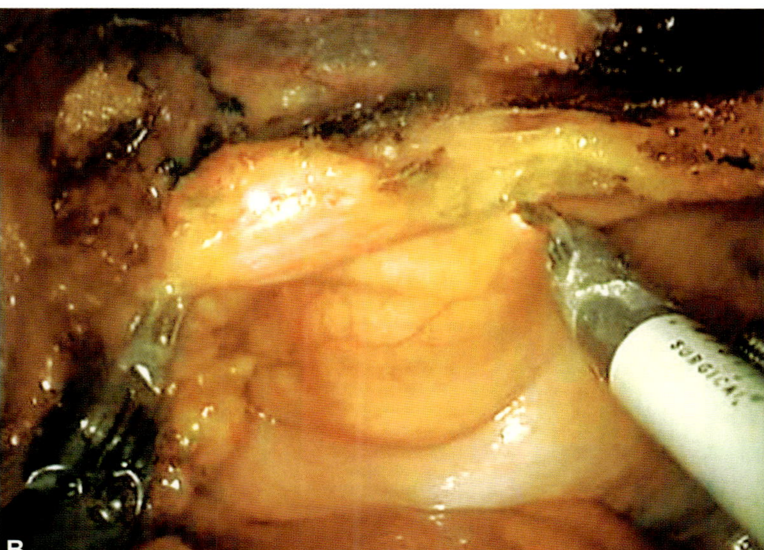

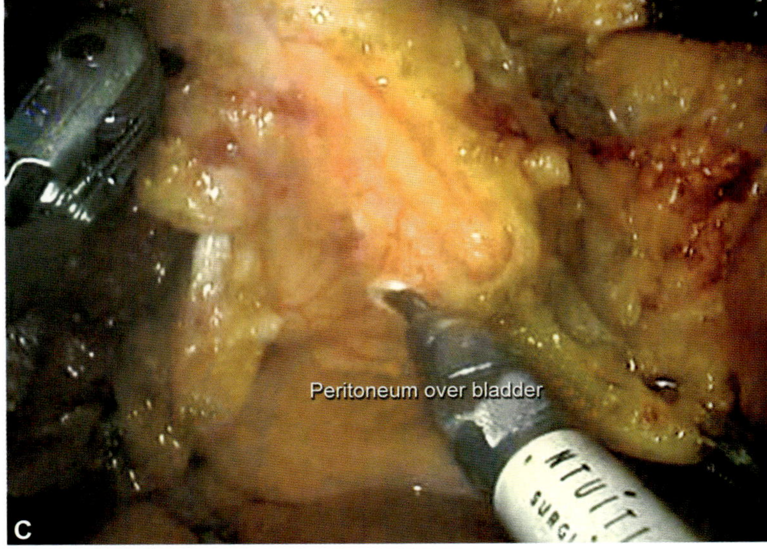

Figs 5A to C: (A) The urachus along with its fat is excised in a plane exposing the underlying muscle fibers; (B) Dissection is carried along the incision line which lies to the lateral aspect of medial umbilical ligament and (C) Posteriorly the incision is carried over to the bladder base on the peritoneum

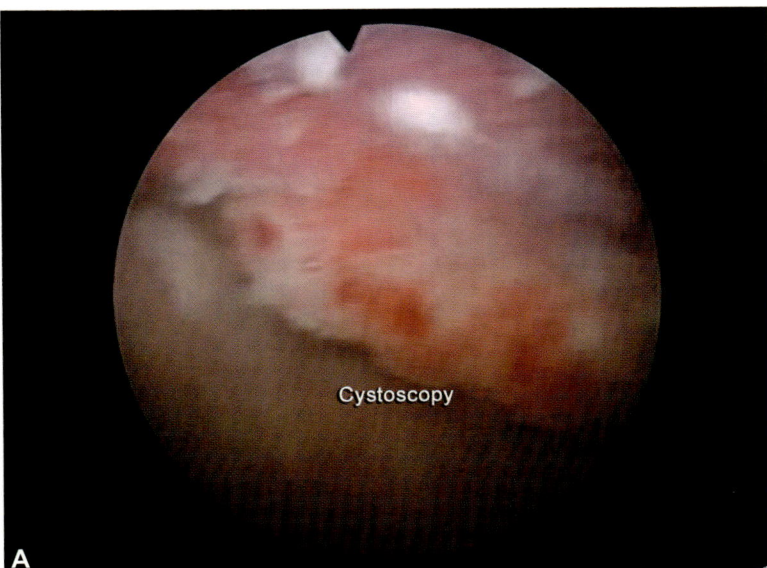

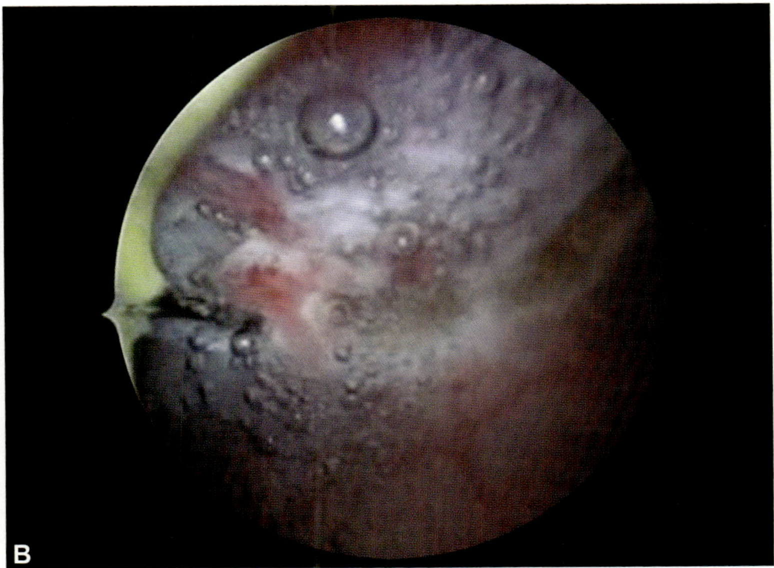

Figs 6A and B: Surgical resection margins are better and more precisely marked in a partially distended bladder. (A) Cystoscopic view of a tumor at bladder dome and (B) A deep incision is made using hot Colling's knife and keeping a margin of greater than 1 cm all around the tumor

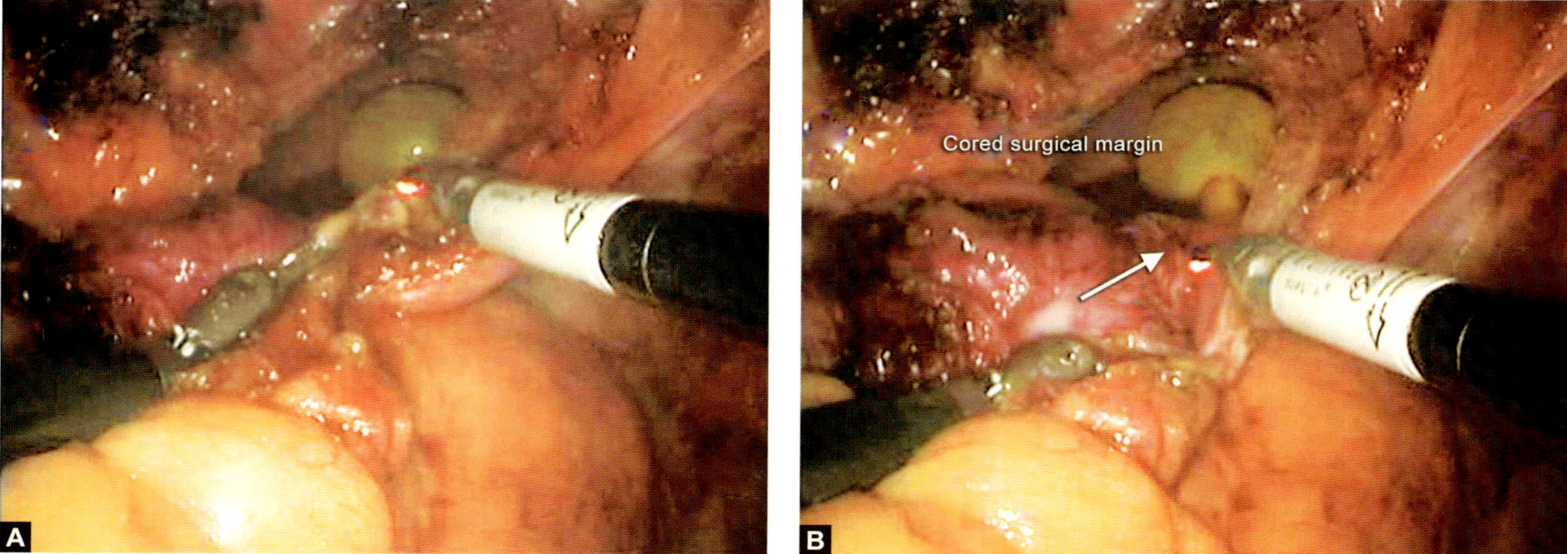

Figs 7A and B: (A) The tumor is excised all around. Hemostasis on the margins is ensured and (B) The initial cystoscopically marked line of incision helps keep proper tumor margin, which may otherwise be difficult to achieve in a collapsed opened up bladder

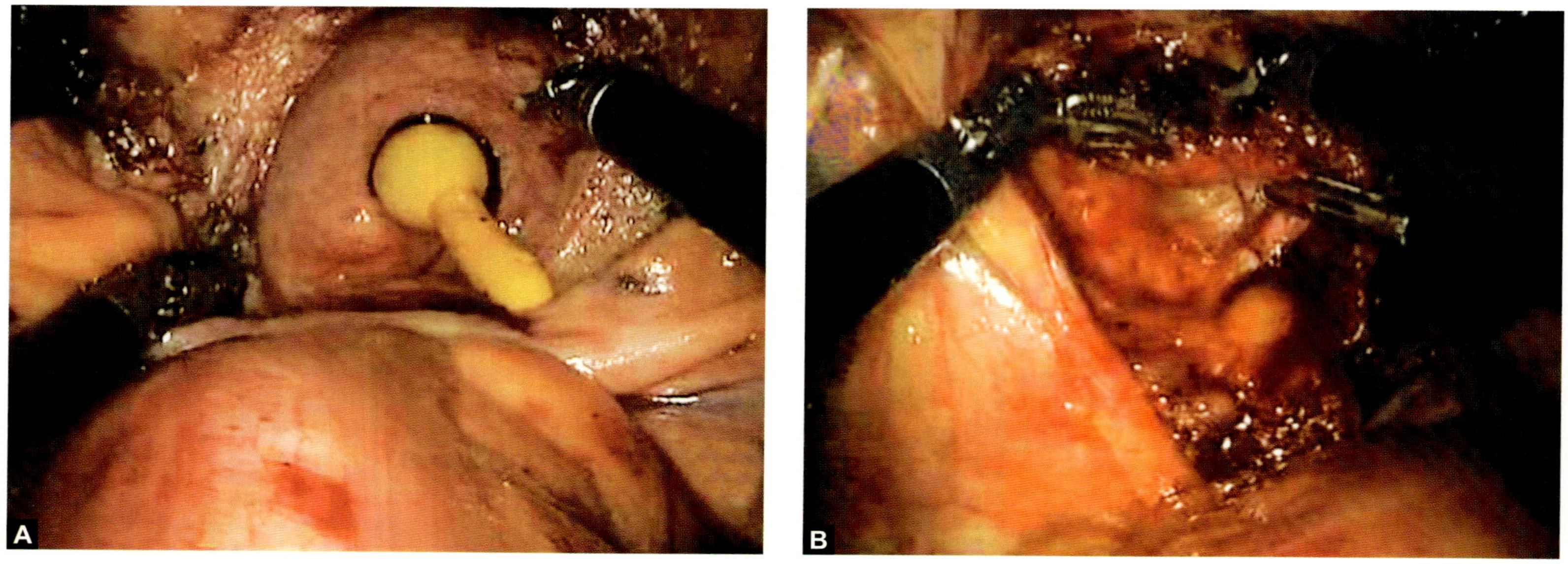

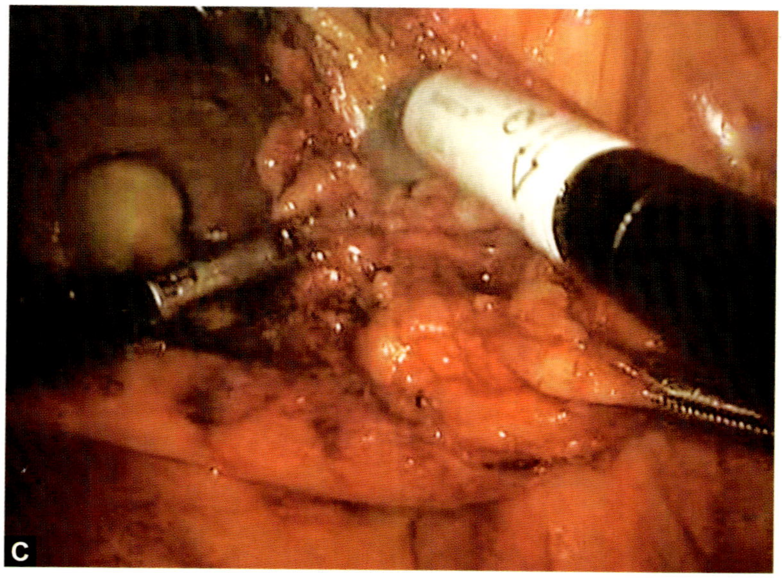

Figs 8A to C: (A) Large bladder opening after complete excision of a big tumor at the dome; (B and C) Mobilization of the lateral bladder walls from the pelvic walls to enable tension-free closure of bladder

(Figs 8A to C). Usually it is easier to sew the posterior margin with the anterior one in a transverse direction, since the posterior margin has relatively more mobility (Figs 9A and B). It is important to be cognizant of the ureteric orifices during the suturing, especially for large tumors where the ureteric openings may come close to the resection margin. Also complete hemostasis should be ensured, as the authors believe in leaving only a urethral catheter. Ureteric reimplantation may be needed in cases where tumor is involving the ureterovesical junction. Reimplantation may be done using extravesical or intravesical technique with or without antireflux mechanisms.[22] A cystogram is done at 10–14 days post surgery to ensure no leakage from the bladder suture line before the catheter is removed (Fig. 10).

Lymphadenectomy

Lymphadenectomy is then performed bilaterally as for standard radical cystectomy in cases of malignancy (Fig. 11).[6,23,24] An extended pelvic lymphadenectomy extends laterally up to the genitofemoral nerve; medially up to the obturator nerve and vessels; inferiorly up to iliacus muscle; proximally up to the level of the aortic bifurcation and ipsilaterally to the level of node of Cloquet distally. Benign diseases may not need a lymphadenectomy.

Drain Placement and Specimen Retrieval

A drain is placed through one of the port sites. The entrapment plastic bag containing the specimen is retrieved (Fig. 12) through one of the port sites or from a periumbilical incision. Port sites are securely closed to complete the procedure.

TOTAL TRANSVESICAL TECHNIQUE (ROBOTIC APPROACH)

A total transvesical technique, without any extravesical dissection has been used by the authors for excision of a symptomatic vesical diverticulum. The ports are placed intravesically after fixing the bladder onto the anterior abdominal wall while in full distention. The diverticulum is excised at its neck and dissected out gradually inverting the diverticulum into the bladder. Maneuvering of laparoscopic instruments may be difficult given the limited availability of space,

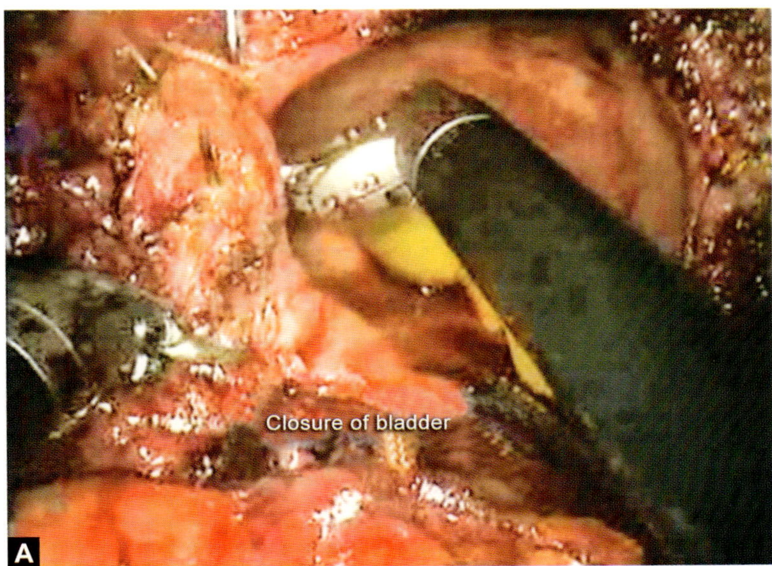

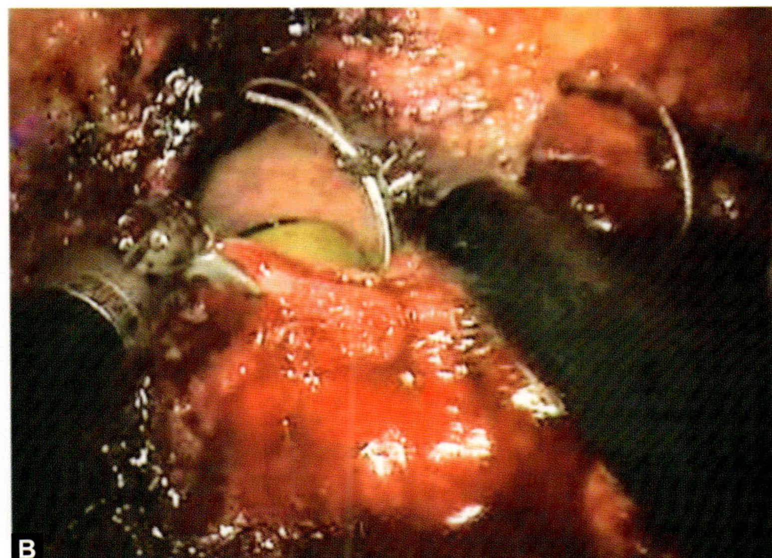

Figs 9A and B: (A and B) Closure of bladder with 2-0 polyglactin continuous interlocking suture in single layer. Adequate hemostasis must be achieved along the resection margins

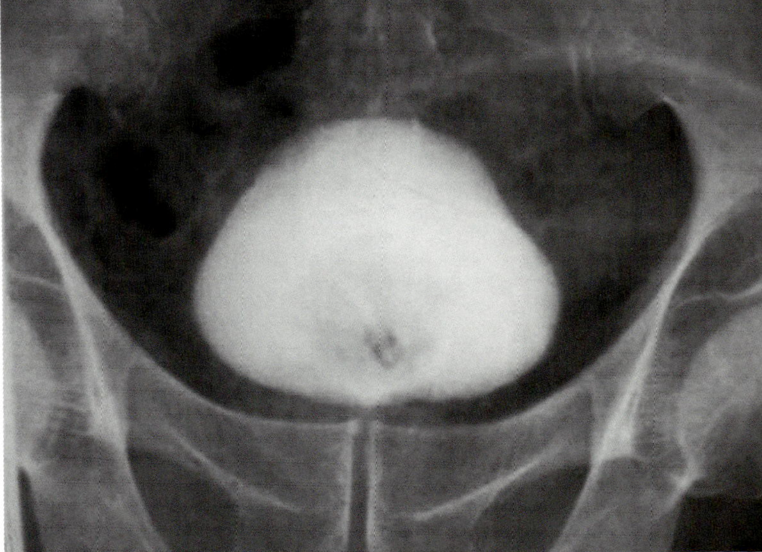

Fig. 10: Postoperative cystogram study after partial laparoscopic cystectomy in a case of urachal tumor

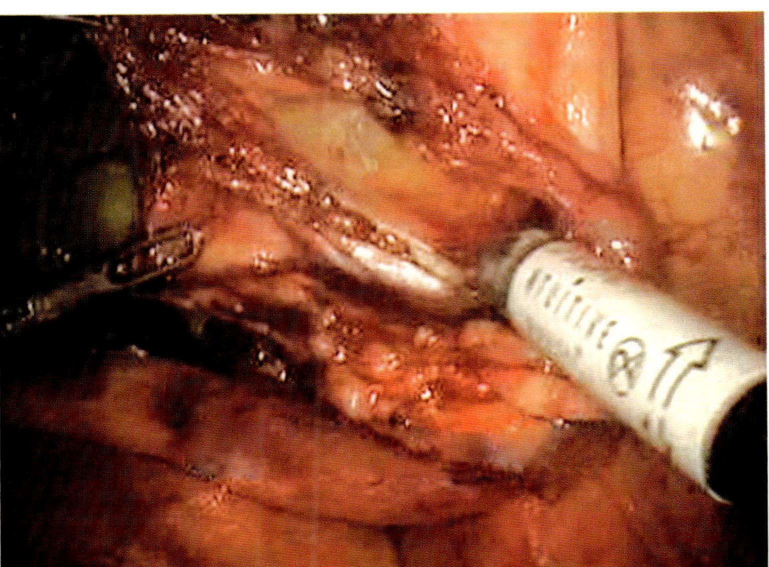

Fig. 11: Standard pelvic lymphadenectomy is done for cases of bladder malignancy as during radical cystectomy, including the obturator, external iliac, Cloquet's and internal iliac nodes bilaterally

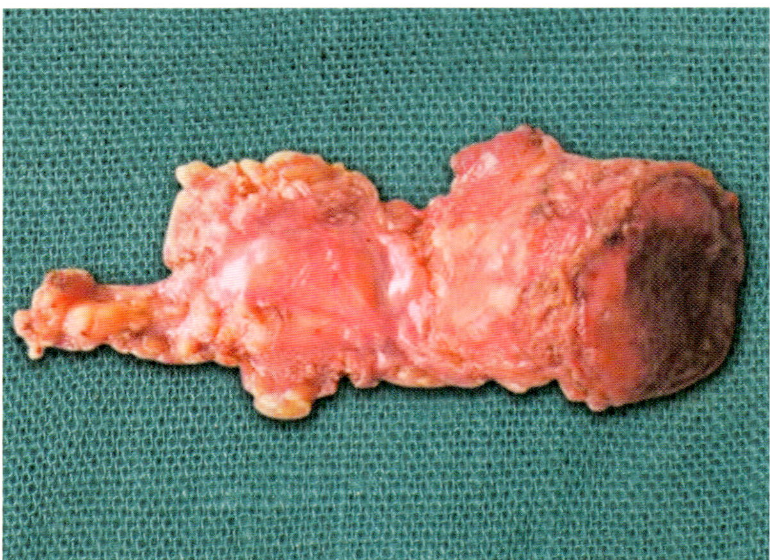

Fig. 12: Specimen of urachal tumor with a major extravesical bulk removed en masse with the entire urachal complex and its surrounding fat

especially for a novice surgeon; hence this approach may not be suitable for the pure laparoscopic approach.

EXISTING LITERATURE ON OUTCOMES

Five-year cancer-specific survival rate of 40–70% may be expected in carefully selected cases of urothelial cancer for partial cystectomy.[2-4] Poor case selection may result in locoregional recurrence and poor survival. Partial cystectomy may be expected in less than 5% cases of bladder cancer as an appropriate management.[25] Clinical stage, grade, margin status and lymph node status are strong predictors of survival.[3,4,26] A regular follow-up is essential for all cases of bladder tumor undergoing partial resection to detect recurrence, if any, at an early stage.

REFERENCES

1. Laufer M. Transurethral resection and partial cystectomy for invasive bladder cancer. Semin Urol Oncol. 2000;18:296-9.
2. Fahmy N, Aprikian A, Tanguay S, et al. Practice patterns and recurrence after partial cystectomy for bladder cancer. World J Urol. 2010;28:419-23.
3. Colombo Jr JR, Desai M, Canes D, et al. Laparoscopic partial cystectomy for urachal and bladder cancer. Clinics. 2008;63(6):731-4.
4. Ashley RA, Inman BA, Sebo TJ, et al. Urachal carcinoma: clinicopathologic features and long-term outcomes of an aggressive malignancy. Cancer. 2006;107(4):712-20.
5. Chammas MF Jr, Kim FJ, Barbarino A, et al. Asymptomatic rectal and bladder endometriosis: a case for robotic-assisted surgery. Can J Urol. 2008;15(3):4097-100.
6. Wadhwa P, Kolla SB, Hemal AK. Laparoscopic en bloc partial cystectomy with bilateral pelvic lymphadenectomy for urachal adenocarcinoma. Urology. 2006;67(4):837-43.
7. Nayyar R, Singh P, Gupta NP. Robotic management of pheochromocytoma of the vesicoureteric junction. JSLS. 2010;14:309-12.
8. Babbar P, Hemal AK. Robot-assisted urologic surgery in 2010 - Advancements and future outlook. Urol Ann. 2011;3(1):1-7.
9. Tai HC, Chung SD, Wang SM, et al. Laparoscopic partial cystectomy for various bladder pathologies. BJU Int. 2007;100(2):382-5.
10. Ansari MS, Hemal AK. A rare case of urachovesical calculus: a diagnostic dilemma and endo-laparoscopic management. J Laparoendosc Adv Surg Tech A. 2002;12(4):281-3.
11. Allaparthi S, Ramanathan R, Balaji KC. Robotic partial cystectomy for bladder cancer: a single-institutional pilot study. J Endourol. 2010;24(2):223-7.
12. Jeon HG, Jeong W, Oh CK, et al. Initial experience with 50 laparoendoscopic single site surgeries using a homemade, single port device at a single center. J Urol. 2010;183:1866-72.
13. Madeb R, Knopf JK, Nicholson C, et al. The use of robotically assisted surgery for treating urachal anomalies. BJU Int. 2006;98(4):838-42.
14. Chelli D, Methni A, Gatri C, et al. Pelvic hydatid (echinococcal) disease. Int J Gynaecol Obstet. 2010;109(1):45-8.
15. Seracchioli R, Mabrouk M, Montanari G, et al. Conservative laparoscopic management of urinary tract endometriosis (UTE): surgical outcome and long-term follow-up. Fertil Steril. 2010;94(3):856-61.
16. Park JW, Jeong BC, Seo SI, et al. Leiomyoma of the urinary bladder: a series of nine cases and review of the literature. Urology. 2010;76(6):1425-9.
17. Spiess PE, Correa JJ. Robotic assisted laparoscopic partial cystectomy and urachal resection for urachal adenocarcinoma. International Braz J Urol. 2009;35(5):609.
18. Nayyar R, Anand A, Gupta NP. Robotic partial cystectomy for urachal adenocarcinoma: results with technique of cystoscopically optimized surgical margins. Urology. 2009;74(4):A1-8, S166.
19. Tareen BU, Mufarrij PW, Godoy G, et al. Robot-assisted laparoscopic partial cystectomy and diverticulectomy: initial experience of four cases. J Endourol. 2008;22(7):1497-500.
20. Pang ST, Chao A, Wang CJ, et al. Transurethral partial cystectomy and laparoscopic reconstruction for the management of bladder endometriosis. Fertil Steril. 2008;90(5):2014.e1-3.
21. Wang CK, Chueh SC. Laparoscopic partial cystectomy with endo-GIA stapling device in bladder diverticular carcinoma. J Endourol. 2007;21(7):772-5.
22. Hemal AK, Nayyar R, Rao R. Robotic repair of primary symptomatic obstructive megaureter with intracorporeal or extracorporeal ureteric tapering and ureteroneocystostomy. J Endourol. 2009;23(12):2041-6.
23. Singh I, Kader K, Hemal AK. Robotic distal ureterectomy with reimplantation in malignancy: technical nuances. Can J Urol. 2009;16(3):4671-6.
24. Richards KA, Hemal AK. Current status and outcomes of robot-assisted laparoscopic radical cystectomy and urinary diversion. Curr Urol Rep. 2011;12(2):107-14.
25. Fedeli U, Fedewa SA, Ward EM. Treatment of muscle invasive bladder cancer: evidence from the national cancer database, 2003 to 2007. J Urol. 2011;185:72-8.
26. Zhang M, Tao R, Zhang C, et al. Lymphovascular invasion and the presence of more than three tumors are associated with poor outcomes of muscle-invasive bladder cancer after bladder-conserving therapies. Urology. 2010;76(4):902-7.

Chapter 19 Robotic Distal Ureterectomy with Ureteroneocystotomy

Kush Patel, Raju Thomas

INTRODUCTION

Traditionally, the gold standard for the treatment of ureteral and renal transitional cell carcinoma (TCC) has been radical nephroureterectomy. In recent years, there has been a recent and increasing trend towards nephron-sparing surgery to preserve renal function and prevent dialysis dependence. Thus, in select patients, removal of the renal unit can be avoided. This can be accomplished with strict adherence to oncologic surgical principles; using lessons learned from laparoscopic versus open surgical technique outcomes. Robotic (da Vinci®, Intuitive Surgical, Sunnyvale, CA) distal ureterectomy with ureteral reconstruction or reimplantation can be accomplished with good short-term oncologic outcomes.[1,2] Unfortunately, this approach is relatively new, long-term oncologic outcome studies are not available. Robotic assistance has greatly aided in decreasing the morbidity of upper and lower urinary tract reconstruction. Appropriate informed consent for each procedure is highly recommended.

DISTAL URETERECTOMY

Indications and Patient Selection

Distal ureterectomy is indicated in patients with low-grade TCC who have failed endoscopic management and high-grade TCC where nephron-sparing surgery is desired. Patient considerations include age, status of renal function, comorbid conditions, and prior abdominal surgery. It is also imperative to have a bedside assistant who is familiar with robotic, laparoscopic and endourologic approaches.

The distal ureterectomy can be easily accomplished after a robotic or pure laparoscopic nephrectomy (a one-stage procedure), and the entire specimen can be removed intact.

Operative Technique

The patient is placed under a general anesthetic. As with all laparoscopic procedures, a nasogastric or orogastric tube is placed by the anesthesia team. The authors' practice is to start with a cystoscopy to identify any bladder lesions. If present, these are appropriately treated, after which a 5-french (Fr) open-ended catheter is placed into the bladder. This catheter is later used to place an indwelling ureteral stent and is secured to a 20-Fr Foley catheter.

The patient is placed in the lithotomy position, with the operating room bed placed in full Trendelenburg. This allows the intraperitoneal contents, namely the bowels, to retract cephelad. A Foley catheter is placed to gravity. The authors' preference is to use a Veress needle to gain safe access to the abdomen. An off-site technique can be utilized, if there is concern for adhesions from prior surgery. To accomplish this, the Veress needle is inserted at least 9 cm away from a prior abdominal scar. Again, care must be taken to avoid the inferior epigastrics and one must stay medial to the White Line of Toldt. Of course, a Hasson technique can be used safely as well.

A periumbilical 12 mm camera port is placed initially. Three 8 mm ports (robotic) and one more 12 mm assistant port are needed for distal ureterectomy and are placed under direct visualization. When done as part of a combined one-stage nephroureterectomy procedure, the trocar configuration is shown and described in Figure 1. The authors' will describe the technique for lower ureterectomy. Once the robot is docked, the ureter is identified as it crosses over the iliac vessels (Fig. 2). The robotic monopolar scissors and bipolar graspers are used for the dissection. The peritoneum overlying the ureter is incised. It must be mentioned that when performing a nephroureterectomy, the ureter is clamped with a clip or tied-off to prevent TCC cells from migration down the ureter during manipulation (Fig. 3). While isolating the ureter, care is taken to leave the periureteral fat on the ureter to preserve the blood supply and

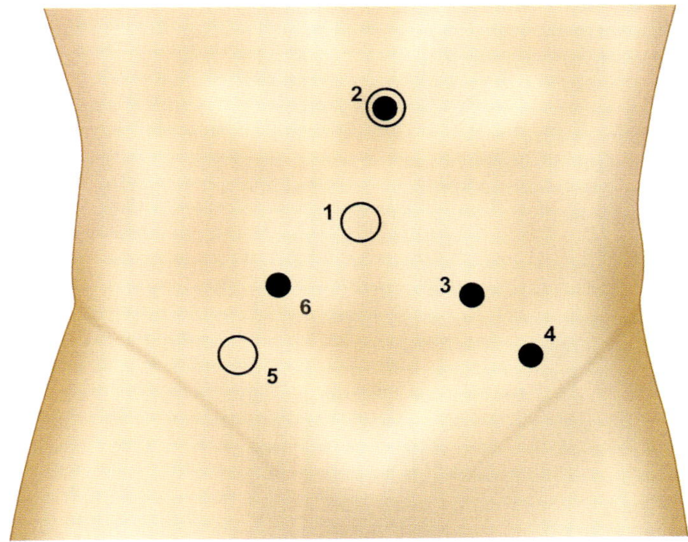

Fig. 1: Trocar placement (A) For combined nephroureterectomy and bladder cuff removal: 1–12 mm Camera Trocar, 2–12 mm Trocar (a robotic trocar can fit inside this), 3–8 mm Robotic Trocar, 4–8 mm Robotic Trocar, 5–12 mm Trocar, 6–8 mm Robotic Trocar; Trocar placement (B) For distal ureterectomy: Use 1, 3, 6 and 5 for left side, Use 1, 6, 3, and 4 for right side

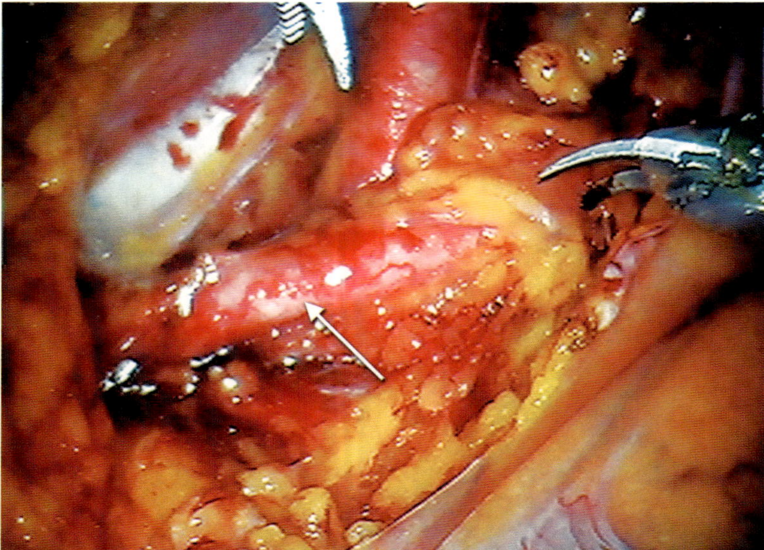

Fig. 2: Identification of the ureter (arrow) as it passes over the left iliac vessels

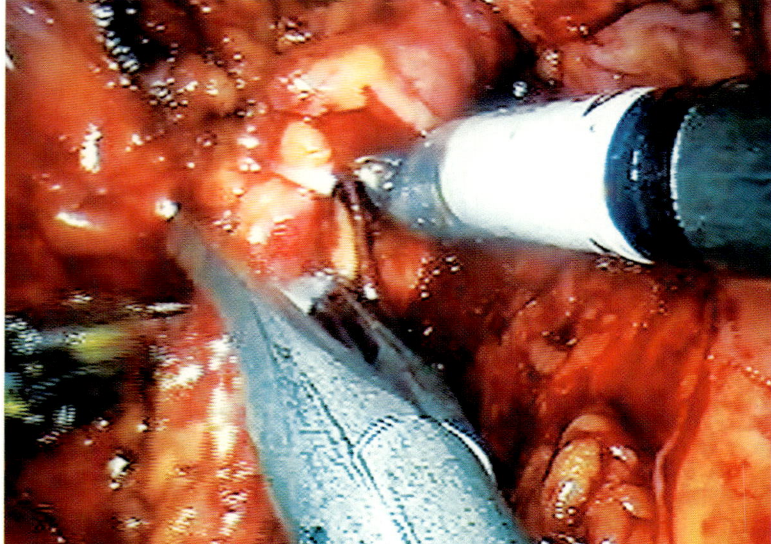

Fig. 3: Clipping of the proximal ureter

protect surgical margins. Placing a vessel loop around the ureter is often helpful to aid in retraction and preventing excessive handling. The ureter is mobilized down to the level of the bladder. During this process, mobilization of the ipsilateral lateral attachments of the bladder may aid in exposure. This dissection may require transection of vas deferens in a male or round ligament in a female. Dissection continues through the detrusor muscle to expose the intramural ureter and mucosa of the bladder at the level of the ureteral orifice. The widening of the mucosa into the wall of bladder can identify the transition from ureteral to bladder mucosa. The bedside surgeon provides retraction to visualize the ureter and place clips, etc.

There is no consensus on the best method to disconnect the distal ureter from its connection to the bladder (Fig. 4). The described techniques are:

a. *Pluck technique:* The distal ureter is initially managed with a transurethral approach and the mucosa and detrusor muscle are incised using electrocautery. Care is taken not to completely perforate the bladder wall to prevent any spillage. A standard transurethral resectoscope is used. This maneuver facilitates disconnecting the ureter from the bladder (pluck technique). After the distal ureterectomy has been completed robotically, the last attachments of the ureter to the bladder are transected and the ureter is literally plucked from the bladder. Once this is complete, the specimen is placed in a specimen retrieval bag and removed. If the distal ureterectomy is in conjunction with a nephroureterectomy, then the entire specimen is placed into an appropriately sized retrieval bag. The opening of the bladder is either sutured with 2-0 polyglactin stay sutures or in some reports, left open. A Foley catheter is left in the bladder for about a week.
b. *Staple technique:* In this scenario, the ureter is dissected and the bladder cuff is identified. An endovascular GIA™ stapler is utilized to staple and disconnect the bladder from the ureter. The specimen is then managed as mentioned above.
c. *Bull-dog clamp at bladder:* In this technique, the ureter is similarly exposed at its junction to the bladder and the bladder portion is clamped using a Bull-dog vascular clamp. If this technique is utilized, the authors' recommend a double clamping and the ureter is then disconnected between the two clamps. The bladder portion is then sutured using 2-0 polyglactin sutures in a standard fashion. The use of stay sutures at the bladder end is recommended for traction as well as to assist in the suturing of the bladder defect. With any of the above-mentioned techniques, the authors' also recommend using intravenous methylene blue to ensure that the contralateral ureter has not been traumatized.

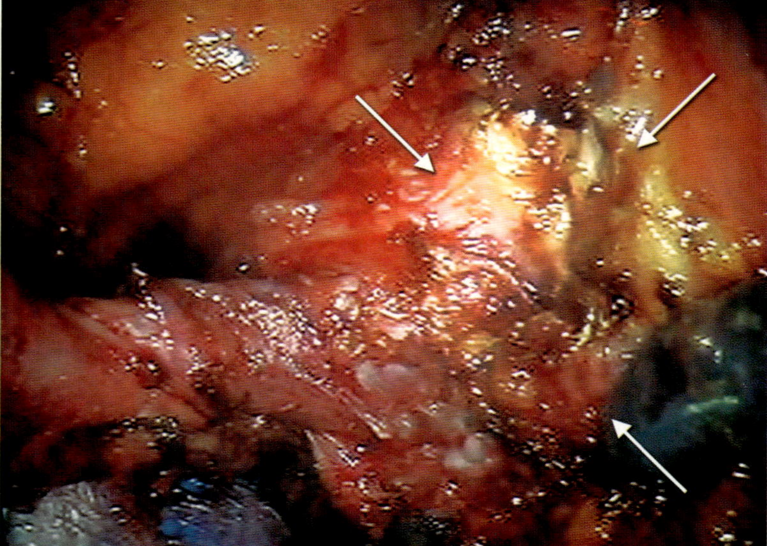

Fig. 4: Dissection of the intramural ureter to expose the bladder cuff (arrows)

To prevent any tumor spillage in the peritoneal cavity, the authors recommend that the ureter be clamped using any of the methods described above. Appropriate frozen-section analyses can be performed to ensure that surgical margins are negative. Additionally, the role of a regional pelvic lymphadenectomy, though not clearly defined for ureteral tumors, needs to be considered before terminating the procedure. The abdomen is examined prior to terminating the procedure. A Jackson-Pratt drain is placed near the sutured bladder incision. The trocar sites are sutured.

The above-mentioned technique for distal ureterectomy is utilized to dissect the distal ureters for robotic radical cystectomy, except that the distal ureter is clamped/transected prior to the radical cystectomy.

URETERONEOCYSTOSTOMY

The indications for ureteroneocystostomy include distal ureteral strictures of various etiologies, distal ureteral tumors, etc.[3-6] The principle of ureteral reconstructive procedures such as ureteroneocystostomy includes: (a) Adequate mobilization of the two ends, (b) Tension-free anastomosis, (c) Adequate stenting and drainage.

Operative Technique

The distal ureter is mobilized, as described above in the previous section. Once the distal ureter has been identified crossing the iliac vessels, the ureter is dissected until the strictured segment of the ureter is identified. The ureter is then transected and the distal end is spatulated. This maneuver will give the robotic surgeon an idea of the distance or the gap between the distal ureteral end and the bladder, thus enabling adequate ureterolysis and bladder mobilization to ensure a tension-free anastomosis.

Prior to placement of the robotic trocars, a cystoscopy is performed and a 5-Fr ureteral catheter is placed and curled in the bladder. This is then retrieved later for retrograde placement of a ureteral stent. Trocar placements are described in Figure 1.

The bladder portion is mobilized similar to a robotic radical prostatectomy and the space of Retzius is entered. The ipsilateral bladder is mobilized more than the contralateral side. The authors recommend a psoas hitch using 0-polyglactin and suturing the ureter onto the psoas muscle using three sutures. The location of the ureteroneocystostomy site is identified and the bladder is filled with approximately 250 cc of normal saline through the indwelling Foley catheter. An incision approximately 1.5–2 cm is made in the bladder and the bladder is drained. The posterior anastomosis between the bladder and the ureter is performed using 4-0 polyglactin sutures in a continuous fashion. Once the cystotomy incision is made, the robotic grasping forceps are used to identify the 5-Fr open-ended catheter in the bladder and this is retrieved through this opening (Fig. 5). Since the posterior anastomosis has been completed, this retrieved ureteral catheter is inserted into the ureter.

Once the 5-Fr open catheter has been placed into the ureter, the bedside surgeon passes a super-stiff guidewire into the 5-Fr catheter and guides us into the renal pelvis (Fig. 6). The 5-Fr open-ended catheter is then off-loaded and an appropriately sized ureteral stent is inserted into the kidney (Fig. 7). The robotic surgeon is visualizing this process and once the stent is in the appropriate location, the guidewire is removed.

The anterior anastomosis is completed in a similar fashion (Fig. 8). Often a two-layer closure is performed using 4-0 polyglactin sutures as well. The bladder can be refilled to test the integrity of the anastomosis and to see if there is any fluid leakage.

If one prefers a nonrefluxing anastomosis, then a longer submucosal tunnel can be created prior to performing the ureteroneocystostomy. The detrusor muscle is incised with the mucosa remaining intact and the ureter is reimplanted into the more distal aspect, using the technique described above. Following this, the detrusor muscle is closed over the ureter duplicating a Lich-Gregoir reimplantation procedure. The peritoneum can be reapproximated over any of the repairs if this is possible. A 7 mm Jackson-Pratt drain is placed through the most lateral 8 mm robotic port and the patients' trocar sites are closed. The patient is admitted over night and usually discharged the following day. The Foley catheter is removed in a week after a negative cystogram. The Jackson-Pratt drain is removed at the same time. If there are concerns about the Jackson-Pratt fluid output then a creatinine level of the fluid is recommended since the drain is intraperitoneal. The ureteral stent is removed in approximately 6 weeks.

CONCLUSION

Distal ureteral surgery such as distal ureterectomy and uretero-neocystostomy can safely be performed using the robotic-assisted

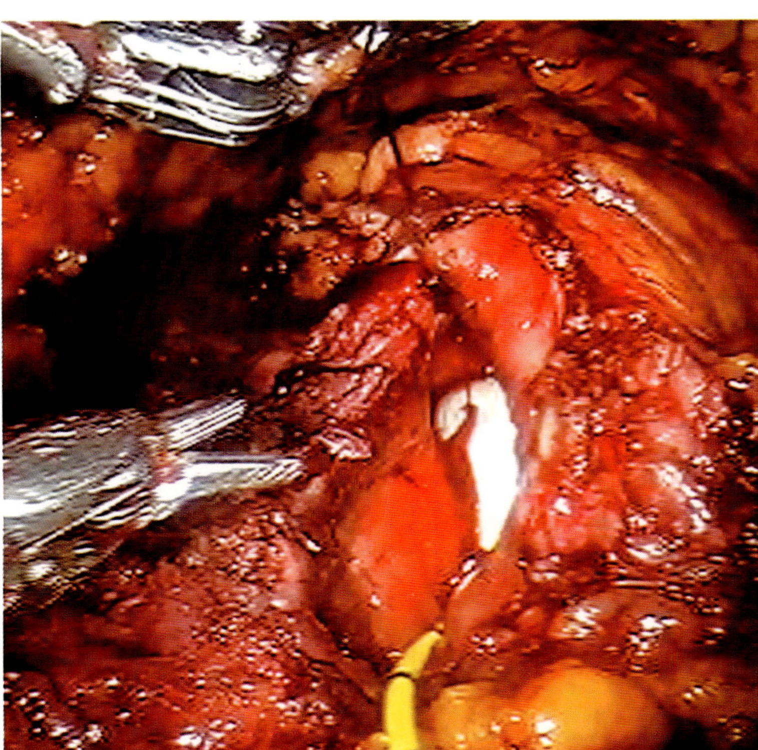

Fig. 5: Cystotomy with previously placed 5-french open-ended catheter brought into the operative field

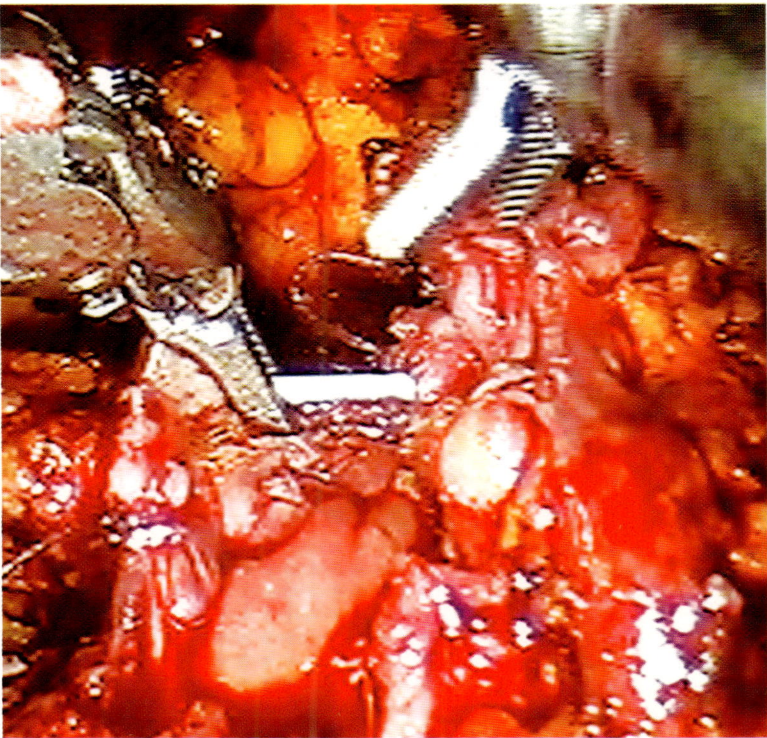

Fig. 6: Removal of 5-french open-ended catheter, leaving the guidewire in place in the ureter

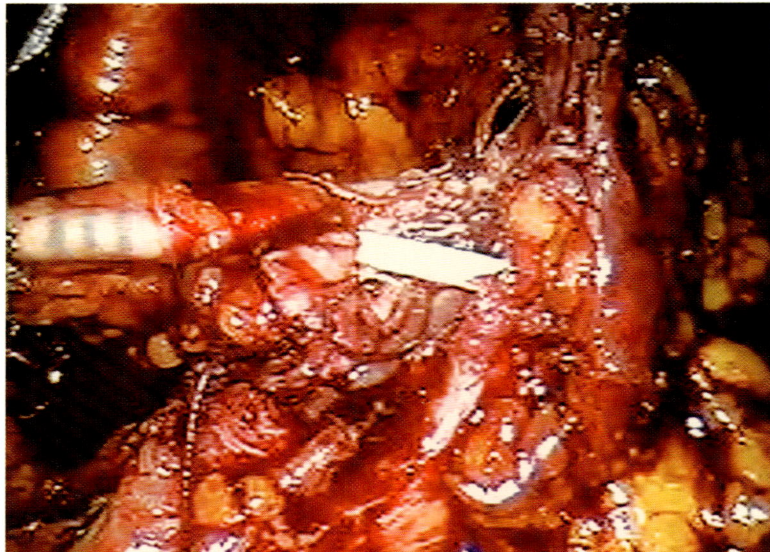

Fig. 7: Passage of the ureteral stent across the anastomosis

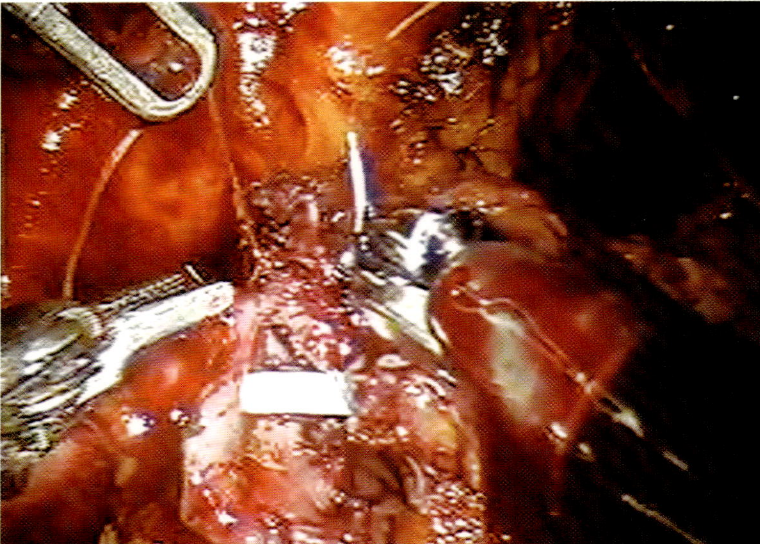

Fig. 8: Completion of vesicoureteral anastomosis

reconstructive techniques. The authors have found this to be safe and can be duplicated in experienced hands. The widespread use of robotic technology has greatly enhanced such reconstructive procedures and it is anticipated that with wider availability, more patients will get the minimally invasive experience with the utilization of robotic surgical techniques.

REFERENCES

1. Allaparthi S, Ramanathan R, Balaji KC. Robotic distal ureterectomy with boari flap reconstruction for distal ureteral urothelial cancers: a single institutional pilot experience. J Laparoendosc Adv Surg Tech A. 2010;20:165-71.
2. Glinianski M, Guru KA, Zimmerman G, et. al. Robotic-assisted ureterectomy and ureteral reconstruction for urothelial carcinoma. J Endourol 2009;23:97-100.
3. Yohannes P, Chiou RK, Pelinkovic D. Rapid communication: pure robot-assisted laparoscopic ureteral reimplantation for ureteral stricture disease: case report. J Endourol. 2003;17:891-3.
4. De Naeyer D, Van Migem P, Schatteman P, et al. Case report: pure robot-assisted psoas hitch ureteral reimplantation for distal-ureteral stenosis. J Endourol. 2007;21:618-20.
5. Uberoi J, Harnish B, Sethi AS, et al. Robot-assisted laparoscopic distal ureterectomy and ureteral reimplantation with psoas hitch. J Endourol. 2007;21:372-3.
6. Singh I, Kader K, Hemal AK. Robotic distal ureterectomy with reimplantation in malignancy: technical nuances. Can J Urol. 2009;16:4671-6.

Chapter 20 Laparoscopic Retroperitoneal Lymph Node Dissection

Brian D Duty, Ornob P Roy, Louis R Kavoussi

INTRODUCTION

Nearly 8,500 new cases of testis cancer were diagnosed within the United States in 2010 making it the most frequently diagnosed solid organ tumor affecting young men.[1] Multimodal therapy, cisplatin-based chemotherapy in particular, has revolutionized the treatment of testicular cancer with long-term survival rates now exceeding 90%.[2] Nevertheless, retroperitoneal lymph node dissection (RPLND) remains a critical component of low-stage, non-seminomatous germ cell tumor (NSGCT) management.

Retroperitoneal lymph node dissection has traditionally been performed via a large midline incision from the xiphoid process to the pubic symphysis. Hulbert and Fraley reported the first case of laparoscopic retroperitoneal lymph node dissection (L-RPLND) in 1992.[2] A meta-analysis of L-RPLND by Rassweiler and colleagues of 34 articles including over 800 NSGCT patients found equivalent staging accuracy and long-term oncologic efficacy compared to open RPLND.[3] Additionally, L-RPLND was associated with decreased length of stay, postoperative pain and overall complication rate.

INDICATIONS

Laparoscopic RPLND is a treatment option for NSGCT patients with Stage I and Stage IIa disease. However, an increasing number of patients with Stage Ia disease are electing for active surveillance given a 70–80% overtreatment rate in this population. Active surveillance is not recommended for patients with Stage Ib disease given the 50% chance of relapse.[4] RPLND remains an excellent treatment option in these patients because the relapse rate outside of the RPLND template is only 1.2%.[3]

Men with low-volume Stage IIb disease may be considered for node dissection.[5] L-RPLND has also been performed following chemotherapy in highly selected patients with seminoma and non-seminoma.[6] However, postchemotherapy L-RPLND is a technically challenging operation, particularly in seminoma patients and should not be entertained early in one's clinical experience.

RPLND is contraindicated in patients with rising tumor markers following radical orchiectomy because rising markers are most commonly associated with systemic disease outside of the retroperitoneal landing zone. Other contraindications to L-RPLND include bleeding diathesis and active infection.

PATIENT PREPARATION

Stage I and IIa NSGCT patients with negative tumor markers following radical orchiectomy have multiple options including active surveillance (Stage Ia), cisplatin-based chemotherapy and RPLND. Consequently, patients should undergo extensive counseling prior to committing to any therapeutic modality. The L-RPLND procedure should be discussed in detail including the risks of hemorrhage requiring transfusion and/or open conversion, damage to adjacent organs (bowel, kidney, ureter, spleen, liver and pancreas), lymph leak and retrograde ejaculation. Patients are offered the option to bank sperm prior to surgery.

Patients who have received chemotherapy require special attention. Adequate time is required to allow normalization of hematological parameters. Referral to a pulmonologist and preoperative pulmonary function testing should be considered in all patients who have received bleomycin given the risk of pulmonary fibrosis.

A type and cross for packed red blood cells is required in all patients. A mechanical bowel preparation should be performed the day prior to surgery. A first-generation cephalosporin is given in the preoperative holding area.

OPERATING ROOM SETUP

The surgeon and assistant stand opposite the side of dissection. The scrub nurse is positioned across from the surgeon at the patient's feet. Monitors are placed on both sides of the patient so all members of the team can observe the procedure. This configuration also allows the surgeon to switch sides should a bilateral dissection be required.

The laparoscopic tray, including laparoscopic vascular instruments, is located at the foot of the operating room table. Additionally, a full laparotomy set with vascular clamps and retractors needs to be present in the room should intraoperative hemorrhage necessitate open conversion.

PATIENT POSITIONING

Following induction of general anesthesia and endotracheal tube placement, a Foley catheter and gastric tube are placed. Both arms are tucked with care being taken to ensure all pressure points are adequately padded. The patient is secured to the operating room table with multiple layers of wide cloth tape. A "test roll" is then performed to ensure the patient is adequately secured to the table. Sequential compression devices are placed on both lower extremities and activated prior to starting the procedure. The operative field (xiphoid process to pubic symphysis) is prepped and draped in a sterile fashion.

LAPAROSCOPIC ACCESS

Transperitoneal access is obtained with either a Veress needle or by the Hasson technique. Pneumoperitoneum to 20 mm Hg is established. Starting 2 cm below the xiphoid process and ending 4 cm about the pubic symphysis, four equally spaced 10/12 mm ports are placed along the midline (Fig. 1). An additional 5 mm lateral port may be placed to facilitate dissection of the spermatic cord (SC) if needed. The first port is placed with an optical trocar using a 0° laparoscope lens. Once intraperitoneal access has been obtained, the 0° lens is exchanged for a 30° scope and the remaining ports are placed under direct vision. Following port placement, the viscera are inspected to rule out injury and the pneumoperitoneum is decreased to 15 mm Hg.

Before starting the dissection, the operating room table is rotated towards the surgeon and the patient is placed in slight Trendelenburg position to passively displace the bowels away from the operative field. A paddle through the most inferior port may be used for active retraction.

Right Template Dissection

The anatomic borders of the right modified RPLND template are the renal helium superiorly, origin of the inferior mesenteric artery (IMA) and right common iliac vessels inferiorly, right ureter laterally, and preaortic nodes medially (Fig. 2). The nodal packets removed during the right-sided dissection include the right iliac, paracaval, interaortocaval and preaortic nodes.

The procedure begins with mobilization of the ascending colon by incising the White Line of Toldt. The colon is mobilized medially from the medial umbilical ligament to the hepatic flexure. Judicious use of electrocautery provides hemostasis while minimizing the risk of thermal injury to the bowel. Following colon mobilization the duodenum is identified and reflected medially thereby exposing the inferior vena cava (Fig. 3). Once the Kocher maneuver has been completed dissection of the SC is performed.

The posterior peritoneum overlying the internal inguinal ring is circumferentially incised exposing the gonadal vessels and vas deferens (Fig. 4). The vas deferens is clipped and divided. With a combination of blunt and sharp dissection the distal SC remnant is retracted out of the inguinal canal until the orchiectomy suture is identified. Once the distal SC has been freed, the dissection proceeds proximally. Care is taken to avoid damaging the iliac vessels posteriorly, inferior epigastric vessels medially and ureter throughout its course. The gonadal vein is clipped and divided at its insertion into the IVC (Fig. 5). Similarly, the gonadal artery is ligated as it originates from the aorta. The SC is then extracted in an entrapment bag.

The lymph node dissection begins following SC removal. The adventitia overlying the IVC is elevated and incised from the renal veins to the bifurcation of the iliac vessels (Fig. 6). Starting where the right ureter crosses the iliac vessels, the paracaval nodes are retracted laterally. The suction-irrigator device is used to bluntly separate the paracaval packet from the underlying psoas fascia (Fig. 7). Exposed vessels and lymphatic channels are controlled with clips. The dissection continues superiorly to the level of the renal hilum.

The preaortic and interaortocaval dissection is then performed (Fig. 8). Proceeding from the aortic bifurcation to renal hilum, the overlying aortic adventitia is "split and rolled" towards the IVC. The right renal artery is identified to prevent injury. As the nodal packet is swept medially off the anterior spinous ligament, multiple lumbar arteries will be encountered that should be divided between clips. The dissection continues down to the IMA. The only remaining nodal attachments to the posterior body wall will be retrocaval.

The IVC is gently elevated as the lumbar veins are identified and divided (Fig. 9). The retrocaval nodes are then freed from the posterior surface of the IVC. The retrocaval dissection is done cautiously to void traction injury to the efferent sympathetic nerve fibers that are located posterior to the IVC.

The lymph nodes are then placed in an entrapment sac and removed. If any nodal packets are grossly positive, then a bilateral template dissection is performed (Fig. 10). Otherwise, the dissection is concluded.

Optional Optional

Fig. 1: Standard trocar placement for laparoscopic retroperitoneal lymph node dissection

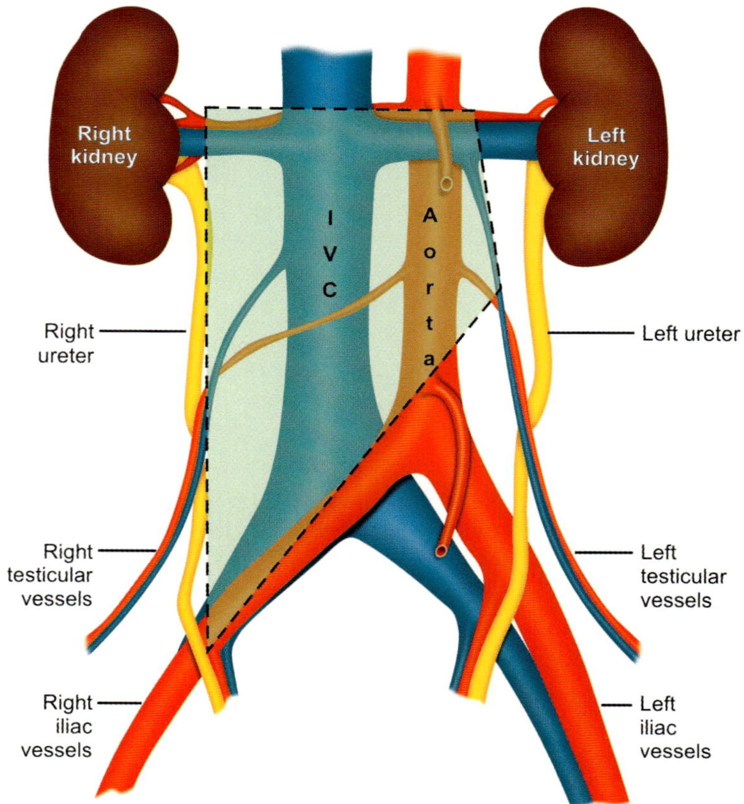

Fig. 2: Modified right retroperitoneal lymph node dissection template

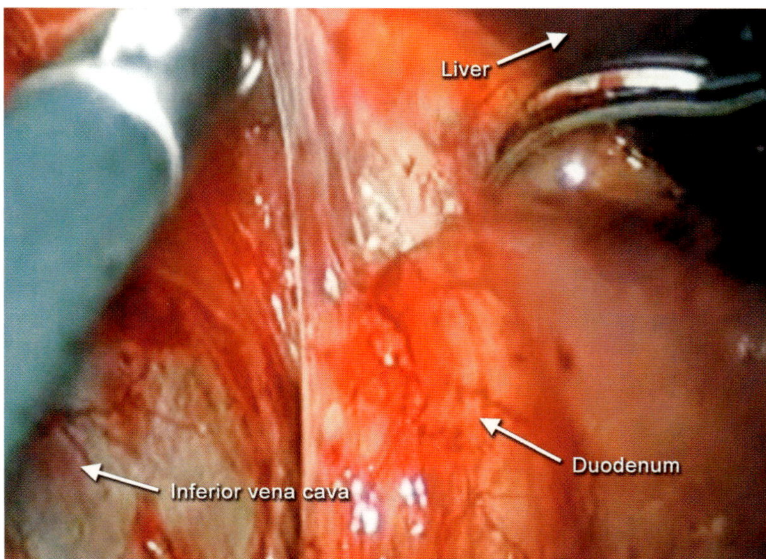

Fig. 3: Kocher maneuver. The duodenum is released from the right kidney and retracted medially off of the inferior vena cava

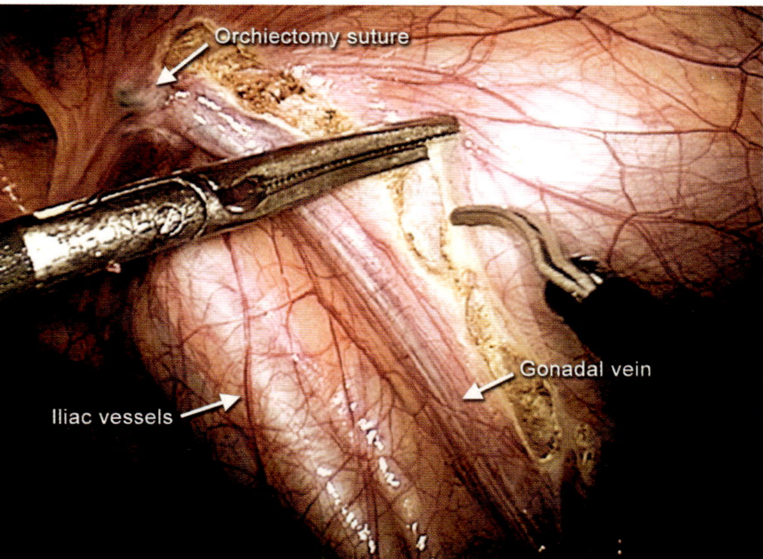

Fig. 4: Incision of the peritoneum overlying the distal spermatic cord

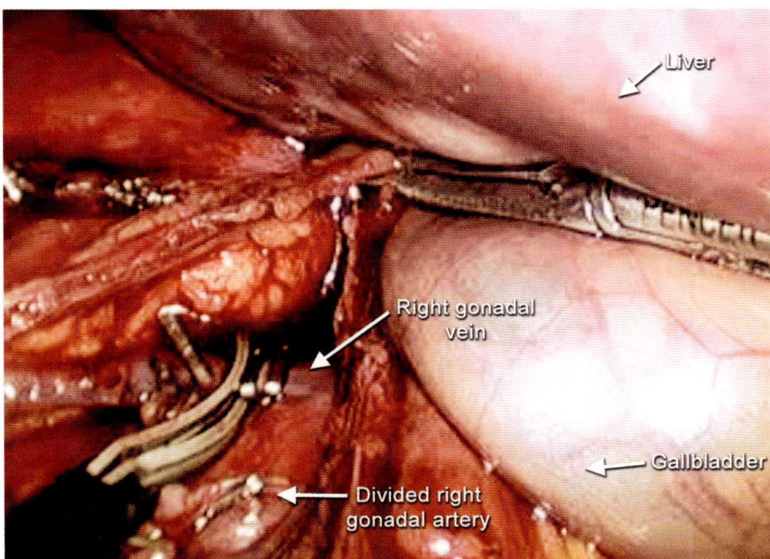

Fig. 5: Division of the proximal right gonadal vein as it enters the inferior vena cava

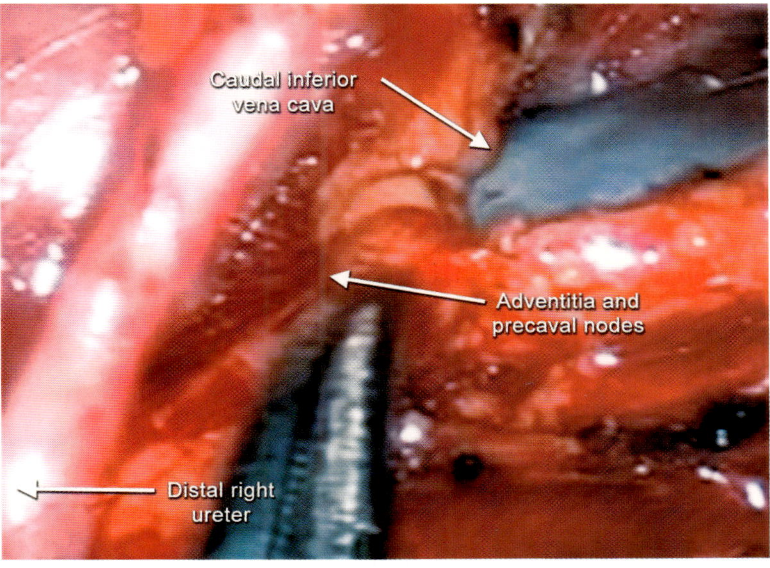

Fig. 6: The adventitia and precaval lymph nodes overlying the inferior vena cava are divided from the renal hilum to the bifurcation of the vena cava. The distal ureter is seen crossing over the pelvic brim

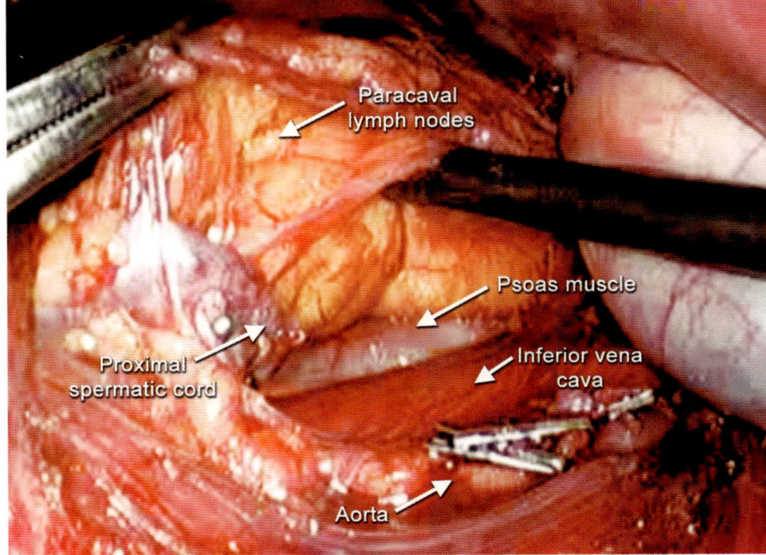

Fig. 7: Dissection of the paracaval lymph nodes away from the inferior vena cava

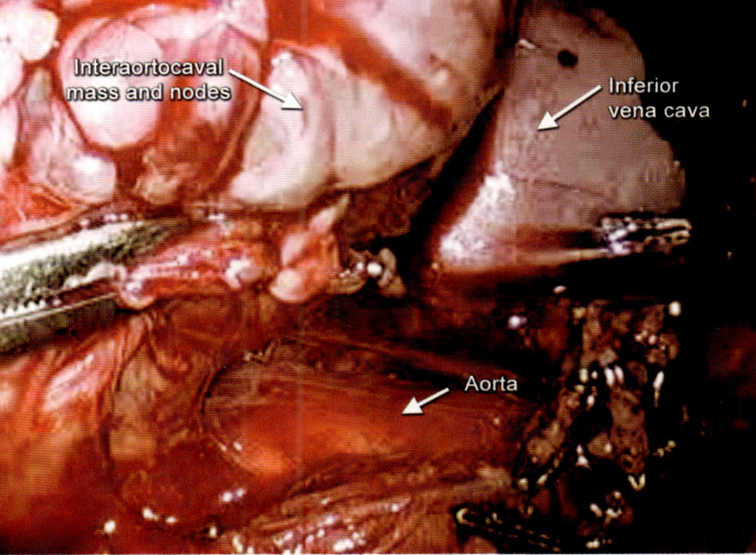

Fig. 8: Dissection of the interaortocaval lymph nodes

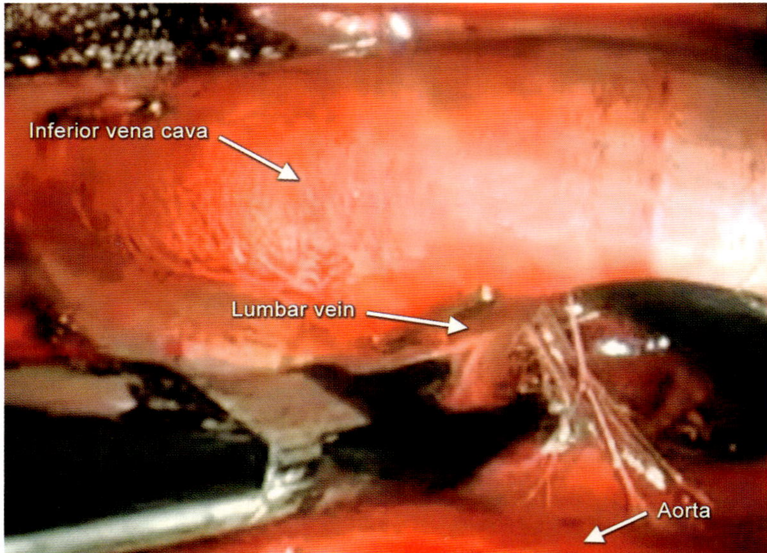

Fig. 9: Retrocaval dissection begins with gentle elevation of the inferior vena cava with ligation of the lumbar veins

The retroperitoneum is carefully inspected for active bleeding or pooling of chylous fluid. A drain is not routinely required. The ports are removed under direct visualization and closed by hand or with a Carter-Thomason (Inlet Medical, Eden Prairie, MN) or EndoClose (US. Surgical, Norwalk, CT) fascial closure device. The port sites are then irrigated and closed with absorbable 4-0 suture.

Left Template Dissection

The anatomic borders of the left modified RPLND template are the renal helium superiorly, origin of the IMA and left common iliac vessels inferiorly, left ureter laterally and IVC medially (Fig. 11). The nodal packets removed during the left-sided dissection include the left iliac, preaortic and para-aortic nodes.

Once again, the procedure begins by incising the White Line of Toldt. The descending colon is freed from the bifurcation of the left iliac vessels to the splenic flexure. Mobilization of the splenic flexure requires division of the splenophrenic and splenorenal ligaments with electrocautery. The tail of the pancreas is identified and gently displaced medially.

The posterior peritoneum over the left internal inguinal ring is incised and the distal SC remnant is freed from the internal inguinal ring. The gonadal vein is traced superiorly and divided as it enters the left renal vein. The gonadal artery is ligated at the aorta. The SC is then extracted. Once again, the ureter is identified early in the dissection to prevent devascularization.

The adventitia overlying the aorta is divided from the renal hilum to the IMA (Figs 12 and 13). The dissection shifts inferolaterally to where the left ureter crosses the iliac vessels. The para-aortic and iliac nodal packets are swept laterally as the dissection continues up to the renal hilum. The preaortic packet from the renal hilum to IMA is wept medially and separated from the aorta and anterior spinous ligament. The right renal artery is identified and preserved.

Lumbar arteries are clipped as the dissection moves inferiorly thereby allowing the aorta to be elevated. The retroaortic dissection is then performed. Once again, care is taken to preserve the efferent sympathetic fibers. Any remaining attachments are divided and the nodal packets are extracted. The abdomen is then exited as previously described.

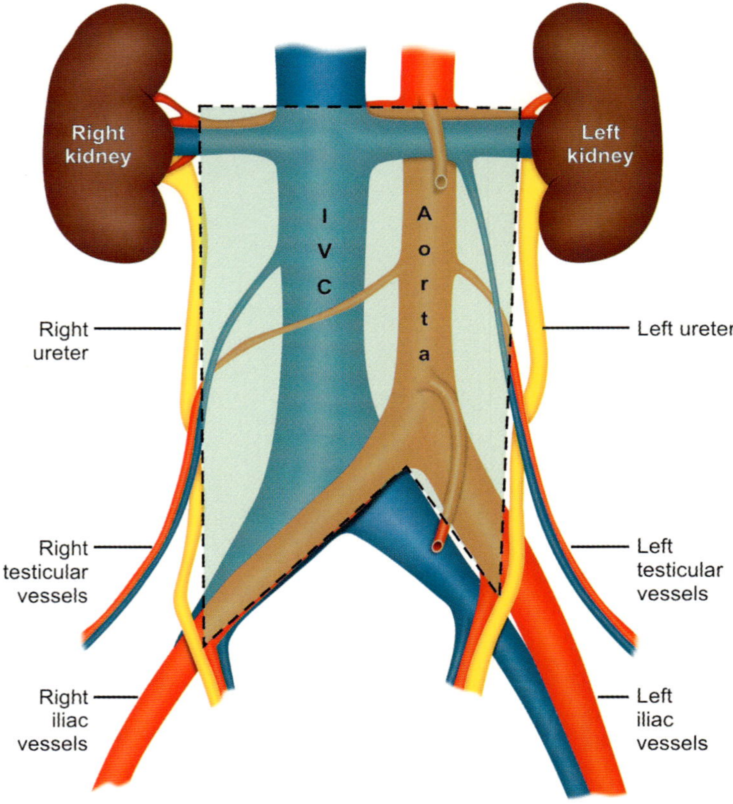

Fig. 10: Bilateral retroperitoneal lymph node dissection template

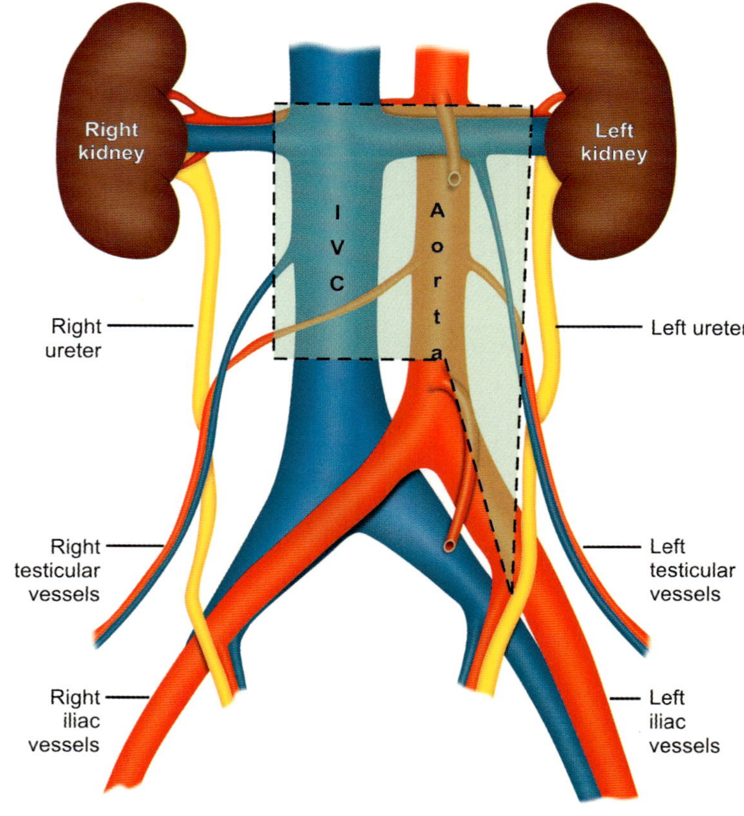

Fig. 11: Modified left retroperitoneal lymph node dissection template

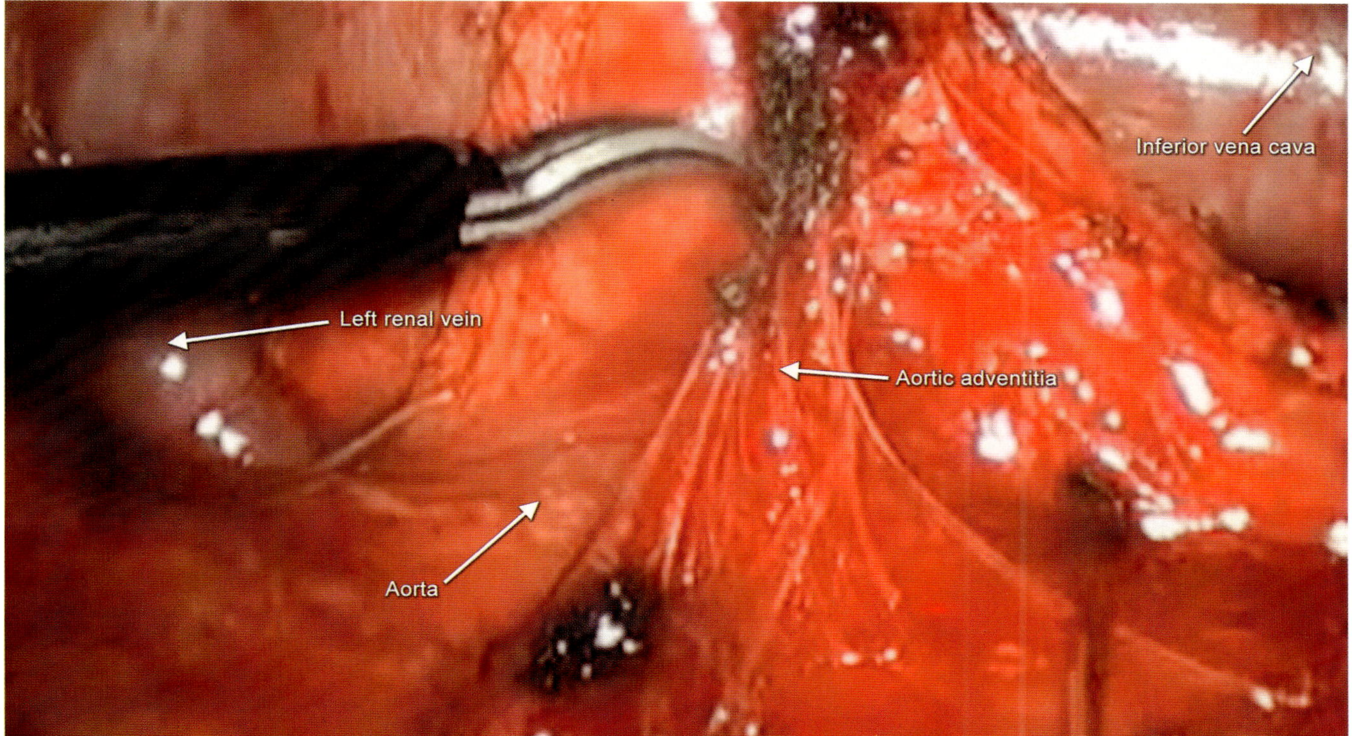

Fig. 12: Division of the adventitia over the aorta from the renal hilum moving distally

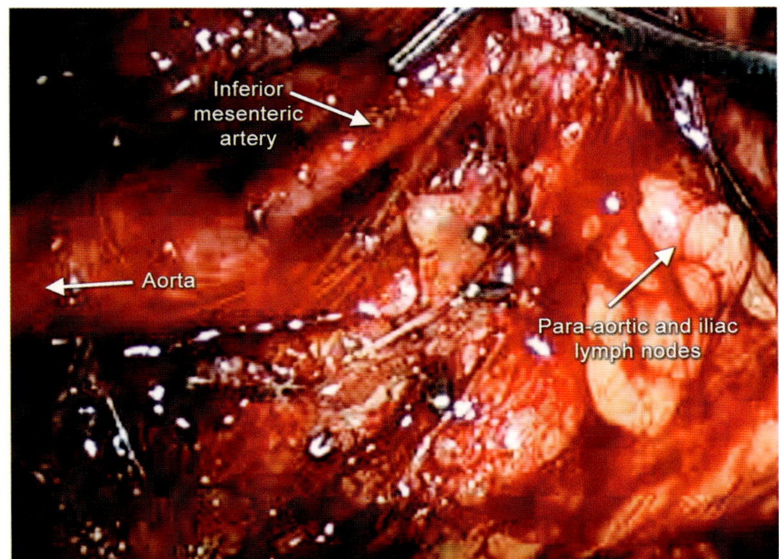

Fig. 13: The adventitia over the aorta is "split and rolled" caudally to the level of the inferior mesenteric artery

POSTOPERATIVE CARE

Unless there is concern for bowel injury, the oro- or nasogastric tube is removed in the operating room. The Foley catheter is removed the morning after surgery. Intra- and postoperative intravenous fluids are minimized in patients who have previously received bleomycin. A liquid diet is started on postoperative day one, which is advanced to a regular diet once gastrointestinal function returns. The patient is discharged home once his pain is under control with oral analgesics, he is ambulating and tolerating a regular diet. This is usually on postoperative day two or three.

COMPLICATIONS

The most serious intraoperative complication is vascular injury, which is more common in the postchemotherapy setting.[6] Venous bleeding can be controlled in the vast majorities of cases with direct pressure and by temporarily increasing the pneumoperitoneum to 20 mm Hg. Unlike venous bleeding, arterial hemorrhage not amenable to clipping will often require intracorporeal suturing. Once controlled, the use of adjunctive hemostatic agents such as Surgicel® (Ethicon, Somerville, NJ.) and FloSeal (Baxter Healthcare Corporation, Fremont, CA) should be considered.

If bleeding cannot be controlled laparoscopically, a vertical midline incision from the xiphoid process to the pubic symphysis should be made quickly. Fortunately, improved instrumentation and hemostatic agents, combined with increasing laparoscopic experience, have dropped the open conversion rate in modern series to 1–5%.[4,7]

Bowel injury remains the most dreaded delayed complication. Trocar placement under direct vision and judicious use of electrocautery help minimize this complication. Minor bowel injuries may be closed in two layers laparoscopically. Larger injuries, or those with extensive thermal damage, may require open repair and diversion. A low index of suspicion for bowel injury should be maintained in all patients with a persistent postoperative ileus, rising or falling white blood cell count, fevers and disproportional pain at a trocar site.

Chylous ascites is a rare complication that usually results from unrecognized injury to the cisterna chyli. Patients may present in a variety of ways, which include prolonged ileus, ascites, chylous leakage from incision sites and/or pleural effusion. Meticulous ligation of lymphatic channels during surgery is critical to prevent this complication. Postoperative treatment consists of a low-fat, medium-chain triglyceride diet. If unsuccessful, hyperalimentation and bowel rest should be used. Lymphangiography has been employed with success rates of 70% in patients with drainage volumes of less than 500 ml per day.[8] Lymphangiography may also aid in preoperative planning in patients who have failed conservative management and require surgical exploration with ligation of open lymphatics.

REFERENCES

1. Jemal A, Center M, DeSantis, C, et al. Global patters of cancer incidence and mortality rates and trends. Cancer Epidemiol Biomarkers Prev. 2010;19:1893-907.
2. Hulbert JC, Fraley EE. Laparoscopic retroperitoneal lymphadenectomy: new approach to pathologic staging of clinical stage I germ cell tumors of the testis. J Endourol. 1992;6:123.
3. Rassweiler JJ, Scheitlin W, Heidenreich A, et al. Laparoscopic retroperitoneal lymph node dissection: does it still have a role in the management of clinical stage I nonseminomatous testis cancer? A European perspective. Eur Urol. 2008;54:1004-15.
4. Jones RH, Vasey PA. Part I: testicular cancer—management of early disease. Lancet Oncol. 2003;4: 730-7.
5. Motzer RJ, Agarwal N, Beard C, et al. National Comprehensive Cancer Network Clinical Practice Guidelines in Oncology: Testis Cancer. J Natl Compr Canc Netw. 2009;6:672-93.
6. Palese MA, Su LM, Kavoussi LR. Laparoscopic retroperitoneal lymph node dissection after chemotherapy. Urology. 2002;60:130-4.
7. Beck SD, Peterson MD. Bihrle R, et al. Short-term morbidity of primary retroperitoneal lymph node dissection in a contemporary group of patients. J Urol. 2007;178:504-6.
8. Alejandre-Lafont E, Krompiec C, Rau WS, et al. Effectiveness of therapeutic lymphography on lymphatic leakage. Acta Radiol. 2011;52:305-11.

Chapter 21

Robotic-Assisted Laparoscopic Retroperitoneal Lymph Node Dissection for Testicular Cancer

Stephen B Williams, David Y Josephson

INTRODUCTION

Robotic technology has enabled urologists to perform a variety of laparoscopic surgeries. Robotic surgery offers enhanced optical magnification and visualization with precise surgical movements. Laparoscopic retroperitoneal lymph node dissection (RPLND) for patients with nonseminomatous germ cell tumors have met with great skepticism with results reported from high-volume laparoscopic surgeons at few dedicated centers.[1] Unfortunately due to the inherent difficulty with dissection, incomplete dissection and limited number of patients there remains insufficient data to suggest superiority to open RPLND.[1] Robotic RPLND has been successfully performed previously and authors believe the robotic approach offers a minimally invasive alternative to conventional laparoscopy.[2,3]

Active surveillance, chemotherapy and open RPLND are currently accepted treatment options for patients with clinical stage (CS) I disease.[4] Indications to perform a robotic RPLND include patients diagnosed with testis cancer and are clinical stage I-IIA.[5] All cases are preoperatively staged with tumor markers (AFP, HCG and LDH), computerized tomography (CT) of the abdomen-pelvis and CT of the chest or chest X-ray. While promising, further application to postchemotherapy patients should be investigated only once additional study for clinical stage I-IIA patients deem it oncologic and functionally equivalent to the open approach.

PROCEDURE

The steps of the procedure are illustrated from Figures 1 to 17. Instrumentation utilized for this procedure is illustrated in Table 1.

A right-sided modified template nerve sparing approach will be described and illustrated which simulates the open experience.[6] The extent of lymph node dissection depends on the side of testis tumor. For right-sided testis tumors, the extent of lymph node dissection includes the interaortocaval region followed by precaval, paracaval, retrocaval and then preaortic and retroaortic nodes. For left-sided tumors, the dissection includes the para-aortic, retroaortic and interaortocaval regions.

Table 1: Instrumentation for Robotic RPLND
da Vinci® surgical system
Robotic ports 8 mm x 3
Excel laparoscopic ports 12 mm x 2
Laparoscopic port 5 mm x 1
Robotic monopolar scissors
Robotic bipolar dissecting forceps
Robotic needle driver
Robotic suture cut needle driver
Assistant instruments
Maryland grasper
Suction and irrigation
Laparoscopic scissors
Laparoscopic needle driver
Hem-o-lok clips
Titanium clips

The colon is reflected medially through an incision along the white line of Toldt and the duodenum is kocherized off the vena cava.

All lymphatic tissue are placed in an endoscopic bag and extracted via the periumbilical camera port. Excised lymph node packets are sent separately from the pericaval, interaortocaval and the para-aortic regions. If metastatic disease is encountered, a bilateral modified template dissection should be carried out.[7] Depending on the patient's body habitus, the contralateral aspect can be dissected without redocking the robot. The use of the 4th arm with the Prograsp may allow enough retraction of the descending bowel to expose the lateral aspect of the aorta. However, if there is any difficulty with the exposure due to redundant bowel, then the patient should be repositioned for better exposure of the contralateral side of the retroperitoneum. No drains are placed for this procedure. 12 mm trocar sites should be closed with a Carter Thomason device. The Foley catheter is removed postoperative day one and discharge home is targeted for postoperative day two.[8]

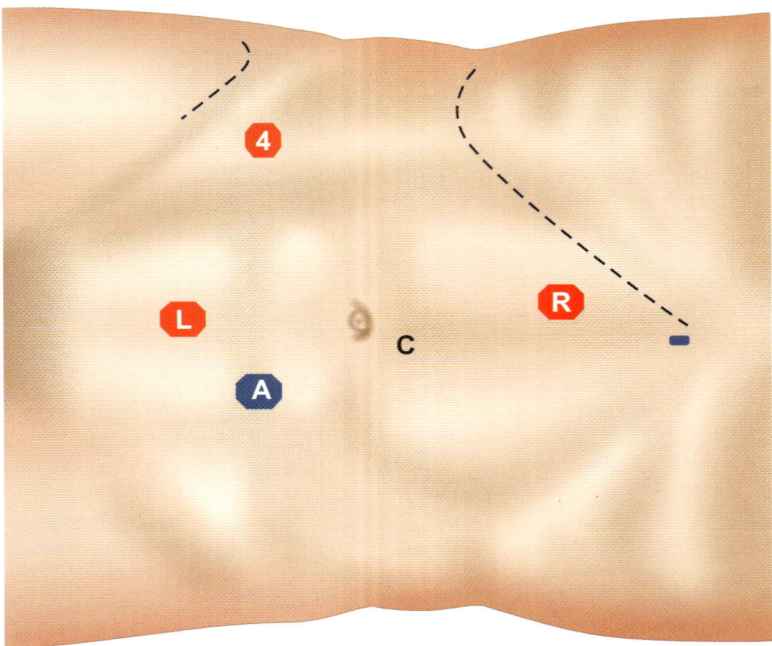

Fig. 1: All procedures are performed transperitoneally with patients placed in the left lateral decubitus position. The patient is placed with the anterior superior iliac spine at the flex of the table and the table is hyperextended. The arms are padded, an axillary roll is placed and the patient is secured to the table at the feet, hips and chest with wide cloth tape. A Veress needle is placed at the umbilicus to establish pneumoperitoneum. A 12 mm optical port is placed just superior to the umbilicus. A total of three additional robotic 8 mm ports are placed in addition to a 12 mm assistant port. With this type of port configuration, a 30 degree down lens is utilized for complete visualization of the operative field. The robot is docked perpendicular to the plane of the table. A monopolar curved scissors is used in the right robotic arm, a fenestrated bipolar in the left robotic arm and a Prograsp in the additional robotic port

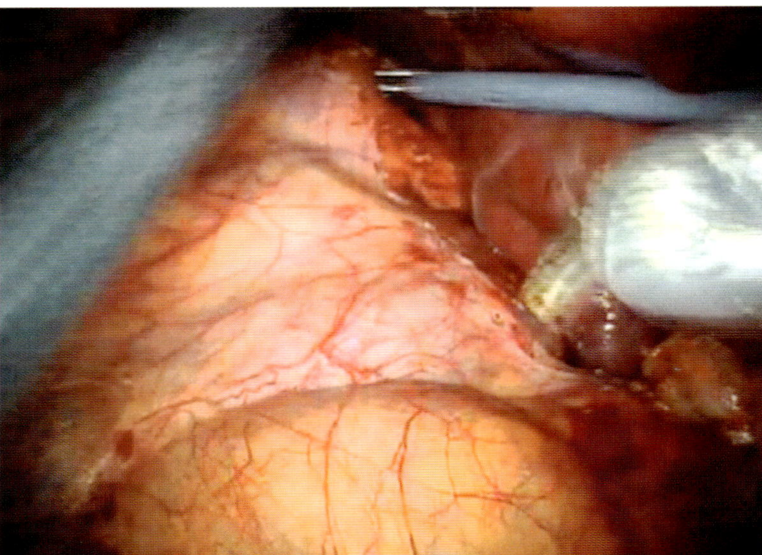

Fig. 2: A self-locking grasper is then used as a liver retractor to expose Gerota's fascia and the right renal hilum

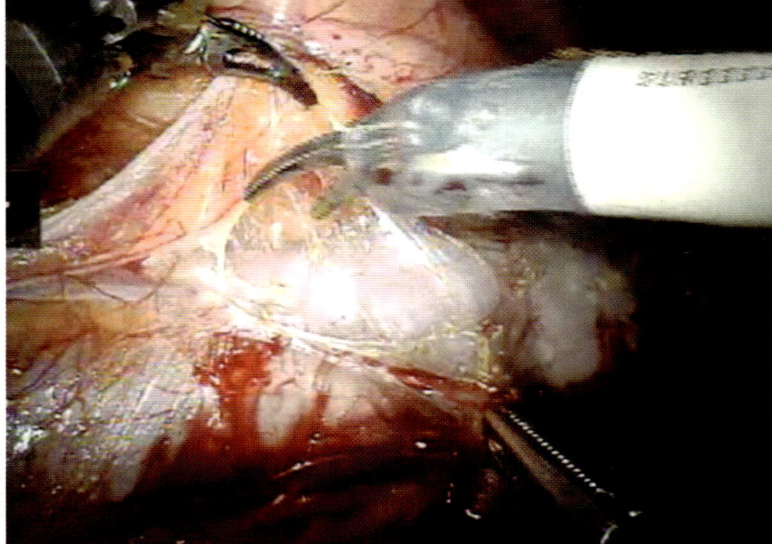

Fig. 3: The fibrinous tissue anterior to the vena cava is divided to identify the insertion of the gonadal vein

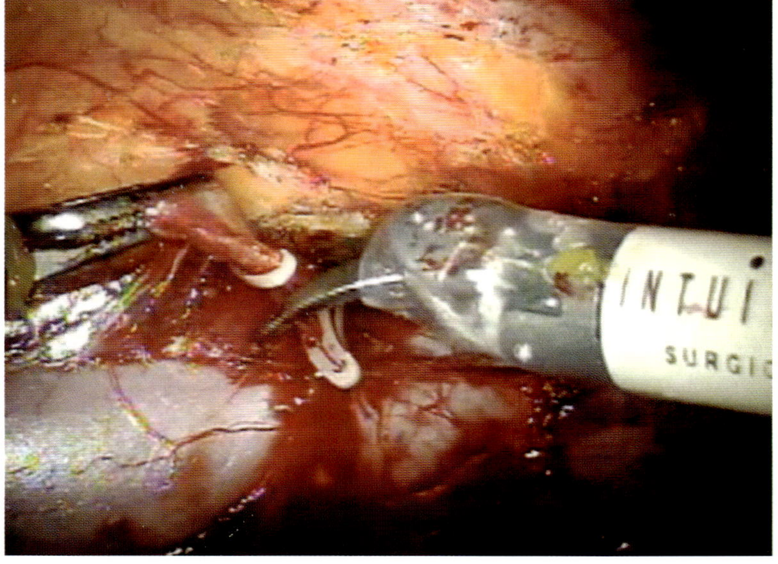

Fig. 4: The gonadal vein is clipped with self-locking Weck clips and divided. The vein is followed and dissected inferiorly to the internal inguinal ring. Care must be taken to identify the ureter and avoid injury as the spermatic vein crosses anterior to it

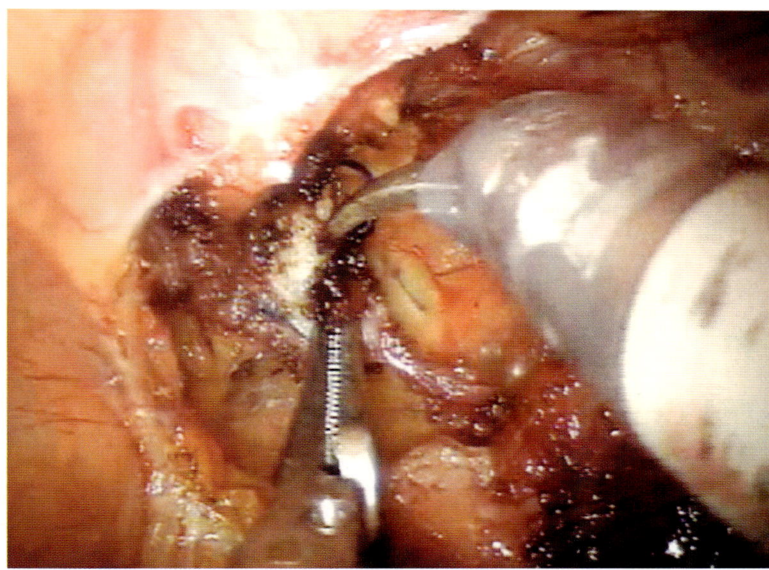

Fig. 5: The posterior layer of the peritoneum is incised and the spermatic cord is removed en bloc at the level of the inguinal ring. The previously used suture for the radical inguinal orchiectomy is identified and taken with the specimen. The ipsilateral vas deferens is identified and divided after clip ligation. Once the spermatic cord has been dissected free from its insertion into the vena cava down to the internal ring, the specimen is placed in an Endocatch™ bag and retrieved through the 12 mm assistant port

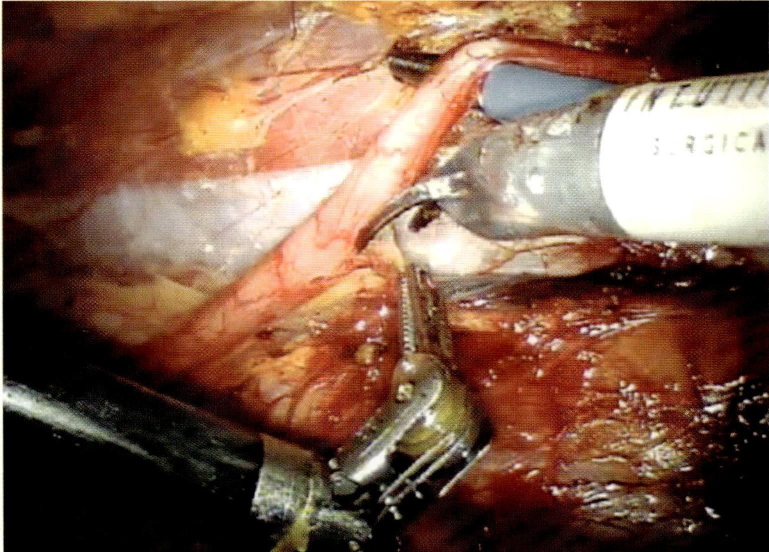

Fig. 6: The ipsilateral ureter is retracted laterally by the assistant to mobilize and skeletonize all lymphatic tissue medial to it, representing the precaval lymph node packet

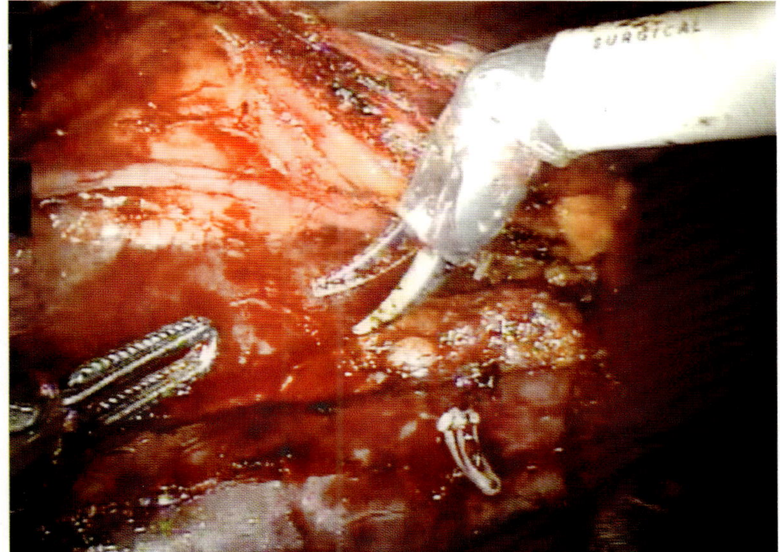

Fig. 7: Once the ureter has been dissected away from the packet, the psoas muscle is identified and serves as a posterior limit. The medial aspect of the precaval lymph node packet is then dissected away from the lateral aspect of the vena cava using a split and roll technique

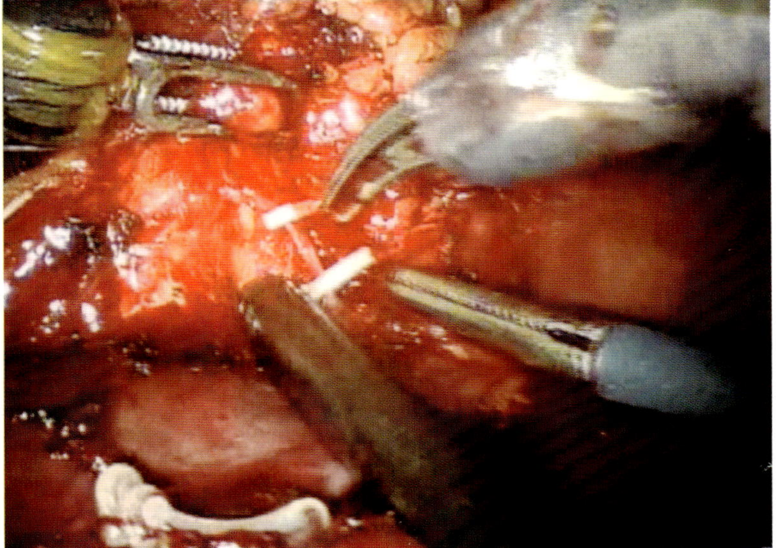

Fig. 8: The assistant utilizes the sucker and/or grasper to retract the vena cava medially. Lumbar veins are then identified and secured with Weck clips before dividing. Additional hemostatic control of small posterior perforators can be achieved with the use of bipolar current. Release of lumbar vein attachments to the vena cava allow for greater mobility of the vena cava to allow for full exposure of tissue posterior to the great vessels and visualization of the anterior spinous ligament

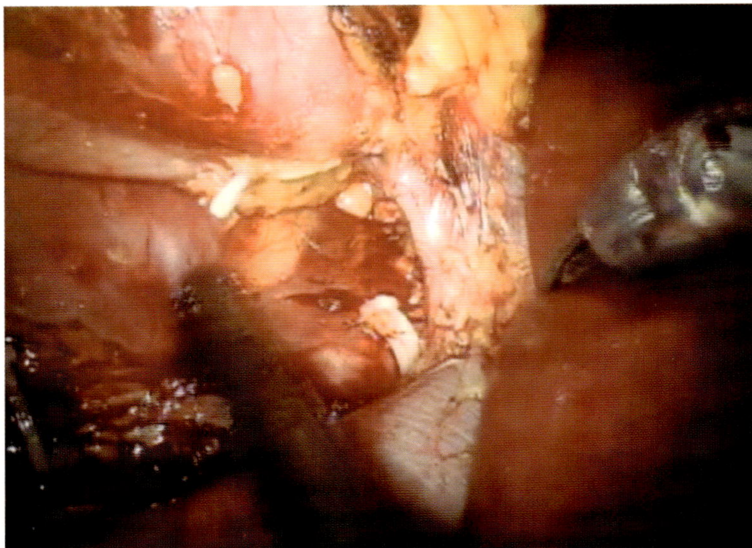

Fig. 9: Lymph node dissection is performed superiorly to the level of the right renal vein and artery and then medially to the greater vessels. Lumbar vessels when encountered are identified and ligated with Hem-o-lok or titanium clips. Depending on the size of the vessels, additional reinforcement is obtained proximal to the clips using 4-0 silk suture since manipulation of the dissected great vessels during the course of the operation can sometime dislodge clips. In addition, the doctors advise to have an adequate end on the divided lumbar artery/vein at its insertion into the great vessels in case a clip dislodges and vascular control needs to be obtained with additional clip or bipolar current

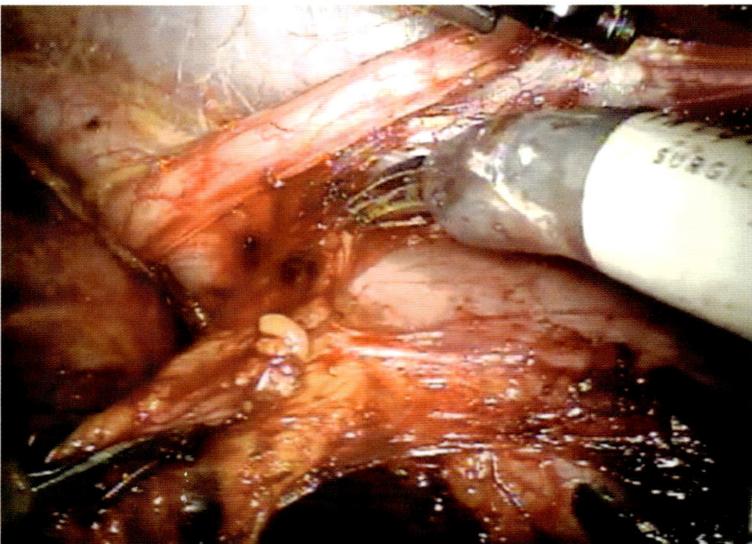

Fig. 10: The paracaval lymphatics are dissected down to the crossing of the ureter over the common iliac artery representing the most inferior extent of the dissection. The packet is sent off as a separate specimen

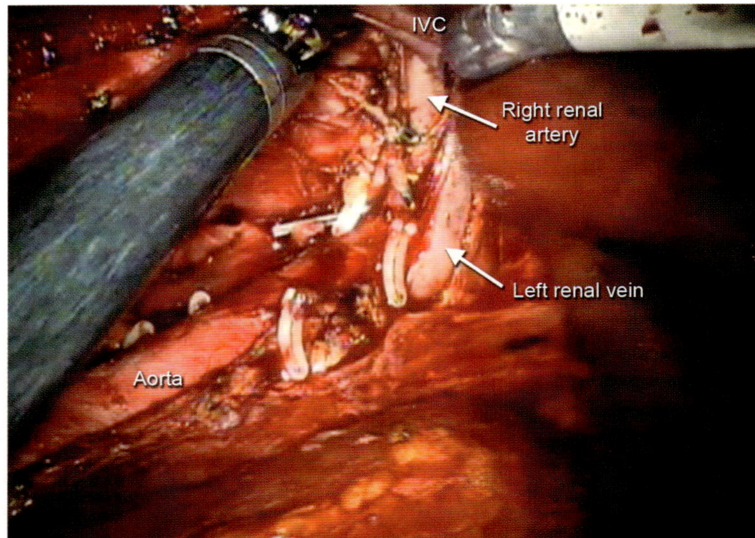

Fig. 11: Lymphatics are ligated at the level of the renal vessels. The right renal artery is seen behind the left renal vein as the left hand provides countertraction on the vena cava to expose lymphatics that are clipped and ligated just medial to the lateral aspect of the aorta

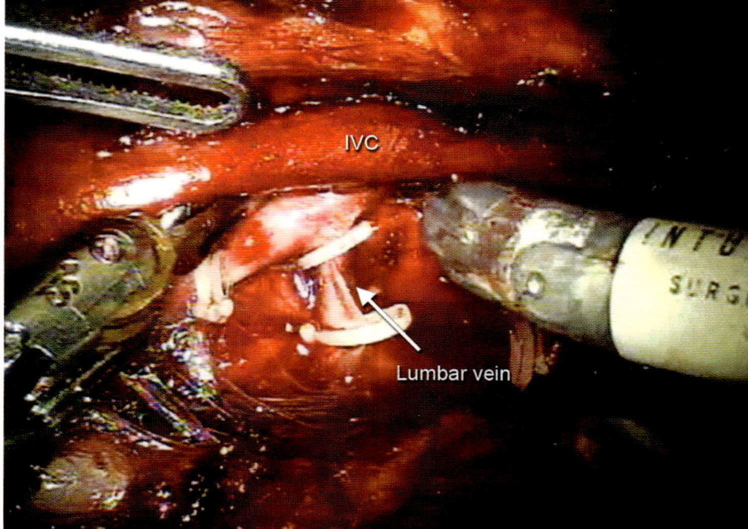

Fig. 12: The medial and posterior aspect of the vena cava is mobilized where additional lumbar vessels are identified and clipped/divided

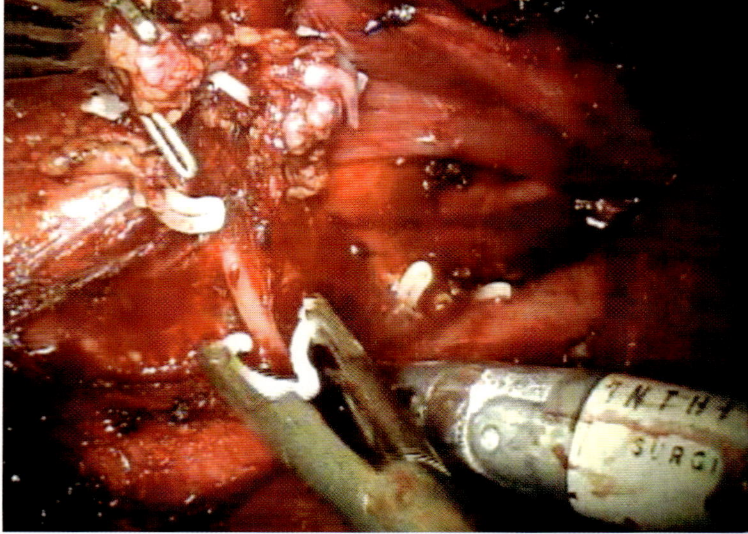

Fig. 13: Arterial lumbar vessels and lymphatics on the medial aspect of the aorta are clipped to provide additional mobility from the aorta to expose the anterior spinous ligament posteriorly

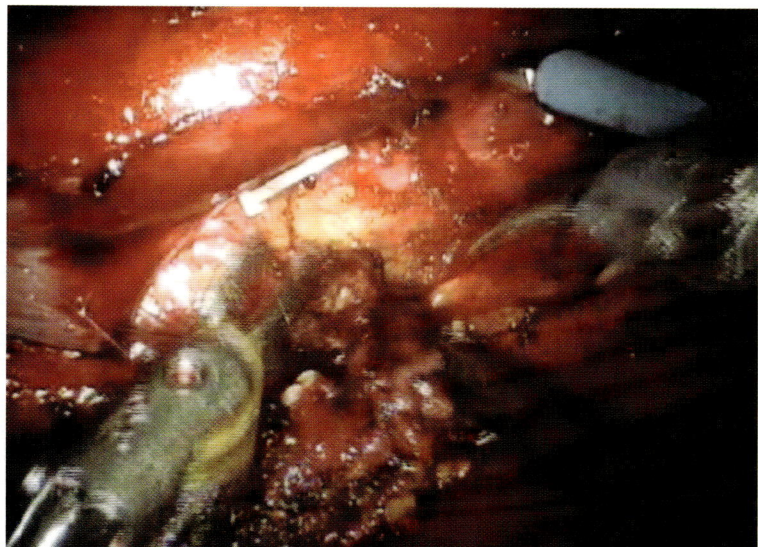

Fig. 14: The assistant provides countertraction laterally on the vena cava to expose the psoas muscle and anterior spin out ligament and free up any remaining attachments to the interaortocaval lymph node packet. The combination of gravity and active retraction by either the fourth arm of the robot or assistant allows complete exposure of the aorta and left common iliac vessels

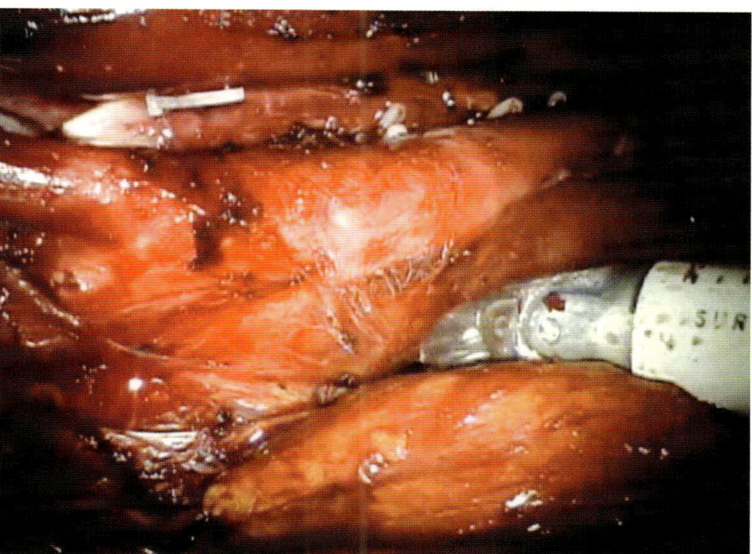

Fig. 15: The preaortics are dissected from the anterior aspect of the aorta from the crossing of the left renal vein cephalad to the insertion of the inferior mesenteric artery and then down the medial aspect of the aorta to the right common iliac artery

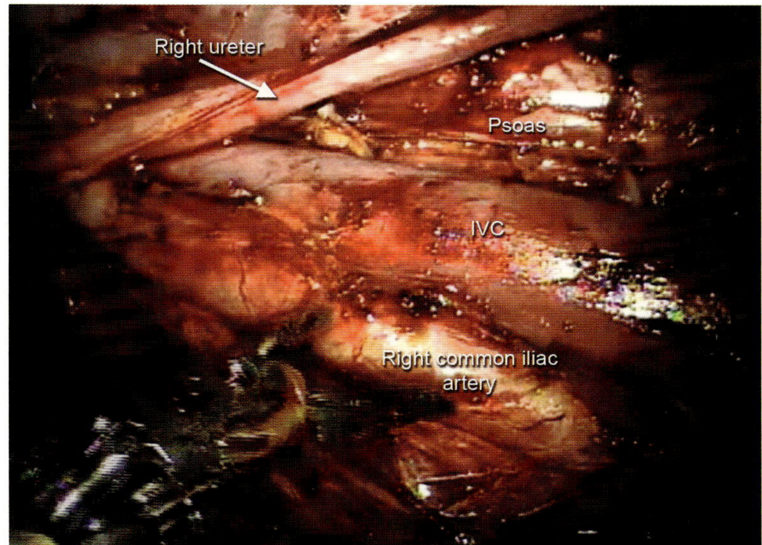

Fig. 16: The right common iliac artery crossing on top of the anterior vena cava is seen to be free of any lymphatic tissue down to the crossing of the ipsilateral ureter

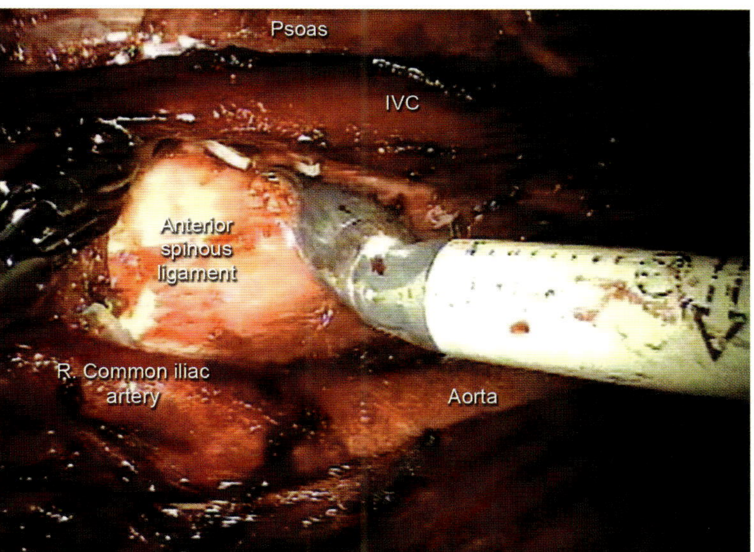

Fig. 17: Upon complete resection of the corresponding lymph node template, the anterior spinous ligament and fascia covering the psoas muscle are meticulously dissected free of lymphatic tissue, and the inferior vena cava (IVC) and abdominal aorta are reflected superiorly off the posterior abdominal wall to ensure complete dissection. Sympathetic chains can be easily identified and preserved. The authors avoid use of monopolar and judiciously use bipolar electrocautery to avoid thermal damage to these and adjacent structures

REFERENCES

1. Rassweiler JJ, Scheitlin W, Heidenreich A, et al. Laparoscopic retroperitoneal lymph node dissection: does it still have a role in the management of clinical stage I nonseminomatous testis cancer? A European perspective. Eur Urol. 2008;54(5):1004-15.
2. Davol P, Sumfest J, Rukstalis D. Robotic-assisted laparoscopic retroperitoneal lymph node dissection. Urology. 2006;67(1):199.
3. Williams SB, Lau CS, Josephson DY. Initial series of robot-assisted laparoscopic retroperitoneal lymph node dissection for clinical stage I nonseminomatous germ cell testicular cancer. Eur Urol. 2011;60(6):1299-302.
4. Krege S, Beyer J, Souchon R, et al. European consensus conference on diagnosis and treatment of germ cell cancer: a report of the second meeting of the European Germ Cell Cancer Consensus Group (EGCCCG): part I. Eur Urol. 2008;53(3):478-96.
5. Stephenson AJ, Bosl GJ, Motzer RJ, et al. Retroperitoneal lymph node dissection for nonseminomatous germ cell testicular cancer: impact of patient selection factors on outcome. J Clin Oncol. 2005;23(12):2781-8.
6. Fossa SD, Klepp O, Ous S, et al. Unilateral retroperitoneal lymph node dissection in patients with nonseminomatous testicular tumor in clinical stage I. Eur Urol. 1984;10(1):17-23.
7. Donohue JP, Zachary JM, Maynard BR. Distribution of nodal metastases in nonseminomatous testis cancer. J Urol. 1982;128(2):315-20.
8. Pizzocaro G, Guarneri A. Consequences of missed nodes during retroperitoneal lymph node dissection and how to avoid them. Eur Urol. 2009;8(5):470-7.

Chapter 22 Complications of Laparoscopic Urologic Surgery

Steve K Williams, Reza Ghavamian

INTRODUCTION

As laparoscopic skills have developed, urologists have been able to perform increasingly more complex urologic procedures previously thought only approachable by open surgery. Most of these procedures offer considerable advantages to patients, including low morbidity, less postoperative pain and shorter convalescence.[1] However, more complex laparoscopic procedures are intuitively associated with a greater risk of intraoperative complications. Fahlenkamp and colleagues reported their review of 2,400 laparoscopic cases and specifically evaluated the complications associated with these procedures.[2] They identified a complication rate of 4.4%, a reintervention rate of 0.8%, and a mortality rate of 0.08%. The authors also found that the complication rate increased in parallel with the difficulty of the procedure but was inversely related to the surgeon's experience. The complications unique to laparoscopic surgery include those related to creation of pneumoperitoneum, patient positioning, and from the surgical procedure itself. Understanding these potential complications and how to avoid them is the purpose of this chapter and is increasingly important for the surgeon.

CLASSIFICATION OF COMPLICATIONS

Standardization of complications in the urologic laparoscopic and robotic literature has been limited.[3] Inconsistent classification of complications makes a review on this topic difficult as most publications do not properly classify complications in a standardized manner. Vigilance for perioperative complications and the definition of a complication may vary among institutions and surgeons. There is still no standard reporting system and, as a result, the quality of complication reports in the surgical literature frequently is poor. Uniform reporting and grading of surgical complications via a standardized classification system may permit more meaningful comparisons among different medical centers and varying surgical techniques.[4] The Clavien complications schema has been recently described and has been used to assess quality outcomes related to disability.[5] This classification offers a convenient and reproducible metric with which to evaluate postoperative complications. This system is not without its limitations however. For example, intraoperative complications that are promptly identified and corrected without any deviation from the normal postoperative course are not graded in the Clavien classification system.

Another classification system in use is the National Cancer Institute Common Toxicity Criteria (NCI-CTC) and in some instances may be a more appropriate tool to assess and compare complications.[6] The NCI-CTC is a five-tiered complication scale for any potential adverse effect resultant from oncological treatment. In contrast to the Clavien scale, which is based on invasiveness of therapy, the NCI-CTC is an exhaustive list that tabulates the complication and then grades it according to specific criteria from one to five. Generally, the five grades represent mild, moderate, severe, life-threatening, and death. Despite their presence in the literature, neither complication classification system has become commonplace in the urological literature. It is imperative that the urologic community reports complications in the literature in a more standardized fashion in order to help further knowledge in improving the standard of care of our patients.

Pneumoperitoneum and Access-related Complications

The establishment of an adequate pneumoperitoneum is critical to successful laparoscopic surgery. Therefore, access-related complications are the first potential site for injury during laparoscopy. A large number of complications specific to laparoscopic surgery occur during access and creation of the pneumoperitoneum.[7] These complications include injuries of the major blood vessels, injuries of the visceral abdominal organs, gas embolism, pneumo-omentum, and subfascial insufflation. Major vascular injuries (MVI) are rare but once inflicted have a reported mortality rate of 15%. Access-related bowel or visceral injuries are relatively more common. Unlike MVI where the risk and presentation are immediate, many bowel injuries go unrecognized at the time of the procedure and may lead to major complications such as sepsis or peritonitis.[8] Overall, the initial phase of any laparoscopic procedure has a mortality rate varying from 0.05–0.2%.[9]

A number of clinical studies evaluated advantages and disadvantages of closed or open methods for the establishment of the pneumoperitoneum, but at present, there is no consensus regarding the best method of gaining access to the peritoneal cavity to create a pneumoperitoneum.[10] The decision to use the Veress needle or perform open Hasson cannulation to establish access is based on the surgeon's preference and individual experience. Open insertion is favorable, however, in the presence intra-abdominal adhesions from prior surgery. Presently, the Veress needle insertion is the most frequently used technique to create a pneumoperitoneum (Fig. 1). The site of insertion depends on the procedure and whether the site is approached trans- or retroperitoneally. To avoid the epigastric vessels, the site is generally located lateral to the rectus abdominus or just below the tip of the 12th rib, respectively, in upper renal tract laparoscopy. In pelvic laparoscopy, the site is para- or infraumbilical according to the type of approach.

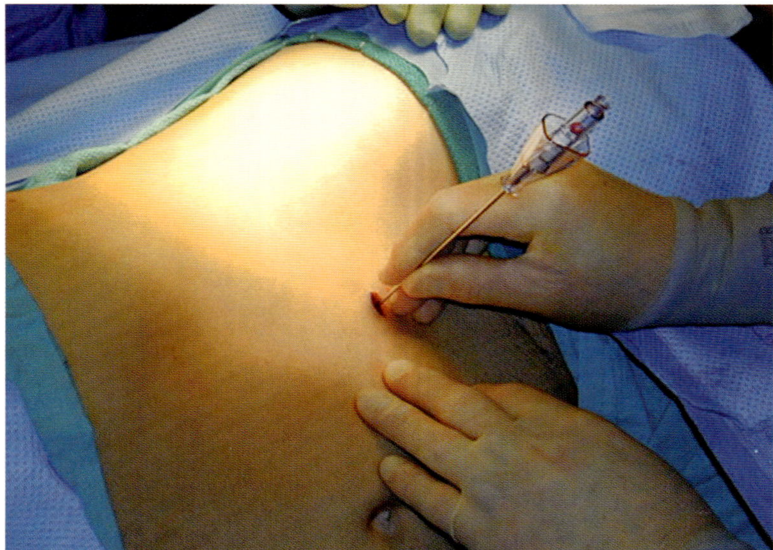

Fig. 1: Veress needle insertion

The Veress needle used to establish the pneumoperitoneum consists of a blunt-tipped, spring-loaded inner stylet and a sharp outer needle. With the Veress needle, appropriate use and placement are imperative to help minimize access injuries. While the needle is passing through the abdominal layers, the stylet retracts to allow penetration. The needle design allows tactile feedback as it passes through various layers of the abdominal wall. Once the peritoneum is entered, the lack of tissue resistance allows the blunt stylet to protrude, preventing perforation of abdominal structures. After initial aspiration to exclude blood or bowel content, various tests confirm the needle's intraperitoneal position (e.g. saline drop) prior to CO_2 insufflation. If appropriate intraperitoneal placement has been confirmed, CO_2 gas is then introduced via the port at the top of the Veress needle. Immediate insufflation pressure should not generally exceed 7–8 mm Hg at a low flow and should remain low as gas insufflates. In addition, visual evaluation of gas distribution is important to ensure proper placement, as uneven distribution of gas indicates preperitoneal placement. Many centers favor the Hasson technique.[11] A 1.5–2 cm skin incision is made, followed by sharp and blunt dissection to visualize the external fascia. The fascia is incised and muscle layers are split, revealing the transversalis fascia and peritoneum, which are grasped with hemostats and opened sharply. A finger is then inserted to confirm presence within the peritoneal cavity. The Hasson blunt tip cannula is then inserted and secured in position by fascial stay sutures, aiming to avoid any gas leak. A blunt tip balloon cannula can also be used.

Port-site related complications may be related to patient and surgeon factors as well as port design. Patient factors include obesity and previous abdominal surgery in the area of interest. The majority of complications related to insufflation are of minimal significance and are usually due to incorrect Veress needle placement. Subcutaneous emphysema may occur secondary to Veress needle placement above the abdominal fascia or carbon dioxide leakage around the trocar ports. It may be diagnosed by palpating crepitus over the abdominal wall. No specific intervention is usually required, and it resolves quickly once the pneumoperitoneum is discontinued. Extensive subcutaneous emphysema may, in rare instances, lead to a pneumothorax, pneumomediastinum, and hypercarbia.[12] If crepitus is palpated extending up the chest wall to the neck, the laparoscopic procedure should be stopped as gas in the subcutaneous tissues can track upward into the neck and then course down into the mediastinum.[13] An undetected pneumothorax or pneumomediastinum and should be evacuated via either a 16-gauge needle placed into the second intercostal space at the midclavicular line or by a tube thoracostomy performed.

In most cases, except with MVI, Veress needle injuries usually heal with conservative management, whereas trocar injuries generally require formal repair. The incidence of MVI from trocars and Veress needles averages around 0.1%.[14] Although these catastrophic injuries are rare, they represent a major reason for mortality from laparoscopic procedures, a major reason for conversion to open procedures, and a significant source of the morbidity associated with any laparoscopic procedure. Approximately 75% of MVI associated with laparoscopy occur while obtaining access and are associated with an 81% mortality rate.[15] The most common vascular injury caused by trocar or Veress needle insertion is damage to the inferior epigastric artery.[16] Kavoussi et al. reported 10 (2.7%) trocar-related injuries in 372 patients undergoing laparoscopic pelvic lymph node dissection.[17] Four of these injuries were laceration of the epigastric vessels and two were due to injury of superficial abdominal wall vessels. The inferior epigastric artery is at risk during initial entrance to the abdomen and during procedures that need a lateral trocar placed. If the inferior epigastric artery is punctured, it can often be easily tamponaded with the cannula. If necessary, a Foley catheter can be passed through the port-site and drawn back to tamponade the vessel. Full thickness sutures may be required for more significant bleeding. Since all subsequent trocars are inserted under direct visualization, it is only the primary trocar and the Veress needle that typically cause such injuries.

In an attempt to overcome some of the risks, trocars have undergone steady improvement, and new techniques for access to the peritoneal cavity have been devised. The main breakthroughs in this search for greater safety have been the development of a protective sleeve for trocars, blunt-tipped trocars, Veress needles, and optical trocars that allow direct recognition of each layer of the abdominal wall during access to the peritoneal cavity.[18] Direct view trocars were designed to avoid injuries by allowing the surgeon to see the tissues as the trocar passes through them. However, MVI and even deaths have been reported to the FDA using these devices. Devices that help control axial force needed to penetrate the trocars have been developed. The most widely studied device uses an expandable sheath that neutralizes the axial force by countertraction on its outer flange. A cone-shaped dilator is pushed through the sheath while forward movement is controlled by the surgeon's non-dominant hand. The sheath stretches and pushes away blood vessels and leaves a smaller wound. Whichever technique is utilized, it is now clear that without a meticulous and cautious technique, none of these safety devices can eliminate the risk of a MVI.[19] Other precautions employed to minimize the risk of injury during initial access include inspection and palpation of the abdomen before placing ports, with avoidance of prior scars or palpable masses. Placement of a nasal or oral gastric tube and Foley catheter before obtaining access may help to minimize hollow organ injuries. Introducing the Veress needle at a 45° angle from the plane of the patient's spine in very thin patients to avoid the aorta while in obese patients, this angle must be increased to as much as 80–90°. In patients who are not obese, a steeper angle is associated with retroperitoneal injury and a shallower angle with preperitoneal placement and subcutaneous insufflation.[16] Very thin patients are potentially at risk of trocar-related injury, mainly with the primary port, as adjacent organs and major vessels are much closer to the abdominal wall. The distance from the skin to the major vessels in thin patients may also be increased by applying traction to the anterior abdominal wall with a forceps.[20]

The Hasson technique should be considered whenever concern exists about injury, particularly if prior scars are present. Access should be obtained away from the quadrant with scars. Once the first port is placed and the abdomen is insufflated, additional ports should be placed only under vision taking care to avoid visible superficial veins, while using surface anatomic landmarks to avoid major vessels. Lateral trocars should be placed lateral to the rectus sheath, and above, the internal ring should minimize the injury to the epigastric vessels.

The incidence of visceral injuries in urological laparoscopy related purely to port placement has not been reported. Reports from the nonurologic literature suggest the reported incidence rate of injury to visceral structures including the alimentary tract, liver, omentum, bladder, uterus, pancreas and ureters of between 0.06–0.12%.[15] Approximately 40% of the iatrogenic bowel injuries reported during laparoscopy were access-related and caused by either a trocar or a Veress needle. These injuries are more likely to occur in patients who have had prior abdominal operations or adhesions to the abdominal wall. The retroperitoneal approach is associated with less visceral injury than is the transabdominal approach, but it does not eliminate this possibility.[21] Many of these injuries are unrecognized at the time of laparoscopy and result in postoperative ileus and peritonitis. Most injuries if recognized intraoperatively are treated with either a conversion or a laparotomy, but laparoscopic repair of the bowel or bladder if the injury is well-visualized is more frequently being applied.[22] It is essential to note that through-and-through injuries may occur that include the back wall of the vessel or bowel and that may not be appreciated laparoscopically. If the bowel or bladder is punctured with the Veress needle, it generally does not require a laparotomy due to the small caliber of the needle. Missed injuries may present postoperatively with persistent pain, drainage from a trocar site, fever, or peritonitis. Rapid radiographic evaluation and surgical exploration are essential because delay in diagnosis will increase the risk of mortality. To reduce the possibility of visceral organ damage, the surgeon should avoid areas where adhesions or scars may exist from previous surgeries.

Positioning Injuries

Proper patient positioning is an often-overlooked, yet critical part of any surgical procedure. It is important that the laparoscopic surgeon be aware of the potential for injuries to occur as a result of patient positioning required for certain laparoscopic approaches. Optimal positioning allows for adequate exposure and access during the case and minimizes the risk of iatrogenic injuries, including peripheral nerve damage and compartment syndrome. Stationary positioning of the patient over long periods of time may place the patient at risk for neurapraxia, rhabdomyolysis, compartment syndrome, and pressure ulcers. Neuromuscular injuries are among the most commonly reported complications after laparoscopic urologic surgery.

Nerve Injuries

Injuries to the nerves of the upper and lower extremities are uncommon but potentially avoidable complications during laparoscopic surgery. A large retrospective study during a 10-year period at a single institution revealed that urologic procedures accounted for 15% of all cases and 13% of the peripheral nerve injuries.[23] Focal compression or stretch injury can lead to elevated intraneural venous pressures, resulting in endoneural edema and impaired axoplasmic transmission. For mild insults, the conduction block may last only a few minutes while more prolonged injuries may lead to Schwann cell damage and demyelination, taking hours to weeks to reverse. More severe injuries can cause axonal loss and/or Wallerian degeneration, causing conduction delay or cessation, depending on the extent of the axonal loss.

The brachial plexus and ulnar and median nerves are the upper extremity nerves most commonly at risk. The brachial plexus is a complex system of nerve roots, trunks, divisions, cords, and branches originating from the anterior nerve roots of C5-T1. Stretch injury to the lower roots of the brachial plexus (C8 and T1) can occur when the arms are abducted on arm boards.[24] This results in a trunk-to-arm angle greater than 90° results in stretch and compression of the brachial plexus between the first rib and the clavicle. The upper roots of the brachial plexus (C5-C7) can be stretched by the use of steep Trendelenburg position, especially when the arm is extended on an arm board.[25] In steep Trendelenburg position, the brachial plexus can be stretched as the body slides cephalad in relation to the arms. Shoulder supports, used to prevent sliding during steep Trendelenburg position, appear to increase the risk of brachial plexus injuries, especially when the arms are extended. The patient may complain of pain, numbness, tingling, or decreased strength as a result of the injured nerve.[26] To minimize the risk of brachial plexus injuries during laparoscopy, the arms should be tucked at the side of the patient. If the arms are extended on arm boards, they should be abducted less than 90°. Both steep Trendelenburg position with the arms extended and shoulder braces should be avoided.

Treatment varies by the symptoms. Patients with postoperative numbness without discomfort can be treated with reassurance alone. Patients who develop motor deficits after laparoscopic surgery require early neurological consultation. Physical therapy should be instituted for muscle weakness. Pain typically responds to non-narcotic analgesics, particularly those used to treat neuralgia, such as gabapentin. The prognosis for position-related nerve injuries resulting in motor deficits is guarded. After such nerve injuries, it can take 10 weeks or more to achieve full recovery of motor function.[27]

Rhabdomyolysis

Rhabdomyolysis results from prolonged pressure to skeletal muscles leading to muscle ischemia, edema, compartment syndrome (Fig. 2), and subsequent muscle necrosis. The tissue necrosis causes metabolic acidosis, and myoglobin is released from the necrotic muscle. High levels of myoglobin in the blood may cause renal tubular obstruction with subsequent acute renal failure requiring temporary or even long-term dialysis. Procedures like laparoscopic nephrectomy (LN), during which patients are placed in the lateral decubitus position, often for long periods, are particularly associated with rhabdomyolysis.[28] Prompt diagnosis is essential for the successful treatment of this potentially debilitating complication. Clinically, the patient may describe severe pain postoperatively in the area of ischemia, such as the legs, or in the dependent flank and gluteal area for patients in the lateral decubitus position.[29] The patient may have dark urine which may look like hematuria. Laboratory testing reveals an elevated level of myoglobin and an elevated serum creatinine phosphokinase. As soon as rhabdomyolysis is suspected, aggressive hydration, diuresis, and urinary alkalization should be initiated. It is important to monitor

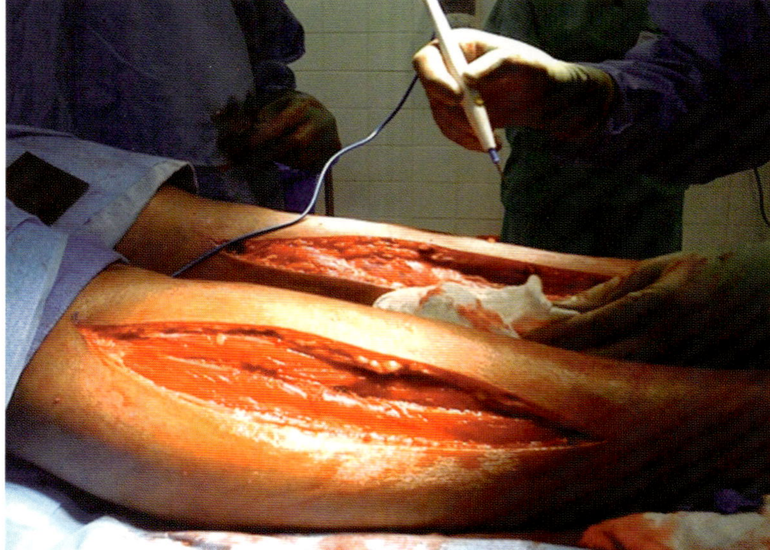

Fig. 2: Fasciotomy performed for compartment syndrome
Courtesy: Raju Thomas

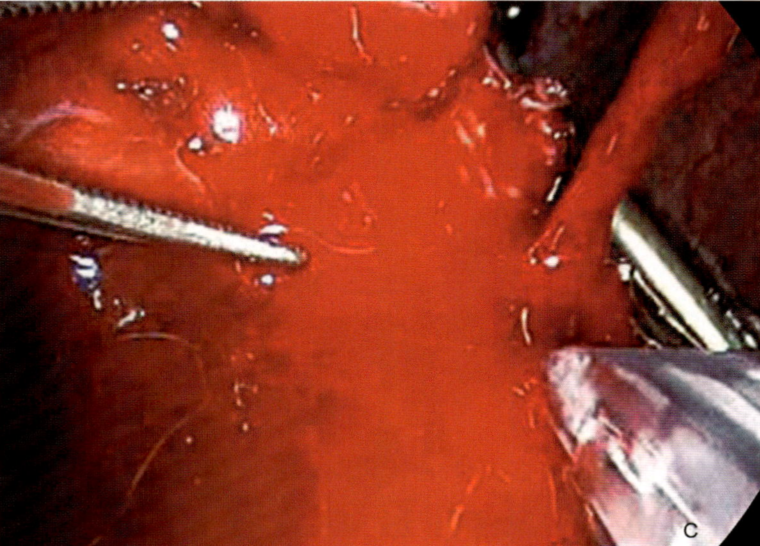

Fig. 3: Major vessel injury

the patient's serum electrolytes actively, including creatinine and potassium, to ensure adequate renal function because hemodialysis may be indicated. A review of postoperative rhabdomyolytic acute renal failure (ARF) case reports suggests several risk factors for this serious complication.[30] These include pre-existing renal disease, obesity, the lateral decubitus position, use of the kidney rest, length of procedure, and extracellular volume depletion/renal hypoperfusion.

Vascular Injuries

Hemorrhagic complications can occur in laparoscopic surgery during the early maneuvers required to enter the peritoneal cavity, or during the surgical dissection required for the specific procedure (Fig. 3). Vascular injuries are the most commonly reported injuries occurring during urologic laparoscopy, occurring in approximately 1.6–4.7% of cases.[31,32] Colombo et al. reviewed 1,867 laparoscopic cases performed for urologic malignancy.[33] The most common intraoperative complication was hemorrhage occurring in 2.3% of patients. Postoperatively, hemorrhage was again the most common complication occurring in 2.7% of patients. Overall, intraoperative and postoperative hemorrhage accounted for 40% of all perioperative complications. Similarly, Permpongkosol et al. reviewed complications in 2,775 laparoscopic urologic procedures and found that the two most common complications were intraoperative vascular injuries (1.98%) and postoperative bleeding requiring blood transfusion (1.76%).[34] In contrast, vascular injury in nonurologic literature appears to be less frequent with rates as low as 0.05–0.9%.[21] The majority of vascular injuries in urologic laparoscopy are dissection injuries, as urologic laparoscopic procedures such as nephrectomy require much more dissection around major vascular structures. They require isolation, clamping and reconstruction of the kidney in the case of partial nephrectomy, a parenchymous organ with a rich blood supply. In contrast, the bulk of the vascular complications in the nonurologic literature are trocar-related injuries.[35] Up to 75% of retroperitoneal vessel injuries at laparoscopy occur during blind placement of the Veress needle or primary trocar through a periumbilical incision.[36] Major vessel injury can also occur during placement of secondary ports or during the operative portion of laparoscopy, in particular when the procedure involves retroperitoneal dissection.

Intraoperative Vascular Complications

It is essential that the laparoscopic surgeon have a thorough knowledge of anatomy relevant to the safe performance of the surgical procedure in order to reduce the possibility of inadvertent vascular injuries. During traditional open surgery, sources of bleeding can be quickly controlled using forceps, clamps, or manual compression. While there have been numerous advances in laparoscopic instruments and improvements in suturing techniques, control of hemorrhage is more difficult in laparoscopic procedures. It is therefore essential that careful preoperative planning with review of all imaging for anomalous vasculature, that meticulous surgical technique be utilized and that the operating room staff be prepared for all eventualities. If a major vessel injury has occurred, conversion to laparotomy can be hampered by lack of preparation or proper equipment. Depending on the surgical facility at which the procedure is being performed, there can be wide variation in the availability of emergency equipment, personnel, blood products, and a surgeon experienced in vascular repair.

Major Vascular Injuries

Major vessels that lie in the retroperitoneal space of the lower abdomen and pelvis include the distal abdominal aorta, the vena cava, the common, external, and internal iliac arteries and the corresponding veins. Injuries to these great vessels are commonly referred to as MVI. In most patients, the aortic bifurcation is located just cephalad to the umbilicus; however, in thin patients, the aorta can lie immediately beneath the umbilicus (Fig. 4). The major veins lie posterior to their corresponding arteries in the lower abdomen and pelvis. It is critical that there is early recognition of any major vessel injury which occurs during the operative portion of laparoscopy. As soon as vascular injury is recognized, the surgeon must determine whether an attempt at controlling the injury laparoscopically is feasible or whether an open conversion would be the best approach.

The first step in the management of any major vascular injury once recognized is to alert anesthesia and nursing staff about the nature of the emergency. This allows the anesthesia team time to call for assistance, ensure adequate vascular access, increase intravenous hydration, and initiate cardiovascular resuscitation. Nursing staff

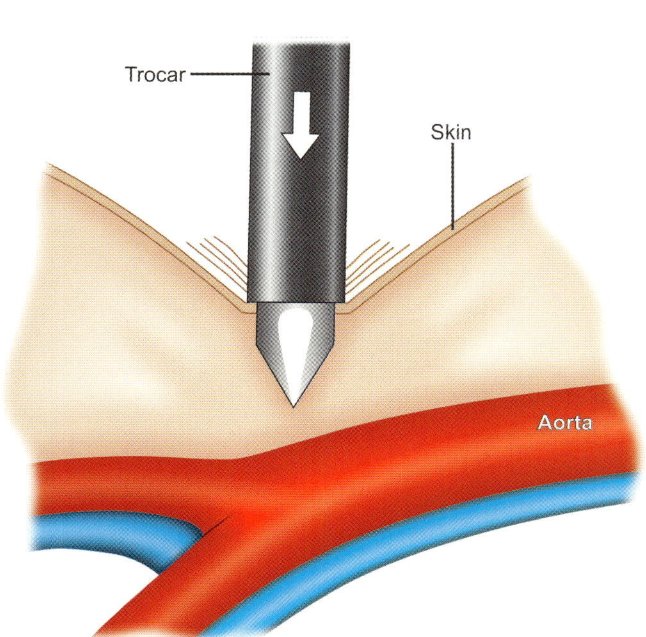

Fig. 4: Schematic demonstrating the relationship of the major vessels and the Veress needle during insertion

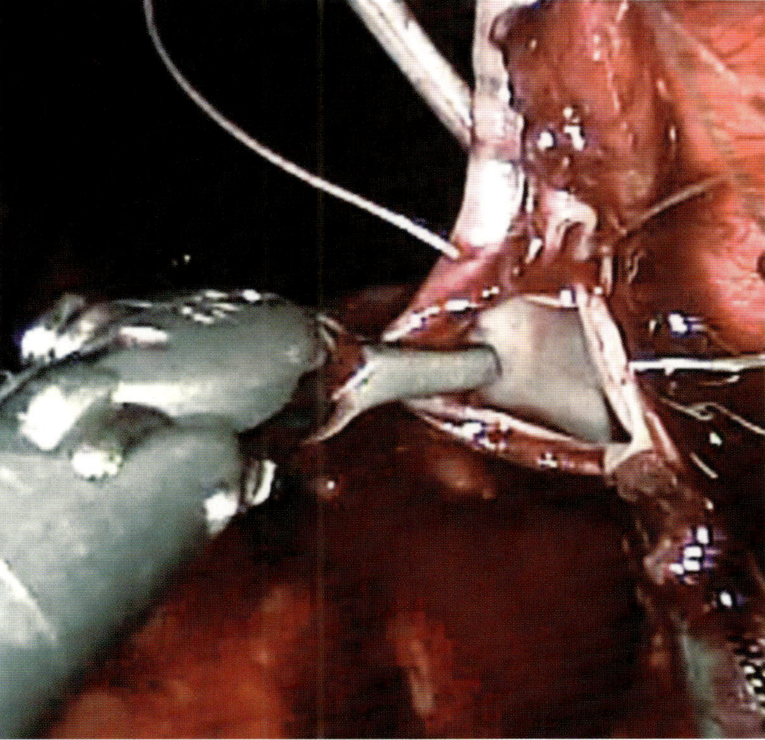

Fig. 5: Intraoperative repair of an iliac vein injury

may also obtain and open ancillary equipment, notify the blood bank to cross-match blood products, and call for assistance from a vascular or trauma surgeon if deemed necessary. The management of individual vascular injuries is best determined by taking the patient's anatomy and collateral circulation as well as the surgeon's experience into consideration. Laparoscopic repair of small injuries to major retroperitoneal veins has been reported, but should only be attempted by experienced laparoscopic surgeons experienced in such repairs (Fig. 5).[37] Adequate exposure is essential in this situation. The suction device is an excellent means of pressure application and exposure. A surgical sponge rolled into a trocar can be expeditiously applied to the bleeding site to get exposure,[35] then the need for additional ports can be assessed and repair attempted with the same principles as in open surgery. Aortic or large vena caval injuries are however rarely attempted laparoscopically and should be repaired at laparotomy.

If laparotomy is to be undertaken, various strategies may be employed by the surgeon to attempt to control or decrease blood loss as much as possible. For venous injuries, increasing insufflation pressure to 20 mm Hg may limit hemorrhage by a tamponading effect as the central venous pressure is normally 8 mm Hg.[38] In some cases, bleeding can be decreased during laparoscopy by applying pressure to the injury site with a laparoscopic Kitner, blunt grasper, or suction cannula.[39] When appropriate equipment is available, the laparoscopic surgeon should perform emergency laparotomy quickly but carefully. A midline incision is recommended for laparotomy as it enables better surgical exposure of the aortic bifurcation and vena cava, which can be important for definitive vascular repair or reconstruction. Injuries to major vessels such as the aorta, common iliac and external iliac should be repaired. If adequate collateral circulation exists, consideration can be given to ligating certain injured vessels such as the celiac axis and inferior mesenteric artery.[40] Superior mesenteric artery injuries are almost universally repaired as its collateral circulation cannot be relied upon. Superior mesenteric trunk injuries have been reported after laparoscopic radical nephrectomy and can lead to devastating outcomes.

Blood Loss in Special Situations

Radical Prostatectomy

Vascular injury has been reported to be a serious complication leading to surgical conversion in laparoscopic prostatectomy series. Hemorrhage requiring blood transfusion occurs more frequently during the learning curve. Reported transfusion rates during the first 100 cases are approximately 18%, but this rate falls to about 6% in more experienced surgeons.[41,42] The main sites of bleeding during laparoscopic prostatectomy are from the dorsal venous complex and inferior epigastric artery. The authors suture the dorsal venous complex with 2-0 or 3-0 vicryl. Occasionally, the suture on the dorsal venous complex may be loose and may cause gradual oozing. By increasing the pneumoperitoneum to 20 mm Hg, it is possible to slow down or stop the bleeding and allow time for appropriate suture repair. In other instances, the 4th arm may be used to clamp the bleeding vessel while the needle holders and sutures are readied for final repair. Injuries may also occur to the external iliac vein particularly during pelvic lymphadenectomy. Even large lacerations of the external iliac vein may be managed by suture repair robotically in expert hands. This is because flow through the vein is sequential and it is decompressed with pneumoperitoneum. At the time of injury, increasing insufflation pressure and temporarily turning off the sequential compression devices on the legs can decrease bleeding and help the repair. The 4th arm and one of the dissecting robotic arms can be used to gain control while the suture is prepared. The repair is then carried out under optimal control. At the end of the repair, the sequential devices are turned on and the pneumoperitoneum is decreased.

Laparoscopic Partial Nephrectomy

Laparoscopic partial nephrectomy (LPN) is a complex procedure which requires transection of multiple blood vessels during renal incision, the need for intracorporeal suturing and bolstering. Bleeding may occur intraoperatively, immediately postoperatively, and at a delayed interval up to several days or weeks after the surgical procedure. It is essential that the operating surgeon be familiar with the renal vascular anatomy by reviewing good quality preoperative imaging. Intraoperative bleeding usually occurs from the cut renal parenchyma, but may also occur from the hilum if the vessels are not carefully dissected during exposure. Parenchymal bleeding during resection may be managed by clamping of the renal artery or vein. Brisk bleeding on renal incision despite clamping can indicate a missed renal artery. If brisk bleeding is noted with the venous clamp is in place, venous hypertension from continued arterial inflow should be suspected. Removal of the venous clamp can reduce bleeding in these instances. Cut renal vessels may be suture ligated with 4-0 absorbable sutures. Coagulative techniques such as with the argon beam coagulator are useful for sealing small transected blood vessels. Increasing the insufflation pressure generally provides adequate slowing of venous ooze to allow effective coagulation. If brisk bleeding occurs after removal of the arterial clamp, venous compression from twisting of the renal pedicle impairing venous outflow should be suspected. If the vein is not compromised, then suture repair of bleeding should be performed while one manually compresses the defect. Reclamping of the artery should be avoided because of the increased risk of ischemic injury following reperfusion.

Postoperative Complications

Vascular complications contribute to a large share of the early postoperative complications after laparoscopic surgery. In a report by Ramani et al. on LPNs, most of the hemorrhagic complications occurred postoperatively and after the patient was discharged.[43] In cases of immediate postoperative bleeding, initial management should be conservative with transfusion, bed rest, and serial monitoring of hematocrit. If multiple transfusions are required, the patient becomes hemodynamically unstable, or the hematocrit is not responsive to transfusion, angiography and selective embolization should be considered given the high likelihood of arteriovenous fistula or pseudoaneurysm (Figs 6 and 7). In this situation, embolization of all visible vessels in the resection bed should be performed even if they are not actively bleeding (Fig. 8). Singh et al. reported a 1.7% incidence of pseudoaneurysm formation after LPN.[44] These patients presented with delayed postoperative hemorrhage at a median of 12 days postoperatively. Arteriovenous fistulae and pseudoaneurysms form when proximate segmental arteries and veins are injured either during resection of renal masses or during suture repair of the parenchymal defect. The deeper the resection as is the case in endophytic tumors, the higher the probability of these complications.

Several measures can be used to decrease the chance of pseudoaneurysms. Careful inspection of the resection bed and ligation of segmental branches when possible can help. In deep tumor resections, the tumor crater should be inspected and in the event of multiple segmental arterial transections, a hemostatic running intracorporeal suture at the crater should be employed with precise needle passes. Sutures for parenchymal repair should not be placed too deeply to risk segmental branch injury. Careful inspection of the repair before laparoscopic exit is mandatory. When clinically suspected and in the scenario of a precipitous decline in the hematocrit, computerized tomography (CT) is indicated. A characteristic blush during the arterial phase is seen.

Urologic Injuries

The overall incidence of urinary tract injury following laparoscopy urologic surgery in large series is under 1%.[36] These injuries include injury to the ureter, urinary leaks after extirpative and reconstructive procedures, bladder injuries, and anastomotic leaks. It is critical to be aware that the initial trauma may go unnoticed (especially if due to cautery damage) and may present as postoperative fever, pain, emesis and nausea. Subsequent imaging will usually reveal a urinoma or hydronephrosis. In the preceding portion of this chapter, the authors attempted to identify the incidence, type, and etiology of some of the urologic complications seen in the performance of various laparoscopic urologic procedures.

Partial Nephrectomy

Laparoscopic partial nephrectomy has emerged as an acceptable alternative to open partial nephrectomy (OPN). LPN is a complex procedure due to the need for laparoscopic hilar vessel clamping and associated warm ischemia time and intracorporeal suturing. Urine leak is second only to hemorrhage in incidence as a complication that can occur after LPN. The reported incidence ranges across various series from 0.5% to a high of 21% for more complex renal tumors.[45,46] Ramani et al. recently reviewed the Cleveland Clinic's experience with complications following 200 LPNs and found an overall urologic complication rate of 9.4%.[46] There were no specific predictors on multivariate analysis. Urine leaks were noted to occur in 4.5% of cases, the majority of which were managed with a double-J ureteral stent (however CT-guided drainage was required for 1% of these). These complication rates were noted to be comparable with or improved

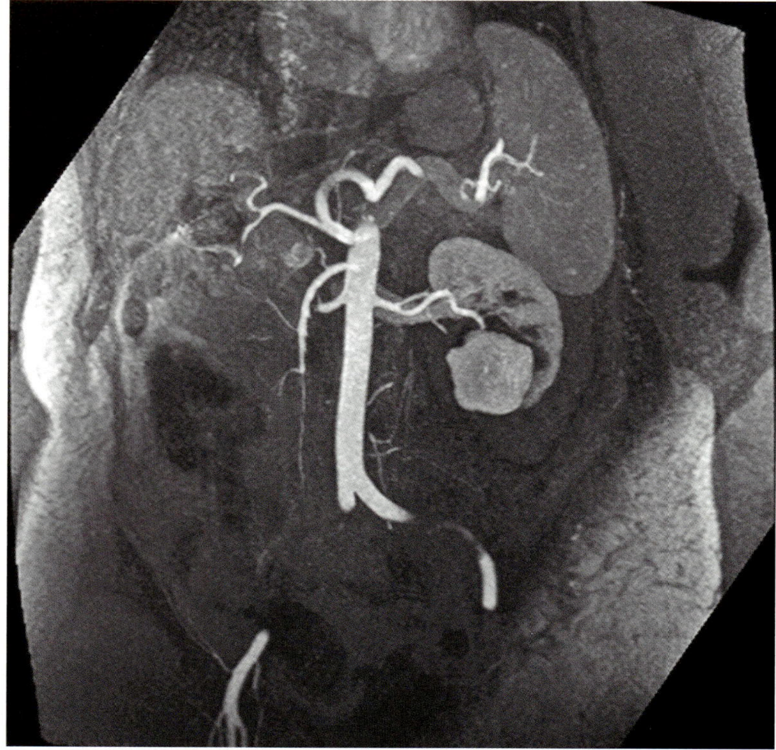

Fig. 6: CT angiogram demonstrating a large pseudoaneurysm
Courtesy: Michael Stifelman

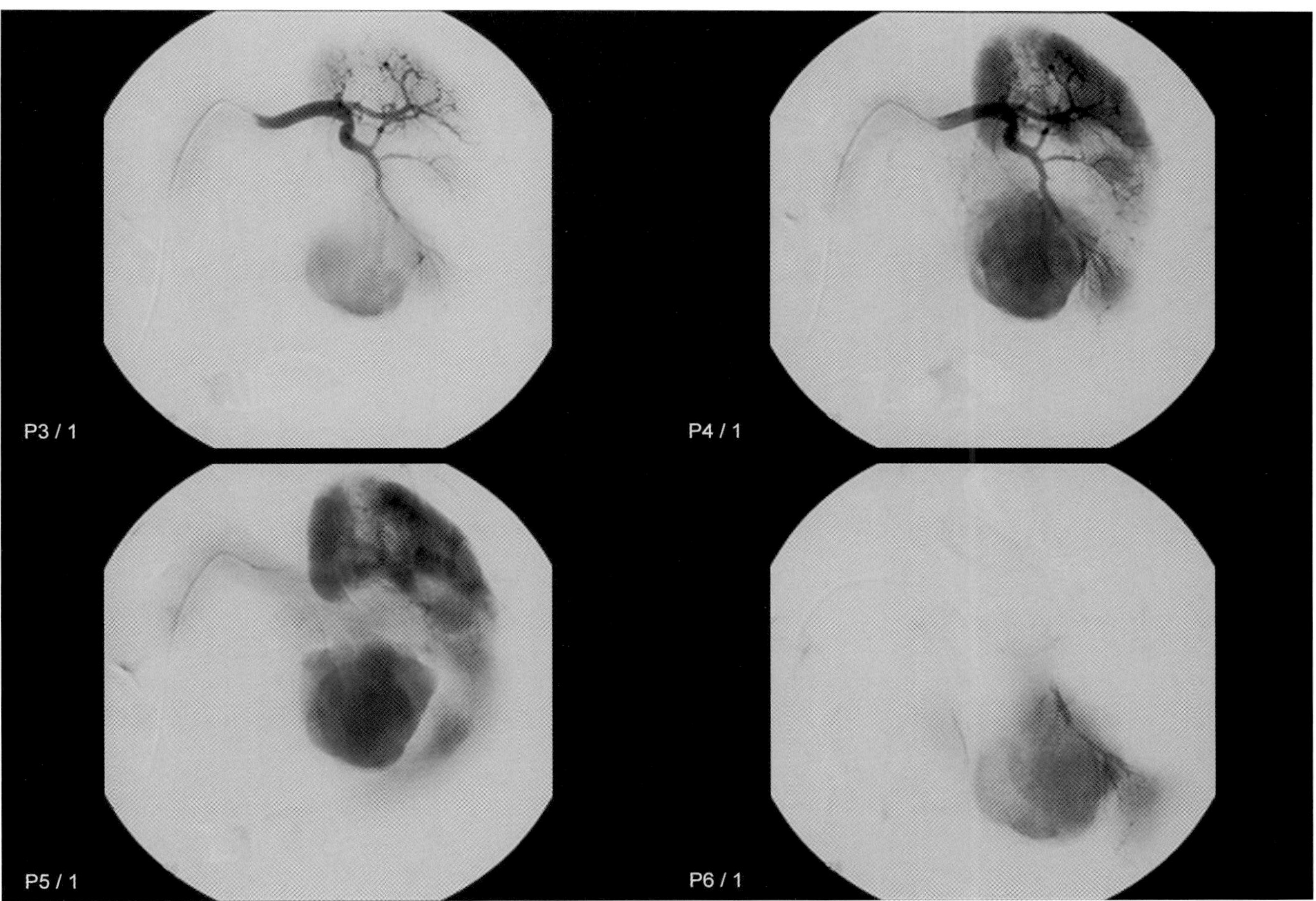

Fig. 7: Angiogram demonstrating a pseudoaneurysm formed after laparoscopic partial nephrectomy (LPN)
Courtesy: Michael Stifelman

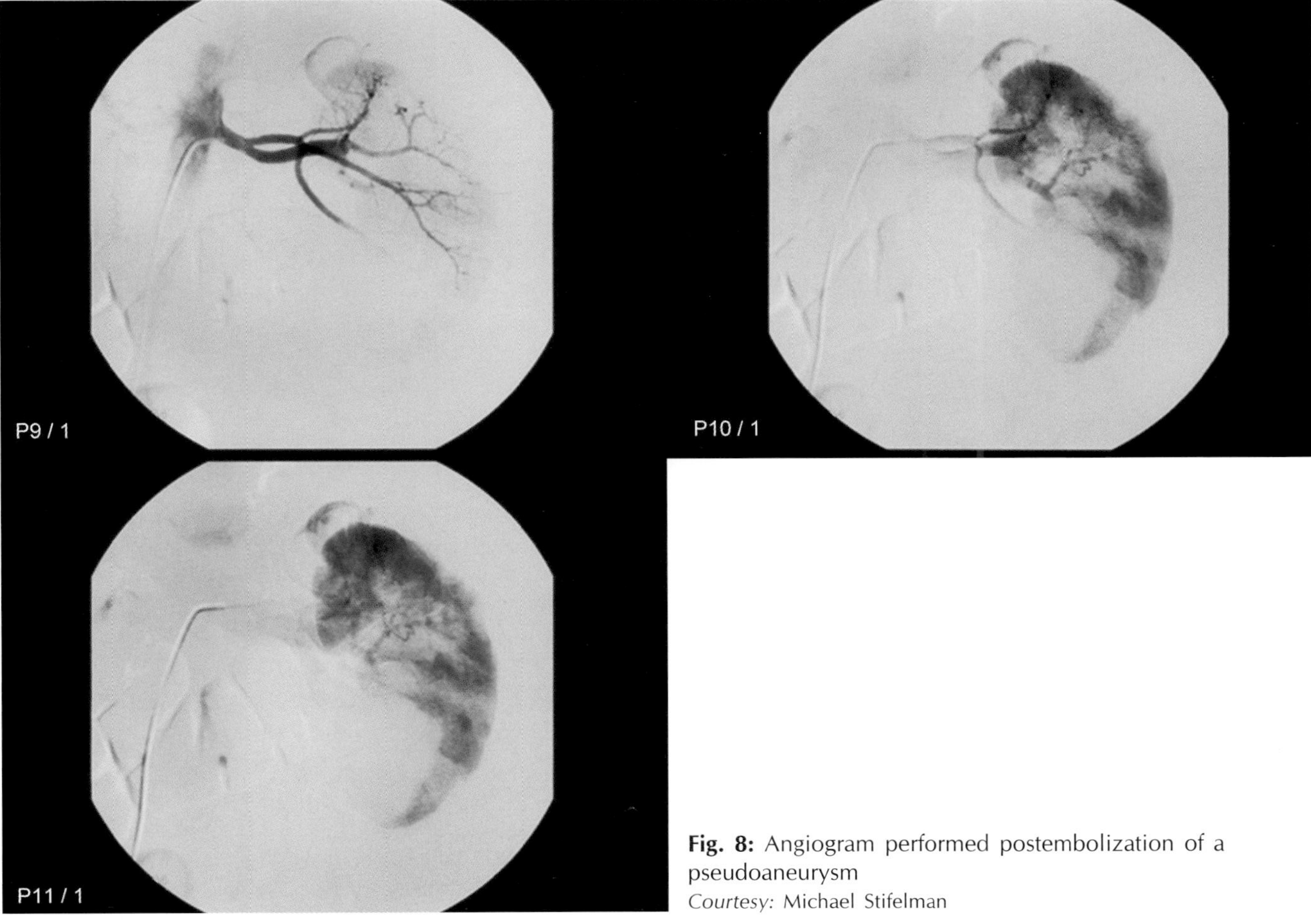

Fig. 8: Angiogram performed postembolization of a pseudoaneurysm
Courtesy: Michael Stifelman

compared with previously reported OPN complication rates. Others, however, have found increased leaks after larger tumors, endophytic masses, and those with collecting system entry.[46]

Renal leak after LPN may be diagnosed in the early or the delayed postoperative setting. In the early postoperative setting, the diagnosis is often made when increased drainage from the perirenal drain is noted. The fluid can be sent for creatinine, which will be markedly elevated and helps distinguish it from serous fluid. Some patients may also present with a low-grade postoperative fever and abdominal distention and/or ileus if the urine tracks into the peritoneum. Most small, nonobstructed renal leaks will resolve spontaneously. Delayed presentations may have a variable clinical picture. Again, if the operated kidney is not obstructed, most leaks tend to resolve spontaneously. If an obstruction is present, the patient may develop increased drainage or nephrocutaneous fistulas often through the drain incision site. This can be confirmed through sampling of the fluid for creatinine or administration of indigo carmine. The ideal imaging modality is an intravenous contrast CT scan with delayed imaging which will help delineate the etiology of the fluid collection (Fig. 9). Left alone, larger collections may form urinomas or abscesses, in which case the patient will often present with urinary tract infections, fevers, abdominal distention, nausea, vomiting, and potentially sepsis.

Generally, the management of renal leaks after LPN is similar at that after OPN. Most leaks can be managed conservatively, especially if the surgical drain remains in place. Many patients will require the drain for several days or even weeks in rare instances. Many surgeons will leave or reinsert a Foley catheter due to the theory that increased bladder pressures can lead to increased upper tract pressures, exacerbating the leak. Most patients who have failed conservative management can be managed with ureteral stent insertion. A retrograde pyelogram performed at the time of stent placement can help define the magnitude and location of the leak and its relation to the location of the drain. If stent insertion does not stop the leakage, the drain can be taken off suction. It should be noted that if the drain is close or abutting the fistula site, it will act as a siphon, keeping the fistula open even if the drain is off suction. In this scenario, the drain can be retracted incrementally. Patients with perinephric abscesses or large urinomas may need additional percutaneous drainage usually performed by interventional radiology.

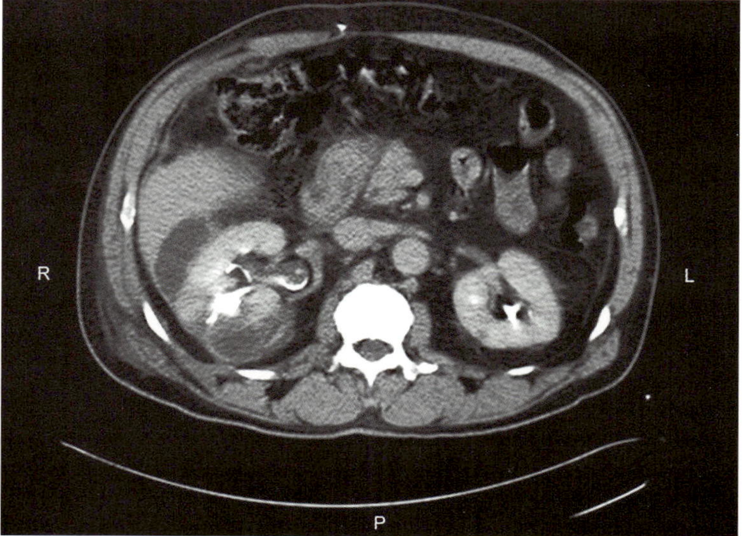

Fig. 9: Urine leak after laparoscopic partial nephrectomy (LPN). Note the extravasation of contrast outside the collecting system on the delayed images

Laparoscopic Pyeloplasty

Laparoscopic pyeloplasty (LP) is a complex procedure due to laparoscopic tailoring and suturing skills which are required. Success rates for reported laparoscopic series are excellent and have met or exceeded published open pyeloplasty results.[47] Urine leak area is rare, but well-documented complications following both open and laparoscopic pyeloplasties. Rassweiler and colleagues reviewed their series of 189 pyeloplasties and found an overall complication rate of 7.9% with a urinary complication rate of 3.1% including four urine leaks and two stent obstructions.[48] Early urine leaks after LP may be due to the use of interrupted sutures. Alternatively, it can occur in the setting of insufficient tension on the continuous suture or if the double-J stent is obstructed with clot or has migrated. The exchange of the JJ stent has to be performed using a hydrophilic guidewire to minimize the trauma on the anastomosis under fluoroscopic guidance. Urinary leakage may also occur after Foley catheter removal due to transmitted voiding pressures. If the drain has been removed already, it should be replaced percutaneously. For this reason, the authors routinely keep the drain in place upon withdrawal of the Foley catheter and strictly monitor output.[49] The management of urinary leakage postpyeloplasty is similar to LPN. Maximum drainage is the key, utilizing JJ stents, drains, and Foley catheter drainage. In refractory cases, nephroureteral or nephrostomy tube drainage can be employed.

Radical Prostatectomy

The true incidence of anastomotic leakage after radical prostatectomy (RP) is difficult to fully assess as there tends to be varying definitions. Clinically, patients with a significant prolonged urine leak may have a prolonged postoperative ileus, fever, an increase in surgical drain output. In more severe instances, patients may present with a complete anastomotic disruption, to urethrocutaneous fistula and urinary tract infection. They are also at long-term risk for development of bladder neck contractures which can lead to voiding difficulties and repeat incisions or dilatations. Quantifying anastomotic leakage after prostatectomy in asymptomatic patients is difficult as most patients are not routinely imaged upon catheter removal. In a novel study of robotic-assisted laparoscopic prostatectomy (RALP), Menon et al. retrospectively reviewed about 450 patients from 2004–2005.[50] Patients routinely underwent cystography 7 days after robotic prostatectomy, while the Foley catheter was still in place. A total of 67 leaks were identified (15.2%). About 60% of the leaks were small, extraperitoneal and confined to the surgical bed. Twenty-one patients had moderate sized leaks limited to the extraperitoneal space, 31% of all leaks or 4.2% of all patients. Six leaks were large, extending into the intraperitoneal space from the extraperitoneal space. Two of these six patients required CT-guided drainage for urinoma (< 0.5% of all patients). One patient had a colovesical fistula requiring revision.

A CT cystogram is critical in evaluation and delineation of the extent of the leak (Fig. 10). It is crucial to ensure that the Foley catheter is adequately draining, as an obstructed catheter can jeopardize the anastomosis. Mild traction should not be employed as it can cause ischemic changes and risk contractures. As with OPN, most anastomotic leaks following LRP or RALP can be managed conservatively with prolonged Foley catheterization and continued surgical drain placement. In cases in which the drain has been removed and the patient presents with a delayed leak, the urinoma if extensive has to be drained. Prolonged extensive leaks have been managed by placing the Foley catheters on suction or placing additional percutaneous drains. Almost all leaks will eventually seal

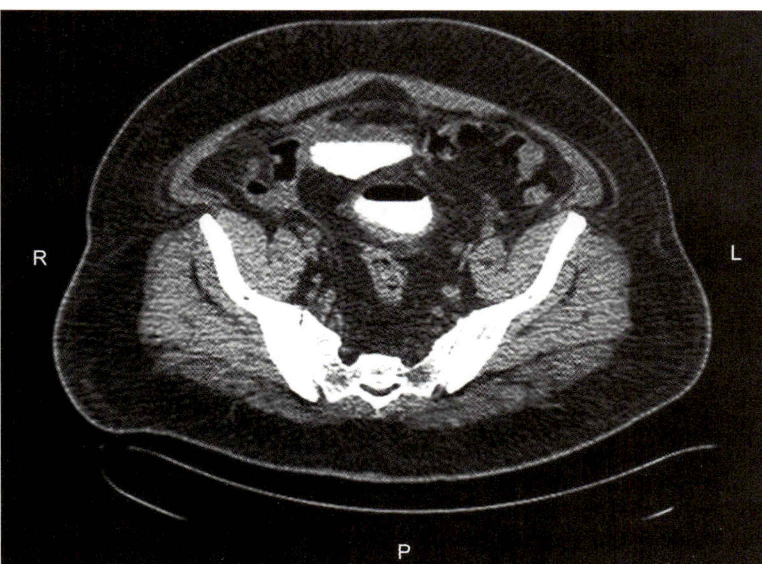

Fig. 10: CT cystogram demonstrating large urine leak

with conservative measures and optimal drainage. Rarely, and only in extreme circumstances, patients require surgical revision of the vesicourethral anastomosis.

CONCLUSION

The advantages of laparoscopic surgery stem from the enhanced surgical precision, miniaturization of the incision, diminished blood loss, reduced pain, and more rapid convalescence. Complications in laparoscopic urology are uncommon, but may have a delayed presentation with variable clinical outcomes resulting in a delay in diagnosis. It is imperative that the surgeon be aware of the various procedure specific complications as well as complications related to laparoscopy in general. Vascular injuries are rare but still comprise the most common major complications in urologic laparoscopy. Neuromuscular and positioning complications can occur as in any operation, with particular body habitus and other patient-related factors as contributors. Urinary complications may be avoided by water-tight intracorporeal suturing and awareness of surrounding structures in order to avoid these injuries. Careful preparation for serious but uncommon laparoscopic emergencies by both the facility and surgeon can be life-saving.

REFERENCES

1. Williams SK, Hoenig DM. Metabolic and Renal Complications and Immunologic Implications of Laparoscopic Urologic Surgery. In: Ghavamian R (Ed). Complications of Laparoscopic and Robotic Urologic Surgery. New York: Springer Science Business Media; 2010. pp. 19-33.
2. Fahlenkamp D, Rassweiler J, Fornara P, et al. Complications of laparoscopic procedures in urology: experience with 2,407 procedures at 4 German centers. J Urol. 1999;162:765-70.
3. Hakimi AA, Faleck DM, Sobey S, et al. Assessment of complication and functional outcome reporting in the minimally invasive prostatectomy literature from 2006 to the present. BJU Int. 2012;109:26-30. doi: 10.1111/j.1464-410X.2011.10591.x. Epub 2011 Sep 27.
4. Gonzalgo ML, Pavlovich CP, Trock BJ, et al. Classification and trends of perioperative morbidities following laparoscopic radical prostatectomy. J Urol. 2005;174:135-9.
5. Clavien PA, Sanabria JR, Strasberg SM. Proposed classification of complications of surgery with examples of utility in cholecystectomy. Surgery 1992;111:518-26.
6. Trotti A. The evolution and application of toxicity criteria. Semin Radiat Oncol. 2002;12:1-3.
7. Leron E, Piura B, Ohana E, et al. Delayed recognition of major vascular injury during laparoscopy. Eur J Obstet Gynecol Reprod Biol. 1998;79:91-3.
8. Soderstrom RM. Bowel injury litigation after laparoscopy. J Am Assoc Gynecol Laparosc. 1993;1:74-7.
9. Nuzzo G, Giuliante F, Tebala GD, et al. Routine use of open technique in laparoscopic operations. J Am Coll Surg. 1997;184:58-62.
10. Larobina M, Nottle P. Complete evidence regarding major vascular injuries during laparoscopic access. Surg Laparosc Endosc Percutan Tech. 2005;15:119-23.
11. Hasson HM. Open laparoscopy: a report of 150 cases. J Reprod Med. 1974;12:234-8.
12. Kent RB. Subcutaneous emphysema and hypercarbia following laparoscopic cholecystectomy. Arch Surg. 1991;126:1154-6.
13. Maunder RJ, Pierson DJ, Hudson LD. Subcutaneous and mediastinal emphysema. Pathophysiology, diagnosis, and management. Arch Intern Med. 1984;144:1447-53.
14. Geers J, Holden C. Major vascular injury as a complication of laparoscopic surgery: a report of three cases and review of the literature. Am Surg. 1996;62:377-9.
15. Bhoyrul S, Vierra MA, Nezhat CR, et al. Trocar injuries in laparoscopic surgery. J Am Coll Surg. 2001;192:677-83.
16. Champault G, Cazacu F, Taffinder N. Serious trocar accidents in laparoscopic surgery: a French survey of 103,852 operations. Surg Laparosc Endosc. 1996;6:367-70.
17. Kavoussi LR, Sosa E, Chandhoke P, et al. Complications of laparoscopic pelvic lymph node dissection. J Urol. 1993;149:322-5.
18. Schaller G, Kuenkel M, Manegold BC. The optical "Veress-needle"—initial puncture with a minioptic. Endosc Surg Allied Technol. 1995;3:55-7.
19. Fruhwirth J, Koch G, Mischinger HJ, et al. Vascular complications in minimally invasive surgery. Surg Laparosc Endosc. 1997;7:251-4.
20. Roviaro GC, Varoli F, Saguatti L, et al. Major vascular injuries in laparoscopic surgery. Surg Endosc. 2002;16:1192-6.
21. Debnath D. Bowel injury as a complication of laparoscopy (Br J Surg 2004; 91: 1253-1258). Br J Surg. 2004;91:1652.
22. Hung CF, Yang CK, Cheng CL, et al. Bowel complication during robotic-assisted laparoscopic radical prostatectomy. Anticancer Res. 2011;31:3497-501.
23. Welch MB, Brummett CM, Welch TD, et al. Perioperative peripheral nerve injuries: a retrospective study of 380,680 cases during a 10-year period at a single institution. Anesthesiology. 2009;111:490-7.
24. Romanowski L, Reich H, McGlynn F, et al. Brachial plexus neuropathies after advanced laparoscopic surgery. Fertil Steril. 1993;60:729-32.
25. Gagnon J, Poulin EC. Beware of the Trendelenburg position during prolonged laparoscopic procedures. Can J Surg. 1993;36:505-6.
26. Wolf JS, Marcovich R, Gill IS, et al. Survey of neuromuscular injuries to the patient and surgeon during urologic laparoscopic surgery. Urology. 2000;55:831-6.
27. Chan JK, Manetta A. Prevention of femoral nerve injuries in gynecologic surgery. Am J Obstet Gynecol. 2002;186:1-7.
28. Brown JA. Lateral gluteal myonecrosis in a patient undergoing partial nephrectomy in the modified flank position. Urology. 2003;61:462.
29. Kuang W, Ng CS, Matin S, et al. Rhabdomyolysis after laparoscopic donor nephrectomy. Urology. 2002;60:911.
30. Kozak KR, Shah S, Ishihara KK, et al. Hand-assisted laparoscopic radical nephrectomy-associated rhabdomyolysis with ARF. Am J Kidney Dis. 2003;41:E5.
31. Gill IS, Kavoussi LR, Clayman RV, et al. Complications of laparoscopic nephrectomy in 185 patients: a multi-institutional review. J Urol. 1995;154:479-83.
32. Siqueira TM, Kuo RL, Gardner TA, et al. Major complications in 213 laparoscopic nephrectomy cases: the Indianapolis experience. J Urol. 2002;168:1361-5.
33. Colombo JR, Haber GP, Jelovsek JE, et al. Complications of laparoscopic surgery for urological cancer: a single institution analysis. J Urol. 2007;178:786-91.
34. Permpongkosol S, Link RE, Su LM, et al. Complications of 2,775 urological laparoscopic procedures: 1993 to 2005. J Urol. 2007;177:580-5.

35. Tare D, Maria P, Ghavamian R. Vascular Complications in Laparoscopic and Robotic Urologic Surgery. In: Ghavamian R (Ed). Complications of Laparoscopic and Robotic Urologic Surgery. New York: Springer Science Business Media; 2010. pp. 45-58.
36. Makai G, Isaacson K. Complications of gynecologic laparoscopy. Clin Obstet Gynecol. 2009;52:401-11.
37. Nezhat C, Childers J, Nezhat F, et al. Major retroperitoneal vascular injury during laparoscopic surgery. Hum Reprod. 1997;12:480-3.
38. Meraney AM, Samee AA, Gill IS. Vascular and bowel complications during retroperitoneal laparoscopic surgery. J Urol. 2002;168:1941-4.
39. Nordestgaard AG, Bodily KC, Osborne RW, et al. Major vascular injuries during laparoscopic procedures. Am J Surg. 1995;169:543-5.
40. Asensio JA, Forno W, Roldan G, et al. Visceral vascular injuries. Surg Clin North Am. 2002;82:1-20.
41. Rassweiler J, Sentker L, Seemann O, et al. Laparoscopic radical prostatectomy with the Heilbronn technique: an analysis of the first 180 cases. J Urol. 2001;166:2101-8.
42. Guillonneau B, Rozet F, Cathelineau X, et al. Perioperative complications of laparoscopic radical prostatectomy: the Montsouris 3-year experience. J Urol. 2002;167:51-6.
43. Ramani AP, Desai MM, Steinberg AP, et al. Complications of laparoscopic partial nephrectomy in 200 cases. J Urol. 2005;173:42-7.
44. Singh D, Gill IS. Renal artery pseudoaneurysm following laparoscopic partial nephrectomy. J Urol. 2005;174:2256-9.
45. Simmons MN, Gill IS. Decreased complications of contemporary laparoscopic partial nephrectomy: use of a standardized reporting system. J Urol. 2007;177:2067-73; discussion 2073.
46. Campbell SC, Novick AC, Streem SB, et al. Complications of nephron sparing surgery for renal tumors. J Urol. 1994;151:1177-80.
47. Bauer JJ, Bishoff JT, Moore RG, et al. Laparoscopic versus open pyeloplasty: assessment of objective and subjective outcome. J Urol. 1999;162:692-5.
48. Rassweiler JJ, Teber D, Frede T. Complications of laparoscopic pyeloplasty. World J Urol. 2008;26:539-47.
49. Hakimi A, Ghavamian R. Urinary and Urologic Complications of Laparoscopic and Robotic Urologic Procedures. In: Reza Ghavamian (Ed). Complications of Laparoscopic and Robotic Urologic Surgery. New York: Springer Science Business Media; 2010. pp. 59-71.
50. Menon M, Shrivastava A, Kaul S, et al. Vattikuti Institute prostatectomy: contemporary technique and analysis of results. Eur Urol. 2007;51:648-57; discussion 657-8. Epub 2006 Nov 3.

23

Chapter

Laparoscopic Nephroureterectomy (With Robotic Distal Ureterectomy and Bladder Cuff Excision)

James S Rosoff, Michael B Marean, Joseph J Del Pizzo

INTRODUCTION

Upper tract urothelial carcinoma (UTUC) is relatively rare, representing only 5% of all urothelial malignancies.[1] Open nephroureterectomy (ONU) remains the gold standard for the treatment of UTUC, although other options include laparoscopic or endoscopic management. Endoscopic management can be considered in cases of low-grade disease in patients with a solitary kidney, poor renal function, or in patients who are poor surgical candidates. Distal ureterectomy with ureteral reimplant is a surgical alternative to nephroureterectomy that has been used in the management of isolated lesions in the distal ureter.

LAPAROSCOPIC NEPHROURETERECTOMY

Laparoscopic nephroureterectomy (LNU) was first described in 1991 by Clayman and colleagues,[2] and has become increasingly accepted as a feasible and effective alternative to ONU. LNU offers the advantages of decreased morbidity associated with minimally invasive surgery, while seemingly preserving oncological efficacy in the treatment of UTUC. Until recently, only short-term data confirmed the oncological equivalence of LNU and ONU. However, new data from the United Kingdom demonstrates similar oncological outcomes between ONU and LNU with a median follow-up of 13.6 years.[3] Previously, a group from the Cleveland Clinic reported oncological outcomes for 100 patients treated with LNU at a median follow-up of 7 years,[4] which appeared comparable to open surgery. A large, multi-institutional study showed no difference in cancer-specific survival between ONU and LNU at a median follow-up of 49 months.[5]

The data comparing LNU to ONU for high-grade, nonorgan confined disease is mixed. A small prospective randomized study of 80 patients showed oncological equivalence between ONU and LNU in patients with low-grade and organ confined disease, but a survival benefit with ONU for pT3 and high-grade tumors.[6] Conversely, a large multicenter study of 773 patients, well-matched for tumor stage and grade, with a median follow-up of 34 months, showed oncological equivalence between ONU and LNU.[7] As more long-term data emerge, LNU remains a favorable alternative to ONU, particularly in cases of organ-confined disease.

One concern regarding LNU frequently cited in the literature is the potential for port-site metastasis. A meta-analysis by Rassweiler et al. reported a 1.6% rate of port-site metastasis, but this was associated (in all cases) with the failure to use a specimen bag or rupture of the specimen bag during organ removal.[8] This highlights the importance of using an organ bag to remove the specimen en bloc in order to prevent tumor spillage.

In cases of both LNU and ONU, there are a variety of different techniques that can be used for the dissection of the distal ureter and bladder cuff. These include open, laparoscopic, robotic, or endoscopic techniques, as well as both intravesical and extravesical approaches. There is no clear consensus on the preferred technique for excision of the distal ureter and bladder cuff. However, many consider mid-to-distal ureteral tumors and coexistent bladder tumors contraindications to an endoscopic approach. That being said, what appears to be most important is that the surgeon adheres to the following oncological principles: avoid opening the urinary tract, avoid direct contact with the tumor, extract the specimen en bloc, and completely excise the intramural ureter and bladder cuff.[9,10]

A recent study by Li et al. compared intravesical, extravesical and transurethral techniques for bladder cuff excision during radical nephroureterectomy.[11] The transurethral technique used in this study was the "pluck" technique in which the ureteral orifice and intramural ureter are resected into the perivesical fat, also known as the transurethral resection of ureteral orifice (TURUO) technique. These authors found no significant differences in cancer-specific survival between the three groups, and no difference in bladder, local, or contralateral upper tract tumor recurrence.

Additional endoscopic or transurethral techniques include ureteral intussusception and cystoscopic unroofing with laparoscopic stapling. The laparoscopic stapling technique is appealing because it avoids opening the urinary tract and minimizes the theoretical risk of tumor spillage. However, laparoscopic stapling is associated with a significantly higher incidence of positive surgical margins (as high as 18–29% in certain studies) and greater local recurrence rates at the site of the resection scar.[10,12,13] It is thought that the stapling technique predisposes patients to positive surgical margins and local recurrence due to incomplete resection of the distal ureter.

A more recently developed technique is the robot-assisted extravesical excision of the distal ureter and bladder cuff. This surgical technique is highlighted in greater detail in the atlas below. The use of the robot offers the advantages of minimally invasive surgery with the possibility of an improved lymph node dissection as compared to a purely laparoscopic approach. To date, only a few case series have been published reporting on the use of the robotic approach. Preliminary results from Hu et al.[14] and Eandi et al.[15] are promising with equivalent short-term oncological outcomes to open or laparoscopic techniques, with median follow-up times of 16.2 months and 15.2 months, respectively.

The role of lymphadenectomy in UTUC remains a topic of controversy. Studies have found that 20–40% of patients with UTUC have lymph node metastasis at the time of diagnosis.[16-18] However, there are no standardized indications for extended lymphadenectomy and no standardized templates have come into widespread use. The landing zones for UTUC need to be better defined in order to develop an effective template for lymph node dissection. Given the lack of consensus on this matter, the steps for extended lymphadenectomy are not included in this chapter.

Instruments

Veress needle
5 mm and 12 mm trocars
5 mm laparoscope with 30° lens
Diamond-Flex liver retractor
Endo GIA™ stapler
Endo Catch™ specimen bag
Harmonic scalpel
Maryland dissector
Right angle dissector
Laparoscopic scissor
Titanium clips
daVinci® Surgical System robot

Procedure (Fig. 1)

1. Prior to the start of the procedure, a Foley catheter is placed under sterile conditions to decompress the bladder.
2. The patient is positioned in 45° flank position on the operating table with adequate padding for the brachial plexus, dependent hip, knees, and ankles. The lower leg is flexed while the upper leg is gently extended with a pillow placed between them. The table is then gently flexed to expose the flank.
3. Once the patient is prepped and draped, a Veress needle is introduced into the peritoneal space just lateral to the umbilicus. The abdomen is insufflated to 15 mm Hg. A 12 mm trocar is introduced into the abdomen at the site of the Veress needle and a 5 mm laparoscope with a 30° lens is introduced through the trocar into the peritoneal cavity. The abdominal contents are carefully inspected for any signs of injury.
4. Under direct vision, a 5 mm trocar is placed two finger breadths below the xiphoid process, just right or left of midline depending on the side of the kidney being removed. The laparoscope is then switched to this 5 mm trocar site. Another 5 mm trocar is then placed under direct vision along the midclavicular line, approximately 2 cm below the umbilicus. In the case of a right-sided nephroureterectomy, a fourth trocar, 5 mm, is placed along the anterior axillary line to assist in retracting the right lobe of the liver. Once the trocars have been placed, the laparoscope is returned to the 12 mm periumbilical port-site.

Once the port placement is completed, the laparoscopic nephrectomy portion of the procedure is performed in the standard fashion as discussed in the laparoscopic radical nephrectomy portion of this text. The following Figures 2 to 13 depict the key steps of the robotic distal ureterectomy portion of a right-sided laparoscopic/robotic nephroureterectomy.

Right Side

1. In a right-sided case, the right triangular ligament is incised while the liver is retracted medially and anteriorly with the assistance of a liver retractor. The coronary ligament is then opened in a lateral-to-medial direction.
2. The ascending colon is mobilized medially by incising the line of Toldt caudally down to the bifurcation of the iliac vessels
3. The hepatic flexure is gently lifted to identify the plane between Gerota's fascia and the mesocolon. Division of renocolic attachments improves mobilization of the ascending colon and provides access to the retroperitoneum.
4. The duodenum is identified and Kocherized to expose the inferior vena cava (IVC) and renal vein. The adventitia surrounding the IVC is lifted with a Maryland dissector and incised, providing better exposure of the vena cava and the renal vein.

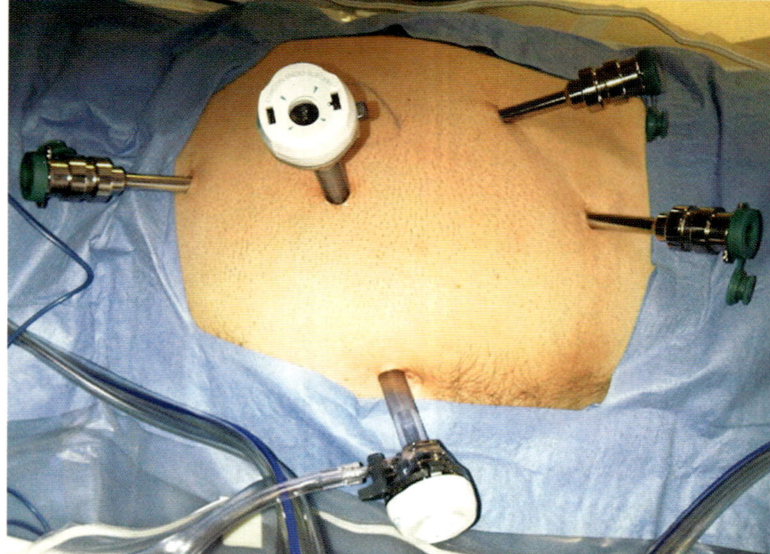

Fig. 1: Port placement for a left-sided robotic/laparoscopic nephroureterectomy. The patient's head is on the left side of the image. The nephrectomy portion of the case is often completed prior to the distal ureterectomy and is performed as a standard laparoscopic radical nephrectomy

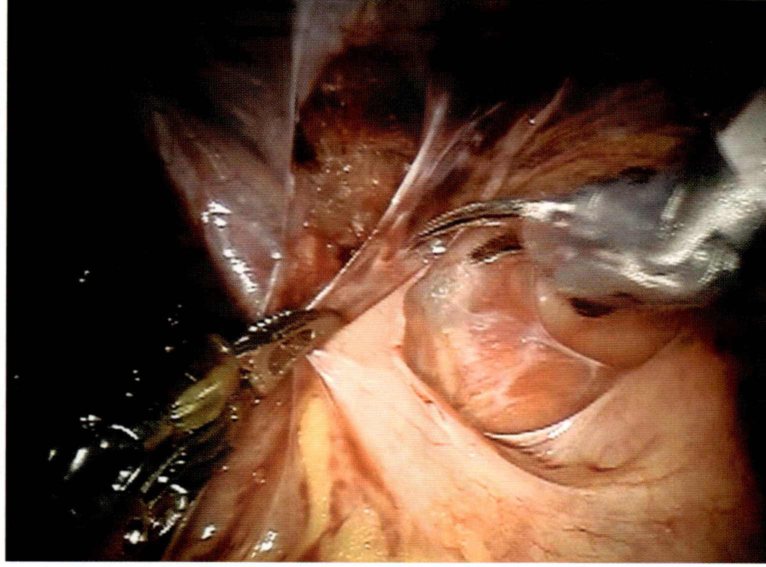

Fig. 2: First, any remaining colonic attachments are divided and the colon is reflected medially

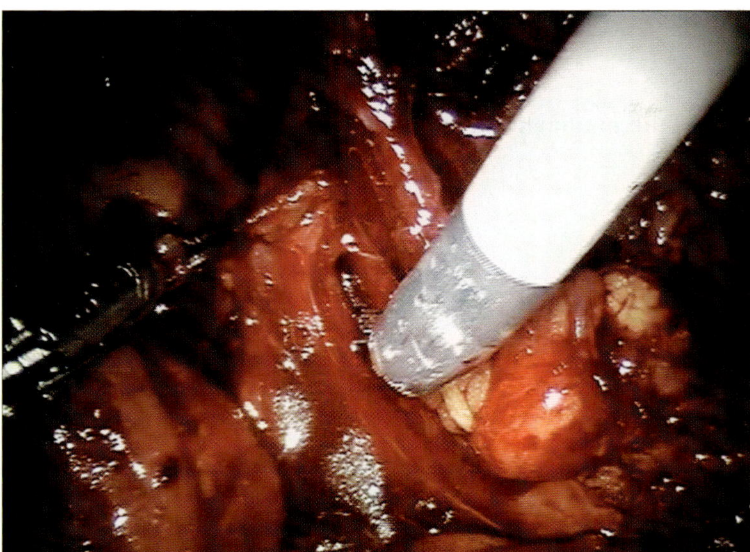

Fig. 3: The ureter is identified as it crosses the iliac vessels. A plane is developed between the vessels and the ureter

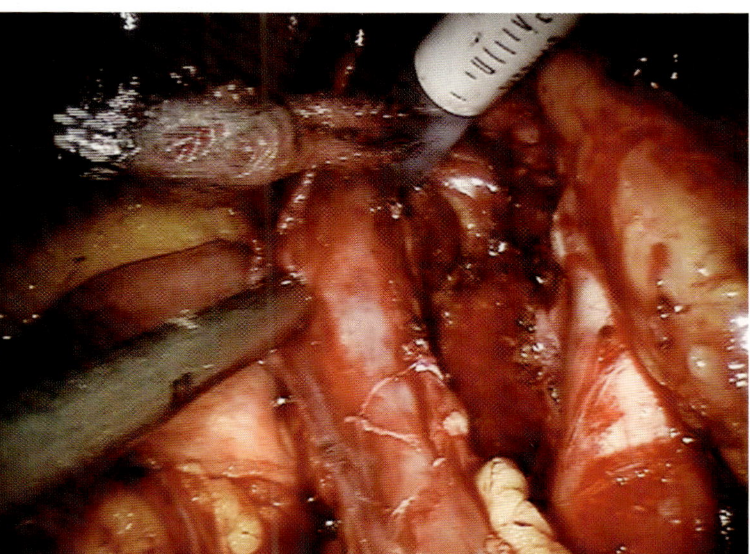

Fig. 4: The ureter is retracted medially as this plane is further developed and the dissection is carried distally

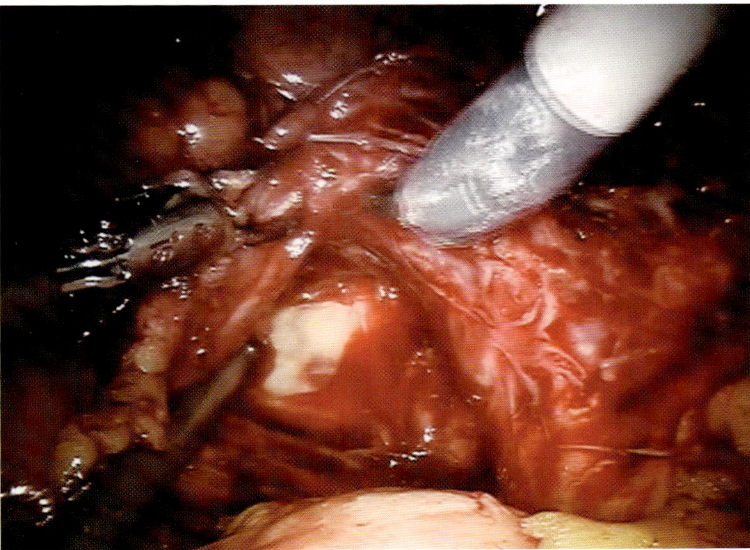

Fig. 5: The ureter is retracted medially and dissected free of the iliac vessels. Small perforating vessels are cauterized and divided

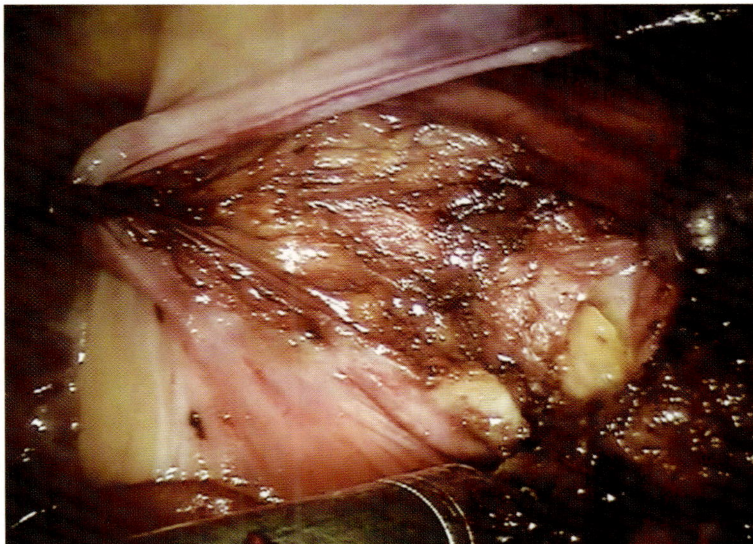

Fig. 6: The peritoneum is retracted medially to expose the ureteral hiatus as the dissection is carried down to the bladder

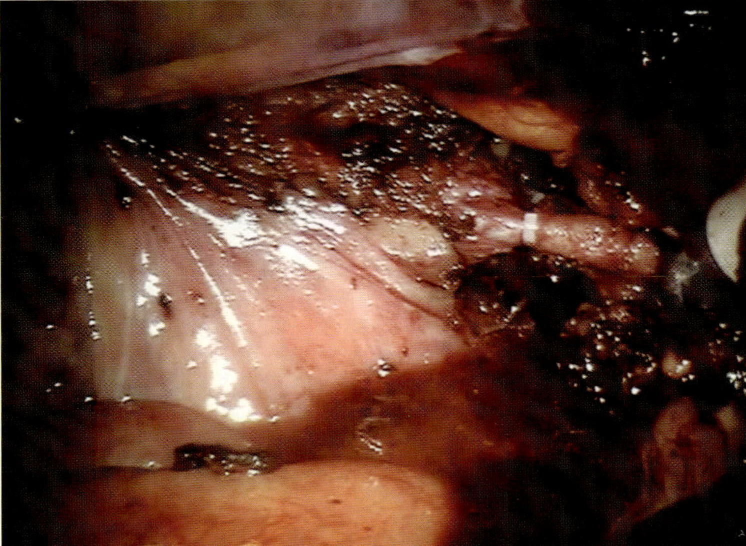

Fig. 7: The ureter is clipped distally prior to dissection of the intramural ureter

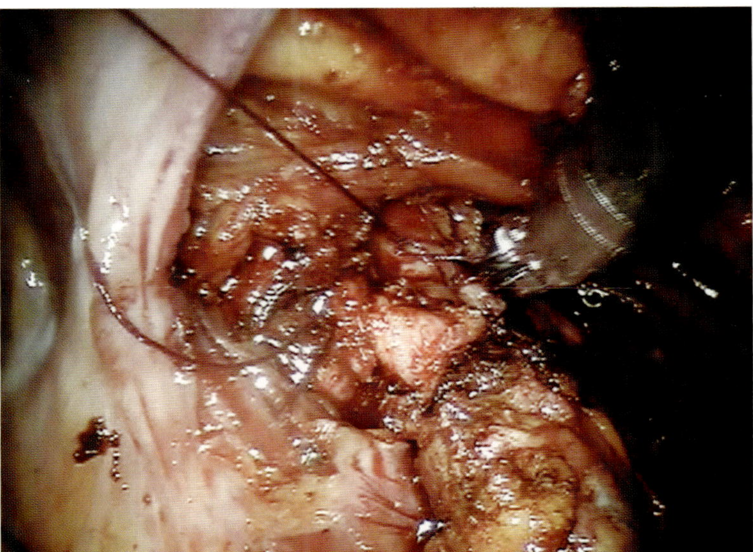

Fig. 8: Sutures are preplaced laterally and medially to the ureter prior to excision. Once the ureter and bladder cuff are excised, these are used to close the cystotomy

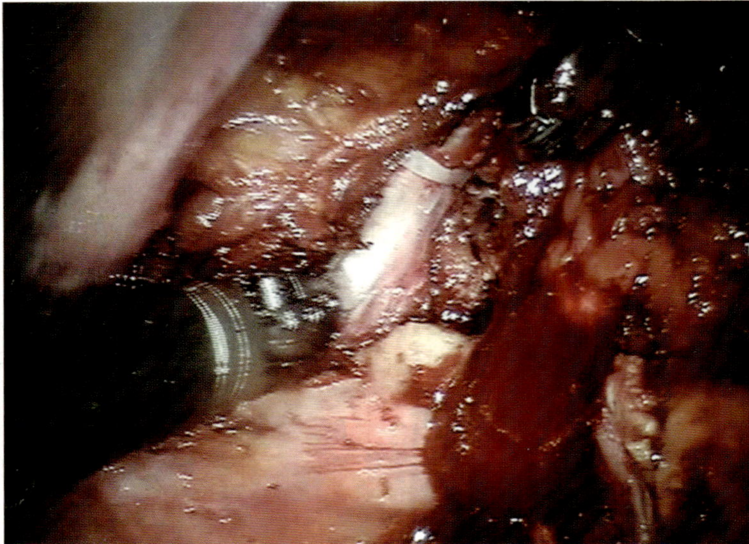

Fig. 9: The intramural ureter is bluntly dissected free from the bladder wall

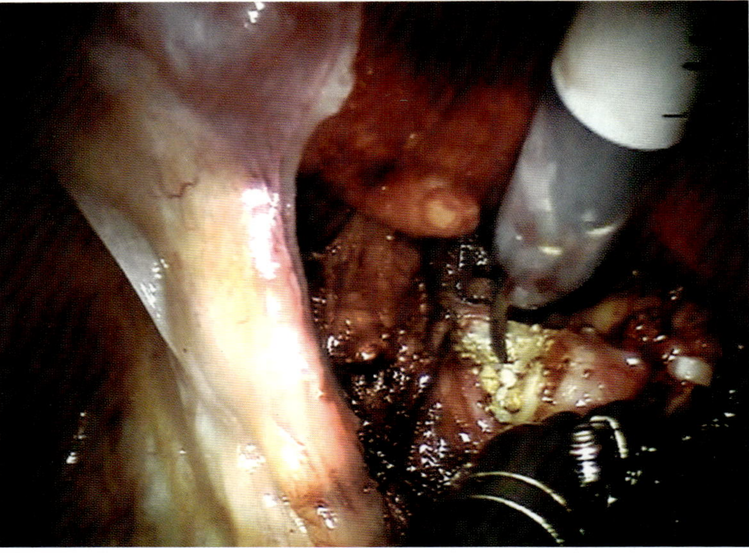

Fig. 10: Once the ureter is dissected down to the level of the ureteral orifice, it is sharply incised anteriorly

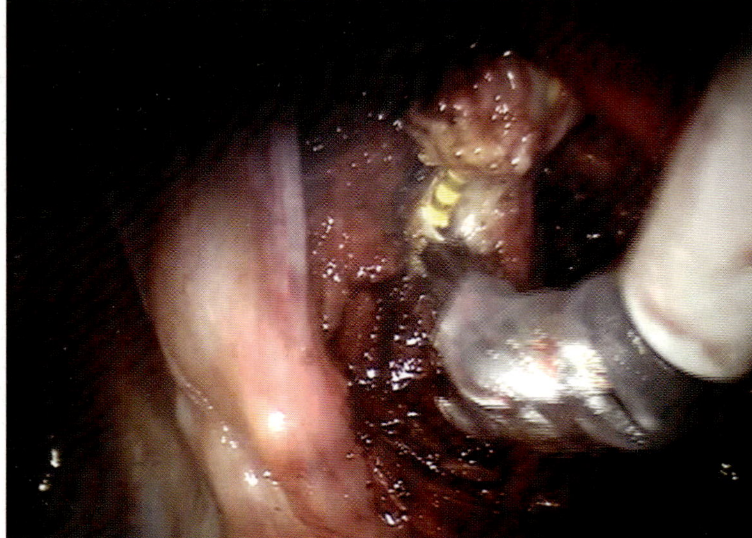

Fig. 11: The ureter is sharply incised circumferentially along with a rim of bladder mucosa. A previously placed ureteral stent is divided along with the ureter

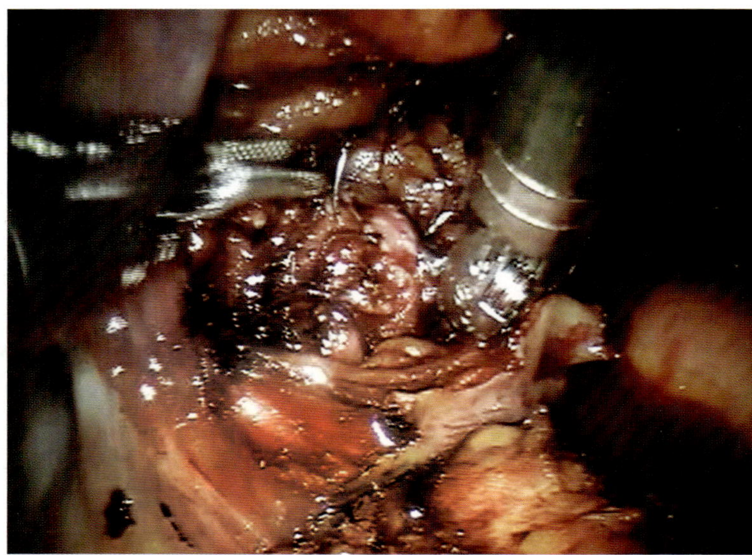

Fig. 12: The cystotomy is then closed in two layers in a running fashion with an absorbable suture. These sutures can be placed prior to excision of the bladder cuff

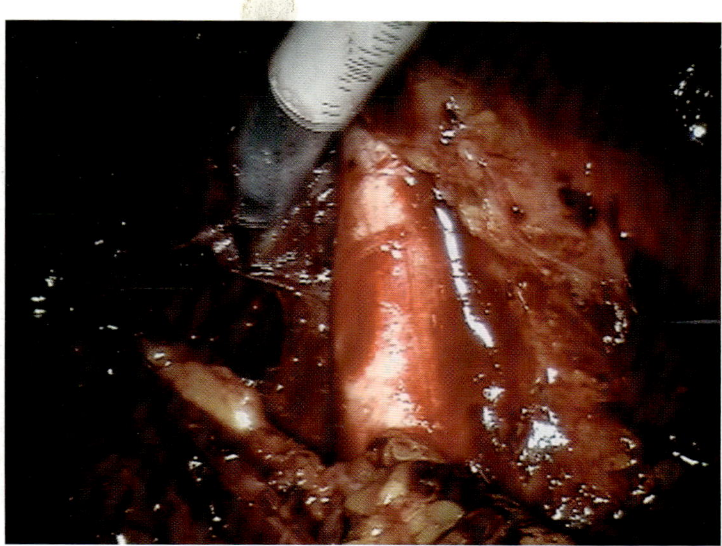

Fig. 13: Lymphatic tissue is dissected off the external iliac vessels

Left Side

1. In a left-sided case, the dissection begins by incising the line of Toldt from the level of the upper sigmoid colon to the splenic flexure. This dissection can be carried further medially by dividing the phrenicocolic and splenorenal ligaments.
2. The descending colon is gently lifted, thereby identifying the plane between Gerota's fascia and the mesocolon. Any renocolic attachments are sharply divided.
3. The pancreas is gently dissected off Gerota's fascia medially.
4. The OR table is rotated medially so as to place the patient in lateral decubitus position at 90°. This helps to mobilize the spleen, pancreas and descending colon medially in order to expose the renal hilum.
5. The investing tissues over the renal hilum are lifted and incised to expose the renal vein. Maryland and right-angle dissectors are used to dissect the tissues off the renal vein and to isolate the adrenal and gonadal veins.

6. The renal artery is identified posterior to the renal vein and dissected free of surrounding tissues close to the vena cava or aorta. This can be done with a Maryland or right-angle dissector.
7. Once the hilar vessels have been identified and dissected from surrounding tissues, the renal artery is transected with an Endo GIA™ stapler. The renal vein is then similarly divided using the Endo GIA™ stapler.
8. Attention is turned towards identifying the ureter in the retroperitoneal fat, medial to the psoas muscle and lateral and posterior to the gonadal vein. The ureter is dissected proximally to the renal hilum and distally into the pelvis to a level just above the bladder. The distal ureter is then clamped with a vascular titanium clip.
9. The psoas muscle is exposed laterally and posteriorly while dissecting cephalad from the lower pole of the kidney towards the upper pole, dividing any inferior and posterior side-wall attachments.
10. The adrenal gland is dissected off the superior medial aspect of the kidney with a harmonic scalpel. Any identified adrenal veins are cauterized and ligated.

DISTAL URETERECTOMY AND BLADDER CUFF

A robotic or open approach can then be used for the distal ureterectomy and bladder cuff excision. The robotic approach is described below.

1. The patient is repositioned from flank position to dorsal lithotomy position without violating the sterile field.
2. The subxiphoid and midclavicular 5 mm trocars are removed and replaced with 8 mm robotic trocars, and the robot is docked.
3. The ureter is dissected free of attachments to the level of the bladder.
4. The intramural ureter is then dissected free from the bladder wall using a combination of sharp dissection and electrocautery. A 1 cm margin of bladder mucosa adjacent to the ureteral orifice is dissected along with the ureter and removed with the entire specimen intact.
5. A lymphadenectomy is performed at the discretion of the surgeon.
6. The bladder mucosal defect is closed with 3-0 chromic sutures and the overlying detrusor muscle is closed with a running 2-0 chromic suture.
7. The bladder is filled via the Foley catheter to test the integrity of the closure.
8. The entire specimen is then placed within an Endo Catch™ bag.
9. A 7 cm Pfannenstiel incision is made to deliver the specimen intact once the robot has been undocked. This fascial incision is closed with a running 0 PDS suture.
10. Pneumoperitoneum is restored to 10 mm Hg and the operative field is closely inspected for hemostasis. The Pfannenstiel skin incision and trocar port sites are then closed in standard fashion.

REFERENCES

1. Munoz JJ, Ellison LM. Upper tract urothelial neoplasms: incidence and survival during the last 2 decades. J Urol. 2000;164:1523-5.
2. Clayman RV, Kavoussi LR, Figenshau RS, et al. Laparoscopic nephroureterectomy: initial clinical case report. J Laparoendosc Surg. 1991;1:343-9.
3. Stewart GD, Humphries KJ, Cutress ML, et al: Long-term comparative outcomes of open versus laparoscopic nephroureterectomy for upper urinary tract urothelial-cell carcinoma after a median follow-up of 13 years. J Endourol. 2011;25:1329-35.
4. Berger A, Haber GP, Kamoi K, et al. Laparoscopic radical nephroureterectomy for upper tract transitional cell carcinoma: oncological outcomes at 7 years. J Urol. 2008;180:849-54.
5. Capitanio U, Shariat SF, Isbarn H, et al. Comparison of oncologic outcomes for open and laparoscopic nephroureterectomy: a multi-institutional analysis of 1249 cases. Eur Urol. 2009;56:1-9.
6. Simone G, Papalia R, Guaglianone S, et al. Laparoscopic versus open nephroureterectomy: perioperative and oncologic outcomes from a randomised prospective study. Eur Urol. 2009;56:520-6.
7. Walton TJ, Novara G, Matsumoto K, et al. Oncological outcomes after laparoscopic and open radical nephroureterectomy: results from an international cohort. BJU Int. 2011;108:406-12.
8. Rassweiler JJ, Schulze M, Marrero R, et al. Laparoscopic nephroureterectomy for upper urinary tract transitional cell carcinoma: is it better than open surgery? Eur Urol. 2004;46: 690-7.
9. Remzi M, Shariat S, Huebner W, et al. Upper urinary tract urothelial carcinoma: what have we learned in the last 4 years? Ther Adv Urol. 2011;3:69-80.
10. Macejko AM, Pazona JF, Loeb S, et al. Management of distal ureter in laparoscopic nephroureterectomy—a comprehensive review of techniques. Urology. 2008;72:974-81.
11. Li WM, Shen JT, Li CC, et al. Oncologic outcomes following three different approaches to the distal ureter and bladder cuff in nephroureterectomy for primary upper urinary tract urothelial carcinoma. Eur Urol. 2010;57:963-9.
12. Busby JE, Matin SF. Laparoscopic radical nephroureterectomy for transitional cell carcinoma: where are we in 2007? Curr Opin Urol. 2007;17:83-7.
13. Gkougkousis EG, Mellon JK, Griffiths TR. Management of the distal ureter during nephroureterectomy for upper urinary tract transitional cell carcinoma: a review. Urol Int. 2010;85:249-56.
14. Hu JC, Silletti JP, Williams SB. Initial experience with robot-assisted minimally-invasive nephroureterectomy. J Endourol. 2008;22:699-704.
15. Eandi JA, Nelson RA, Wilson TG, et al. Oncologic outcomes for complete robot-assisted laparoscopic management of upper-tract transitional cell carcinoma. J Endourol. 2010;24:969-75.
16. Roscigno M, Brausi M, Heidenreich A, et al. Lymphadenectomy at the time of nephroureterectomy for upper tract urothelial cancer. Eur Urol. 2011;60:776-83.
17. Kondo T, Hashimoto Y, Kobayashi H, et al. Template-based lymphadenectomy in urothelial carcinoma of the upper urinary tract: impact on patient survival. Int J Urol. 2010;17:848-54.
18. Brausi MA, Gavioli M, De Luca G, et al. Retroperitoneal lymph node dissection (RPLD) in conjunction with nephroureterectomy in the treatment of infiltrative transitional cell carcinoma (TCC) of the upper urinary tract: impact on survival. Eur Urol. 2007;52:1414-8.

24 Chapter

Laparoscopic Renal Thermal Ablation

Phillip Mucksavage, Achim Lusch, Joseph Graversen, Chris R Kelly, Jaime Landman

INTRODUCTION

The incidence of small renal masses has steadily increased over the past few decades, primarily due to the widespread use of newer axial abdominal imaging technologies.[1] It is estimated that over 60 thousand new cases of renal tumors will be detected in the United States in 2011.[2] Additionally, over half of the patients with incidentally found renal masses are expected to be older than 65 years.[3] These patients typically have more severe medical comorbidities, which has led to an increased interest in minimally invasive methods for the managements of small renal masses (SRM).[4]

Currently, nephron sparing approaches, such as open, laparoscopic, or robotic-assisted laparoscopic partial nephrectomy are the considered the standard of care in the treatment of SRM.[5] Nephron sparing surgery reduces the risk of end stage renal disease and potential cardiac death when compared to radical nephrectomy with equivalent overall cancer survival rates; however, the surgery is associated with significant risk of morbidity.[6] Thermal ablative therapies, such as cryotherapy and radiofrequency ablation, offer a less invasive option, with reduced risk of surgical complications, and can be a reasonable alternative to surgical extirpation.[7]

CRYOTHERAPY

The era of modern cryoablation was initiated in 1961, when automated cryosurgical units that pump liquid nitrogen through the tip of the cryoprobe were introduced. This innovation led to the investigation of cryoablation for different diseases, but cumbersome cryoprobes and a lack of control over the freezing process made the widespread use impractical. Modern cryoprobes coupled with computer modulators have eliminated these problems. Current cryoprobes utilize high-pressure ambient-temperature argon gas through small needles ranging from 1.47–5.0 mm diameter.[8] These probes also incorporate alternative gases, such as helium, that warm rather than cool when expanded. Accordingly, helium can and has been incorporated into cryogenic systems to rapidly warm the cryoprobe in order to arrest the freezing process or thaw the ice ball. Computer modulated regulators also precisely control the flow of argon or helium to maximize freezing and thawing capabilities.

Cryoablation results in tumor destruction via multiple mechanisms. Tissue destruction occurs as a result of intra- and extracellular ice crystal formation and microcirculatory failure through the controlled process of freezing and thawing.[9] Rapid freezing leads to increase in the osmolarity of the extracellular space, which results in an abrupt loss of intracellular fluid and cellular dehydration. Ice crystals also mechanically disrupt the cell membrane leading to changes in cellular pH and protein denaturation.[10] These events lead to immediate cell death, while microvascular injury results in widespread thrombosis, coagulative necrosis and apoptosis that occur over the course of hours to days.[11]

Chosey and colleagues demonstrated that a temperatures of -20°C must be reached to reliably kill benign or malignant cells[12]; however, recent data suggests that a temperature of at least -40°C lead to more consistent tumor ablation.[13] Further research suggests that the ice ball visualized by ultrasonography should at least extend 3.1 mm beyond the outer edge of a lesion to achieve a target temperature of less than -20°C[14] and extending up to 1 cm will ensure temperature less than -40°C at the tumor margin. To guarantee complete homogenous necrosis of tissue, thermocouples can also be used to monitor temperatures. Renal artery occlusion does not appear to significantly alter the freezing process and provides no practical advantage during cryoablation[14]; however, maximizing cell death in the target lesion can be achieved utilizing 2 freeze-thaw cycles.[9]

RADIOFREQUENCY ABLATION

Radiofrequency ablation (RFA) was first used for the treatment of renal tumors in 1997.[15] RFA creates thermal injury by resistive heating. High frequency alternating electrical current is delivered to the target tissue through a needle creating electrical resistance and molecular friction that is transformed into heat.[16] The heat generated causes direct cellular toxicity and coagulative necrosis which is characterized by protein denaturation, cellular membrane disruption and local microvascular injury. The size of the ablation zone is limited by the resistive properties of the tissue and local blood flow. The rapid rise in temperature results in a direct cytotoxic effect that occurs over 4–6 minutes at temperatures above 50°C, but occurs instantaneously at temperature between 60–100°C.[17,18] Temperatures over 105°C result in immediate tissue vaporization and Eschar formation that can reduce the efficacy of RFA; therefore, temperatures are generally kept between 50–100°C to achieve the maximal ablative zone.[7]

Radiofrequency ablation (RFA) can be performed using needles placed directly into the target (dry RFA) or aided by the use of ionic solutions perfused directly into the tissue (wet RFA).[7] Similar to cryotherapy, the zone of ablation must be extended 1 cm beyond the edge of the tumor to ensure the adequacy of treatment; however, unlike cryoablation, the ablation zone cannot be visually monitored using ultrasound guidance. The zone of ablation can be estimated using temperature based or impedance based systems, which employ sensors to ensure the adequacy of treatment and estimate the extent of the thermal injury. While the majority of RFA is performed percutaneously, RFA can also be performed laparoscopically.

INDICATIONS FOR THERMAL ABLATION

Size of the renal tumor is one of the only important limitations to thermal ablation. Renal masses > 4 cm can be successfully treated with cryosurgery; however, there is an increased risk of complications, length of hospitalization and potential risk of bleeding when treating larger tumors.[19] Laparoscopic cryoablation is generally reserved for anterior located tumors, or tumors that cannot be adequately treated percutaneously due to anatomic limitations.[20]

The current American Urological Association (AUA) Guidelines for the treatment of small renal masses (Clinical T1) recommends the use of thermal ablation (cryoablation or radiofrequency ablation) either percutaneously or laparoscopically for the high surgical risk patient who wants active treatment and accepts the need for long-term radiologic surveillance.[5] The guidelines include recommendation that biopsies (core biopsies) should be performed and that each patient should be thoroughly counseled about the risks and benefits of thermal ablation compared to surgical excision. Larger tumors (> 3.5 cm) and those tumors that have an irregular shape and or infiltrative appearances may also be associated with increased risk of local recurrence after thermal ablation.[21]

INSTRUMENTATION

Disposable Equipments

- 5 mm Ace Harmonic Curved forceps (Ethicon)
- Trocars
  - 12 mm (2) [axially dilating clear ports (Ethicon)] and 5 mm (1) [axially dilating clear ports (Ethicon)]
  - 12 mm Airseal Port (Surgiquest)
- Veress needles (150 mm) (Covidien)
- CO_2 Insufflation Tubing/Airseal Tubing (Surgiquest)
- 10 Sponges (Raytex)
- Bard MaxCore Disposable Core Biopsy Instrument, 18-gauge × 25 cm (Bard)
- BD Spinal Needle, 22-gauge × 3.5 in (BD Medical)

Nondisposable Equipments

- Endoholder (Bookwalter Endoscopic Instrument)
- Suction Irrigator, extra long, 5 mm (Nezhat system: K Storz)
- Laparoscopes: 10 mm 0° and a 10 mm 30° lens (K Storz)
- 8666-RF Laparoscopic Ultrasound Transducer (BK Medical Systems Inc.)
- Pro Focus UltraView (BK Medical Systems Inc.)
- 2, Atraumatic, nonlocking 5 mm smooth tip (duckbill) grasping forceps (K Storz)
- 4, traumatic (toothed), locking, 5 mm grasping forceps (K Storz)
- 5 mm and 10 mm PEER retractors (J Jamner Inc.)
- 5 mm Needleholders (Aesculap) (2; one straight, one curved)
- 5 mm Bipolar Macro Forceps (Aesculap)
- 10 mm Spoon Forceps (K Storz)
- 10 mm soft curved angled forceps (Maryland dissector) (K Storz)
- 10 mm right angle dissector (K Storz or J Jamner)

Available But Not Opened Equipments

- 10 mm Clip Appliers with 9 mm and 11 mm clips (Ethicon)
- Disposable Roticulating Endoshears (Covidien)
- Endostitch and all types of suture used (0, 2-0, 4-0, Polysorb, Polydac and Prolene) (Covidien)
- Disposable Hasson Trocar 12 mm Blunt Tip (Bluntport, Covidien)
- 3-0 cardiovascular silk (RB-1 needle) and 0-Vicryl suture for fascial closure
- 1 rack of LAPRA-TY clips and 10 mm LAPRA-TY clip applier (Ethicon)
- 1 rack of Hem-o-loc clips and 5 mm Hem-o-loc clip applier (Weck)
- Gauze rolls (5) (Carefree Surgical Specialties)
- 10 mm Satinsky clamp with flexible port (Aesculap)
- 1 set of laparoscopic bulldog clamps (Klein Inc., San Antonio, TX)
- 12 mm Multifire EndoGIA: Vascular stapler with reloads available (Covidien or Ethicon)

Additional Equipment for Cryoablation

- IceRod Cryoneedles, 1.47 mm 17-gauge (Galil)
- Precise® Cryoablation System (Galil)

Additional Equipment for Radiofrequency Ablation

- HABIB 4X™ Laparoscopic RFA device (Angiodynamics)
- RITA Model 1500X RF Generator (Angiodynamics)

ATLAS OF PROCEDURAL STEPS

The following figures (Figs 1 to 26) are derived from the cryosurgical ablation of a right-sided, 2.0 cm, interpolar, anterior located renal mass. All of the steps for cryoablation are similar to RFA, except ultrasound monitoring is not utilized during RFA.

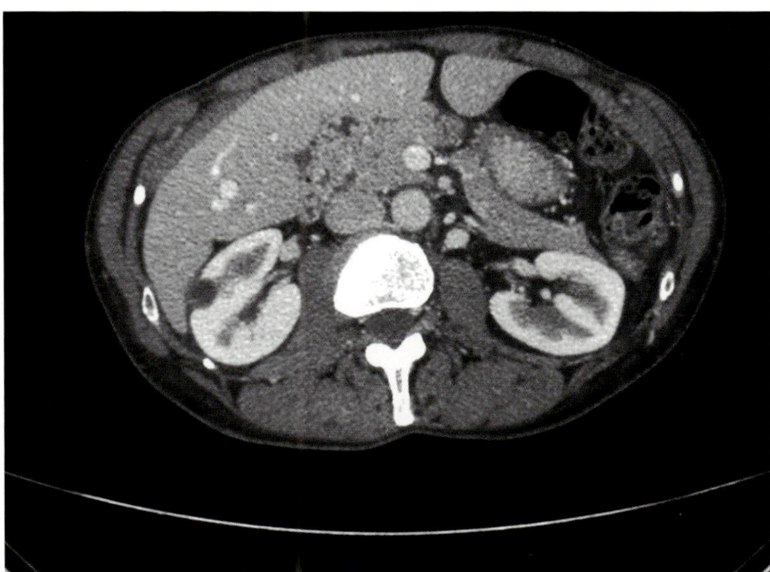

Fig. 1: CT image of the lesion prior to cryoablation. The right-sided lesion measures 2.0 cm x 1.8 cm x 1.5 cm. The anterior location of the tumor and overlying liver edge precluded safely treating the mass percutaneously

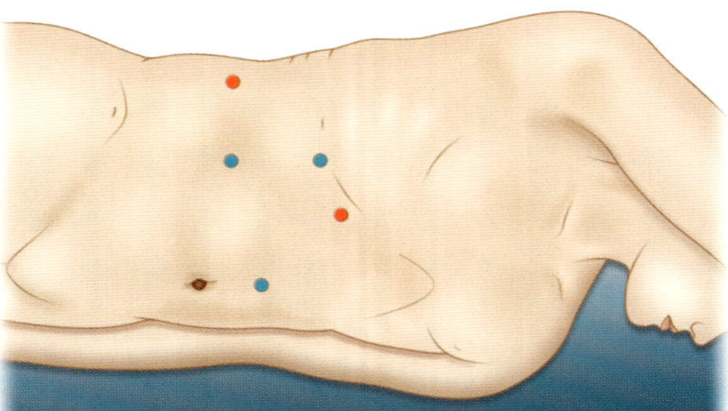

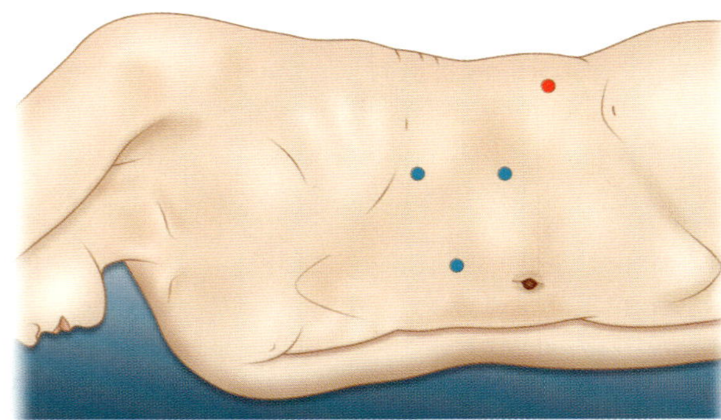

Fig. 2: Patient positioning and port placement. The patient is placed in the lateral decubitus position. Two working ports placed just above the paramedian line, approximately 10 cm apart. The superior port is placed a finger breath off the costal margin. A camera port (10 mm) is placed in the midline half way between the working ports. An additional 5 mm port is placed laterally off the anterior superior iliac spine if a kidney retractor is needed. Finally, on the right side, and additional 5 mm port is generally placed at the midline just below the xiphoid process and is used to retract the liver

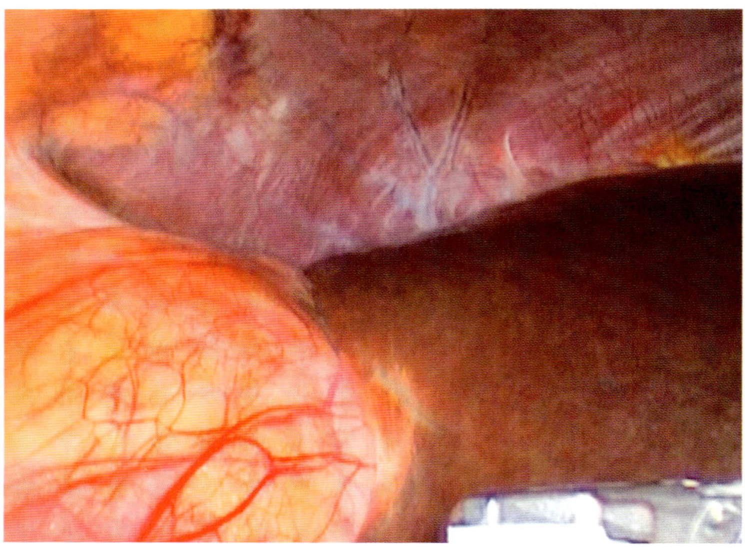

Fig. 3: Initial image once all the trocars are in place. The liver is seen draping just over the upper pole of the right kidney. The colon is located medially to the kidney and is not seen on this image

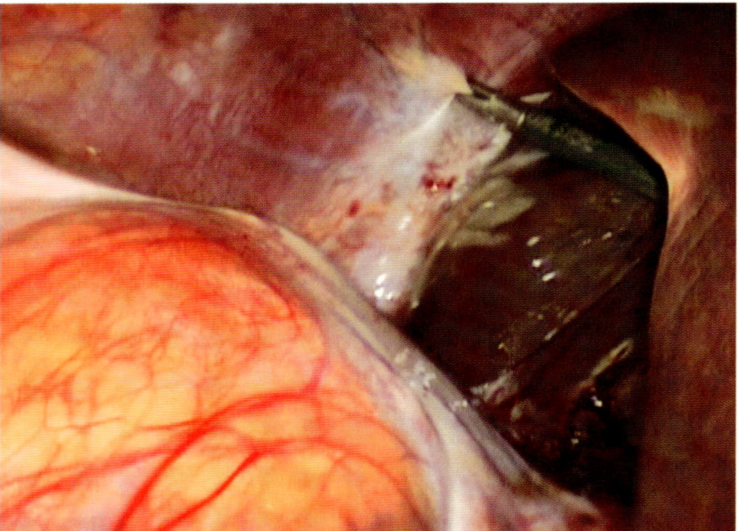

Fig. 4: Placement of the liver retractor. Once the posterior coronary ligaments and triangular ligaments of the liver have been transected, a locking toothed grasper is placed through a 5 mm port that placed in the midline just below the xiphoid process. The anterior abdominal wall is grasped, thereby tenting up the liver off of the kidney and hilum

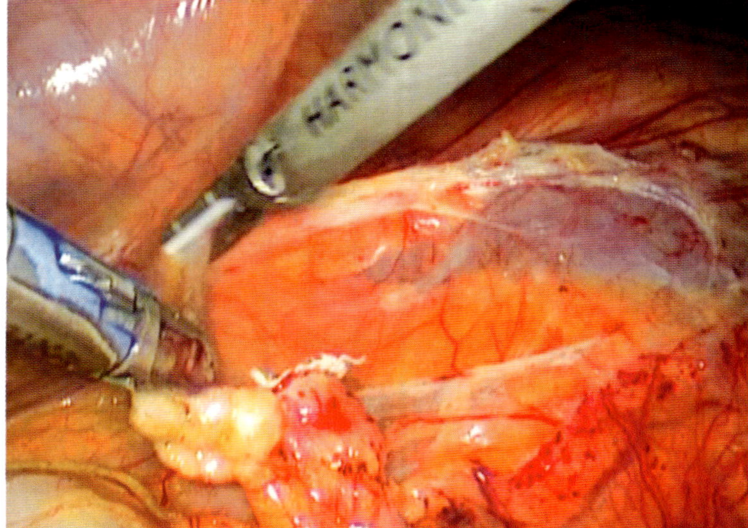

Fig. 5: Medial reflection of the colon. The peritoneum overlying Gerota's fascia is incised. There is a notable difference in the color of the fat within Gerota's fascia (pale yellow), differentiating it from mesenteric fat (bright yellow). The plane between Gerota's fascia and the colonic mesentery is generally bloodless, providing a useful landmark for dissection. The colon is seen on the bottom left corner as it is reflected medially

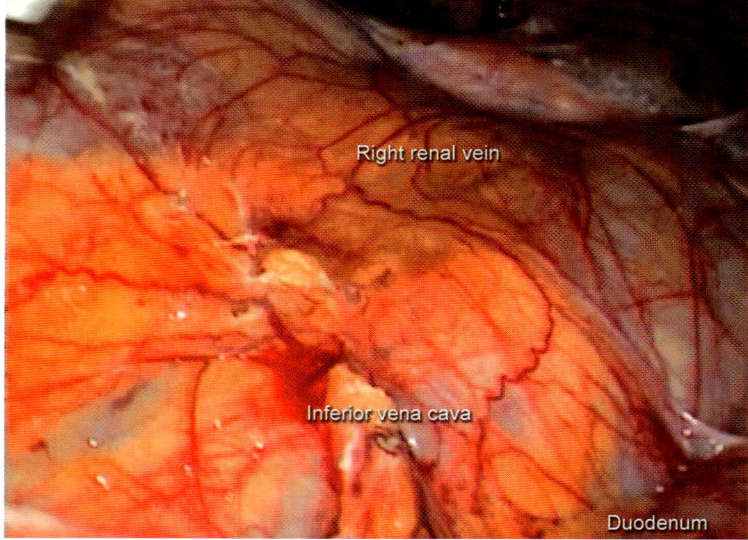

Fig. 6: The duodenum is reflected medially (Kocher Maneuver), revealing the inferior vena cava and the right renal vein. Complete hilar dissection is generally not necessary for smaller endophytic masses. Large or exophytic tumors may require exposure of the hilum if there is a risk of serious hemorrhage after cryoablation and immediate access to the renal vasculature is needed

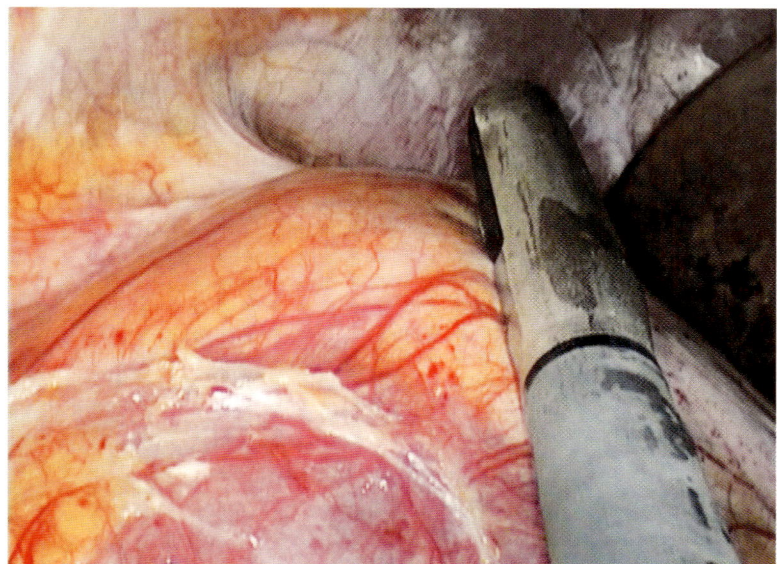

Fig. 7: Intraoperative ultrasound of the renal tumor. Intraoperative ultrasound of the kidney is performed in order to identify the location of the tumor and inspect the kidney for other abnormalities

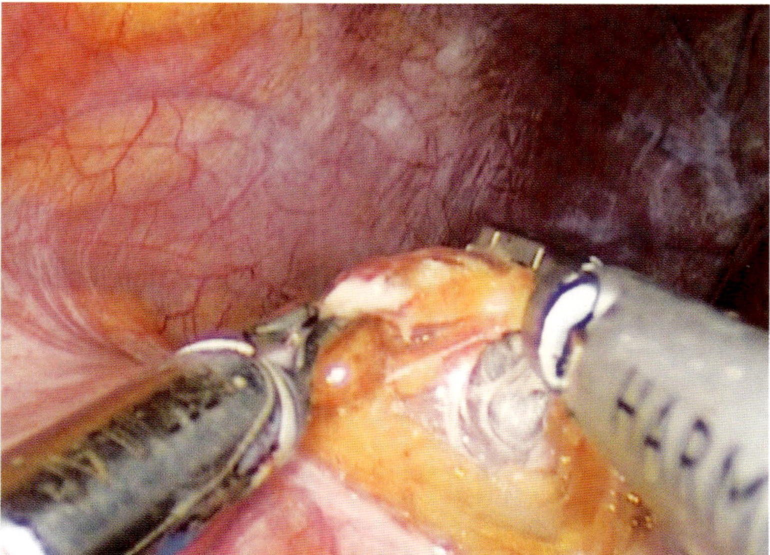

Fig. 8: Dissection of peritumoral fat. The fat overlying the tumor is carefully dissected off of the tumor and surrounding normal renal parenchyma. The normal renal capsule can be seen here underneath the perinephric fat. Mobilization of the fat is not mandatory as ablation can be performed under ultrasound guidance with the fat and Gerota's fascia intact. Removal of the fat and direct visualization of the renal lesion facilitates targeting. If the fat is removed, it is extracted and sent for histopathological evaluation for staging purposes

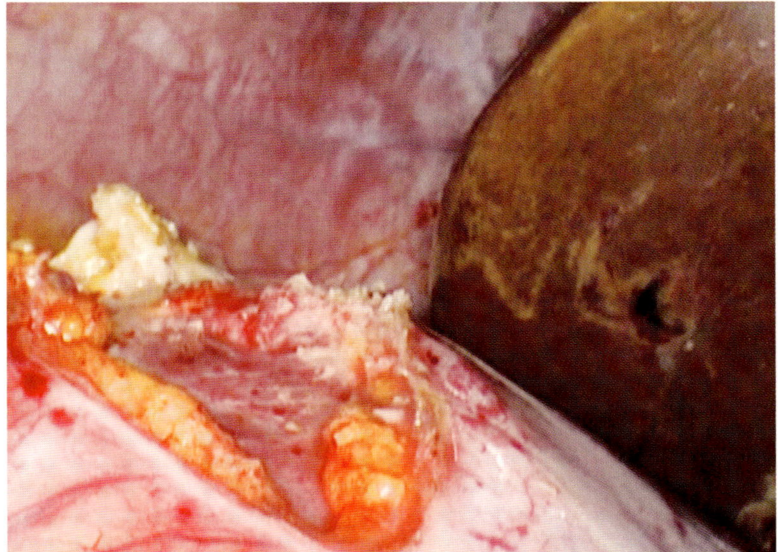

Fig. 9: Exposure of the renal tumor. The peritumoral fat is removed and extracted from the abdomen. The tumor is now completely exposed

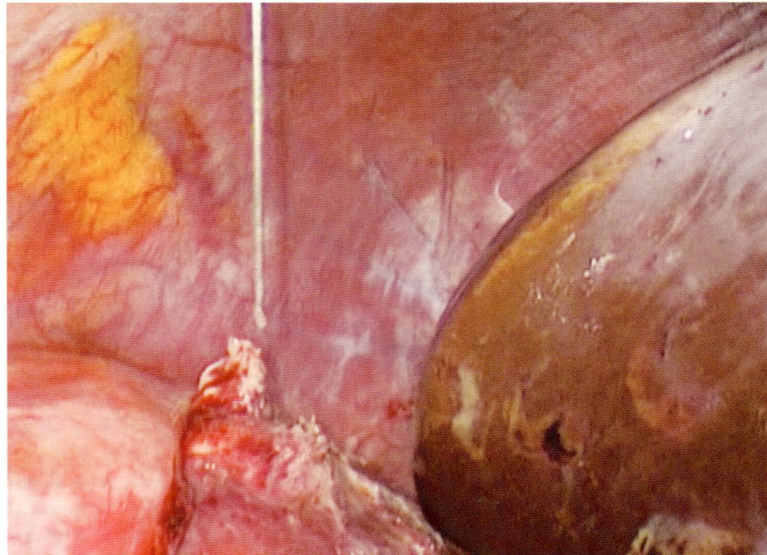

Fig. 10: Placement of the finder needle. A long spinal needle is used as a 'finder' needle. This needle in small caliber is used to identify the ideal angles for biopsy and cryoneedle deployment. In this situation, the kidney is not adequately positioned to place the cryoneedle with good visualization

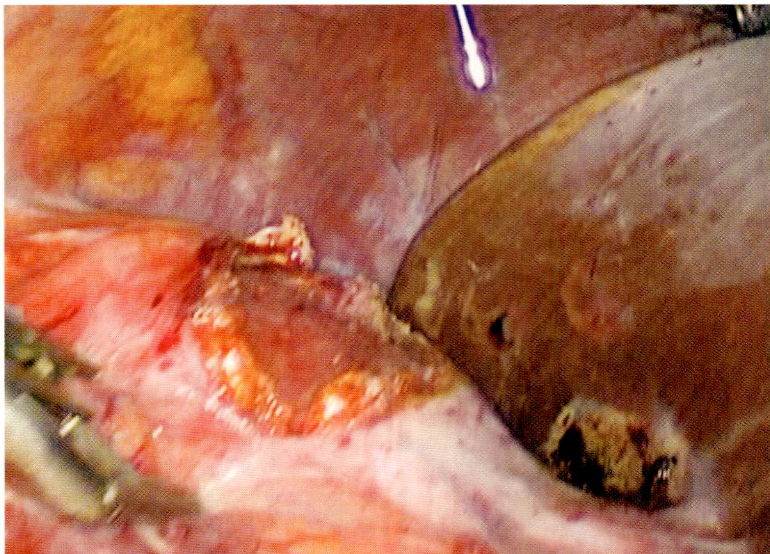

Fig. 11: Positioning of the kidney with the PEER retractor. The PEER retractor can be used to mobilize and reposition the kidney during cryoablation or as a fixed retractor under the kidney during dissection of the hilum. In this situation, the kidney is repositioned so the tumor faces medially for better visualization during cryoablation

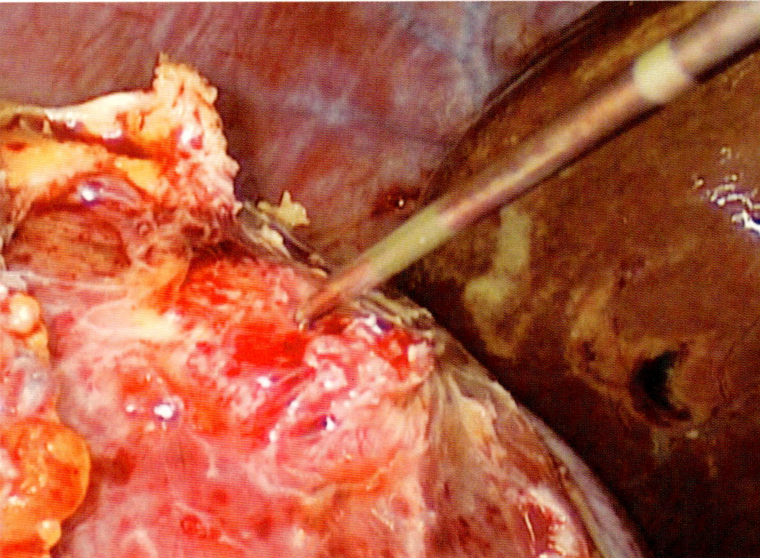

Fig. 12: Biopsy of the renal mass. A finder needle was again used to confirm proper position the kidney prior to biopsy. The tumor is now well visualized after repositioning the kidney with the PEER retractor. In this image, three biopsies are taken directly from the renal mass

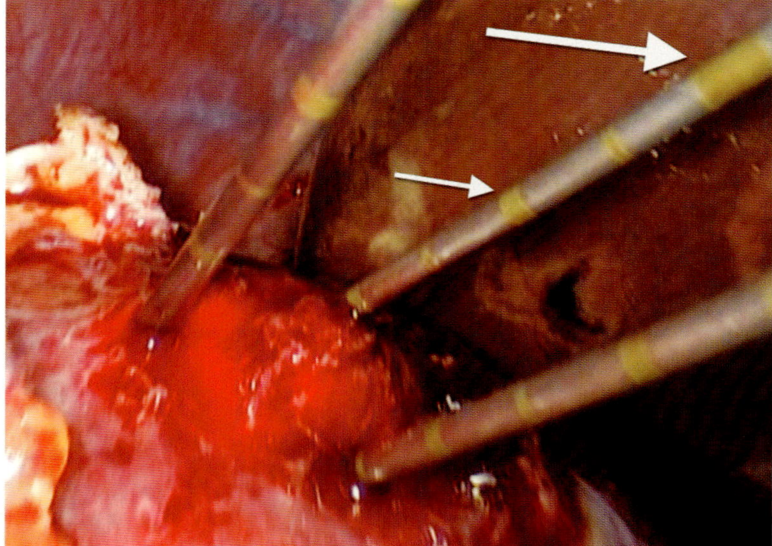

Fig. 13: Placement of the cryoneedles. Three cryoneedles are placed into the periphery of the renal tumor. Each is separated by approximately 1.5 cm. Note the marking on the cryoneedles that indicate the depth of the tip of the needle in the kidney. Individual markings are 1 cm apart (small arrow) and a thicker marking occurs at the 5 cm depth point (large arrow). The depth for each needle deployment is determined based on preoperative CT and intraoperative ultrasound imaging

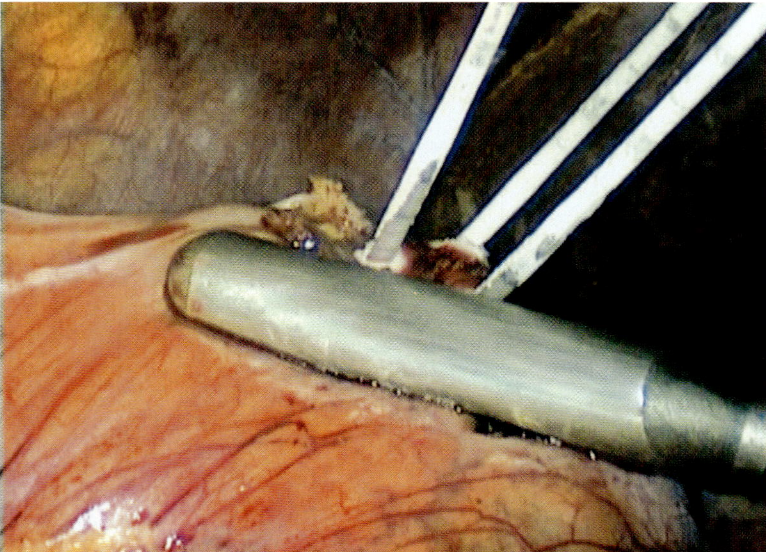

Fig. 14: Ultrasound confirmation of needle placement and ice ball monitoring. The placement of the needles in the correct position is confirmed using ultrasound. The freeze cycle is also monitored on ultrasound to ensure the ice ball extends at least 1 cm beyond the tumor margin

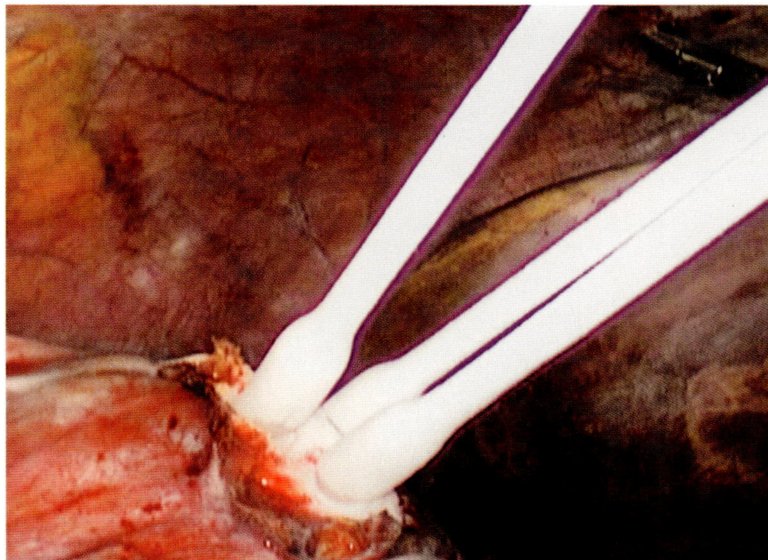

Fig. 15: Freeze cycle. The freeze cycle is then performed. Ice forms on the rods, as well as on the surface of the kidney and tumor. A double freeze thaw is used, with freeze cycles typically lasting between 4–10 minutes depending on the appearance of the ice ball on ultrasound. The cryoablation system is activated until the ice extends beyond the tumor margin, and the time of deployment is not relevant

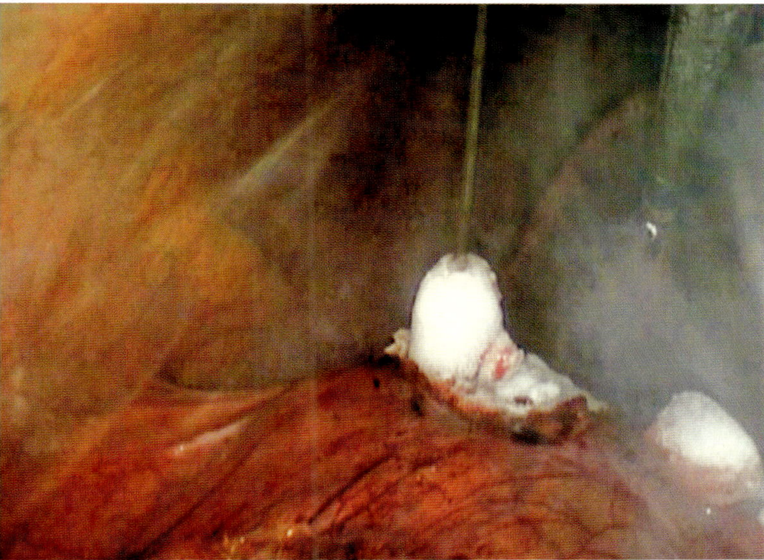

Fig. 16: Removal of the cryoneedles. Each needle is carefully removed during an active thaw cycle. Prior to removal of the needles, they are carefully twisted and checked to ensure that they can be safely removed (tissue does not move with rotation of the needle). If any resistance is noted, the needle is left in place until they can be thawed well enough to safely remove

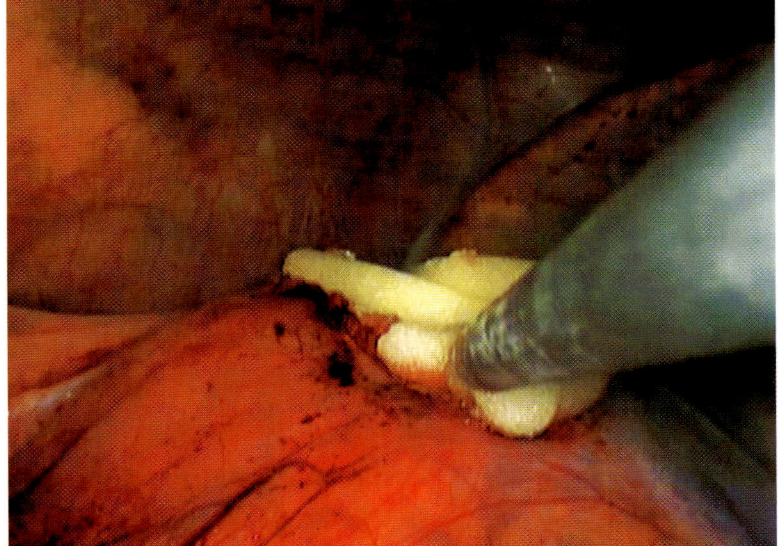

Fig. 17: Placement of hemostatic agents. FLOSEAL is placed at the site of tumor ablation. Care is taken to ensure that FLOSEAL is placed over the location of the cryoneedles in the kidney and any potential source of bleeding

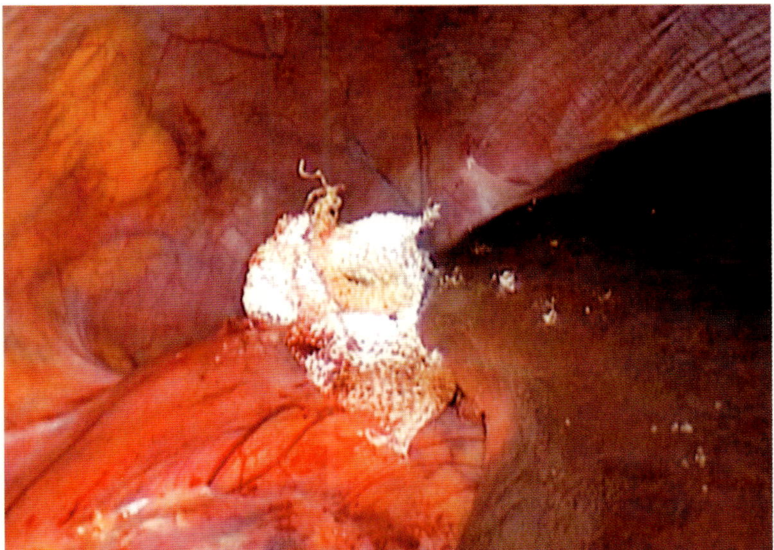

Fig. 18: Placement of hemostatic agents. After the placement of FLOSEAL, the liver retractor is removed and the ablation zone is covered with Surgicel®. The entire area is then inspected under low intra-abdominal pressure (5 mm Hg) for at least 10 minutes for any signs of bleeding. If no bleeding is noted, the ports are removed and the operation is complete

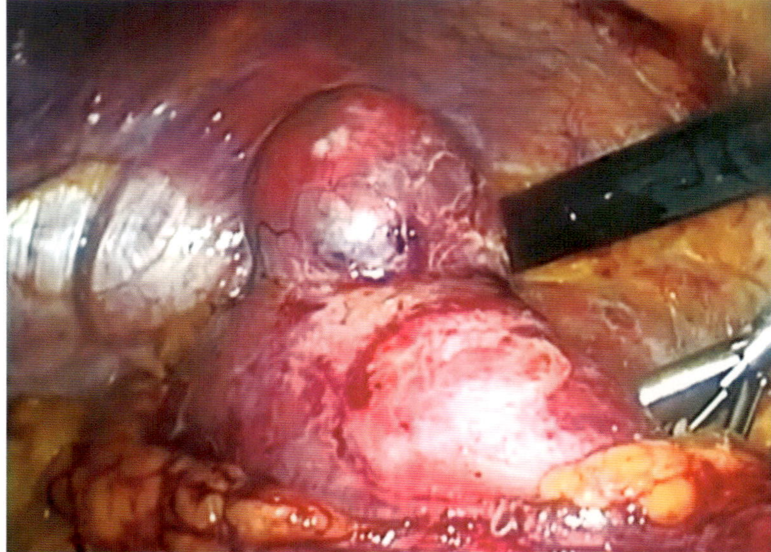

Fig. 19: A large 4 cm exophytic renal mass prior to cryoablation. In this situation, the renal vessels are completely exposed during the dissection in case there is bleeding which cannot be controlled with hemostatic agents and pressure and a partial nephrectomy must be performed (different case)

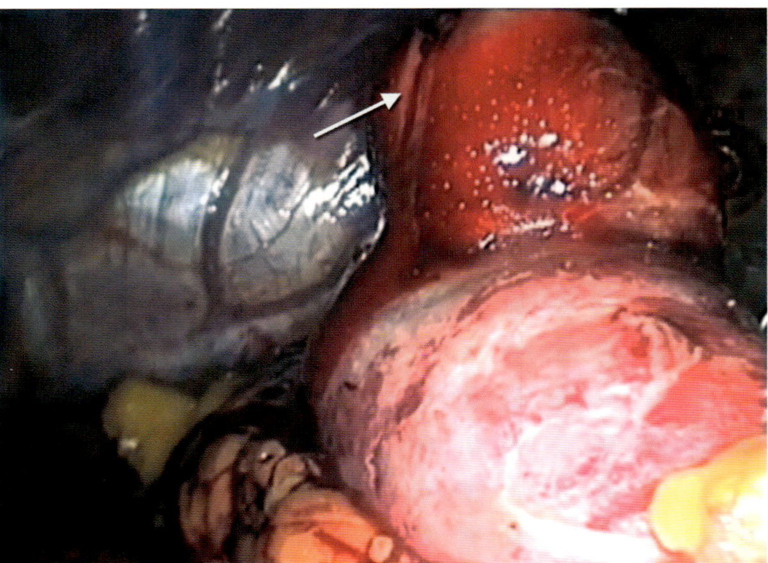

Fig. 20: A large fracture (white arrow) of the tumor is noted along the inferior border of the mass during the first thaw cycle (needles are barely seen at the superior border of the tumor) (different case)

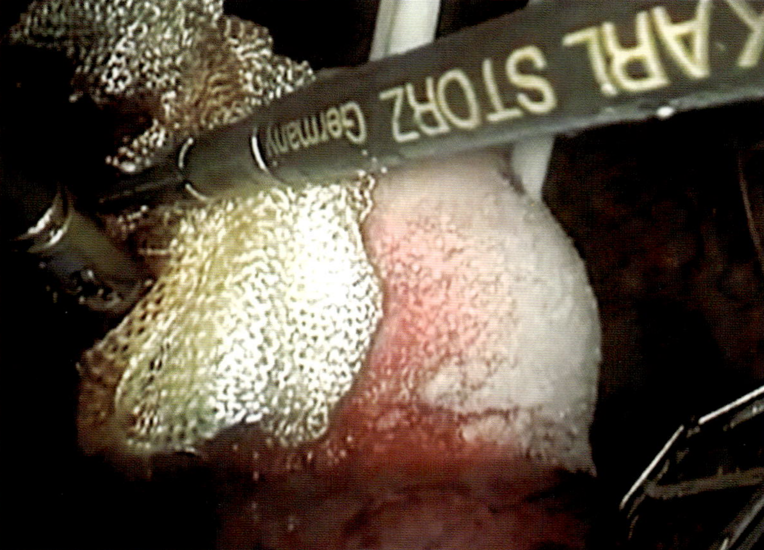

Fig. 21: The cryoablation continues and the bleeding is controlled with gentle pressure and surgical. The ice is already forming on the outside of the mass as seen here. After all needles were removed, FLOSEAL and surgical controlled the bleeding adequately (different case)

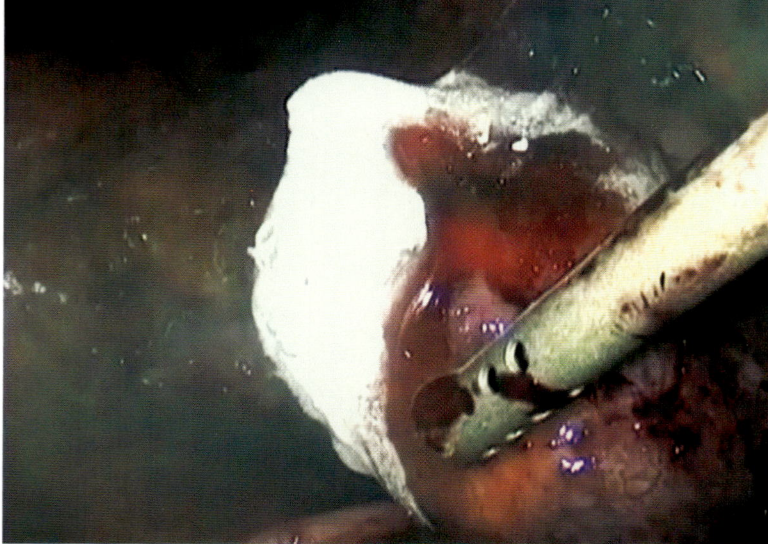

Fig. 22: Another large (3.5 cm) exophytic mass with noted cracking and bleeding after removal of the cryoneedles. Surgicel® and FLOSEAL are applied with gentle pressure to the area of bleeding (different case)

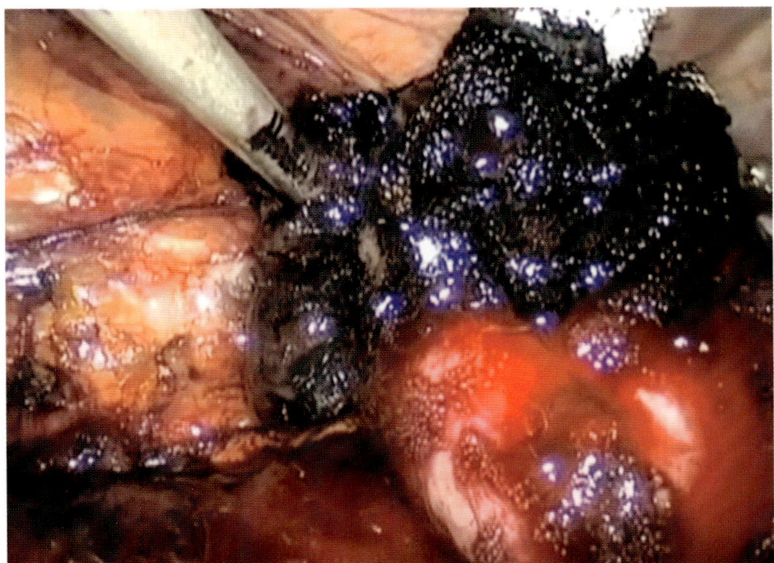

Fig. 23: Bleeding is persistent despite multiple hemostatic attempts. Note the large pool of blood at the base of the tumor and the saturated Surgicel® (different case)

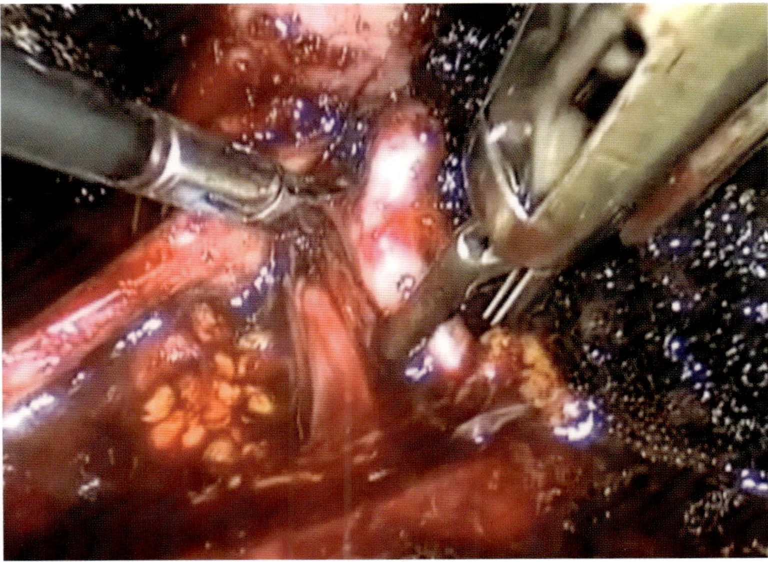

Fig. 24: The renal artery is clamped at this point in preparation for a partial nephrectomy secondary to inability to control the bleeding. As the tumor was large and the risk of significant ice ball fracture anticipated, the surgeon had completely dissected the renal vasculature, administered mannitol, and had all equipment prepared for partial nephrectomy prior to initiating the cryoablation procedure (different case)

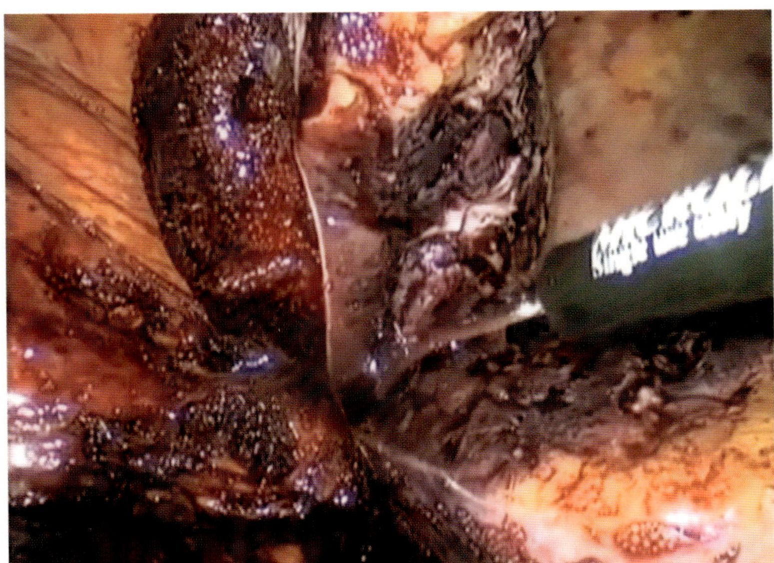

Fig. 25: Once the artery is clamped, the tumor is excised with sharp dissection (different case)

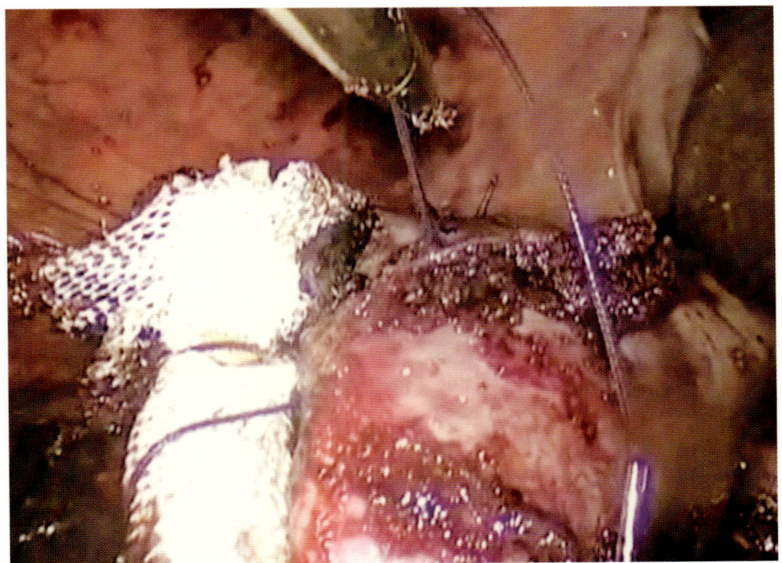

Fig. 26: The defected is then closed using a bolster as in a standard partial nephrectomy (different case)

REFERENCES

1. Jayson M, Sanders H. Increased incidence of serendipitously discovered renal cell carcinoma. Urology. 1998;51:203-5.
2. American Cancer Society: Cancer Facts and Figures 2011. Atlanta GACS, 2011.
3. Luciani LG, Cestari R, Tallarigo C: Incidental renal cell carcinoma - age and stage characterization and clinical implications: study of 1092 patients (1982–1997). Urology. 2000;56:58-62.
4. Hollingsworth JM, Miller DC, Daignault S, et al. Rising incidence of small renal masses: a need to reassess treatment effect. J Natl Cancer Inst. 2006;98:1331-4.
5. Campbell SC, Novick AC, Belldegrun A, et al. Guideline for management of the clinical T1 renal mass. J Urol. 2009;182:1271-9.
6. Fergany AF, Hafez KS, Novick AC. Long-term results of nephron sparing surgery for localized renal cell carcinoma: 10-year follow-up. J Urol. 2000;163:442-5.
7. Raman JD, Hall DW, Cadeddu JA. Renal ablative therapy: radiofrequency ablation and cryoablation. J Surg Oncol. 2009;100:639-44.
8. Wen CC, Nakada SY. Energy ablative techniques for treatment of small renal tumors. Curr Opin Urol. 2006;16:321-6.
9. Gage AA, Baust JM, Baust JG. Experimental cryosurgery investigations in vivo. Cryobiology. 2009;59:229-43.
10. Gage AA, Baust J. Mechanisms of tissue injury in cryosurgery. Cryobiology. 1998;37:171-86.
11. Baust JG, Gage AA. The molecular basis of cryosurgery. BJU Int. 2005;95:1187-91.
12. Chosy SG, Nakada SY, Lee FT, et al. Monitoring renal cryosurgery: Predictors of tissue necrosis in swine. J Urol. 1998;159:1370-4.
13. Gill IS, Novick AC. Renal cryosurgery. Urology. 1999;54:215-9.
14. Campbell SC, Krishnamurthi V, Chow G, et al. Renal cryosurgery: experimental evaluation of treatment parameters. Urology. 1998;52: 29-33.

15. Zlotta AR, Wildschutz T, Raviv G, et al. Radiofrequency interstitial tumor ablation (RITA) is a possible new modality for treatment of renal cancer: ex vivo and in vivo experience. J Endourol. 1997;11:251-8.
16. Goel RK, Kaouk JH. Probe ablative treatment for small renal masses: cryoablation vs. radio frequency ablation. Curr Opin Urol. 2008;18:467-73.
17. Hsu THS, Fidler ME, Gill IS. Radiofrequency ablation of the kidney: acute and chronic histology in porcine model. Urology. 2000;56:872-5.
18. Rehman J, Landman J, Lee D, et al. Needle-based ablation of renal parenchyma using microwave, cryoablation, impedance- and temperature-based monopolar and bipolar radiofrequency, and liquid and gel chemoablation: laboratory studies and review of the literature. J Endourol. 2004;18:83-104.
19. Lehman DS, Hruby GW, Phillips CK, et al. Laparoscopic renal cryoablation: efficacy and complications for larger renal masses. J Endourol. 2008;22:1123-7.
20. Mues AC, Okhunov Z, Haramis G, et al. Comparison of percutaneous and laparoscopic renal cryoablation for small (< 3.0 cm) renal masses. J Endourol. 2010;24:1097-100.
21. Matin SF, Ahrar K, Cadeddu JA, et al. Residual and recurrent disease following renal energy ablative therapy: a multi-institutional study. J Urol. 2006;176:1973-7.

Index

Page numbers followed by *f* refer to figure and *t* refer to table.

S

T

U

V

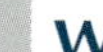

W